ADDICTIONS – FROM PATHOPHYSIOLOGY TO TREATMENT

Edited by **David Belin**

Addictions – From Pathophysiology to Treatment
Edited by David Belin

Contributors

Aude Belin-Rauscent, David Belin, José Vicente Negrete-Díaz, Gonzalo Flores, Talvinder S. Sihra, Antonio Rodríguez-Moreno, Edgar Antonio Reyes-Montaño, Edwin Alfredo Reyes-Guzmán, Ezio Carboni, Roberto Cadeddu, Anna Rosa Carta, Sonia Luz Albarracín Cordero, Bernd Robert Stab II, Felipe Guillen, Edgar Antonio Reyes Montano, Alfredo Ramos-Miguel, María Álvaro-Bartolomé, M. Julia García-Fuster, Jesús A. García-Sevilla, Marta Rodríguez-Arias, María Asunción Aguilar, Karen M. von Deneen, Yijun Liu, M.L. Laorden, M. V. Milanés, P. Almela, Zheng-Xiong Xi, Jennifer E. Murray, Jérôme Lacoste, David Belin, Cynara Teixeira Ribeiro, Andréa Hortélio Fernandes, Andrea Leonardi, Sonia Scavelli, Gianluca Ciuffardi, Paolo Stocco, Alessandra Simonelli, Nicoletta Capra, Francesca De Palo, Philippe Chossegros

Published by InTech

Janeza Trdine 9, 51000 Rijeka, Croatia

Copyright © 2012 InTech

Notice

Publishing Process Manager Masa Vidovic
Technical Editor InTech DTP team
Cover InTech Design team

Additional hard copies can be obtained from orders@intechopen.com

Addictions – From Pathophysiology to Treatment, Edited by David Belin
p. cm.
ISBN 978-953-51-0783-5

For EU product safety concerns:
IN TECH d.o.o., Prolaz Marije Krucifikse Kozulić 3, 51000 Rijeka, Croatia,
info@intechopen.com or visit our website at intechopen.com.

Meet the editor

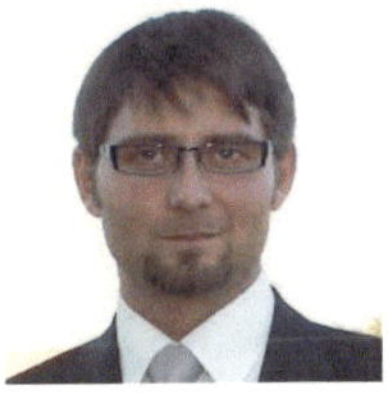

After completing an undergraduate course in cellular and molecular biology in 2003, David Belin entered a PhD program in Neurosciences and Neuropharmacology at Université Bordeaux 2 in Michel Le Moal's INSERM laboratory under the supervision of Véronique Deroche-Gamonet. During his PhD, David Belin developed the so-called addiction-like behaviour model for cocaine. In January 2006, he was recruited as a post-doctoral research associate to Barry Everitt's laboratory at the Department of Experimental Psychology at the University of Cambridge where he studied intrastriatal processes subserving habitual cocaine seeking. In 2008 he became senior research associate and entered the INSERM in 2009 where he established his team in Poitiers focusing on the psychobiology of compulsive disorders such as addictions and OCD.

Contents

Preface XI

Section 1 General Considerations 1

Chapter 1 **Drug Addictions: An Historical and Ethological Overview 3**
Aude Belin-Rauscent and David Belin

Chapter 2 **Animal Models of Drug Addiction 21**
Aude Belin-Rauscent and David Belin

Section 2 Pathophysiology of Addictions 65

Chapter 3 **Addictive Drugs and Synaptic Plasticity 67**
José Vicente Negrete-Díaz, Gonzalo Flores,
Talvinder S. Sihra and Antonio Rodríguez-Moreno

Chapter 4 **Cocaine Addiction: Changes in Excitatory and Inhibitory Neurotransmission 103**
Edgar Antonio Reyes-Montaño and Edwin Alfredo Reyes-Guzmán

Chapter 5 **Role of Prefrontal Cortex Dopamine and Noradrenaline Circuitry in Addiction 129**
Ezio Carboni, Roberto Cadeddu and Anna Rosa Carta

Chapter 6 **A Molecular Mechanism of Ethanol Dependence: The Influence of the Ionotropic Glutamate Receptor Activated by N-Methyl-D-Aspartate 169**
Sonia Luz Albarracín Cordero, Bernd Robert Stab II,
Felipe Guillen and Edgar Antonio Reyes Montano

Chapter 7 **Role of Multifunctional FADD (Fas-Associated Death Domain) Adaptor in Drug Addiction 201**
Alfredo Ramos-Miguel, María Álvaro-Bartolomé,
M. Julia García-Fuster and Jesús A. García-Sevilla

Chapter 8 **Polydrug Use in Adolescence 227**
Marta Rodríguez-Arias and María Asunción Aguilar

Chapter 9 **Food Addiction, Obesity and Neuroimaging 259**
Karen M. von Deneen and Yijun Liu

Chapter 10 **Pathways Involved in the Cardiac Adaptive Changes Observed During Morphine Withdrawal 291**
M.L. Laorden, M. V. Milanés and P. Almela

Section 3 Addiction Treatment – Pharmacology 309

Chapter 11 **Medication Development for the Treatment of Cocaine Addiction – Progress at Preclinical and Clinical Levels 311**
Zheng-Xiong Xi

Chapter 12 **N-Acetylcysteine as a Treatment for Addiction 355**
Jennifer E. Murray, Jérôme Lacoste and David Belin

Section 4 Therapeutic Strategies – Behavioural, Social and Analytical Approaches 381

Chapter 13 **Proposals for the Treatment of Users of Alcohol and Other Drugs: A Psychoanalytic Reading 383**
Cynara Teixeira Ribeiro and Andréa Hortélio Fernandes

Chapter 14 **The Interactional Approach in the Treatment of Cocaine Addicts 403**
Andrea Leonardi, Sonia Scavelli and Gianluca Ciuffardi

Chapter 15 **Research and Intervention for Drug-Addicted Mothers and Their Children: New Perspectives 425**
Paolo Stocco, Alessandra Simonelli, Nicoletta Capra and Francesca De Palo

Chapter 16 **HCV and Drug Use – What Can Be Learned from the Failure to Control This Epidemic? 453**
Philippe Chossegros

Preface

Addiction is the psychiatric disorder for which the definition has evolved the most in the last thirty years. From the DSM-III in which addiction was defined as tolerance and withdrawal to the current clinical definition in the DSM-IV and upcoming DSM-V, with five out of seven criteria referring to loss of control over, and compulsive use of, drugs, the social and medical views of addictions have dramatically changed.

Drug addiction is no longer a question of altered "psychophysical need" of the drug. It is beyond this, an alteration of both the basic, i.e., reward, and sophisticated systems of the brain, including attention, behavioural control, decision making, memory, and even insight.

Despite this updated neurological understanding, drug addicts remain considered by the general public as mere criminals with very weak willpower. This general wisdom must change especially in the face of the current trends towards increasing recreational use of drugs worldwide, and the emergence of the easy access to online casinos and gaming Indeed, most of us, if not all, have already been exposed to a stimulus with addictive properties, thereby having gambled with a potential fall into the vicious cycle that is addiction. As such, it is important to keep in mind that tobacco and alcohol, including wine, are among the most dangerous addictive drugs, causing the majority of drug-related deaths.

Behind the legal status of drugs and the relative failure in law enforcement management, remains our lack of understanding of the psychological, neurobiological, and environmental factors that contribute to the transition from controlled recreational drug use to compulsive drug use. In other words, to date, we still do not know why some people exposed to addictive stimuli will develop an addiction while others will be able to use these drugs recreationally throughout their life without succumbing to the negative personal, societal, and legal side effects of drug consumption. Hence, we have no effective prevention strategies nor do we have effective individual-based therapeutic treatments to offer.

In the search for an effective treatment, as a psychobiologist, I suggest that addiction is a loss of prefrontal executive control over a maladaptive incentive habit process that bridges limbic pavlovian impulses originating from the amygdala and the insula to a rigid habit system dependent upon the dorsolateral striatum. We therefore must find a way to counteract this between-systems adaptation, with the most promising approach being pharmacological tools. However, this psychobiolgical model does not capture key aspects of the pathology, such as the economic status of the addict, his current social and personal environment, the unique history that drove him to the use of a particular drug, whether his addiction involves the use of several different drug classes and so on.

Since the now well-accepted claim that addiction is a brain disease has opened the potential development of pharmacological treatment based on a better understanding of addiction pathophysiology, many researchers have focused on the understanding of the neurobiological adaptations to drug exposure. They have forgotten that the neurobiological adaptations to exposure to addictive drugs are common to all that are exposed to drugs, whether they be addicted or not. It is only recently that the interest in inter-individual vulnerability to compulsive drug use has emerged in the field of neuroscience, and the additional potential role of environmental conditions is only emerging.

Several outstanding books have now been published covering the neurobiology of drug addiction and aiming to provide a rather exhaustive overview of the current state of addiction research integrating these issues.

Here, we offer an alternative point of view focusing on the complexity and heterogeneity of treatment management of addictions involving players from the legal, medical, social, psychological, neurobiological, psychiatric, and psychoanalytical fields.

None of these fields and associated management strategies has so far proven to have developed effective treatment to prevent relapse of compulsive drug use in drug addicts. This lack of success may stem from the fact that there are several forms of addiction with specific etiologies and pathophysiologies that we have no insights into, but it may also be explained by a lack of interaction and understanding among the different approaches involved in the management of addiction. Indeed, not only a brain disease, addiction should be additionally considered in terms of comorbidity, both at the psychiatric and somatic levels. By emphasizing how much the definition of addiction and the foreseen potential treatments differ among biologists, psychologists, psychoanalysts, or GPs, this book provides an original framework whereby one can reach beyond an initial area of interest regarding addictions.

This book also provides insights into the experimental approaches of drug addiction, both in preclinical models and in humans, as well as the neurobiological mechanisms that may be associated with addictions. It provides a synthesis of the current and emerging pharmacological tools for the management of addiction to different drugs and opens new perspectives on various management strategies of drug addicts. Gathering experts in different fields, from basic research to the clinic, involved in the care of drug addicts, the present book aims at providing the reader with an original overview of the strategies implemented to treat drug addiction. This may be of interest for those who share the wisdom that refined and more effective treatments lie in the adequate combination of pharmacological and psychological/psychosocial strategies.

I am extremely grateful to the authors of the various chapters for the quality of their contribution to this book. I would like to acknowledge Ms Masa Vidovic, the patient project manager at InTech, for her support and Ms Gorana Scerbe for initiating this book project. I would like to thank the members of my research team for their support. Finally, I would like to dedicate this book to the two pillars of my research and personal life: my mentor, Barry Everitt, and the one to whom I am addicted, my wife, Aude Belin-Rauscent.

David Belin, PhD
INSERM European Associated Laboratory
Psychobiology of Compulsive Habits,
U1084 - LNEC & University of Poitiers,
France

Section 1

General Considerations

1

Drug Addictions: An Historical and Ethological Overview

Aude Belin-Rauscent and David Belin
INSERM U 1084, LNEC, Université de Poitiers,
INSERM AVENIR Team "Psychology of Compulsive Disorders", Poitiers,
France

1. Introduction

1.1 Preliminary considerations: Focus on cocaine and heroin

It is well established that several psychoactive substances can lead to addiction. These include legal drugs such as alcohol and nicotine which generate the major part of the addiction-related social and economical costs to modern societies (1), and a pleiad of illegal drugs amongst which cannabis, cocaine and heroin are the most commonly used.

When one wants to consider the harmful consequences of an addictive drug, both the dependence and physical harm potencies of the drug should be considered for these two aspects contribute to the deterioration of the user's life. A recent classification of the major classes of addictive drugs reveals that heroin and cocaine are clearly the most dangerous ones since both their addictive properties and physical harm potency are high (2). Cocaine and heroin are followed by barbiturates and street methadone, but tobacco is shown to have addictive property of the same magnitude as cocaine, thereby demonstrating that the legal status of a substance is not a predictive factor of least addictive properties.

In the present chapter, we will consider exclusively cocaine and heroin addictions, not only because these two drugs are clearly the most dangerous ones, but mainly because cocaine and heroin use have been increasing among western countries populations in the last ten years. This focus is one limitation of the general conclusions that will be provided in the following chapters that will also address alcoholism and food addiction that will be joined by another addiction, namely pathological gambling, in the clinical definition of addictions in the upcoming DSM-V. Thus, addictions are increasingly recognised as abnormal persistent maladaptive behaviours driven by specific, initially reinforcing, stimuli in the environment that are not anymore restricted to psychoactive substances.

1.2 Drug use: A behaviour as old as humankind?

Drug use seems to have entered human customs as early as the emergence of human societies. Evidences that recreational drug use has emerged early on after human sedentarisation, perhaps with the development of religious rites, can be found for several drugs and routes of administration.

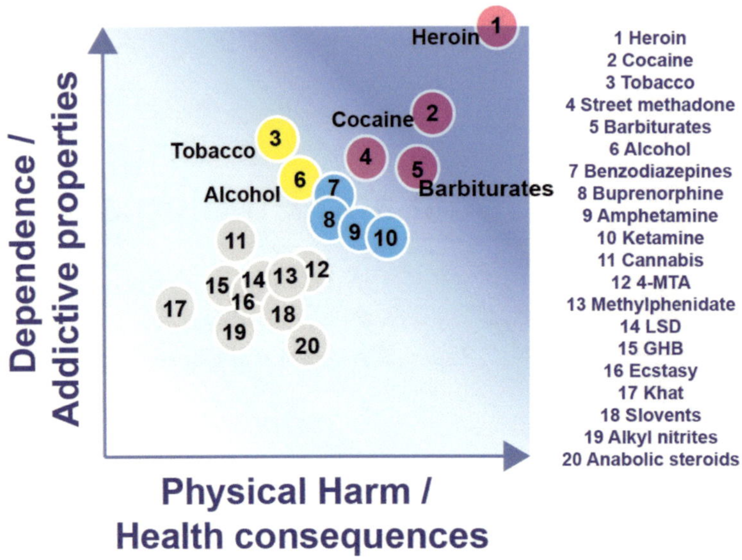

Fig. 1. Rational scale to assess the harm of drugs of potential misuse, after (2).

The addictive potential of a drug varies from substance to substance, and from individual to individual. Dose, frequency, pharmacokinetics of a particular substance, route of administration, and time are critical factors for physical harm and addictive potency. Heroin and cocaine are clearly the most dangerous ones since both their addictive properties and physical harm potency are high.

Thus, 5000 B.C. the sumerians used opium, as suggested by the fact that they had an ideogram for it which has been translated as HUL, meaning « joy » or « rejoicing » (3). A 3500 B.C. egyptian papyrus provides the earliest historical record of the production of alcohol in the description of a brewery (4).

Interestingly, 3000 B.C. is also the approximate date of the supposed origin of the use of tea in China. It is likely that coca leaf chewing began in the Andes at the same time since traces of coca have been found in mummies dating 3000 years back (5). The cocaine content of coca leaf is under 1% but after 1859, when cocaine was first isolated from coca leaf by Albert Niemann, cocaine was available legally in concentrations that were nearly 100% pure. Cocaine was first used recreationally in the 1860s, almost as soon as it was synthesised. A few years after its synthesis by Richard Willstätter in 1898 (6), cocaine appeared in cigarettes, ointments, nasal sprays, and tonics. The most popular cocaine-based product was Mariani Wine (Vin Mariani). It was a wine and cocaine mixture that was launched in 1863. Nearly all popular personalities of the day, including Queen Victoria, Thomas Edison and Pope Leon XIII endorsed it. Cocaine has also been popularised by Sigmund Freud who prescribed it for the treatment of digestive disorders, asthma, depression or opiate and alcohol dependence (7).

At the same time, more precisely in 1898, heroin (diacetylmorphine) was synthesized by Felix Hoffmann, 23 years after a first academic synthesis by Alder Wright. Akin to the launch of cocaine as a medicine, heroin was then introduced by Bayer as "safe preparation free from addiction-forming properties".

The broad availability of the pure form of cocaine and heroin has contributed to the marked development of addiction to these substances which, in their primary forms and routes of administration, were far less addictive. This phenomenon has been suggested to stem from a discrepancy between our brain and our modern environment, i.e, Nesse and Berridge wrote in 1997: «We are vulnerable to such fitness-decreasing incentives because our brains are not designed to cope with ready access to pure drugs, video games, and snack foods. Hundreds of generations of exposure would likely shape resistance to their allure and their deleterious effects» (8). This interesting consideration suggests that drug addiction may be a matter of mismatch between Human evolution and the recent revolution of human environment, a problem to which Evolution may be the best solution.

	All illicit drugs	Cannabis	Amphetamine-type stimulants		Cocaine	All opiates	Heroin
			Amphetamines	Ecstasy			
Number of users (in millions)	185.0	147.4	33.4	7.0	13.4	12.9	9.20
Proportion of global population (%)	3.1	2.5	0.6	0.1	0.2	0.2	0.15
Proportion of population 15 years and above (%)	4.3	3.5	0.8	0.2	0.3	0.3	0.22

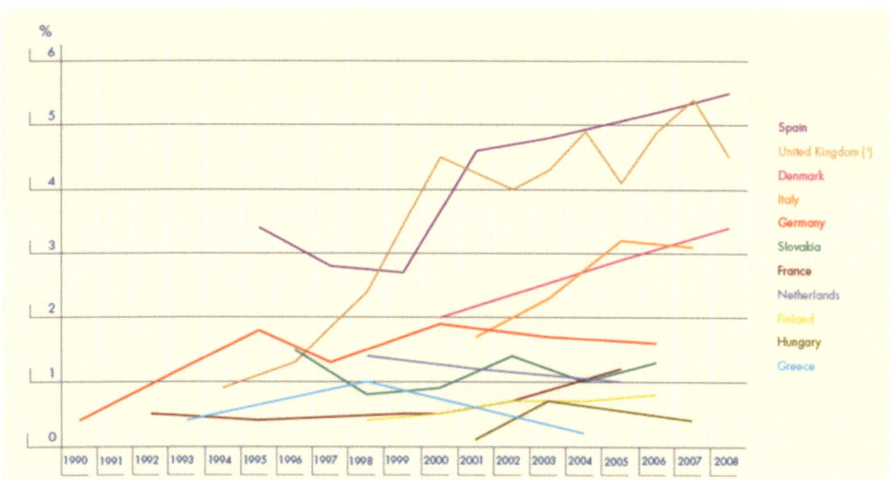

Fig. 2. Illicit drug use state at the beginning of the 21st century

Top panel: Annual prevalence of global, worldwide, illicit drug use over the period 1998-2001 (11). Bottom. A trend to increased cocaine use in European countries (10).

However, before these evolutionary, and rather fatalistic considerations, human societies have developed social and legal strategies to cope with addiction, as early as 10 years following the synthesis of heroin and cocaine. Indeed, the United States prohibited the importation of smoking opium (9) and the manufacture of heroin in 1909 and 1924, respectively, while the Harrison Narcotics Act of 1914 prohibited the use of cocaine. Since then law enforcement has limited, but not eradicated, heroin and cocaine use, as illustrated by figure 2 (EMCDDA) (10), the bottom panel of which shows a general increase in cocaine use within European countries over the past 20 years. Such a trend may induce an increase in the prevalence of drug-related health problems, and most importantly, of drug addiction.

1.3 Drug use: An evolutionary feature of animal kingdom

Drug use seems inherent to animal behaviour, perhaps because of the evolutionary selection of a reward system developed to maintain species survival, bringing animals towards sources of reinforcement. Thus spontaneous drug use has been observed in several species in the wild. Elephants would intoxicate with alcohol contained in ripe fruits and baboons would readily eat over-ripe fruits from the marula tree until they cannot walk anymore. Birds also use alcohol in that song thrush, for instance, struggle to fly after eating ripe grapes.

An exhaustive list of examples of spontaneous drug use in animal kingdom is beyond the scope of this chapter, but a last example should be enough to emphasise how broad are sources of intoxication in mammals: in the south of the United States, sheep and horses eat astragalus and then show hyperactive behaviour akin to human beings.

In experimental settings, it has been demonstrated that all drugs abused by humans are reinforcing in many species including planarians (12) and flies (13, 14), and they are readily self-administered by vertebrates such as mice (15-21) or rats (22-26), dogs (27, 28) and non human primates (29, 30).

Thus not only is drug used common to several species of the animal kingdom but the demonstration that pure forms of psychoactive drugs have reinforcing properties in animals under experimental conditions suggests that drug taking is not a specific behavioural feature of human beings. Drug use in animals seems rather to be the evidence that the neurobiological substrates of primary motivational and reinforcement processes selected by evolution have been shaped early on and maintained from planarians to human beings, and that drugs highjack these systems.

However, it remains unclear the extent to which these findings help inform our understanding of drug addiction in humans since it is a brain disorder that is clearly far removed from primary reinforcement mechanisms.

2. Drug addiction: A human-specific disorder?

2.1 What is drug addiction?

Drug addiction is a complex brain disorder (31), affecting the motivational (32, 33), learning (34-37) and behavioural control systems of the brain (38-40). Several definitions of drug addiction, ranging from the psychiatric to the social view have been presented by Koob and Le Moal (1) and will not be discussed any further.

Drug addiction is defined as a chronic relapsing compulsive habit characterised by loss of control over drug intake, maintained drug use despite adverse consequences (36, 41, 42) and the development of negative psycho-affective distress when access to the drug is prevented (42, 43).

Because the aetiology and pathophysiology of drug addiction remain unknown, this prominent psychiatric disorder is best defined by the clinical features of the DSM-IV (44) (figure 3). The diagnostic of drug addiction is currently based on a categorial dichotomous approach in that the patient must present at least three out of the seven clinical criteria listed in figure 5 to be said addicted to a substance.

DSM-IV diagnostic criteria for drug addiction
(adapted from the DSM-IV, American Psychiatric Association, 2000)

1. Need for markedly increased amounts of a substance to achieve intoxication or dedired effect, or markedly diminished effect with continued use of the same amount of the substance

2. The presence of a characteristic withdrawal syndrome or use of a substance (or closely related substance) to relieve or avoid withdrawal symptoms

3. Persistence desire to use drugs or one or more unsuccessful efforts to cut down or control substance use

4. Substance used in larger amounts or over a longer period of time than the person intended

5. Important social, occupational, or recreational activities given up or reduced because of substance use

6. A great deal of time spent in activities necessary to obtain, to use or to recover from the effects of substance used

7. Continued substance use despite knowledge of having a persistent or recurrent physical or psychological problem that is likely to be caused or exacerbated by continued use

Fig. 3. Clinical features of drug addiction according to the DSM-IV-R (44).

The subject is diagnosed addicted to the substance if they show at least three out of the 7 clinical criteria over the last 12 months.

However, all addicted patients are not equally severely affected and a dimensional addiction severity scale has been developed to assess general behavioural, health and social drug-induced impairments (45-49).

Indeed, drug addicts do not only take drugs, they spend great amounts of time foraging for their drugs, compulsively take drugs, lose control over drug intake, and persist in taking drugs despite the many adverse consequences of doing so, including compromising their health, family relationships, friendships and work. Many drug addicts resort to criminal behaviour to obtain the funds necessary to sustain their compulsive drug use and the great majority eventually relapse to drug use even after prolonged periods of abstinence.

This negative behavioural picture illustrates how drug addiction is not merely a drug taking disorder. Indeed, among the individuals exposed to drugs, and there are many who occasionally drink only a glass or two of an alcoholic beverage, or smoke a cigarette or two, only 15 to 30% overall will switch from casual, 'recreational' drug use to drug abuse and drug addiction (1, 50) (figure 4).

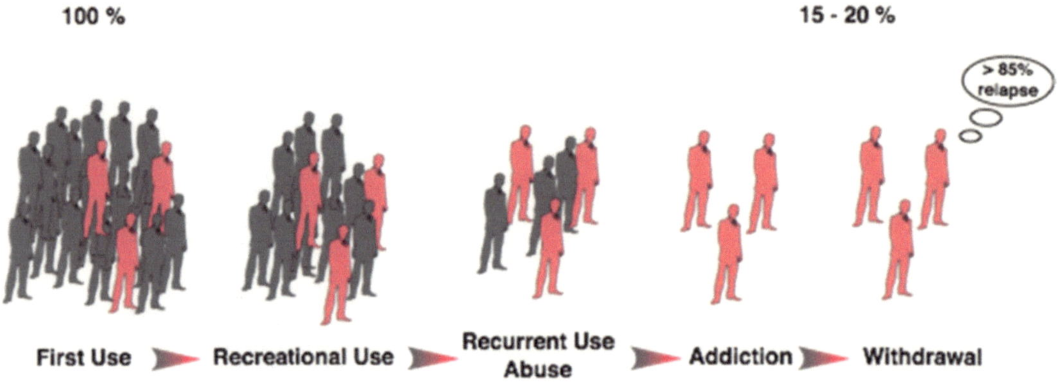

Fig. 4. We are not equally vulnerable to drug addiction

A substantial proportion of the general population experiences drugs at least once in a lifetime. Of the recreational users who control their drug intake, some will shift to more chronic drug use. Only a subgroup of these individuals will develop drug abuse and eventually drug addiction. Epidemiological studies reveal that of the individuals who have been exposed to addictive drugs, 15 to 20 % eventually develop addiction.

Despite considerable research we still do not understand why some individuals develop a compulsive use of drugs nor do we have effective treatments (51) to reduce the substantial social and economic burden (52); for review, see (1) of drug addiction (figure 5). Nevertheless, there is increasing evidence suggesting that drug addiction results from gradual adaptation processes in the brain of vulnerable subjects in response to chronic drug exposure. Not only do these between-systems adaptations trigger an emotional allostatic state (hedonic allostasis) (1, 53-55) characterised for instance by increased anxiety, irritability and depression but they may ultimately lead to a shift in the psychological mechanisms that govern drug seeking and drug taking behaviours, including habits (36, 37, 41, 42, 56, 57) as aberrant instrumental learning mechanisms controlled by Pavlovian cues, altered behavioural control (39, 58-60), decision-making and self-monitoring processes (61, 61).

Similarly, Everitt and colleagues have argued that, during the development of drug addiction, drug seeking is initially goal-directed but becomes habitual, and ultimately compulsive, thereby emphasizing the potential importance of maladaptive automatic instrumental learning mechanisms and their control by Pavlovian incentive processes, so called incentive habits (37, 42), in the emergence of compulsive drug use (35, 37, 42, 59). Additionally, drug-induced adaptations may also facilitate the shift from impulsivity to compulsivity that has been suggested to occur in the development of drug addiction (figure 6) whereby only vulnerable subjects would show a transition from impulse-related recreational drug use to compulsive drug intake (1).

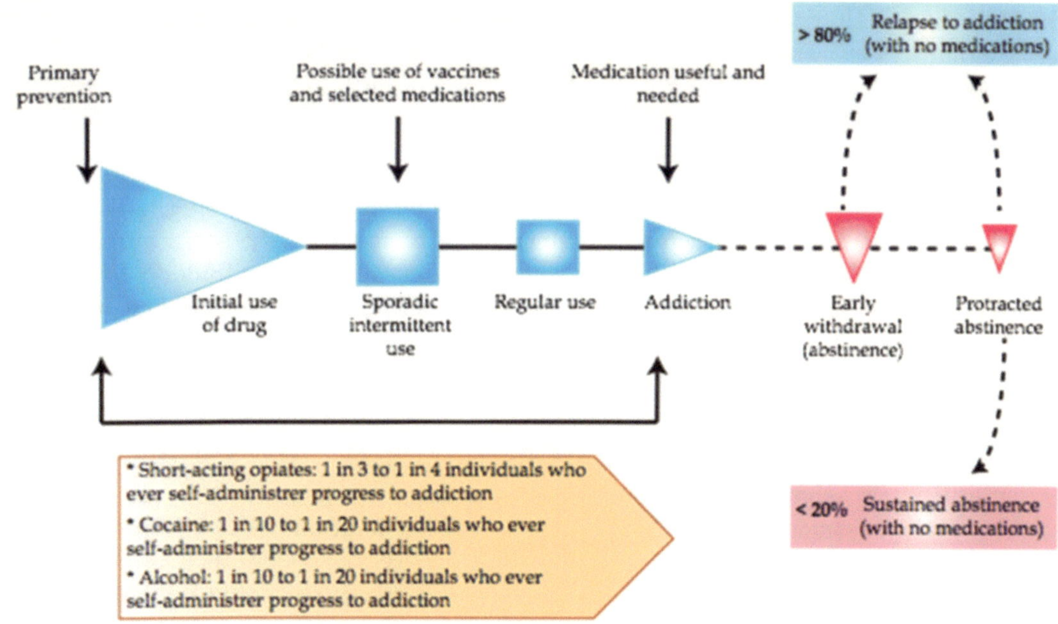

Fig. 5. Strategic targets of therapeutic treatment in the course of drug addiction (reproduced from (51))

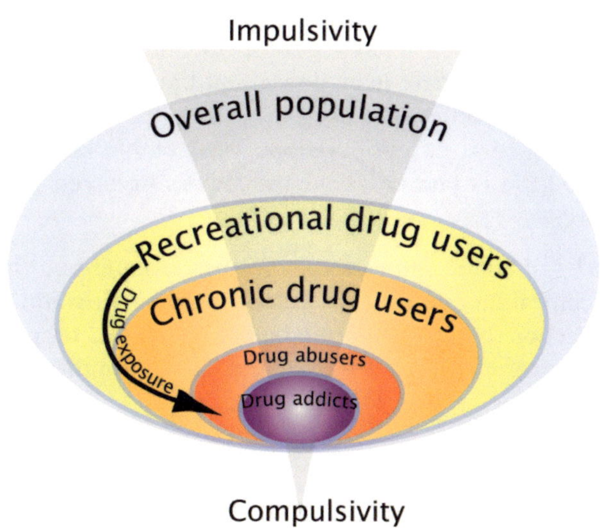

Fig. 6. A progressive shift from impulsivity to compulsivity in the development of drug addiction (42)

2.2 Behavioural and psychological profile of drug addicts

Besides their disinterest for alternative sources of reinforcement and their focus on the drug, drug addicts are characterised by several behavioural and cognitive deficits including impaired inhibitory control (62-67), decision making (68-75) and insight (76-78).

However, major differences can be observed between addicts depending on their preferred drug of abuse. For instance, although opiate and stimulant addicts both display increased sensation seeking (79-81) and impulsivity (82-87), they nevertheless differ in other respects, with heroin addicts showing greater anxiety than cocaine addicts (88), while the latter display higher impulsivity (62, 89, 90).

Thus not only are several personality traits, including sensation seeking, anxiety and impulsivity, associated with increased vulnerability to use drugs (91-94), but different personality traits are preferentially associated with use (95) and addiction to specific drugs (91, 92, 94, 96-103). It is therefore possible that heroin and cocaine addicts may self-medicate different personality characteristics or affective states (104-107), with impulsivity being preferentially self-medicated by cocaine use. However, as discussed in chapter 2 of this book, the relative contribution of a behavioural trait to the choice of a drug does not necessarily predict its implication in the transition to compulsive drug use.

Drug addicts also show several comorbid psychiatric disorders (108-111), as stated by O'Brien (112): «Psychiatric disorders commonly coexist with addictive disorders. These include anxiety disorders, psychotic disorders, and affective disorders such as depression. Although some of these so-called "dual diagnosis" cases are simply a coincidental occurrence of common disorders, the overlap is greater than would be expected by chance on the basis of population prevalences (109)». However, it remains unknown whether comorbid elements contribute to increased vulnerability to drug addiction (113) or whether chronic drug exposure facilitates the emergence of psychiatric comorbidity (for discussion see (112)). Similarly, while some personality, or behavioural, traits are triggered by chronic drug use, there is evidence that personality variables are associated with increased vulnerability to develop drug addiction (92, 114). This rather blur picture not only suggests that several sub-populations exist within drug addicts (115), but it clearly illustrates how little is known about the factors involved in the vulnerability to develop drug addiction.

To date a triadic model of contributing factors has been established that accounts well for both clinical and preclinical literature. Thus, vulnerability to drug addiction is suggested to result from the interaction between a vulnerable phenotype, or personality (being the interaction between genes and history), the drug and the environment (figure 7).

There is clearly a genetic vulnerability to addiction. Genetic factors may contribute up to 40% to the development of drug addiction (51). This estimation gives genetic factors a limited contribution to the vulnerability to drug addiction and highlights the importance of both the drug and the environment in the development of the pathology. There is indeed compelling evidence that life experiences and environments highly influence the effects of drugs of abuse and play a critical role in the transition from controlled to compulsive drug use (116, 117). For instance, drug addiction seems to be more frequent in people living in degraded areas or in people that undergo difficult experiences during their childhood. Such specific environmental conditions at either perinatal, developmental or adulthood stages may alter one's personality construction so that they become more vulnerable to use or abuse drugs (118). On the other hand, positive family relationships, friendships, involvement and attachment appear to somehow protect against the development of drug addiction (119, 120).

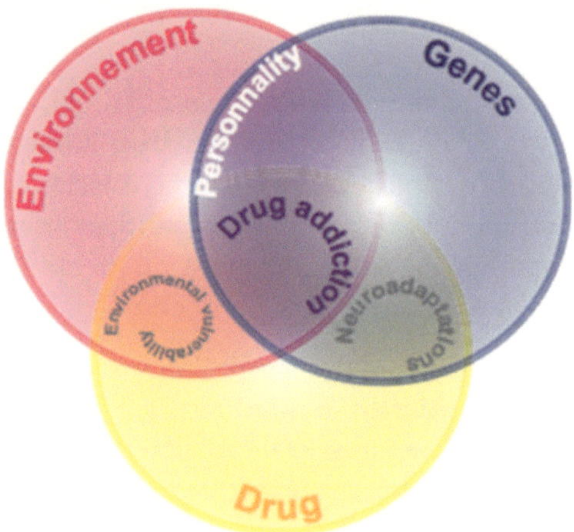

Fig. 7. Triad of influences underlying vulnerability to drug addiction

A number of interacting factors are hypothesised to influence the pathway to addiction, including biological determinants (genes), drug exposure and the environment. Genetic influences may account for up to 40% of the vulnerability for drug addiction

Thus, the present general strategies developed to treat addictions should perhaps be re-oriented towards a more patient-based medication strategy once better insights are gained in the understanding of the etiological and neurobiological substrates of individual vulnerabilities to addictions.

2.3 Biological correlates of drug addiction in humans: Insights from imaging studies

An exhaustive synthesis of the neurobiological correlates of drug addiction is beyond the scope of this chapter. Overall, drug exposure impacts both brain structure and function. Thus at the morphological level, drug addicts have decreased grey matter volumes in prefrontal (121-125) and cerebellar regions of the brain (126). Functionally, when presented with drug-related cues that induce craving, drug addicts show abnormal activation of limbic structures including the amygdala (127, 128), the insular (40, 129) and orbitofrontal cortices (39, 130) as well as cognitive prefrontal areas such as the cingulate (127, 128, 131) and dorsolateral prefrontal cortices (74).

Moreover, drug addicts are characterised by decreased levels of striatal D2/3 dopamine receptors (132-134) and reduced metabolism in the orbitofrontal cortex (132). These two alterations are highly correlated (132), thereby providing the orbitofrontal-limbic striatum circuit a prominent implication in addiction (134, 135), even though other networks, including the thalamo-cortical systems, have been identified to be impaired in drug addicts (136).

Interestingly, a growing body of evidence points towards an implication of non limbic striatal areas in the pathophysiology of drug addiction since dopamine transmission is specifically increased in the dorsal striatum of cocaine addicts experiencing craving in response to presentation of drug-associated cues (137, 138), providing a neurobiological evidence for a progressive involvement of dorsal striatum-dependent habits (139-141) in drug addiction (35-37, 41, 42).

A major limitation of human studies is that the data obtained, though clearly informative, are based on the comparison of current or former drug addicts and drug naive control subjects. Thereby, human studies cannot control for the effects of protracted drug exposure on the brain nor can they define whether the abnormalities observed in drug addicts are a pathological biological adaptation to drug exposure or predated drug use and hence are instead endophenotypes of vulnerability to drug addiction.

This is where the case for animal experimentation in addiction research is revealed compelling. Besides the aforementioned limitations, studies in human addicts are often prone to interpretative issues not least due to inter-subject variability in drug exposure, the frequent co-abuse of several drugs often in combination with alcohol, cannabis and nicotine, the regular occurrence of co-morbid brain disorders such as depression, conduct disorder and attention-deficit/hyperactivity disorder (ADHD) and the difficulty in controlling pre-morbid cognitive and intellectual abilities.

3. References

[1] Koob G, Le Moal M. Plasticity of reward neurocircuitry and the 'dark side' of drug addiction. Nat Neurosci. 2005; 8: 1442-1444.
[2] Nutt D, King LA, Saulsbury W, Blakemore C. Development of a rational scale to assess the harm of drugs of potential misuse. Lancet. 2007; 369: 1047-1053.
[3] Lindesmith AR. Addiction and opiates. Chicago: Aldine Pub. Co.; 1968: vii, 295.
[4] Fort J. The pleasure seekers; the drug crisis, youth, and society. Indianapolis: Bobbs-Merrill; 1969: 255.
[5] Rivera MA, Aufderheide AC, Cartmell LW, Torres CM, Langsjoen O. Antiquity of coca-leaf chewing in the south central Andes: a 3,000 year archaeological record of coca-leaf chewing from northern Chile. J Psychoactive Drugs. 2005; 37: 455-458.
[6] Humphrey AJ, O'Hagan D. Tropane alkaloid biosynthesis. A century old problem unresolved. Nat Prod Rep. 2001; 18: 494-502.
[7] Freud S. Uber coca. 1884; Centralbl Gesamte Ther: 289-314.
[8] Nesse RM, Berridge K. Psychoactive Drug Use in Evolutionary Perspective. Science. 1997; 278: 63-66.
[9] Kolb LC. Drug addiction. Bulletin of the New York Academy of Medicine. 1965; 41: 306.
[10] EMCDDA. The state of the drugs problem in Europe (annual report 2009).
[11] WHO. Neuroscience of psychoactive substance use and dependence. Geneva: World Health Organization; 2004
[12] Kusayama T, Watanabe S. Reinforcing effects of methamphetamine in planarians. Neuroreport. 2000; 11: 2511-2513.
[13] Li H, Chaney S, Roberts IJ, Forte M, Hirsh J. Ectopic G-protein expression in dopamine and serotonin neurons blocks cocaine sensitization in Drosophila melanogaster. CurrBiol. 2000; 10: 211-214.
[14] Wolf F, Heberlein U. Invertebrate models of drug abuse. J Neurobiol. 2002; 54: 161-178.

[15] Carney JM, Landrum RW, Cheng MS, Seale TW. Establishment of chronic intravenous drug self-administration in the C57BL/6J mouse. Neuroreport. 1991; 2: 477-480.

[16] Grahame NJ, Phillips TJ, Burkhart-Kasch S, Cunningham CL. Intravenous cocaine self-administration in the C57BL/6J mouse. Pharmacol Biochem Behav. 1995; 51: 827-834.

[17] Highfield DA, Mead AN, Grimm JW, Rocha BA, Shaham Y. Reinstatement of cocaine seeking in 129X1/SvJ mice: effects of cocaine priming, cocaine cues and food deprivation. Psychopharmacology (Berl). 2002; 161: 417-424.

[18] Cain ME, Denehy ED, Bardo M. Individual Differences in Amphetamine Self-Administration: The rôle of the Central Nucleus of the Amygdala. Neuropsychopharmacology. 2007; 33: 1149-1161.

[19] Thomsen M, Caine SB. Intravenous drug self-administration in mice: practical considerations. Behav Genet. 2007; 37: 101-118.

[20] van der Veen R, Piazza PV, Deroche-Gamonet V. Gene-environment interactions in vulnerability to cocaine intravenous self-administration: a brief social experience affects intake in DBA/2J but not in C57BL/6J mice. Psychopharmacology (Berl). 2007; 193: 179-186.

[21] Thomsen M, Han DD, Gu HH, Caine SB. Lack of cocaine self-administration in mice expressing a cocaine-insensitive dopamine transporter. J Pharmacol Exp Ther. 2009

[22] Pickens R, Harris WC. Self-administration of d-amphetamine by rats. Psychopharmacologia. 1968; 12: 158-163.

[23] Ettenberg A, Pettit HO, Bloom FE, Koob GF. Heroin and cocaine intravenous self-administration in rats: Mediation by separate neural systems. Psychopharmacology. 1982; 78: 204-209.

[24] Collins RJ, Weeks JR, Cooper MM, Good PI, Russell RR. Prediction of abuse liability of drugs using IV self-administration by rats. Psychopharmacology (Berl). 1984; 82: 6-13.

[25] Koob G, Le HT, Creese I. The D1 dopamine receptor antagonist SCH 23390 increases cocaine self-administration in the rat. NeurosciLett. 1987; 79: 315-320.

[26] Weissenborn R, Yackey M, Koob GF, Weiss F. Measures of cocaine-seeking behavior using a multiple schedule of food and drug self-administration in rats. Drug Alcohol Depend. 1995; 38: 237-246.

[27] Risner ME, Goldberg SR. A comparison of nicotine and cocaine self-administration in the dog: fixed-ratio and progressive-ratio schedules of intravenous drug infusion. J Pharmacol Exp Ther. 1983; 224: 319-326.

[28] Shannon HE, Risner ME. Comparison of behavior maintained by intravenous cocaine and d-amphetamine in dogs. JpharmacolExpTher. 1984; 229: 422-432.

[29] Deneau G, Yanagita T, Seevers MH. Self-administration of psychoactive substances by the monkey. Psychopharmacologia. 1969; 16: 30-48.

[30] Goldberg SR, Woods JH, Schuster CR. Morphine: Conditioned Increases in Self-Administration in Rhesus Monkeys. Science. 1969

[31] Leshner AI. Addiction is a brain disease, and it matters. Science. 1997; 278: 45-47.

[32] Robinson T, Berridge K. The psychology and neurobiology of addiction: an incentive-sensitization view. Addiction. 2000; 95: S91-S117.

[33] Kalivas P, Volkow N. The Neural Basis of Addiction: A Pathology of Motivation and Choice. American Journal of Psychiatry. 2005; 162: 1403-1413.

[34] Everitt B, Parkinson JA, Olmstead M, Arroyo M, Robledo P, Robbins TW. Associative processes in addiction and reward. The role of amygdala-ventral striatal subsystems. Ann NYAcadSci. 1999; 877: 412-438.

[35] Everitt BJ., Dickinson A, Robbins TW. The neuropsychological basis of addictive behaviour. Brain Research Reviews. 2001; 36: 129-138.

[36] Everitt BJ., Robbins TW. Neural systems of reinforcement for drug addiction: from actions to habits to compulsion. Nat Neurosci. 2005; 8: 1481-1489.

[37] Belin D, Jonkman S, Dickinson A, Robbins TW, Everitt BJ.. Parallel and interactive learning processes within the basal ganglia: Relevance for the understanding of addiction. Behavioural Brain Research. 2009; 199(1): 89-102.

[38] Volkow N, Fowler J. Addiction, a Disease of Compulsion and Drive: Involvement of the Orbitofrontal Cortex. Cerebral Cortex. 2000

[39] Goldstein RZ, Volkow ND. Drug addiction and its underlying neurobiological basis: neuroimaging evidence for the involvement of the frontal cortex. Am J Psychiatry. 2002; 159: 1642-1652.

[40] Goldstein RZ, Alia-Klein N, Tomasi D et al. Anterior cingulate cortex hypoactivations to an emotionally salient task in cocaine addiction. Proc Natl Acad Sci U S A. 2009; 106: 9453-9458.

[41] Robbins TW, Everitt BJ. Drug addiction: bad habits add up. Nature. 1999; 398: 567-570.

[42] Belin D, Everitt BJ. The Neural and Psychological Basis of a Compulsive Incentive Habit. In: Steiner H, tseng K, editors. Handbook of basal ganglia structure and function, 20. Elsvier, ACADEMIC PRESS; 2010.

[43] Koob G, Le Moal M. Addiction and the Brain Antireward System. Annu Rev Psychol. 2008; 59: 29-53.

[44] APA. Diagnostic and Statistical Manual of Mental Disorders fourth edition, Text revision (DSM-IV TR). Washington DC: American Psychiatric Association; 2000

[45] Mclellan A, Kushner H, Metzger D, Peters R. The Fifth Edition of the Addiction Severity Index. J Subst Abuse Treat. 1992

[46] McLellan AT, Cacciola JC, Alterman AI, Rikoon SH, Carise D. The Addiction Severity Index at 25: origins, contributions and transitions. Am J Addict. 2006; 15: 113-124.

[47] Rikoon S, Cacciola J, Carise D, Alterman A, Mclellan A. Predicting DSM-IV dependence diagnoses from Addiction Severity Index composite scores. Journal of Substance Abuse Treatment. 2006; 31: 17-24.

[48] Krenz S, Dieckmann S, Favrat B et al. French version of the addiction severity index (5th Edition): validity and reliability among Swiss opiate-dependent patients. French validation of the Addiction Severity Index. Eur Addict Res. 2004; 10: 173-179.

[49] Cacciola J, Alterman A, O'Brien CP, Mclellan A. The Addiction Severity Index in clinical efficacy trials of medications for cocaine dependence. NIDA ResMonogr. 1997; 175: 182-191.

[50] Anthony JC, Warner LA, Kessler RC. Comparative epidemiology of dependence on tobacco, alcohol, controlled substances, and inhalants: Basic findings from the National comorbidity Survey. Exp Clin Psychopharmacol. 1994; 2: 244-268.

[51] Kreek M, Laforge K, Butelman E. Pharmacotherapy of addictions. Nat Rev Drug Discov. 2002; 1: 710-726.

[52] Uhl G, Grow RW. The burden of complex genetics in brain disorders. Arch GenPsychiatry. 2004; 61: 223-229.

[53] Koob G, Moal ML. Drug Abuse: Hedonic Homeostatic Dysregulation. Science. 1997; 278: 52-58.

[54] Koob G, Le Moal M. Drug addiction, dysregulation of reward, and allostasis. Neuropsychopharmacology. 2001; 24: 97-129.

[55] Koob GF, Le Moal M. Review. Neurobiological mechanisms for opponent motivational processes in addiction. Philos Trans R Soc Lond B Biol Sci. 2008; 363: 3113-3123.

[56] Tiffany ST. A cognitive model of drug urges and drug-use behavior: rôle of automatic and nonautomatic processes. Psychol Rev. 1990; 97: 147-168.

[57] O'Brien CP, Mclellan A. Myths about the treatment of addiction. Lancet. 1996; 347: 237-240.

[58] Jentsch JD, Taylor JR. Impulsivity resulting from frontostriatal dysfunction in drug abuse: implications for the control of behavior by reward-related stimuli. Psychopharmacology. 1999; 146: 373-390.

[59] Everitt BJ, Belin D, Economidou D, Pelloux Y, Dalley J, Robbins TW. Neural mechanisms underlying the vulnerability to develop compulsive drug-seeking habits and addiction. Philos Trans R Soc Lond B Biol Sci. 2008; 363: 3125-3135.

[60] Kalivas PW. Addiction as a pathology in prefrontal cortical regulation of corticostriatal habit circuitry. Neurotox Res. 2008; 14: 185-189.

[61] Baumeister RF, Heatherton TF, Tice DM. Losing Control: How and Why People Fail at Self-Regulation. 1994.

[62] Kirby KN, Petry NM. Heroin and cocaine abusers have higher discount rates for delayed rewards than alcoholics or non-drug-using controls. Addiction. 2004; 99: 461-471.

[63] Mitchell C, Flaherty C. Differential effects of removing the glucose or saccharin components of a glucose–saccharin mixture in a successive negative contrast paradigm. Physiology & Behavior. 2005; 84: 579-583.

[64] Baler RD, Volkow ND. Drug addiction: the neurobiology of disrupted self-control. Trends Mol Med. 2006; 12: 559-566.

[65] Dom G, D'haene P, Hulstijn W, Sabbe B. Impulsivity in abstinent early- and late-onset alcoholics: differences in self-report measures and a discounting task. Addiction. 2006; 101: 50-59.

[66] Verdejo-Garcia A, Benbrook A, Funderburk F, David P, Cadet JL, Bolla KI. The differential relationship between cocaine use and marijuana use on decision-making performance over repeat testing with the Iowa Gambling Task. Drug Alcohol Depend. 2007; 90: 2-11.

[67] Verdejo-Garcia A, Lawrence AJ, Clark L. Impulsivity as a vulnerability marker for substance-use disorders: review of findings from high-risk research, problem

gamblers and genetic association studies. Neuroscience and biobehavioral reviews. 2008; 32: 777-810.

[68] Grant S, Contoreggi C, London ED. Drug abusers show impaired performance in a laboratory test of decision making. Neuropsychologia. 2000; 38: 1180-1187.

[69] Monterosso J, Ehrman R, Napier KL, O'Brien CP, Childress AR. Three decision-making tasks in cocaine-dependent patients: do they measure the same construct? Addiction. 2001; 96: 1825-1837.

[70] Bechara A, Damasio H. Decision-making and addiction (part I): impaired activation of somatic states in substance dependent individuals when pondering decisions with negative future consequences. Neuropsychologia. 2002; 40: 1675-1689.

[71] Bechara A, Dolan S, Hindes A. Decision-making and addiction (part II): myopia for the future or hypersensitivity to reward? Neuropsychologia. 2002; 40: 1690-1705.

[72] Hester R, Garavan H. Executive dysfunction in cocaine addiction: evidence for discordant frontal, cingulate, and cerebellar activity. J Neurosci. 2004; 24: 11017-11022.

[73] Bechara A. Decision making, impulse control and loss of willpower to resist drugs: a neurocognitive perspective. Nat Neurosci. 2005; 8: 1458-1463.

[74] Verdejo-Garcia A, Vilar-Lopez R, Perez-Garcia M, Podell K, Goldberg E. Altered adaptive but not veridical decision-making in substance dependent individuals. J Int Neuropsychol Soc. 2006; 12: 90-99.

[75] Vassileva J, Petkova P, Georgiev S et al. Impaired decision-making in psychopathic heroin addicts. Drug Alcohol Depend. 2007; 86: 287-289.

[76] Goldstein RZ, Craig AD, Bechara A et al. The neurocircuitry of impaired insight in drug addiction. Trends Cogn Sci. 2009; 13: 372-380.

[77] Naqvi NH, Bechara A. The hidden island of addiction: the insula. Trends Neurosci. 2009; 32: 56-67.

[78] Naqvi NH, Bechara A. The insula and drug addiction: an interoceptive view of pleasure, urges, and decision-making. Brain Struct Funct. 2010

[79] Allcock CC, Grace DM. Pathological gamblers are neither impulsive nor sensation-seekers. Aust N Z J Psychiatry. 1988; 22: 307-311.

[80] Gerra G, Angioni L, Zaimovic A et al. Substance use among high-school students: relationships with temperament, personality traits, and parental care perception. Subst Use Misuse. 2004; 39: 345-367.

[81] Maremmani I, Pacini M, Popovic D et al. Affective temperaments in heroin addiction. J Affect Disord. 2009; 117: 186-192.

[82] Madden GJ, Petry NM, Badger GJ, Bickel WK. Impulsive and self-control choices in opioid-dependent patients and non-drug-using control participants: drug and monetary rewards. Exp Clin Psychopharmacol. 1997; 5: 256-262.

[83] Kirby KN, Petry NM, Bickel WK. Heroin addicts have higher discount rates for delayed rewards than non-drug-using controls. J Exp Psychol Gen. 1999; 128: 78-87.

[84] Coffey SF, Gudleski GD, Saladin ME, Brady KT. Impulsivity and rapid discounting of delayed hypothetical rewards in cocaine-dependent individuals. Exp Clin Psychopharmacol. 2003; 11: 18-25.

[85] Bornovalova MA, Lejuez CW, Daughters SB, Zachary Rosenthal M, Lynch TR. Impulsivity as a common process across borderline personality and substance use disorders. Clin Psychol Rev. 2005; 25: 790-812.
[86] Clark L, Robbins TW, Ersche KD, Sahakian BJ. Reflection impulsivity in current and former substance users. Biol Psychiatry. 2006; 60: 515-522.
[87] Verdejo-Garcia AJ, Perales JC, Perez-Garcia M. Cognitive impulsivity in cocaine and heroin polysubstance abusers. Addict Behav. 2007; 32: 950-966.
[88] Lejuez CW, Paulson A, Daughters SB, Bornovalova MA, Zvolensky MJ. The association between heroin use and anxiety sensitivity among inner-city individuals in residential drug use treatment. Behav Res Ther. 2006; 44: 667-677.
[89] Bornovalova M, Daughters S, Hernandez G, Richards J, Lejuez C. Differences in impulsivity and risk-taking propensity between primary users of crack cocaine and primary users of heroin in a residential substance-use program. Experimental and Clinical Psychopharmacology. 2005; 13: 311-318.
[90] Lejuez CW, Bornovalova MA, Daughters SB, Curtin JJ. Differences in impulsivity and sexual risk behavior among inner-city crack/cocaine users and heroin users. Drug Alcohol Depend. 2005; 77: 169-175.
[91] Zuckerman M. Sensation seeking and the endogenous deficit theory of drug abuse. NIDA Res Monogr. 1986; 74: 59-70.
[92] Franques P, Auriacombe M, Tignol J. [Addiction and personality]. Encephale. 2000; 26: 68-78.
[93] Sher KJ, Bartholow BD, Wood MD. Personality and substance use disorders: a prospective study. J Consult Clin Psychol. 2000; 68: 818-829.
[94] Terracciano A, Lockenhoff CE, Crum RM, Bienvenu OJ, Costa PTJ. Five-Factor Model personality profiles of drug users. BMC Psychiatry. 2008; 8: 22.
[95] Adams JB, Heath AJ, Young SE, Hewitt JK, Corley RP, Stallings MC. Relationships between personality and preferred substance and motivations for use among adolescent substance abusers. Am J Drug Alcohol Abuse. 2003; 29: 691-712.
[96] Gossop M. Drug dependence, crime and personality among female addicts. Drug Alcohol Depend. 1978; 3: 359-364.
[97] Labouvie EW, McGee CR. Relation of personality to alcohol and drug use in adolescence. J Consult Clin Psychol. 1986; 54: 289-293.
[98] Greene RL, Adyanthaya AE, Morse RM, Davis LJ. Personality variables in cocaine- and marijuana-dependent patients. JpersAssess. 1993; 61: 224-230.
[99] Clapper RL, Martin CS, Clifford PR. Personality, social environment, and past behavior as predictors of late adolescent alcohol use. J Subst Abuse. 1994; 6: 305-313.
[100] Schinka JA, Curtiss G, Mulloy JM. Personality variables and self-medication in substance abuse. JpersAssess. 1994; 63: 413-422.
[101] Ball SA, Kranzler HR, Tennen H, Poling JC, Rounsaville BJ. Personality disorder and dimension differences between type A and type B substance abusers. J Pers Disord. 1998; 12: 1-12.
[102] Conway K, Swendsen JD, Rounsaville BJ, Merikangas KR. Personality, drug of choice, and comorbid psychopathology among substance abusers. Drug Alcohol Depend. 2002; 65: 225-234.

[103] Gerra G, Bertacca S, Zaimovic A, Pirani M, Branchi B, Ferri M. Relationship of personality traits and drug of choice by cocaine addicts and heroin addicts. Subst Use Misuse. 2008; 43: 317-330.

[104] Khantzian EJ, Mack JE, Schatzberg AF. Heroin use as an attempt to cope: clinical observations. AmJPsychiatry. 1974; 131: 160-164.

[105] Khantzian EJ. Addiction: self-destruction or self-repair? JsubstAbuse Treat. 1989; 6: 75.

[106] Khantzian EJ. Self-regulation factors in cocaine dependence--a clinical perspective. NIDA ResMonogr. 1991; 110: 211-226.

[107] Khantzian EJ. The self-medication hypothesis of substance use disorders: a reconsideration and recent applications. HarvRevPsychiatry. 1997; 4: 231-244.

[108] Khantzian EJ. Psychiatric illness in drug abusers. NenglJMed. 1980; 302: 869-870.

[109] Kessler RC, Nelson CB, McGonagle KA, Edlund MJ, Frank RG, Leaf PJ. The epidemiology of co-occurring addictive and mental disorders: implications for prevention and service utilization. Am J Orthopsychiatry. 1996; 66: 17-31.

[110] Skinstad AH, Swain A. Comorbidity in a clinical sample of substance abusers. Am Jdrug Alcohol Abuse. 2001; 27: 45-64.

[111] Gum AM, Cheavens JS. Psychiatric comorbidity and depression in older adults. Curr Psychiatry Rep. 2008; 10: 23-29.

[112] O'Brien CP. A Range of Research-Based Pharmacotherapies for Addiction. Science. 1997; 278: 66-70.

[113] Khantzian EJ. The self-medication hypothesis of addictive disorders: focus on heroin and cocaine dependence. Am J Psychiatry. 1985; 142: 1259-1264.

[114] Franques P. Sensation seeking as a common factor in opioid dependent subjects and high risk sport practicing subjects. A cross sectional study. Drug and Alcohol Dependence. 2003; 69: 121-126.

[115] Gunnarsdottir ED, Pingitore RA, Spring BJ et al. Individual differences among cocaine users. Addict Behav. 2000; 25: 641-652.

[116] Swadi H. Individual risk factors for adolescent substance use. Drug and Alcohol Dependence. 1999; 55: 209-224.

[117] Batts K, Grabill T, Galvin D, Schlenger W. Contextual and other factors related to workplace-based substance abuse prevention and earl intervention for adolescents and young adults [dissertation]. 2004.

[118] Khantzian EJ. A contemporary psychodynamic approach to drug abuse treatment. AmJDrug Alcohol Abuse. 1986; 12: 213-222.

[119] Jessor R, Jessor S. A social-psychological framework for studying drug use. NIDA Res Monogr. 1980; 30: 102-109.

[120] Jessor R, Chase JA, Donovan JE. Psychosocial correlates of marijuana use and problem drinking in a national sample of adolescents. Am J Public Health. 1980; 70: 604-613.

[121] Bartzokis G, Beckson M, Lu PH et al. Increased CSF volumes are associated with diminished subjective responses to cocaine infusion. Neuropsychopharmacology. 2000; 23: 468-473.

[122] Bartzokis G, Beckson M, Lu PH et al. Age-related brain volume reductions in amphetamine and cocaine addicts and normal controls: implications for addiction research. Psychiatry Res. 2000; 98: 93-102.

[123] Bartzokis G, Beckson M, Lu PH et al. Cortical gray matter volumes are associated with subjective responses to cocaine infusion. Am J Addict. 2004; 13: 64-73.
[124] Liu J, Liang J, Qin W et al. Dysfunctional connectivity patterns in chronic heroin users: an fMRI study. Neurosci Lett. 2009; 460: 72-77.
[125] Tanabe J, Tregellas JR, Dalwani M et al. Medial orbitofrontal cortex gray matter is reduced in abstinent substance-dependent individuals. Biol Psychiatry. 2009; 65: 160-164.
[126] Andersen BB. Reduction of Purkinje cell volume in cerebellum of alcoholics. Brain Res. 2004; 1007: 10-18.
[127] Childress AR, Mozley PD, McElgin W, Fitzgerald J, Reivich M, O'Brien CP. Limbic activation during cue-induced cocaine craving. Am J Psychiatry. 1999; 156: 11-18.
[128] Childress AR, Ehrman R, Wang Z et al. Prelude to Passion: Limbic Activation by "Unseen" Drug and Sexual Cues. PloS ONE. 2008; 3: e1506.
[129] Gray MA, Critchley HD. Interoceptive basis to craving. Neuron. 2007; 54: 183-186.
[130] Goldstein RZ, Tomasi D, Rajaram S, Cottone LA, Zhang L, Maloney T, Telang F, Alia-Klein N, Volkow ND. Role of the anterior cingulate and medial orbitofrontal cortex in processing drug cues in cocaine addiction. Neuroscience. 2007; 144: 1153-1159.
[131] Kaufman JN, Ross TJ, Stein EA, Garavan H. Cingulate hypoactivity in cocaine users during a GO-NOGO task as revealed by event-related functional magnetic resonance imaging. Jneurosci. 2003; 23: 7839-7843.
[132] Volkow ND, Fowler J, Wang G, Hitzemann R. Decreased dopamine D2 receptor availability is associated with reduced frontal metabolism in cocaine abusers. Synapse. 1993; 14: 169-177.
[133] Volkow ND, Chang L, Wang GJ, Fowler JS, Ding YS, Sedler M, Logan J, Franceschi D, Gatler J, Hitzemann R, Gifford A, Wong C, Pappas N. Low level of brain dopamine D2 receptors in methamphetamine abusers: association with metabolism in the orbitofrontal cortex. Am J Psychiatry. 2001; 158: 2015-2021.
[134] Koob GF, Volkow ND. Neurocircuitry of Addiction. Neuropsychopharmacology. 2009
[135] Fowler JS, Volkow ND, Kassed CA, Chang L. Imaging the addicted human brain. Sci Pract Perspect. 2007; 3: 4-16.
[136] Tomasi D, Goldstein R, Telang F, Maloney T, Alia-Klein N, Caparelli EC, Volkow ND. Thalamo-cortical dysfunction in cocaine abusers: implications in attention and perception. Psychiatry Res. 2007; 155: 189-201.
[137] Garavan H, Pankiewicz J, Bloom A, Cho JK, Sperry L, Ross TJ, Salmeron BJ, Risinger R, Kelley D, Stein EA. Cue-Induced Cocaine Craving: Neuroanatomical Specificity for Drug Users and Drug Stimuli. American Journal of Psychiatry. 2000; 157: 1789-1798.
[138] Volkow ND. Stimulant medications: how to minimize their reinforcing effects? Am J Psychiatry. 2006; 163: 359-361.
[139] Yin H, Mulcare S, Hilário MR, Clouse E, Holloway T, Davis MI, Hansson AC, Lovinger DM, Costa RM. Dynamic reorganization of striatal circuits during the acquisition and consolidation of a skill. Nat Neurosci. 2009; 12: 333-341.

[140] Yin H, Knowlton B. The role of the basal ganglia in habit formation. Nat Rev Neurosci. 2006; 7: 464-476.

[141] Yin H, Zhuang X, Balleine B. Instrumental learning in hyperdopaminergic mice. NeurobiolLearnMem. 2006

2

Animal Models of Drug Addiction

Aude Belin-Rauscent and David Belin
INSERM U 1084, LNEC, Université de Poitiers,
INSERM AVENIR Team "Psychology of Compulsive Disorders", Poitiers,
France

1. Introduction

The study of drug addiction integrates a broad range of research fields including social sciences, psychology, psychiatry, behavioural neurosciences, pharmacology or genetics, each of which being represented in the different chapters of this book. Preclinical studies involving behaving animals have been pivotal for our increasing insights into the psychobiological substrates of addiction and so for about 100 years. Even today, our understanding and knowledge of addiction increase in parallel with the refinement of animal models of this pathology.

1.1 Necessity for animal models in drug addiction research

Whilst animal models can never reproduce the complex social and often personal reasons why people abuse drugs they nevertheless provide a rigorous means to precisely control environmental context, drug exposure as well as assessing behavioural and cognitive performance prior to drug administration. They also allow neural manipulations (e.g., using selective ligands) and so establish the causal influences of putative neural loci and, in turn, the cellular and molecular substrates, of drug addiction. Thus, to date, animal models provide a valuable means to investigate the different stages of the drug addiction cycle including especially the initiation of drug taking, the maintenance phase, which is often accompanied by binges and escalation of drug intake, and finally the switch to compulsive drug intake defined operationally by an increased motivation to take the drug, an inability to inhibit drug seeking and continued dug use despite negative or adverse consequences.

1.2 Definition and validity criteria of animal models

1.2.1 Definition of an animal model

An animal model is a preparation in one organism that allows for the study of one or several aspects of a human condition. Thus a model of drug addiction must provide insights into the neurobiological, psychological or etiological mechanisms of the pathology in humans, at least mimicking some aspects of the pathology.

Two strategies are generally used when designing animal models of drug addiction. Firstly, the model can address a specific symptom, a neurobiological or psychological feature or a behavioural / neurobiological construct associated with the pathology (figure 1).

DSM-IV diagnostic criteria for drug addiction	Psychobiological dimension	Monodimensional animal model	Polydimensional animal model
1 Need for markedly increased amounts of a substance to achieve intoxication or desired effect, or markedly diminished effect with continued use of the same amount of the substance	Pharmacological tolerance		
2 The presence of a characteristic withdrawal syndrome or use of a substance (or a closely related substance) to relieve or avoid withdrawal symptoms	Negative affect/mood depression, anheonia, anxiety		
3 Persistent desire to use drugs or one or more unsuccessful efforts to cut of control substance use	Impulsivity / **compulsivity** behavioural control failure	Reinstatement {1-4} Relapse {5}	3-criteria model of drug addiction: inability to refrain from drug-seeking {14-16}
4 Substance used in larger amounts or over a longer period time than the person intented	Impulsivity / **compulsivity** behavioural control failure	Escalation of drug intake {6-7}	3-criteria model of drug addiction: escalation of drug intake during long access to cocaine {14-16}
5 Important social, occupational, or recreational activities given up or reduced because of substance use	Impulsivity / **compulsivity** behavioural control failure	Resistance to punishment {8} Resistance to conditioned suppression {9}	
6 A great deal of time spent in activities necessary to obtain, to use or to recover from the effects of substance used	Habit / **compulsivity**	Progressive ratio seeking-taking and second order schedule of reinforcement {10-13}	3-criteria model of drug addiction: increased break points in a progressive ratio schedule of reinforcement {14-16}
7 Continued substance use despite knowledge of having a persistent or recurrent physical or psychological problem that is likely to be caused or exacerbated by continued use	**Compulsivity**	Resistance to punishment {8} Resistance to conditioned suppression {9}	3-criteria model of drug addiction: resistance to punishment or adverse consequences {14-16}

Fig. 1. Animal models of drug addiction in reference to the DSM IV diagnostic criteria for drug addiction (adapted from the DSM-IV [97]))

{1} Stewart J. & De Wit H. (1987). *Methods of assessing the reinforcing properties of abused drugs*, (M.A.Bozarth, Ed.). 211-227. Springer-Verlag, New-York.
{2} Shaham Y., Erb S. & Stewart J. (2000). *Brain research review*, 33: 13-33
{3} Grimm J.W., Hope B.T., Wise R.A. & Shaham Y. (2001). *Nature*, 412: 141-142
{4} Bossert J.M., Liu S.Y., Lu L. & shaham Y. (2004). *J. Neurosci.*, **24**(47): 10726-30
{5} Fuchs R.A., Branham R.K. & See R.E. (2006). *J. Neurosci.*, **26**(13): 3584-8
{6} Ahmed S.H. & Koob G.F. (1998). *Science*, **282**(5387): 298-300
{7} Ahmed S.H., Walker J.R. & Koob G.F. (2000). *Neuropsychopharmacology*, **22**(4):413-421
{8} Pelloux Y., Everitt B.J. & Dickinson A. (2007). *Psychopharmacology*, **194**(1): 127-137
{9} Vanderschuren L.J. & Everitt B.J. (2004). *Science*, **305**(5686): 1017-1019
{10} Goldberg S.R., Morse W.H. & Goldberg D.M. (1976). *J Pharmacol Exp Ther*, **199**(1): 278-286
{11} Arroyo M., Markou A., Robbins T.W. & Everitt B.J. (1998). *Psychopharmacology*, **140**(3): 331-344
{12} Everitt B.J. & Robbins T.W. (2000). *Psychopharmacology*, **153**(1): 17-30
{13} Olmstead M.C., Parkinson J.A., Miles F.J., Everitt B.J. & Dickinson A. (2000). *Psychopharmacology*, **152**(2): 123-131
{14} Deroche-Gamonet V., Belin D. & Piazza P.V. (2004). *Science*, **305**(5686): 1014-1017
{15} Belin D., Mar A.C., Dalley J.W., Robbins T.W. & Everitt B.J. (2008). *Science*, **320**(5881):1352-1355
{16} Belin D., Balado., Piazza P.V. & Deroche-Gamonet V. (2009). *Biological psychiatry* 65:863-868
{17} Amhed S.H. (2010). *Neurosci Biobehav Rev*, **35**(2): 172-84

These models have been widely developed the last 40 years and have provided substantial informations about the molecular targets of addictive drugs as well as the neurobiological and psychological adaptations resulting from either acute or chronic drug exposure. Indeed, models that focus on defined features of drug addiction provide a powerful heuristic framework for determining the brain mechanisms underlying the pathology. However, they rarely address other clinical dimensions of the disorder such as behavioural predictive factors or interactions between different symptoms of the pathology. Thus, the second type of models are those that try to incorporate several symptoms of the pathology in humans, thereby providing powerful tools for longitudinal studies or even testing pharmacological treatments, but are somewhat limited in the identification of underlying mechanisms. Indeed, the behavioural complexity of these models makes it difficult to implement causal investigative studies where the end-point is well defined. We discuss the general utility and application of both modelling approaches as complementary tools to investigate the neurobiological and psychological mechanisms of drug addiction and its vulnerability.

1.2.2 Validity criteria of animal models

The validation of animal models of addiction is based upon the same principles that have been established for models in general, namely fulfilling standard criteria amongst which reliability and predictive validity are the most important [1]. However, there are other criteria that have been used widely in validating animal models of drug addiction, including face validity and construct validity [1]. Briefly, reliability refers to the consistency and stability with which the independent and the dependent variables are measured. Thus a reliable model of drug addiction must allow for a precise and reproducible manipulation of the independent variable and an objective and reproducible measure of the dependent variable in standard conditions. A further key criterion for the validation of an animal model is its predictive validity. A valid animal model should predict either the therapeutical potential of a compound in humans (pharmacological isomorphism) or a variable that may influence both the dependent variable of the model and the process under investigation in humans.

Face validity refers to the similarities between the dependent variable of the model, i.e., behaviour in the case of drug addiction, and the human condition, i.e. the symptoms of the pathology. Thus face validity may be important in designing the model but is unlikely an objective criterion to actually assess its validity. Indeed, it is very difficult, if not impossible, to provide an objective criterion to evaluate the similarities between the behavioural output of a rat preparation and drug addiction in humans when the behavioural repertoire of the two species is so different.

Construct validity has been increasingly considered in animal models of drug addiction. It refers to the ability of a model to take into account psychological or neurobiological constructs that characterise the specific pathological processes in humans. Thus, incentive sensitisation, habit formation or top-down prefrontal executive control failure are examples of constructs which have been investigated in animal models.

2. Reinforcing effects of drugs of abuse, abuse liability

As previously mentioned all addictive substances show reinforcing properties in animals. Indeed, the abuse liability of a substance is often measured by its ability to support self-administration and a conditioned place preference [2]. In this section are reviewed the experimental designs that have been developed to investigate the reinforcing properties of addictive drugs. These procedures, combined with molecular biology and pharmacology, have been crucial in the identification and functional characterisation of the molecular targets of addictive drugs.

The seminal discovery by Olds and Milner of intra-cranial self-stimulation (ICSS) in 1954 marked a major turning point for research on the neural mechanisms of addiction [3]. The discovery that dopaminergic projections from the ventral tegmental area (VTA) to limbic cortico-striatal structures (nucleus accumbens, Acb), olfactory tubercle, amygdala, orbitofrontal cortex (OFC), medial prefrontal cortex (mPFC) were effective substrates for ICSS sparked considerable interest in the brain dopamine systems as neural substrates for the rewarding properties of both natural [food] and drug reinforcers. A few years later Weeks developed an operant procedure to deliver intravenous morphine infusions to relatively unrestrained rats [4], a method still widely used in many pre-clinical research laboratories today. That research continued on the opioid drugs morphine and heroin for some considerable time thereafter was no surprise given the strong emphasis at that time in the DSM-III on the symptomatology of opioid dependence and withdrawal [5].

Since then it has been established that addictive substances exert powerful effects on primary and secondary (i.e. conditioned) reinforcement mechanisms. As instrumental reinforcers they strongly encourage behaviours that lead to the availability of a drug, a process subserved by stimulus-response associative mechanisms (instrumental conditioning). Abused drugs also facilitate Pavlovian conditioning whereby previously neutral stimuli in the environment become conditioned to the drug, and can predict it, or even act as conditioned reinforcers.

In operational terms, a reinforcer is a stimulus that increases the probability of a response consequent upon its presentation. Thus, all addictive drugs are reinforcers since they are self-administered by animals and humans and support conditioned place preference (a form of contextual Pavlovian conditioning). Pavlovian conditioned stimuli can act as conditioned reinforcers when presented contingently. Then they can have powerful motivational effects and support long sequences of instrumental drug-seeking behaviour by bridging delays to future drug reinforcement [6-8].

2.1 Conditioned place preference

Conditioned place preference (CPP), has been used extensively to probe the psychological [9] and neurobiological [10-11] mechanisms underlying the rewarding properties of addictive drugs [10;12], as well as negative emotional states associated with drug withdrawal [13-15]. Indeed, through Pavlovian conditioning, the negative affective state caused by drug withdrawal can induce a reliable conditioned place aversion [13-15].

The first study based on the modern paradigm of CPP was reported by Rossi and Reid in 1976 [16] although earlier demonstration of preference for a drug paired environment was published as early as the 1940's [10]. In this procedure two different unconditioned stimuli (US) are paired with two distinct environments. These contextual cues differ in their spatial configuration, colour, flooring, and sometimes even olfactory cues. Briefly, the CPP procedure involves injecting animals with either the drug in question or a control solution, each being administered in a different environment often over successive days. The conditioning phase may combine several pairings, ideally according to a Latin square and unbiased design such that every pairing does not predict subsequent pairings, and that any spontaneous bias or preference for a compartment is initially controlled for. CPP is then tested during a drug-free choice phase where subjects are given access to both compartments. Preference for the drug-paired environment is indicative of the rewarding properties of the drug. CPP can be established not only for addictive drugs but also for natural rewards such as food, water, sexual partner and novelty [10]. Based on a plethora of studies, it is widely accepted that increased dopamine transmission is necessary for the establishment of CPP [17]. Although some authors suggest that CPP is a model of drug seeking behaviour [or drug craving], being essentially dependent upon Pavlovian associations, CPP alone cannot account for the instrumental nature of drug seeking and drug taking behaviour, which is perhaps better modelled by drug self-administration procedures.

2.2 Drug self-administration models

Drug self-administration procedures lie at the core of the most sophisticated preclinical models of drug addiction that have been developed over the last twenty years, ranging from relapse to drug taking [18-20], to loss of control over intake [21-22], compulsive drug taking [23-25] and addiction-like behaviour [8;26-28].

Addictive drugs act as reinforcers, in that they increase the probability of a behavioural response that leads to their presentation, through instrumental conditioning. Thus, animals can readily detect the contingency between an instrumental response and the delivery of a particular drug (e.g., an intravenous infusion of heroin, cocaine, nicotine or THC, or a small volume of alcohol in a magazine) and respond in an instrumental manner to obtain such drugs. The acquisition of drug self-administration is a behavioural marker of its reinforcing properties and abuse liability [2]. Indeed, apart from LSD, all drugs abused by human are self-administered by animals.

Drugs of abuse can be self-administered by a variety of routes across preclinical models, including intramuscular, intranasal, oral, and intravenous [29].

Drug self-administration was initially developed in non human primates, however since the pioneering work of Weeks (1962), rats have extensively been used to investigate the psychological, neural and cellular mechanisms underlying drug self-administration.

Self-administration procedures can be arranged according to different schedules of reinforcement [29]. In fixed ratio schedules, the drug is delivered after the completion of a fixed number of responses by the animal, thereby providing a direct relationship between the actual response and drug delivery. By contrast, in fixed interval schedules, the animal is trained to seek the drug for prolonged periods of time.

Different schedules allow for the investigation of different processes of drug taking or drug seeking behaviour which are beyond the scope of this chapter. However, insightful descriptions of, and discussions about, these schedules can be found in [6;29-32].

The acquisition of drug self-administration is widely considered to depend on the functional integrity of the olfactory tubercle and the shell of the nucleus accumbens (AcbS) [7]. An important role for mesolimbic dopamine in this process was inferred by findings in freely moving rats that dopamine concentration is greatly increased in the striatum, and especially the Acb, following the self-administration of drugs commonly abused by humans [33]. This important study supported the influential hypothesis at that time that addictive drugs exert their primary reinforcing effects and addictive properties through activation of the mesolimbic dopamine system [34-37]. Although it is now clear that increased dopamine release in the Acb does not provide a sufficient account for the addictive properties of drugs such as cocaine, alcohol and heroin, dopamine still remains one of the most important neurotransmitters in the aetiology and pathophysiology of drug addiction, a role underscored by its proposed involvement in salience detection and learning [7;38-52].

In its classic form, the drug self-administration paradigm has provided valuable insights into the brain substrates mediating drug taking behaviour, which differ somewhat according to the particular drug under investigation [53-56]. Addictive drugs not only influence the function of the mesolimbic dopamine system [33] they also trigger a variety of between-systems anatomical [57-62] and functional neuroadaptations [63-66] as well as changes in gene transcription and function in a number of brain systems including the hypothalamus [67], the VTA [68], the amygdala [69-74], Acb [75-79], dorsal striatum [80], orbital [81-82] and prefrontal cortices [83-85], with important effects on stress responsivity [86-88] and epigenetic processes in the limbic system [77;89-92].

However, even though these data have increased our knowledge about the neurobiological substrates of the reinforcing effects of addictive drugs and the neurobiological adaptations to drug self-administration, they provide only limited insights into the neurobiology of drug addiction. As very well brought to remembrance by Serge Ahmed [93], intravenous (intrajugular) self-administration of saline had been demonstrated in water-deprived monkeys [94] a year before the pioneer morphine self-administration work in rats of Weeks (1962), thereby demonstrating that drug self-administration is a measure of instrumental conditioning, but not really a model of drug addiction.

Thus, when one considers working on drug addiction one has to keep in mind that studying drug taking behaviour is not a way of studying drug addiction. This was already stated long ago by Wise and Bozart [95] and quoted by Robinson & Berridge [96]: "To assert that all addictive drugs are reinforcers is to do little more than redefine the phenomenon of addiction."..."To identify a drug as reinforcing goes no further than to identify the drug as addicting"; indeed, there is an obvious gulf between taking a drug on a social basis, as most of us often do, at least when one considers a glass of wine, and compulsively taking drugs. Nevertheless, even after the publication of the DSM-IV in 1994 [97] and the new diagnostic criteria for compulsive drug use that now form the hallmark of the clinical features of drug addiction many, if not all, of the early animal models focused on the "rewarding" properties of addictive drugs and their acute and chronic neurobiological effects.

Thus, during the last ten years pre-clinical research in drug addiction has attempted to better integrate one or more clinical features of the pathology according to the DSM-IV diagnostic criteria. New phenotypes have been identified based on craving or either reinstatement [20;98-99] or relapse to drug seeking [100], a loss of control over drug taking [21-22], habitual / compulsive cocaine seeking and taking [6;23-25;101] and inter-individual vulnerability to addiction-like behaviour [8;26-28].

3. Monodimensional animal models of addiction

3.1 Craving and relapse

Drug addicts show a high propensity to relapse, even after protracted abstinence [102]. This hallmark feature of addiction can be modelled in animals using two main procedures: extinction-reinstatement, initially developed by Stewart and colleagues [18-19] and abstinence-relapse [103]. Reinstatement of responding for drug can be induced by stress, low doses of the drug itself and by the presentation of drug-associated cues [20;104-112]. In the extinction-reinstatement procedure [18-19], animals experience a series of extinction sessions following a short period of drug self-administration, leading to a progressive decline in responding. Following extinction, responding for drug is reinstated by a stressful stimulus, a priming injection of drug, a presentation of a conditioned stimulus (CS) or by placing the animal in a drug-associated environment.

Reinstatement of drug seeking depends upon a broad neurobiological network which subsets are recruited based on the nature of the trigger of reinstatement, be it stress, the drug or drug associated cues and context [105]. Overall, reinstatement to drug seeking depends upon the extended amygdala, prefrontal cortex and dopaminergic neurons [105;113-114]. A large impetus has recently been put on the prominent role of glutamate homeostasis in reinstatement to drug seeking, especially focusing on prefrontal - accumbens pathways [111;115-116].

Interestingly, it has been shown that levels of reinstatement induced by contingent presentations of drug-associated cues increase with prolonged time of withdrawal. This observation suggests that drug craving increases with withdrawal duration [117-118], an adaptation that was specifically related to increase dopamine transporter (DAT) and N-Methyl-D-Aspartate receptor 1 (NMDA R1) protein levels in respectively the prefrontal cortex and the mesolimbic system [118]. However, incubation process has also been reported for food and fear, thereby suggesting that it is a common neurobehavioural adaptation to cessation of stimulation, whatever the nature of the unconditioned stimulus, rather than a specific neurobiological substrate of drug addiction.

In the abstinence-relapse procedure [103], animals are given a forced abstinence period after a brief period of drug self-administration. They are then maintained in their home cage until they are exposed again to the self-administration chamber where they are tested under extinction.

Whereas the reinstatement procedure clearly involves the Acb and both its dopaminergic and glutamatergic inputs, relapse to drug seeking depends upon the dorsolateral striatum [100;103]. Thereby, this neurobiological dissociation suggests that parallel, not necessarily mutually exclusive, neurobiological systems are involved in relapse to drug seeking. However, their respective contribution to the human craving and relapse situation remains unclear, especially the one of reinstatement since the situation in which human addicts go through extinction before responding to drug-associated stimuli or stress is very unfrequent.

3.2 Escalation of drug taking

The first well-established animal model of loss of control over drug intake, namely escalation of drug self-administration, is based on the fourth diagnostic criterion of drug addiction and was developed by Serge Ahmed and George Koob in 1998 for cocaine [21] and 2000 for heroin [22]. Short access ("ShA") to addictive drugs generally results in stable levels of self-administration such that plasma drug levels are controlled within an optimal level of reinforcement [119]. As mentioned previously, this pattern of self-administration does not account for the clinical features of drug addiction in humans. Ahmed and Koob thus gave extended access to cocaine to a group of animals ("LgA", or long access) following a period of moderate exposure (ShA, fixed ratio 1, one hour a day). A second group of rats received short access to cocaine throughout the experiment.

Introduction of the long access was immediately associated with higher drug intake, as compared to ShA rats. In other words, the LgA rats escalated their rate of cocaine self-administration compared with ShA rats, which maintained a constant level of cocaine intake. LgA rats also exhibited higher rates of cocaine self-administration during the first hour of each session. Escalation of cocaine intake has been associated with an upward shift in the intracranial self-administration threshold (ICSS), indicative of reward dysfunction [21] that has been postulated by the hedonic allostasis theory [2;86-88]. However, escalation of cocaine self-administration is not associated with psychomotor sensitisation but, instead, with a sensitization of the incentive motivational properties of cocaine [120], thereby suggesting a dissociation between loss of control over drug intake and behavioural sensitisation.

Escalation of drug intake has also been associated with higher resistance to shock-induced suppression of drug self-administration and conditioned suppression [24;121], and therefore might contribute to the instantiation of addiction.

However, all rats subjected to extended access to heroin do not necessarily escalate their intake [122]. Thus, when the upper and lower quartile of a population of Lister-Hooded rats are selected on the basis of the escalation slope (a direct measure of the magnitude of escalation of drug intake over time), marked differences can be observed [122]. Whereas low escalation (LE) rats show a marked increase in their intake when extended access is introduced and then reach a plateau in their daily drug intake, high escalation (HE) rats tend to show a slower adaptation to extended access, in that they do not increase their intake as quickly as LE rats, but progressively lose control over heroin self-administration (figure 2). This first formal description of inter-individual differences in the propensity to escalate heroin intake lead to the investigation of the behavioural markers of loss of control over heroin and cocaine intake (see "Vulnerabilities to drug addiction" section). This observation may resonate well with the demonstration that escalation of drug intake does not necessarily render rats insensitive to alternative reinforcers, i.e., despite escalation of cocaine self-administration rats have been reported to prefer a saccharine solution when given the choice between this reinforcer and the drug [123]. This suggests that schedule-induced escalation of drug intake, when considered without the individual dimension, does capture one criterion of drug addiction, namely, drug is used in larger amounts, but not necessarily extends to other criteria. However, inter-individual differences can also be observed in the resistance to alternative reinforcers after extended access to cocaine [93].

3.3 Animal models of drug seeking: The distinction between drug seeking and drug taking behaviour: Second-order and two-link heterogeneous chained schedules of reinforcement

Drug addiction does not involve only taking drugs, drug addicts spend most of their time foraging for the drug. It is therefore vital to dissociate drug taking from drug seeking. In trying to separate drug seeking from drug taking, schedules of reinforcement must be implemented in which operant responding for the drug during the drug seeking phase is not affected by the drug itself, i.e., so that drug seeking behaviour can be measured without interference by stimulant or sedative actions of the self-administered drug.

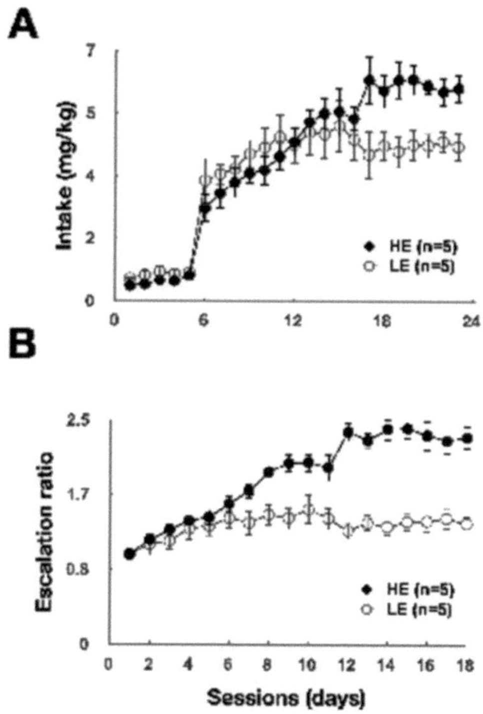

Fig. 2. Inter-individual propensity to lose control over heroin intake, after (122)
Marked inter-individual differences were revealed when the upper (high-escalation rats, HE, n=5) and lower quartile (low-escalation rats, LE, n=5) of a population of lister hooded rats were selected based on the slope of drug intake over all 18 days of the LgA phase [group: $F_{1,8} = 59.44$, $P < 0.001$]. Thus, HE and LE rats displayed a different profile both in terms of heroin intake (A) and escalation ratio (B) [group x session interaction: $F_{22,176} = 8.26$, $P < 0.001$ and $F_{16,128} = 10.20$, $P < 0.001$, respectively]. Post-hoc analysis confirmed that HE rats displayed a daily increase in both intake and escalation ratio from the 4th and 6th day of extended access, respectively (vs. LgA d1, all Ps < 0.05), whereas LE rats showed no escalation at all.

Two-link heterogeneous chained schedules of reinforcement aim to dissociate spatially, temporally, and instrumentally drug seeking from drug taking behaviour. Second-order schedules of reinforcement allow the investigation of cue-controlled drug seeking over prolonged periods of time.

3.3.1 Two-link heterogeneous chain schedules of reinforcement

In this procedure completion of the first link of the chain, designated as the seeking link, results in access to the second link, or taking link, which permits, once performed, the delivery of the reinforcer. Acquisition of the chain schedule is achieved through successive steps of increasing complexity which start with introduction of the taking lever. A lever press is then reinforced under a fixed ratio (FR) 1 schedule so that each lever press produces drug reinforcement accompanied by the withdrawal of the taking lever. After several sessions of stable responding, the seeking lever is introduced while the taking lever is retracted. The first press on the seeking lever initiates a random interval (RI) schedule with the first seeking lever press occurring after the RI has elapsed terminating the first link of the chain; this results in retraction of the seeking lever and insertion of the taking lever to initiate the second link. One press on the taking lever results in the presentation of the reinforcer followed by a time-out period. Thereafter, the seeking lever is reinserted to start the next cycle of the schedule. The effects of experimental manipulation can thus be assessed through measures of seeking responding (latency, number or response rate) as well as taking responding (latency). The interest in dissociating seeking and taking behaviour is obvious when considering that the two instrumental components are influenced by dissociable processes since they are differentially sensitive to devaluation, incentive learning or Pavlovian manipulations [124]. In addition, cocaine seeking performance is monotonically related to the dose of drug with a relatively long time out [125]. Whereas early cocaine seeking performance is profoundly affected by extinction of the taking link [126-127] but not by inactivation of the dorsolateral striatum [127], after extended training it becomes automatic, i.e., insensitive to extinction of the taking lever and sensitive to inactivation of the dorsolateral striatum [127], thereby suggesting a shift in both the psychological and neurobiological mechanisms governing drug seeking when it becomes well established [128].

3.3.2 Second-order schedule of cocaine reinforcement

In the street, drug seeking behaviour is stimulus-bond in that drug addicts forage for their drug under the control of stimuli in the environment, acting as conditioned reinforcers, that support long sequences of behaviour in the absence of the outcome. More formally, conditioned reinforcers are stimuli that have themselves acquired rewarding properties after repeated associations with unconditioned rewards. Conditioned reinforcers bridge delays between seeking and obtaining the drug. Psychostimulants, opiates, speedball, cannabis, or nicotine-associated CSs act as powerful conditioned reinforcers since they greatly enhance drug seeking behaviour when presented contingently, but not non-contingently, upon instrumental responding during, usually, interval schedules of reinforcement [6;30;32;129-130]. Conditioned reinforcers can also support the acquisition of a new instrumental response [131-132]. Such properties are clearly demonstrated in procedures where animals work to obtain presentation of a conditioned stimulus, often in the absence of the unconditioned reward.

In second-order schedules of reinforcement, the CS is presented response-contingently usually under a fixed ratio schedule, during an overall fixed interval or fixed ratio schedule for the primary reinforcer, and markedly enhances and maintains responding for long periods of time (figure 3). Thus, under a second-order schedule of reinforcement, a strong contingency exists between the instrumental response and the presentation of the CS (under a fixed ratio) as well as the relatively weaker contingency that is arranged between instrumental performance and the outcome (the drug) that is reinforced only after completion of the first ratio after each interval has elapsed. Such schedules therefore facilitate the development of stimulus-response (S-R) control over instrumental responding. In addition, it has been shown that omission of CS presentation in second-order schedules of reinforcement disrupts cocaine seeking more than food seeking behaviour [130], suggesting that prolonged psychostimulant seeking is particularly dependent upon conditioned reinforcement.

Thus, instrumental responding during the first interval of a second-order schedule of reinforcement shows face and construct validity with regards to the behavioural features of drug seeking in humans: stimulus-bound, somewhat dissociated from the unconditioned effects of the drug and long lasting.

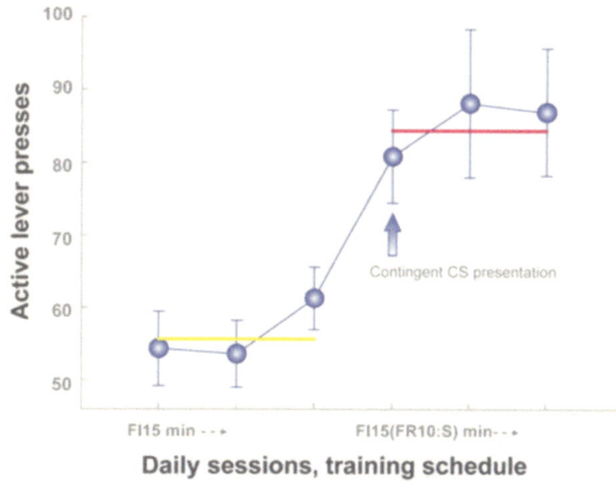

Fig. 3. Acquisition of cocaine seeking under a second-order schedule of reinforcement. Instrumental performance of a population of 24 Lister Hooded rats during the first interval of a FI15 and FI15(FR10:S) schedule of reinforcement (see text for explanation). Once animals have acquired self-administration under continuous reinforcement, the reinforcement schedule is switched to fixed intervals, with daily increments: FI1 min, FI2 min, FI4 min, FI8 min, FI10 min, and FI15 min. After 3 days of training under the FI15 schedule (*left part of the figure*), contingent presentations of the CS are introduced under a FR10 schedule such that rats are now trained under a FI15(FR10:S) second-order schedule of reinforcement. This acquisition procedure provides a direct measure of the potentiation of responding during interval schedules by the contingent presentation of the CS since they are introduced only once responding under fixed interval has stabilized. Thus, although the average response rate is 50 during the first interval of a FI15 schedule, it reaches 90-100 when the CS is contingently presented (Belin-Rauscent & Belin, unpublished).

Second-order schedules of cocaine and heroin self-administration were initially developed by Goldberg and colleagues in non human primates to assess the influence of environmental stimuli upon drug self-administration [30;129-130]. Everitt and colleagues have also established second-order schedules of drug reinforcement in rats [133]. In the study by Arroyo and colleagues (1998), rats were initially required to learn cocaine to self-administer under continuous reinforcement, i.e., FR1. After stabilisation of responding, (5 to 7 daily 2 hours sessions), a second-order schedule with fixed ratio components of the type FRx(Fry:S) was introduced, with initial values of x and y set to 1, so that each active lever press resulted in the presentation of the CS and and the delivery of 0.25 mg of cocaine. Then x and y values were progressively increased with increments in response requirements starting with x i.e., FR5(FR1:S) and FR10(FR1:S), then y, i.e., FR10(FR2:S), FR10(FR4:S), FR10(FR7:S) and FR10(FR10:S). After stabilisation of responding under this FR10(FR10:S) schedule of reinforcement which therefore requires 100 active lever presses and 10 one second presentations of the CS to obtain a cocaine infusion, a final fixed interval schedule FI15(FR10:S) was introduced such that a cocaine infusion was delivered only following the tenth active lever press that occurred when the 15 min interval had elapsed. Finally rats were allowed to perform cocaine seeking behaviour under this schedule for ten days. This acquisition procedure produces robust and stable CS-dependent rates of responding [133] and has been used extensively to probe the neural mechanisms involved in the acquisition, and the performance of, cue-controlled cocaine-seeking [101;134-135].

It is also possible to decrease the acquisition period to 11 days [101;136] (figure 3). In this case the training phase consists of three days of FR1 training, 2 hour daily sessions, 30 infusions (0.25 mg cocaine / infusion) followed by the introduction of interval schedules, with daily increments: FI1 min, FI2 min, FI4 min, FI 8 min, FI10 min, FI15 min. After three days of training under the FI15 schedule, contingent presentations of the CS are introduced under a FR10 schedule such that rats are now trained under a FI15(FR10:S) second-order schedule of reinforcement. This acquisition procedure provides a direct measure of the potentiation of responding during interval schedules by the contingent presentation of the CS since they are introduced only once responding under fixed interval has stabilised.

Thus, although the average response rate is 50-70 during the first interval of a FI15 schedule, it reaches 100-150 when the CS is contingently presented (figure 3), as described in several studies from Everitt's laboratory [101;137-138]. Indeed, short and long-term training under second-order schedules of reinforcement for cocaine have been very useful for investigating the neural mechanisms involved in the transition from newly acquired to well established or habitual cue-controlled cocaine seeking. Thus, acquisition of cue-controlled cocaine seeking depends upon the core of the Acb (AcbC) and its functional relationships with the basolateral amygdala [139] as well as dopamine transmission into the posterior dorsolateral striatum [137]. However, when it is well established, or habitual, cue-controlled cocaine seeking rather depends upon dopamine transmission into the dorsolateral striatum and its functional relationship with the AcbC, as demonstrated by functional disconnections between these two structures [101].

A dorsomedial to dorsolateral striatal shift in the control over drug seeking has recently been demonstrated to occur in alcohol self-administration after eight weeks of training [140a] and cocaine seeking after two weeks of training under an FI15(FR10:S) schedule of reinfocement [140b], a stage at which alcohol seeking was shown to be impervious to devaluation, i.e., was habitual. Thus addiction to both stimulants and alcohol may be dependent upon a shift from goal-directedness to habits that parallels, at the neural systems level, a progressive recruitment of the dorsolateral striatum. These data obtained in preclinical models resonate well with the recent demonstration of dorsal striatum implication cue-induced in alcohol [141] or cocaine [142] craving in humans.

3.4 Animal models of compulsive drug seeking and drug taking

As emphasised previously, addicted individuals not only consume large amounts of drugs but are also unable to repress their drug use regardless its consequences. Thus addiction shares common features with other compulsive disorders which are characterised as the uncontrollable and irresistible urge to performance an act, often to relieve anxiety or stress, but regardless of the rationality of the motivation.

The compulsive aspect of drug use in addicted subjects is even more obvious when similarities between addiction and obsessive compulsive disorder (OCD) are considered. Indeed, compulsive behaviour in the 4th version of the DSM [97] as a criterion for OCD is defined by the repetitive behaviours or mental acts that the person feels driven to perform in response to an obsession, or according to rules that must be applied rigidly aiming at preventing or reducing distress or some dreaded event or situation; but are either not connected to the issue or are excessive. Similarities between addiction and OCD have led, based on a modified version of the Yale–Brown Obsessive Compulsive Scale (Y-BOCS-hd) [143-144], to the development of the Obsessive Compulsive Drinking Scale (OCDS), a self-rated questionnaire which is able accurately to discriminate between alcoholic out-patients and social drinkers with high sensitivity and specificity [145], suggesting that obsessionality and compulsivity are key features of the heavily addicted individual [145].

Clinical data on abstinence from cocaine use suggest that the negative consequences directly related to use are a major reason for cessation [146]. Indeed, drug use is a high risk behaviour as it often compromised health, work and social relationships [147-148].

Preclinical models of drug addiction might therefore attempt to resemble in several respects the human conditions of compulsivity and fulfil some important features of the pathology in order to meet the necessary requirements of construct, face and predictive validity essential for the clinical application of data obtained from animal studies [1]. Of course, in animals it is extremely difficult to exactly reproduce compulsive drug seeking and taking as seen in human drug addicts because of obvious limitations including the absence of direct personal costs such as family or society problems associated with drug abuse, or limited alternative reinforcement choices.

However, despite such limitations, compulsivity in preclinical models of drug addiction should and must be defined as an inability to cease drug seeking and taking under conditions in which the drug is constantly available but its obtainment is associated with adverse consequences.

In recent years, progress has been made in an attempt to mimic human conditions of compulsive drug use.

3.4.1 Maintained drug use despite adverse consequences

1. Resistance to devaluation / adulteration

In addition to their reinforcing properties, most addictive drugs have toxic effects, which after repeated use can lead to severe health complications. Such aversive properties would normally progressively devalue any reinforcer, and facilitate the engagement of the subject in alternative responses, incompatible with the pursuit of the initial reinforcer. However, despite often acknowledging the deleterious outcome of drug use, addicts rarely achieve spontaneous voluntary abstinence, and when they manage to do so, often relapse to compulsive drug use.

Similarly, rats differentially respond to devaluation of drugs of abuse and natural reinforcers. Performance for food is markedly affected by pairing its ingestion with illness produced by injection of lithium chloride. In contrast, devaluation of orally administered alcohol and cocaine does not greatly decrease drug seeking performance [140;149-150].

Similarly, extended access to free choice between drug solutions and water interrupted by periods of withdrawal in rats results in high levels of drug intake even when solutions are adulterated with bitter tasting quinine, evidencing the compulsive pattern of alcohol drinking after protracted exposure to the drug [151-153].

2. Conditioned suppression

Until drug users explicitly experience the aversive consequences of drug use, drug taking is mainly moderated through warnings rather than actual punishment. Once experienced, aversive stimuli temporally distant from drug intake can appear, thereby rendering aversive contingencies less distinguishable. Moreover, the aversive consequences of drug use are counter-conditioned by previously extended drug presentation, which has been described as retarding the development of the conditioned emotional response [154]. All these processes may facilitate the attribution of aversive consequences to irrelevant stimuli. Adding a stimulus previously associated with an aversive outcome to the training context should normally reduce the frequency of a conditioned response. Indeed, although the aversive stimuli are not directly associated with drug use itself, a conditioned suppressor may be viewed as 'devaluing' the drug reinforcer since subjects would be required to respond for the drug in a state of conditioned fear [121].

However, Vanderschuren and Everitt (2004) found that the presentation of a Pavlovian conditioned fear stimulus after an extended self-administration training history failed to suppress cocaine self–administration, whereas after a brief cocaine taking history it did. These data support the view that while instrumental behaviour directed at obtaining drugs is initially a flexible, goal-directed form of behaviour, following prolonged drug exposure, drug seeking becomes insensitive to signals of punishment, thereby indicating its compulsive nature. However, it remains unclear whether in the multi-operant environment that drug addicts are normally exposed to, presentation of aversive conditioned stimuli may favour avoidance rather than abstinence.

4. Punishment

Aversive stimuli might eventually be perceived as directly associated with drug use. Punishment has often been debated as a treatment procedure, both in terms of its ethical acceptability and its efficacy. Nevertheless, it remains an undoubtedly important component of the every day life of drug addicts.

In animals, even though differing in many procedural parameters such as the locus or intensity of punishment, foot shock-induced punishment has been used in several recent models of compulsive drug seeking and drug taking behaviour. Thus we will focus here on this punisher, although foot shock-induced suppression may not easily be generalised to the human condition.

In most of the studies on drug taking despite adverse consequences, mild foot shocks, set at a constant intensity, are applied contingently upon a response reinforced by a constant dose of drug. In this case resistance to punishment is assessed through the persistence of the instrumental response despite contingent delivery of the punisher. Alternatively, the degree of response suppression is both dependent upon the magnitude of the reinforcer, the intensity of the punishment event, the schedule of their respective presentation and the delay between the instrumental responses and their consequences [155].

Consequently, Cooper et al. [156] increased daily by 0.04 mA the intensity of a shock that was initially set to 0.25 mA until rats stopped responding (lever pressing) during the 30 min daily sessions for three consecutive days. Whereas such a procedure has the advantage of assigning for each rat the final shock intensity that led to self-imposed abstinence, it constrains the opportunity for repeated testing when required.

The punishment contingency has been used at different loci of the instrumental drug taking action. Thus taking [157] or seeking behaviour [24] have been specifically punished. Since preparatory and consummatory responses have been shown to be under the influence of dissociable processes [158], it is conceivable they are differentially sensitive to punishment. In order to assess the sensitivity of seeking and taking responses to punishment Pelloux et al. used punishment in the seeking taking task that spatially and temporally dissociates the "preparatory" and "consummatory" behaviours [125]. Pelloux et al. conducted a study where either 50% of the seeking sequences where associated with the delivery of a shock instead of the activation of the taking lever or 50% of the instrumental responses on the taking lever were punished. With this probabilistic schedule of punishment both types of punishment induced a progressive suppression in performance but punishment of the taking response resulted in less suppression than punishment of the seeking response.

Finally, the efficacy of the punishment of drug seeking or taking seems to greatly depend on drug history. After short exposure to amphetamine or an opiate (remifentanil) punishment produces robust suppression of self-administration that resumed for the opiate in all subjects approximately 5 days after punishment was discontinued [159]. However, the punishment effect obtained for amphetamine lasted much longer [157]. After extended access to cocaine, punishment produced suppression of a seeking response except in a subgroup of animals (about 25%). Thus, compulsive drug seeking appears, as in humans, only after extended exposure to the drug in a small proportion of subjects conferring on these models good predictive validity.

5. Multidimensional animal model of drug addiction: addiction-like behaviour

As previously presented, there are two main strategies when developing preclinical models of drug addiction. The first category refers to models developed to understand the psychobiological, neurological, cellular and molecular processes involved in a particular aspect of the pathology. Therefore, these models specifically address one aspect of the pathology, whether a diagnostic criterion, such as escalation of intake, resistance to punishment, high motivation for the drug, habitual instrumental performance, vulnerability to relapse, or impaired cognitive flexibility. They may also be relevant to influential theories such as behavioural sensitisation [44;96;160-161] and hedonic allostasis [2;86-88]. Such models generally assume that drug exposure triggers rather similar behavioural, neural or molecular effects in all the subjects tested.

However, these models cannot address other crucial aspects of drug addiction, such as inter-individual differences in the vulnerability to develop the pathology and their behavioural and biological correlates. They also fail to capture the multi-symptomatic nature of drug addiction. Thus, the second category of animal models of drug addiction takes into accounts both inter-individual differences and the complementary strategy of meeting diagnostic criteria of the pathology in humans according to the DSM-IV. Thus, to be diagnosed as 'addicted' an individual must fulfil three out of seven diagnostic criteria of drug addiction over the last 12 months. This approach forms the basis of a new pre-clinical animal model based on vulnerability to addiction-like behaviour in the rat [26].

In this model, three diagnostic criteria, namely [i] an inability to refrain from drug seeking, [ii] high motivation for the drug, and [iii] maintained drug use despite negative consequences, have been operationalised by, respectively, [i] drug seeking during periods when the drug is not available and signalled as so, [ii] break points during progressive ratio schedules of reinforcement, and [iii] persistence of self-administration despite punishment by contingent electric foot-shocks.

When the population is large enough, as it has been the case in several of our studies [26;28], a systematic analysis of the distributions of each of the three addiction-like behaviours revealed that the distribution of the motivation for the drug and the persistence of drug seeking (n=40) were best fitted by a log-normal regression (Khi^2 and K-S: $p>0.05$, $R^2 = 0.96$ and 0.99, respectively) (figure 4, left and middle panel). In contrast the distribution of resistance to punishment was bimodal, composed of a first log-normal distribution (n=27 or 67.5% of the total population, K-S: d = 0.22451, p>0.1), and a second normal sub-distribution (n=13 or 32.5% of the total population, K-S: d = 0.15604 p>0.1) (figure 4, right panel) which general regression fit can be described as a 3 order polynomial equation $y=3.24x^3 + 37.33x^2 +130.86x +146.67$ [28].

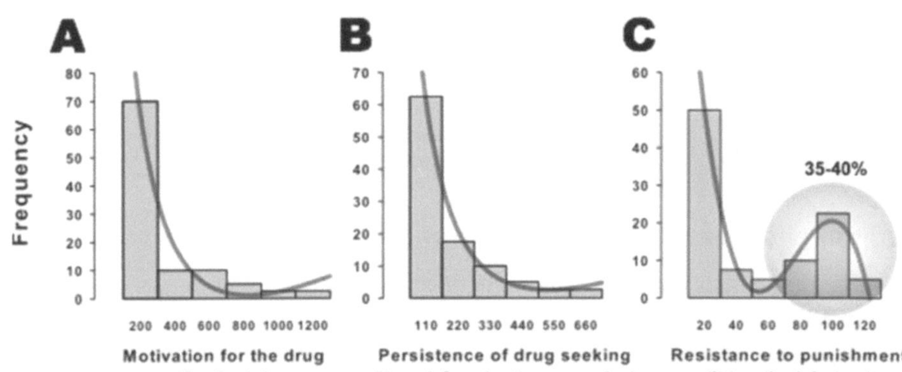

Fig. 4. Distribution of each of the addiction-like criteria, after (28)
The distribution of motivation for the drug and persistence of drug seeking (left and middle panel, respectively) (n=40) were best fitted by a log-normal regression (Khi2 and K-S: P>0.05). In contrast the distribution of resistance to punishment was bimodal, composed of a first log-normal distribution (n=27 or 67.5% of the total population, K-S: d=0.22451, p> 0.1) , and a second normal sub-distribution (n=13 or 32.5% of the total population, K-S: d=0.15604, p>0.1) (right panel) which general regression fit can be described as a 3 order polynomial equation: y=3.24x3+37.33x2+130.86x+146.67

The bimodal nature of the distribution of resistance to punishment we demonstrated in this study is in agreement with the observation of Pelloux et al. [24]. Bimodal distributions are very common in life science literature, especially during speciation process [162] whereby one whole population is somehow giving birth to two independent populations [163]. Rare in behavioural neuroscience, bimodal distributions have however been observed for drug-induced behaviours [164], suggesting that the neurobiological substrates of behavioural inter-individual differences need in some cases to be challenged in order to reveal bimodal distribution. Our results suggest that a specific subpopulation in the rat has diverged so that it has become specifically more vulnerable to maintain drug use despite averse consequences, as measured as resistance to punishment, when chronically exposed to the drug. This hypothesis, although speculative, when transferred to the human situation may actually resonate well with the Nesse and Berridge's suggestion that the vulnerability to drug addiction is a matter of evolution [165].

In practical terms, this bimodal distribution is particularly handy because it provides us with an objective criterion to determine a threshold in the population in order to carry out a dichotomous, categorial, strategy to identify animals that show addiction-like behaviour, i.e., 30-40% highest part of the population, depending on the study. Thus, for each of these three addiction-like criteria animals are ranked according to their score. If a rat's score is included in the 30-40% highest percentile of the distribution, this rat is considered positive for that addiction-like criterion and is given an arbitrary criterion score of 1. Then the arbitrary criteria scores for each of the three addiction-like criteria are added, and consequently four distinct groups are identified according to the number of positive scores: 0 criteria, 1 criterion, 2 criteria and 3 criteria rats (figure 5).

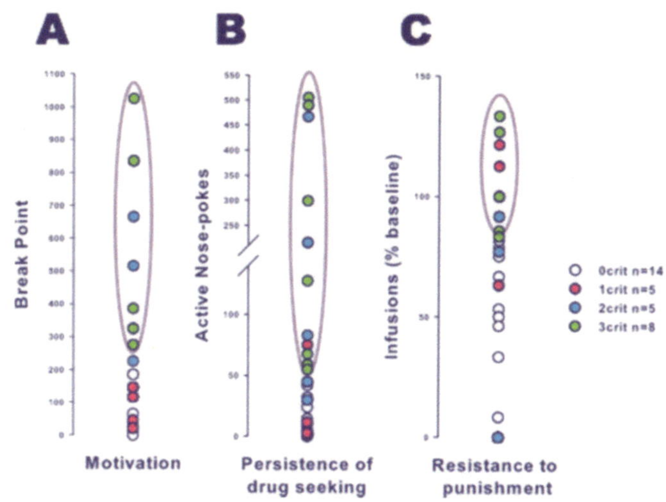

Fig. 5. Selection strategy of rats addicted (3crit rats) and rats resistant (0crit rats) to cocaine
Data analysed from (11). For each of these three addiction-like criteria animals are ranked according to their score. If a rat's score is included in the 30-40% highest percentile of the distribution, this rat is considered positive for that addiction-like criterion and is given an arbitrary criterion score of 1. Then the arbitrary criteria scores for each of the three addiction-like criteria are added, and consequently four distinct groups are identified according to the number of positive scores: 0 criteria, 1 criterion, 2 criteria and 3 criteria rats

Behaviourally, the categorial selection is associated with a criteria-dependent magnitude in each of the addiction-like criteria (figure 6). Our model is based on the comparison of three criteria (3crit) and 0 criteria (0crit) rats. 3crit rats show high scores for each of the three addiction-like criteria and are therefore considered "addicted", whereas 0crit rats are considered resistant to addiction. 3crit rats represent approximately 20% of the population exposed to cocaine, an incidence observed in several independent studies with Lister-

Hooded or Sprague-Dawley rats as well as either nose-poke or lever press as instrumental response [26;28;101;166], that is remarkably similar to that reported in humans [167].

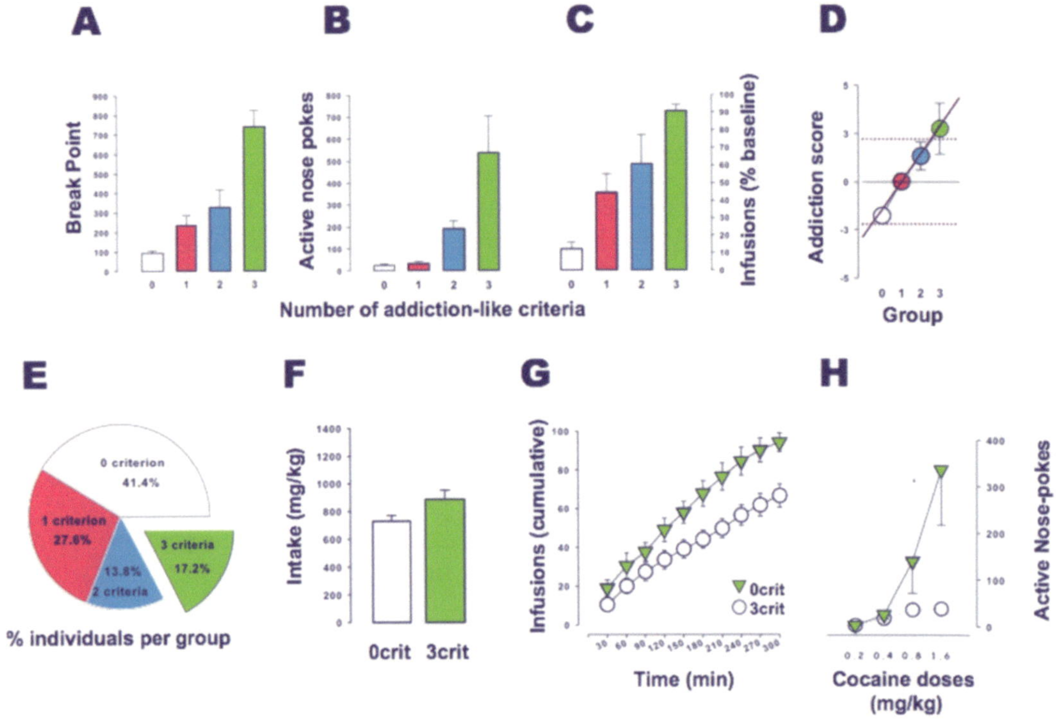

Fig. 6. Behavioural characterisation of addiction-like behaviour in the rat

A dichotomous approach to the diagnosis of addiction-like behaviour can be implemented in preclinical models of addiction on the understanding that some, but not all, animals chronically exposed to drug self-administration eventually develop one or more behavioural features resembling a clinical criterion for drug addiction as defined in the DSM-IV (see table 13.1). Thus we have operationally defined three addiction-like criteria, namely, (i) an inability to refrain from drug seeking (A), (ii) maintained drug use despite aversive consequences (B) and (iii) increased motivation to take the drug (C). Rats positive for none of the three criteria (0 criteria rats) are resistant to addiction, whereas rats that have three addiction-like criteria (3 criteria rats) are considered "addicted," and represent 15 to 20% of the population initially exposed to cocaine (D). Importantly these behavioural differences are not attributable to differential levels of cocaine intake, since throughout protracted exposure 3 criteria and 0 criteria rats do not differ in this measure (E). Although selected on three addiction-like criteria, 3criteria rats display complementary features of drug addiction, such as inability to limit drug intake when offered extended access to cocaine (F) and high vulnerability to relapse, as measured by reinstatement of cocaine seeking behaviour by increasing doses of non contingent cocaine infusions (G). A-E: after (11), F: after (8)

Although 3crit rats do not differ significantly from 0crit rats in terms of cocaine self-administration [26;28;166], 3crit rats eventually develop higher motivation for the drug, an inability to refrain from drug-seeking, and resistance to punishment [8;26;28;101;166].

More importantly, although selected on three addiction-like behaviours, 3crit rats also display enhanced escalation of cocaine self-administration as compared to 0crit rats (figure

6F). 3crit rats therefore fulfil a fourth criterion of addiction, namely an inability to control drug intake [26] classically established after extended access to the drug [21]. This results demonstrate that loss of control over drug intake does not necessarily follow extended access to the drug, but instead develops in some vulnerable subjects exposed to cocaine self-administration for prolonged periods of time.

The predictive validity of the model is further supported by de demonstration that 3crit rats also show a high vulnerability to relapse in response to non-contingent infusions of cocaine (figure 6G) [8] or contingent presentations of a drug-associated stimulus [26]. Thus, even though selected on three addiction-like criteria, after chronic exposure to cocaine, 3crit rats display important features of clinical addiction as defined in the DSM-IV. These observations provide the model with both construct and predictive validities.

Moreover, since addiction-like behaviour emerges in three criteria rats only after extended exposure to the drug, i.e., after at least 50 daily self-administration sessions, these results highlight the importance of the interaction between a vulnerable phenotype and chronic drug exposure in the development of compulsive drug self-administration.

6. Vulnerabilities to drug addictions

Like many other psychiatric disorders, we are not all equally vulnerable to develop drug addiction. Epidemiological studies have revealed that between 15 to 35% of the population exposed to addictive drugs will develop compulsive drug use [167]. The results described in the previous section illustrate very well that inter-individual differences in vulnerability to develop compulsive cocaine self-administration can also be observed in rats. Thus, in any given population of rats exposed to cocaine only some develop addiction-like behaviour, thereby demonstrating that animal models provide a realistic estimate of risk for addiction in humans [41;166;169].

As already discussed, the underlying aetiology of the different pathways to addiction are likely to involve interactions between a vulnerable phenotype, environmental influences and drug exposure itself [170-171]. It is therefore important to identify the psychobiological substrates of vulnerability to develop compulsive drug use both in drug naive subjects and drug experienced individuals, thereby being able to develop preventive and therapeutic strategies at different stages of drug use history.

6.1 Psychobiological factors of vulnerability to drug addiction: contribution of behavioural traits

Epidemiological studies in human populations have revealed striking associations between drug use [172-173b], and certain behavioural traits [174-189] such as anxiety [190-193], impulsivity [187;194-195] and sensation-seeking [176;183;196-199]. The relevance of these traits for animal models of addiction is discussed below.

6.1.1 Anxiety

Anxiety can be assessed in preclinical models using various procedures which include the elevated plus maze (EPM) [200-201]. During the classic 5-min test session on the EPM a variety of behaviours are measured including the ratio of open and closed arms entries, time spent in the open and closed arms, as well as self-grooming which are all indices of anxiety. High levels of anxiety including high grooming behaviour and a low percentage of time spent in the open arms of the EPM have been associated with an enhanced propensity to acquire cocaine CPP [202] as well as an increased motivation to self-administer cocaine [203], but see [204]. Trait anxiety has also been associated with an enhanced preference for alcohol [205-206], consistent with the notion that alcohol use may self-medicate underlying mood disorders related to anxiety and stress [207-208].

We have recently established that high anxiety in the EPM predicts escalation of cocaine, but not heroin self-administration in the rat (figure 7) [209].

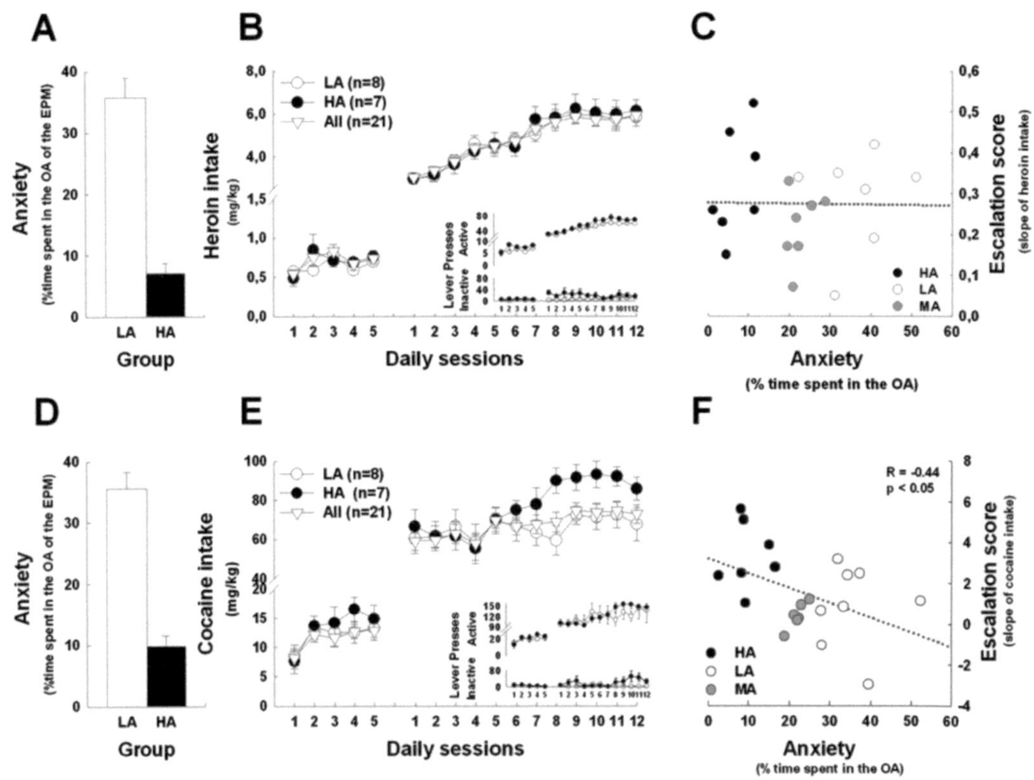

Fig. 7. High anxiety trait predicts loss of control over cocaine, but not heroin, self-administration in the rat, after (122)

High anxious (HA) and low anxious (LA) rats were selected in the upper and lower 33% of a Lister Hooded population (A & D). Whereas HA did not differ from either LA and the overall population in their escalation of heroin intake throughout 12 sessions of 6 h extended access to the drug (B) HA rats showed a marked increase in their cocaine intake as compared to LA or the overall population (E). Thus, high anxiety is related to the magnitude of cocaine escalation (F) whereas it is not related to the slope of escalation of heroin intake (C).

These data suggest that if high anxiety trait may contribute to the choice of the drug used, i.e., preference for alcohol or opiates [210], it does not necessarily contribute to the development of compulsive use when the drug is initially used as a self-medication [211]. However, the striking relationship between high anxiety levels in the EPM and subsequent vulnerability to escalate cocaine intake suggest that high anxiety may facilitate a tolerance to anxiogenic properties of cocaine [212] perhaps because of a ceiling effect, or, instead enhance the potential anxiolytic properties of cocaine that have been suggested for low doses of the drug [213].

6.1.2 Sensation seeking / Novelty-seeking

Sensation- and novelty-seeking traits have been the focus of a large number of pre-clinical studies on addiction vulnerability (for review, see [12]).

In preclinical studies, sensation/novelty seeking trait has been suggested to be modelled both by high locomotor reactivity to a new inescapable environment (high responder phenotype, HR) [214-215], and high propensity to visit a new environment in a free-choice, novelty-induced CPP, paradigm (high novelty preferring phenotype, HNP) [12;216].

Piazza and colleagues were the first to investigate the role of sensation-seeking in this context by measuring the locomotor response of rats to an inescapable novel environment [217]. In this model, rats are placed for two hours in a new environment and their horizontal activity is monitored. Based on inter-individual differences in locomotor response animals are either selected as high (HR) or low responders (LR) according to a median division [217]. HR rats show a greater propensity to acquire psychostimulant self-administration [217] since they more readily self-administer low doses of amphetamine than LR rats [2;217]. Moreover, HR rats show a greater propensity for drug-induced neural plasticity [218-219] and increased stress-evoked dopamine release in the Acb than LR rats [220].

However, sensation seeking does not predict the acquisition of CPP for addictive drugs, which instead is predicted by novelty-seeking [12;216;221-223], the latter being a behavioural trait dissociable from the former [9;28;224].

Novelty-seeking is normally assessed by measuring the preference of rats for a novel versus familiar compartment using a procedure quite similar to CPP [225], although broad methodological differences are observed in the literature that can impact onto the nature of the behavioural construct one is investigating. Indeed, depending on the study, novelty preference has been measured as (1) the number and time duration of visits of a new arm in a Y-maze during the first 2 or 5 min, respectively, of a test session taking place 30 min after the habituation to the other two arms of the set-up [226], (2), novelty-induced place preference tested for 15 min on the third day of a protocol during which animal were exposed 30 min daily to one compartment of a CPP box [223-224] whereas locomotor reactivity to novelty has been measured in (1) circular corridors [226-227], playground maze [228] or (2) activity chambers [216;229], each environment differing from one other in terms of light intensity, openness and area.

Overall, animals selected as novelty-seekers, or novelty-preferring (HNP), are those that fall in the upper quartile range. Unlike animals selected from the lower quartile of the population, high novelty seekers readily develop a conditioned place preference to amphetamine [224;228] and self-administration of cocaine under an autoshaping procedure [230].

Thus, although both traits are dependent upon the dopaminergic system [12], they are mutually exclusive [12;216], but see [231] and therefore may predict different dimensions of vulnerability to drug addiction [12].

We have investigated the respective role of HR and HNP phenotypes in inter-individual vulnerability to switch from controlled to compulsive cocaine SA. A cohort of rats were tested for their locomotor response to inescapable novelty and, subsequently for their preference propensity to express novelty-induced CPP.

After extended cocaine self-administration these rats were tested for each of the three addiction-like criteria. Whereas LR and HR rats were highly represented in the 0 and 1crit populations, 60% of the LNP rats were included in the 0crit population as opposed to 70% of the HNP rats that showed 2 or 3 addiction-like criteria, none belonging to the 0crit population (figure 8A). This asymmetric distribution specific to LNP and HNP rats was further investigated, as illustrated in figure 8B-D which depict the representativity of LR, HR, LNP and HNP rats within the distributions for each of the addiction-like criteria. Importantly, HNP rats, as opposed to LNP rats, represented the great majority of the subpopulation resistant to punishment (figure 8D).

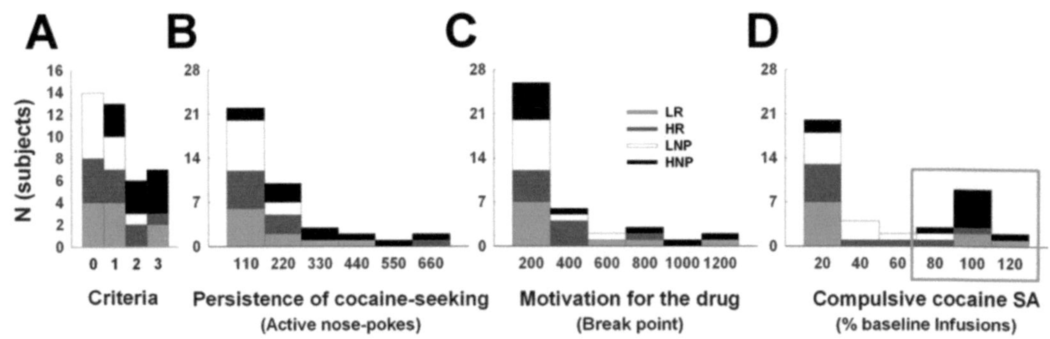

Fig. 8. High novelty preference (HNP) and sensation seekers (HR) rats are not equally distributed within the different addiction-like criteria.

A. Addiction score.The great majority of HNP rats are represented in the 2 and 3crit subgroups of the population whereas HR rats are equally distributed throughout the different groups. B-C. HNP and LNP rats are distributed asymmetrically within the population relative to persistence of drug seeking (**B**) and motivation for the drug (**C**). LNP rats are clustered on the right side of the distribution whereas HNP rats are also represented in the right part of the distribution. Such asymmetry is not observed for LR and HR rats which are equally distributed throughout the overall population for these two criteria. **D**. Distribution of LNP, HNP, LR and HR rats for compulsive cocaine self-administration. Whereas LR and HR rats did not show any difference in their distribution throughout the population, HNP rats were highly clustered in the compulsive subpopulation as emphasised by the encircling square. Thus HNP rats may be highly vulnerable to compulsive cocaine self-administration. Analysis of data from (28)

Thus although no differences were observed between HR and LR rats for their scores in each of their addiction-like criteria, HNP rats displayed higher scores than LNP rats in each of the addiciton-like criteria, namely resistance to punishment, inability to refrain from cocaine-seeking even if the drug is not available since they persisted, responded, more on the active nose-poke than LNP rats during "no-drug" periods and motivation for cocaine (figure 9D).

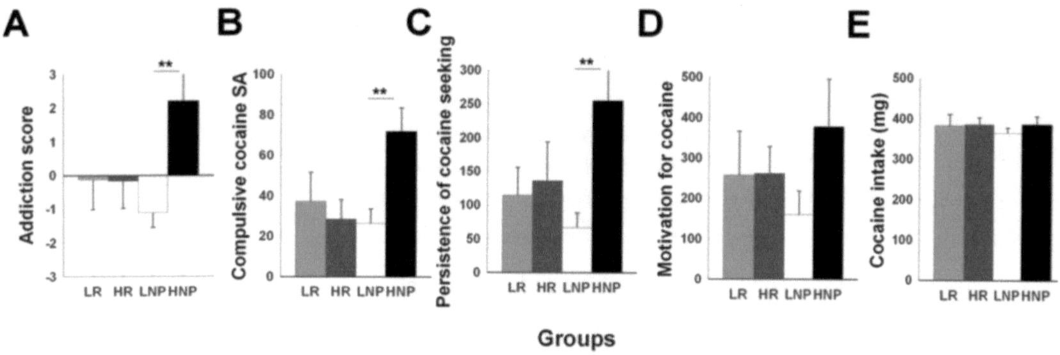

Fig. 9. Novelty Preference, but not locomotor reactivity to novelty predicts the switch to compulsive cocaine self-administration.
ANOVAs with HNP/LNP groups as between-subject factors revealed that HNP rats showed higher addiction score than LNP rats [$F_{1,18}$=10.59, p<0.01] (A). Compared to LNP rats, HNP rats developed compulsive cocaine SA as measured by high level of resistance to punishment [$F_{1,18}$=11.16, p<0.01] (B) and were unable to stop seeking cocaine when it was not available and signaled as so [$F_{1,18}$=9.03, p<0.01] (C). HNP rats tend to show higher motivation for cocaine than LNP though this difference did not reach statistical significance (D). These behavioral differences between HNP and LNP rats could not be attributable to differential cocaine intake since the two groups have been exposed to the same amount of cocaine throughout the experiment [$F_{1,18}$<1] (E). When compared to LR rats, HR rats showed no difference in the addiction-like behavioral measures. These two groups had behavioral scores similar to those of LNP rats, thereby illustrating that locomotor reactivity to novelty, as opposed to novelty preference, doesn't predict addiction-like behavior for cocaine.

The relationship between high novelty preference trait and vulnerability to switch to compulsive cocaine SA was further supported by a clear relationship assessed with a non parametric Spearman correlation analysis R=0.32, p<0.05, with the percentage of time spent in the new environment of the novelty-induced place preference procedure and the percentage of infusions compared to baseline when punished contingently by electric foot shocks as variables. However, no relationship was observed between locomotor reactivity to novelty and resistance to punishment (Spearman R=-0.15, p=0.36). Importantly, the behavioural differences observed between HNP and LNP rats cannot be attributed to a difference in the total amount of cocaine intake since the two groups did not differ for their total cocaine intake during the 60 days preceding the assessment of the addiction-like criteria [$F_{1,18}$<1] (figure 9E).

Since a great majority of the HNP, and none of the LNP, rats was clustered in the compulsive subpopulation, HNP rats, even though identified from a normally distributed population, may represent a specific sub-population vulnerable to compulsive cocaine intake after protracted exposure to the drug. Thereby the high novelty preference trait in the rat, as identified as the upper quartile of the population tested with the present paradigm is a promising behavioural tool for the study of the neurobiological substrates of vulnerability to compulsive cocaine intake.

While providing the first evidence for a causal relationship between novelty preference and compulsive cocaine use, this study confirms that locomotor reactivity to novelty does not predict the vulnerability to develop cocaine addiction, but does rather predict the propensity to self-administer drugs [27;217]. Altogether, these data suggest that the HR phenotype and its underlying neurobiological mechanisms may be involved in facilitating cocaine use, but not in the transition to switch from controlled to compulsive cocaine use, the hallmark of cocaine addiction [97].

Thus two different behavioural measures suggested to reveal a putative sensation/novelty seeking trait in rats [12], namely novelty-induced locomotor activity and novelty preference, are differentially predictive of inter individual propensity to self-administer cocaine and to switch from controlled to compulsive cocaine use, respectively.

These preclinical data suggest that the correlates of the increased propensity shown by human sensation seekers to use addictive drugs [175] should be dissociated from those associated with the transition from controlled to compulsive drug use. Indeed, not only is sensation seeking a heterogeneous, multifaceted, construct [232] but it is quantified according to different, not necessarily overlapping [233], personality scales including the Zuckerman, Eysenck, Arnett and Cloninger's scales. A factorial analysis of the different items of the sensation seeking scale developed by Zuckerman [197] revealed four dimensions [234] namely Thrill and Adventure Seeking [TAS], Experience Seeking [ES], Disinhibition [Dis], and Boredom Susceptibility [BS], of which the TAS and DIS sub-scales have been suggested to refer to sensation seeking whereas the ES and BS sub-scales would refer to novelty seeking [234-235]. Further research is needed to investigate which of these sub-scales is the most predictive of the vulnerability to switch to compulsive cocaine use, thereby clearly refining the relationships between sensation seeking trait and vulnerability to cocaine addiction.

6.1.3 Impulsivity

A popular paradigm used to assess impulsivity in rodents is the 5-choice serial reaction time task (5-CSRTT), which was developed originally as an analogue of the human continuous performance task of sustained attention [236]. The 5-CSRTT requires animals to detect brief flashes of light presented pseudo-randomly in one of five holes and to make a nose-poke response in the correct spatial location in order to receive a food reward. The rat is thus required to monitor a horizontal array of apertures and to withhold from responding until the onset of the stimulus. Generally, the accuracy of stimulus discrimination provides an index of attentional capacity, while premature responses - made before the presentation of the stimulus - are regarded as a form of impulsive behaviour and hence a failure in impulse control [237-238]. The neural and neurochemical basis of impulsivity on the 5-CSRTT has been extensively investigated, involving important contributions from the anterior cingulate cortex (ACC), infralimbic cortex, Acb, medial striatum and by the ascending monoaminergic systems [239-240].

More recently, the 5-CSRTT has been used to screen for spontaneously high levels of impulsivity in rats, a phenotype associated with increased cocaine, sucrose and nicotine self-administration [241-243]. Interestingly, Dalley and colleagues have recently shown using microPET brain imaging that high impulsive rats have lower dopamine D2/3-binding levels in the ventral striatum as compared to low impulsive littermates [241], thereby suggesting that alteration of dopamine D2/3-receptors in the Acb may contribute to high impulsivity and vulnerability to drug addiction.

We have used the animal model of addiction-like behaviour for cocaine described in previous sections to investigate whether high impulsivity trait predicts the switch to compulsive cocaine SA.

A cohort of 40 Lister Hooded rats was screened in the 5-CSRTT for their impulse control. These rats were then tested for their locomotor response to a new, inescapable environment. Thus, prior to cocaine exposure, rats were identified as high (HI) and low (LI) impulsive or HR and LR (figure 10).

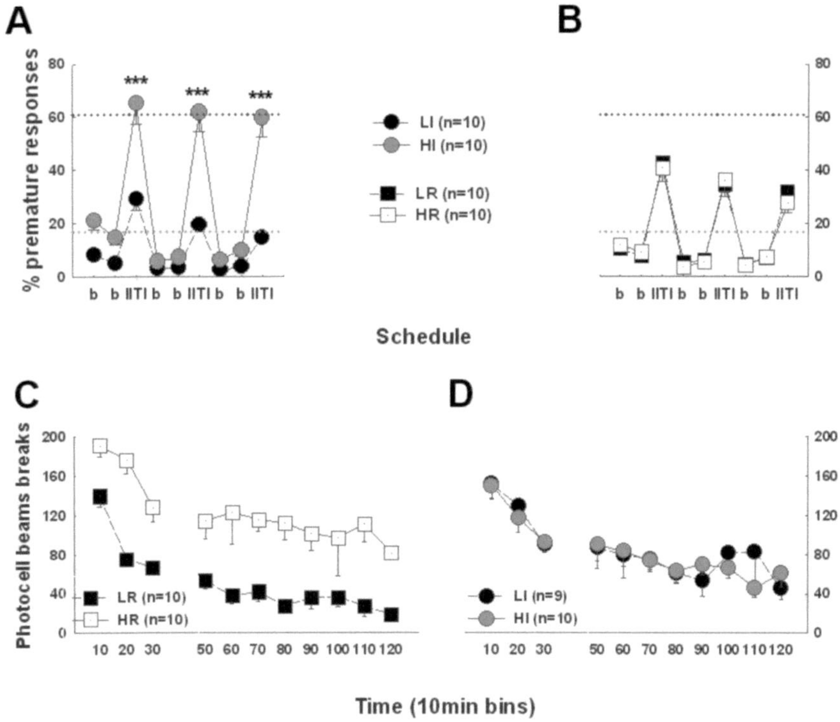

Fig. 10. Impulsivity and novelty-induced locomotor activity: two distinct phenotypes. After (27)

On two baseline days (B), premature responses in the 5_CSRTT were measured. (A and B) During long intertrail intervals (LITIS), HI rats showed more premature responses than LI rats (Group: $F_{3,36} = 14.4$, $p<0.01$; scedule: $F_{8,288} = 130.22$, $p<0.01$; Schedule x Group: $F_{24,288} = 7.01$, $p<0.01$) (***$p<0,001$) (A) and HR ($p<0.01$) or LR rats ($p<0.05$) (B). HR rats did not differ from LR rats or from LI subjects (B). (C and D) HR rats were more reactive to novelty tha LR rats ($F_{3,35} = 17.63$, $p<0.01$). HI and LI subjects never differed from each other. *Comparison with HR: *$p<0.05$, **$p<0.01$, ***$p<0.001$. (D) Pink and blue dotted lines represent the average premature responses during the last two intertrial intervals for HI and LI rats, respectively.

High impulsivity trait and locomotor response to novelty were demonstrated to be independent behavioural traits. We then tested whether high locomotor response to novelty and high impulsivity traits predicted higher propensity to acquire cocaine self-administration. We allowed animals to acquire cocaine SA with daily increasing doses of the drug. We demonstrated that HR rats acquire cocaine self-administration at doses at which

LR rats do not, thereby confirming that HR rats are more prone to acquire stimulants self-administration than LR animals [217]. However, HI rats did not differ from LI in their propensity to acquire cocaine SA (figure 11).

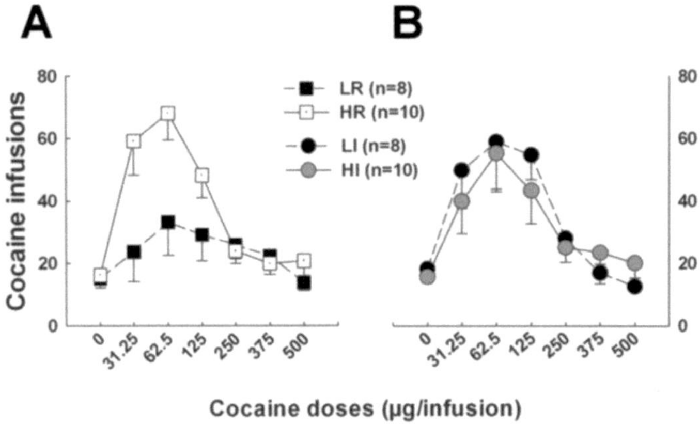

Fig. 11. Novelty-induced locomotor activity predicts the propensity to acquire cocaine self-administration, after (27)
(A) HR rats showed an upward shift of the cocaine dose-response curve compared with LR littermates (Group: $F_{1,16} = 4.9$, $p<0.05$; Dose: $F_{6,96} = 11.73$, $p<0.01$; Group x Dose: $F_{6,96} = 4.39$, $p<0.01$). HR rats infused more cocaine at the lowest three doses than vehicle ($p<0.01$). (B) HI and LI subjects did not differ in the number of self-administered cocaine infusions (Group: $F_{1,16}<1$; Dose: $F_{6,96} =10.79$, $p<0.01$; Group x Dose: $F_{6,96}<1$)

When subsequently exposed to protracted cocaine self-administration and tested for their addiction-like behaviour, rats were identified as 0, 1, 2 and 3crit rats and each animal was given an addiction score (figure 12). We then retrospectively compared HI vs LI and HR vs LR rats for their addiction score and revealed that HI rats had higher addiction score than LI whereas HR did not differ from LR rats.

This increased addiction score observed in HI rats was specifically attributed to the development of compulsive cocaine SA in these rats since they maintained cocaine SA despite punishment to the same extent as 3crit rats did. However, HR and LR rats did not differ in this behavioural criterion. The specific relationship between high impulsivity and compulsivity was further demonstrated by a correlational analysis between the percentage of premature responses in the 5-CSRTT and resistance to punishment, as assessed by a non parametric correlation analysis (figure 12).

This evidence suggests that the predisposition to initiate drug use is independent of the vulnerability to shift from controlled to compulsive drug taking, and therefore provides new insights into the various behavioural and psychological factors that influence the pathways to addiction. In particular, the demonstration that the high impulsive trait predicts the shift to compulsive drug taking behaviour is of major interest since a shift from impulse control failure to compulsivity has been suggested to play a major role in the development of drug addiction in humans [87;244] (figure 13).

Together with the demonstration that novelty preference predicts addiction-like behaviour for cocaine [28] the present data suggest that further investigations should focus on the additive or interactive contribution of high impulsivity and novelty seeking traits to the vulnerability to switch to compulsive cocaine SA.

This suggestion is timely since we [245] have recently demonstrated that high impulsive rats, as identified in the 5-CSRTT, prefer a novel compartment in a novelty-induced CPP procedure [245] (figure 14).

Thus both novelty preference and impulsivity, but not locomotor response to novelty, contribute to inter-individual propensity to switch from controlled to compulsive cocaine SA.

However, this conclusion may be taken with caution since it might be true only for stimulants. Indeed, we [122] have recently demonstrated that high impulsivity trait does not predict inter-individual differences in escalation of heroin self-administration (figure 15). This propensity was instead predicted by pharmacological flexibility in response to extended access to heroin, i.e., increased titration in response to increased availability of the drug.

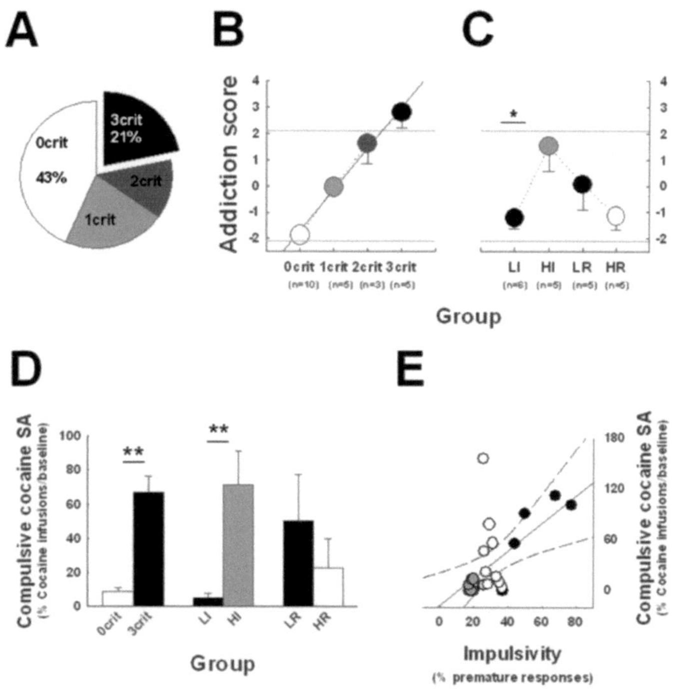

Fig. 12. Impulsivity predicts the transition to compulsivity

After extended exposure to cocaine SA 0, 1, 2 and 3crit rats were identified and were distributed similarly to previously described (A) in that 3 crit rats represented 20% of the overall population. When ranked on a linear addiction scale ($R^2 = 0.99$, Group: $F_{3,19}=34.43$, $p<0.01$), three-criteria rats had addiction scores (2.8 ± 0.6) above the standard deviation (2.1), and higher than all the other groups (B). (C) HI rats displayed higher addiction score than LI rats ($F_{1,9} = 7.55$, $*p<0.05$), whereas HR rats did not differ from LR rats. (D) HI rats (n=5) displayed higher resistance to punishment than LI rats (n=6) ($F_{1,9} = 12.79$, $p<0.01$), whereas HR (n=5) rats did not differ from LR rats (n=5). (E) Impulsivity predicts compulsive cocaine self-administration ($R= 0.42$, $p<0.05$). Gray and black shadings represent LI and HI rats, respectively.

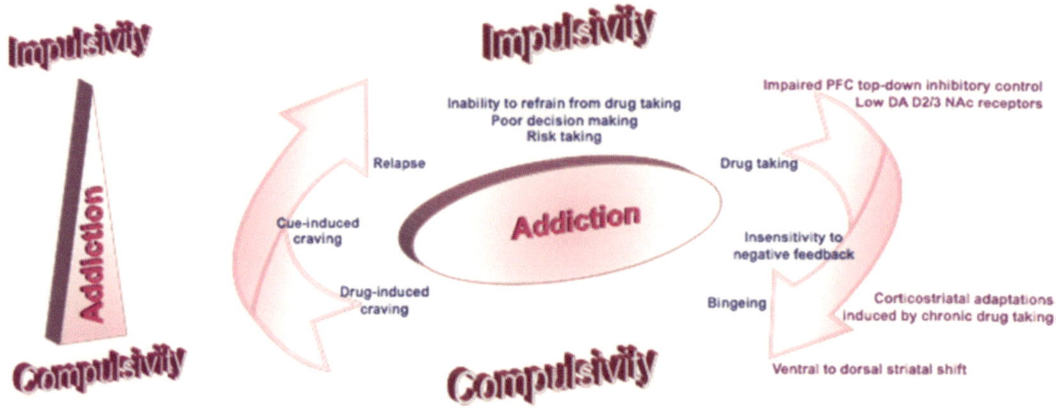

Fig. 13. Impulsivity and compulsivity in drug addiction.
It has been suggested that a shift occurs from impulsivity to compulsivity in the control over drug seeking during the development of drug addiction (left). According to this theoretical framework, drug use is initially controlled by the positive reinforcing properties of drugs. However, when addiction develops drug taking is no longer controlled by positive reinforcement but, instead, is controlled by negative reinforcement and the need to avoid the negative consequences of withdrawal. Other theoretical frameworks suggest a contribution of both impulsivity and compulsivity to different stages of the addiction cycle (right). Impulsivity might then be associated with drug taking and relapse, whereas compulsivity might be associated with craving, bingeing and insensitivity to negative feedback.

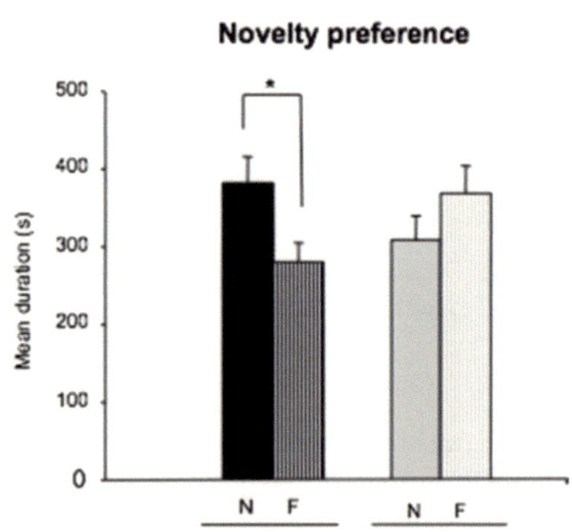

Fig. 14. High impulsive rats seek novelty
HI rats explored the novel compartment of the CPP apparatus for significantly longer period of time compared with the familiar compartment, a preference that was not observed in LI rats (group x compartment interraction: $F_{1,24} = 6.53$, p=0,017; post hoc t-test p=0.031). Howerver, there was no significant difference between HI and LI rat in the total time spent in the novel compartment. LI rats showed a trend increase in time spent in the familiar compartment compared with HI rats (p=0.059).

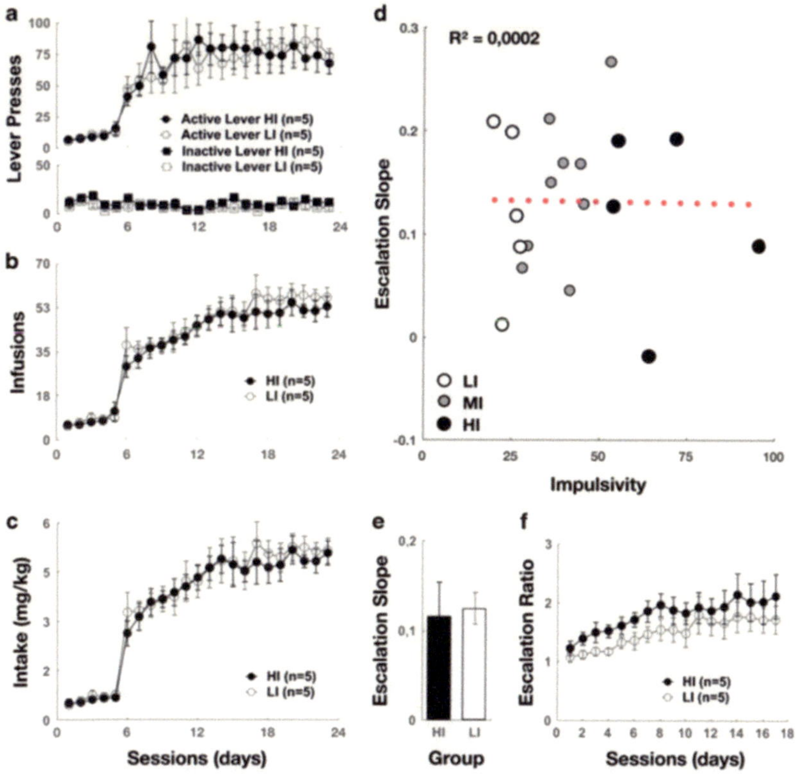

Fig. 15. High impulsivity trait does not predict a greater propensity to escalate heroin SA. After (122)

Extended access to heroin resulted in escalation of heroin SA over time in both HI and LI rats (a-d). After 5 days of 1-hour access to heroin, an 18-day 6-hour daily self-administration period was introduced. Following initiation of the LgA sessions, HI rats (n=5) and LI rats (n=5) did not differ in their time-dependent increase in active lever presses (a), heroin infusion (b), and intake (calculated as the amount of heroin self-administered by each rat in milligrammes per kilogramme bidy weight) (c). A dimentional analysis based on the overall population tested (n=19) did not reveal any correlation between the individual level of impulsivity (percentage of premature responses during the last two 7 s-LITI sessions) and the propensity to escalated heroin SA (escalation score; calculated as the slope of intake over 18 days od LgA for each subject) (d). Consequently, HI and LI rats differed neither in their escalation slope (e) not in the increase of their ER (intake for each LgA day divided by intake for day 1) over the 18 LgA sessions (f).

This observation is of interest since it suggests that pharmacological flexibility in response to changes in drug availability and individual propensity to titrate drug intake according to drug availability may protect against loss of control over heroin SA. Nevertheless, the marked dissociation between high impulsivity trait and individual propensity to lose control over heroin intake is in marked contrast with the demonstration that high impulsivity predicts increased vulnerability to lose control over cocaine SA [241]. Such dissociation suggests that heroin and cocaine addiction may not necessarily share common etiological factors, or, since impulsivity is a multifaceted construct [246], that other forms of impulsivity predict vulnerability to opiates addiction.

7. Conclusions

Major advances in the understanding of the neurobiological substrates of addictive drugs and their short and long-term consequences on the brain have been provided by CPP or self-administration models. Refined preclinical models, that go beyond drug reinforcement or neurobiological adaptations to repeated exposure to addictive drugs, hence with heuristic value with regards to the compulsive nature of drug seeking in drug addicts, have provided new insights into the aetiology and pathophysiology of drug addiction. Nevertheless, to date several critical behavioural aspects of drug addiction remain under-investigated, including the influence of alternative reinforcers during self-administration sessions and the role of environmental conditions, and especially environmental enrichment in inter-individual vulnerability to switch to compulsive drug use. Additionally, the recent data we have acquired on inter-individual differences in loss of control over heroin intake and the marked dissociation between high impulsivity trait and escalation of heroin SA reveal the necessity to develop preclinical models of addiction-like behaviour for other classes of drugs than stimulants. Only then will we be able to determine whether drug addiction is one pathology characterised by common etiological and pathophysiological factors or whether it should instead be considered as multifaceted, with different etiological and pathophysiological pathways, depending, at least, on the drug [56].

8. Acknowledgements

This work was supported by the INSERM AVENIR program, the IREB, the Fondation pour la recherche Médicale (FRM) and the University of Poitiers. Aude Belin-Rauscent was supported by the AXA research fund and an INSERM post-doctoral fellowship. The authors would like to thank Drs Yann Pelloux, Daina Economidou and Pr Barry Everitt for previous work on contents of this chapter.

9. References

[1] Geyer MA, Markou A, Bloom FE, Kupfer DJ. Animal models in psychatric disorders. 1995. p. 787-798.

[2] Koob G, Le Moal M. Plasticity of reward neurocircuitry and the 'dark side' of drug addiction. Nat Neurosci. 2005; 8: 1442-1444.

[3] Olds J, Milner P. Positive reinforcement produced by electrical stimulation of septal area and other regions of rat brain. Jcomp Physiol Psychol. 1954; 47: 419-427.

[4] Weeks JR. Experimental Morphine Addiction: Method for Automatic Intravenous Injections in Unrestrained Rats. Science. 1962; 138: 143-144.

[5] DSMIII. Diagnostic and Statistical Manual of Mental Disorders [Third Edition]. American Psychiatric Association.; 1985

[6] Everitt BJ, Robbins TW. Second-order schedules of drug reinforcement in rats and monkeys: measurement of reinforcing efficacy and drug-seeking behaviour. Psychopharmacology. 2000; 153: 17-30.

[7] Everitt BJ, Robbins TW. Neural systems of reinforcement for drug addiction: from actions to habits to compulsion. Nat Neurosci. 2005; 8: 1481-1489.

[8] Belin D, Balado E, Piazza PV, Deroche-Gamonet V. Pattern of intake and drug craving predict the development of cocaine addiction-like behavior in rats. Biol Psychiatry. 2009; 65: 863-868.

[9] Pelloux Y, Costentin J, Duterte-Boucher D. Differential effects of novelty exposure on place preference conditioning to amphetamine and its oral consumption. Psychopharmacology. 2004; 171: 277-285.

[10] Bardo M, Bevins RA. Conditioned place preference: what does it add to our preclinical understanding of drug reward? Psychopharmacology [Berl]. 2000; 153: 31-43.

[11] Kusayama T, Watanabe S. Reinforcing effects of methamphetamine in planarians. Neuroreport. 2000; 11: 2511-2513.

[12] Bardo M, Donohew RL, Harrington NG. Psychobiology of novelty seeking and drug seeking behavior. Behavioural Brain Research. 1996; 77: 23-43.

[13] Frenois F, Cador M, Caille S, Stinus L, Le Moine C. Neural correlates of the motivational and somatic components of naloxone-precipitated morphine withdrawal. Eur J Neurosci. 2002; 16: 1377-1389.

[14] Frenois F, Le Moine C, Cador M. The motivational component of withdrawal in opiate addiction: rôle of associative learning and aversive memory in opiate addiction from a behavioral, anatomical and functional perspective. Rev Neurosci. 2005; 16: 255-276.

[15] Frenois F, Stinus L, Di Blasi F, Cador M, Le Moine C. A specific limbic circuit underlies opiate withdrawal memories. J Neurosci. 2005; 25: 1366-1374.

[16] Rossi NA, Reid LD. Affective states associated with morphine injections [dissertation]. Bradley University.; 1976.

[17] Tzschentke T. Behavioral pharmacology of buprenorphine, with a focus on preclinical models of reward and addiction. Psychopharmacology. 2002; 161: 1-16.

[18] De Wit H, Stewart J. Reinstatement of cocaine-reinforced responding in the rat. Psychopharmacology [Berl]. 1981; 75: 134-143.

[19] De Wit H, Stewart J. Drug reinstatement of heroin-reinforced responding in the rat. Psychopharmacology [Berl]. 1983; 79: 29-31.

[20] Bossert JM, Ghitza UE, Lu L, Epstein DH, Shaham Y. Neurobiology of relapse to heroin and cocaine seeking: an update and clinical implications. Eur J Pharmacol. 2005; 526[1-3]:36-50.

[21] Ahmed SH, Koob G. Transition from Moderate to Excessive Drug Intake: Change in Hedonic Set Point. Science. 1998; 282: 298-300.

[22] Ahmed SH, Walker JR, Koob G. Persistent Increase in the Motivation to Take Heroin in Rats with a History of Drug Escalation. Neuropsychopharmacology. 2000; 22: 413-421.

[23] Vanderschuren L, Everitt BJ. Behavioral and neural mechanisms of compulsive drug seeking. European Journal of Pharmacology. 2005; 526: 77-88.

[24] Pelloux Y, Everitt BJ, Dickinson A. Compulsive drug seeking by rats under punishment: effects of drug taking history. Psychopharmacology [Berl]. 2007; 194: 127-137.

[25] Economidou D, Pelloux Y, Robbins TW, Dalley JW, Everitt BJ. High Impulsivity Predicts Relapse to Cocaine-Seeking After Punishment-Induced Abstinence. Biol Psychiatry. 2009; 65: 851-856.

[26] Deroche-Gamonet V, Belin D, Piazza P. Evidence for addiction-like behavior in the rat. Science. 2004; 305: 1014-1017.

[27] Belin D, Mar A, Dalley J, Robbins TW, Everitt BJ High Impulsivity Predicts the Switch to Compulsive Cocaine-Taking. Science. 2008; 320: 1352-1355.
[28] Belin D, Berson N, Balado E, Piazza PV, Deroche-Gamonet V. High-Novelty-Preference Rats are Predisposed to Compulsive Cocaine Self-administration. Neuropsychopharmacology. 2011; 36: 569-579.
[29] Spealman RD, Goldberg SR. Drug Self-Administration by Laboratory Animals: Control by Schedules of Reinforcement. Annual Reviews in Pharmacology and Toxicology. 1978; 18: 313: 339.
[30] Goldberg SR, Kelleher RT, Morse WH. Second-order schedules of drug injection. Fed Proc. 1975; 34: 1771-1776.
[31] Stafford D, LeSage MG, Glowa JR. Progressive-ratio schedules of drug delivery in the analysis of drug self-administration: a review. Psychopharmacology. 1998; 139: 169-184.
[32] Schindler CW, Panlilio LV, Goldberg SR. Second-order schedules of drug self-administration in animals. Psychopharmacology [Berl]. 2002; 163: 327-344.
[33] Di Chiara G, Imperato A. Drugs abused by humans preferentially increase synaptic dopamine concentrations in the mesolimbic system of freely moving rats. ProcNatlAcadSciUSA. 1988; 85: 5274-5278.
[34] Bozarth MA, Wise RA. Intracranial self-administration of morphine into the ventral tegmental area in rats. Life Sci. 1981; 28: 551-555.
[35] Bozarth MA, Wise RA. Neural substrates of opiate reinforcement. Prog Neuropsychopharmacol Biol Psychiatry. 1983; 7: 569-575.
[36] Bozarth MA, Wise RA. Anatomically distinct opiate receptor fields mediate reward and physical dependence. Science. 1984; 224: 516-517.
[37] Bozarth MA, Wise RA. Toxicity associated with long-term intravenous heroin and cocaine self-administration in the rat. JAMA. 1985; 254: 81-83.
[38] Di Chiara G, Tanda G, Bassareo V, Pontieri F, Acquas E, Fenu S, Cadoni C, Carboni E. Drug addiction as a disorder of associative learning. rôle of nucleus accumbens shell/extended amygdala dopamine. Ann N Y Acad Sci. 1999; 877: 461-485.
[39] Everitt BJ, Parkinson JA, Olmstead M, Arroyo M, Robledo P, Robbins TW. Associative processes in addiction and reward. The rôle of amygdala-ventral striatal subsystems. Ann NYAcadSci. 1999; 877: 412-438.
[40] Everitt BJ, Dickinson A, Robbins TW. The neuropsychological basis of addictive behaviour. Brain Research Reviews. 2001; 36: 129-138.
[41] Everitt BJ, Belin D, Dalley J, Robbins TW. Dopaminergic mechanisms in drug-seeking habits and the vulnerability to drug addiction. In: Leslie Iversen SI, Stephen Dunnett, and Anders Bjorklund, editor. Dopamine Handbook. New York: Oxford University Press; 2010.
[42] Robbins TW, Everitt BJ. Drug addiction: bad habits add up. Nature. 1999; 398: 567-570.
[43] Robbins TW, Everitt BJ. Limbic-Striatal Memory Systems and Drug Addiction. Neurobiology of Learning and Memory. 2002; 78: 625-636.
[44] Robinson T, Berridge K. Incentive-sensitization and addiction. Addiction. 2001; 96: 103-114.
[45] Everitt BJ, Wolf ME. Psychomotor Stimulant Addiction: A Neural Systems Perspective. Journal of Neuroscience. 2002; 22: 3312-3320.

[46] Jones S, Bonci A. Synaptic plasticity and drug addiction. Curr Opin Pharmacol. 2005; 5: 20-25.
[47] Hyman SE, Malenka RC, Nestler EJ. Neural mechanisms of addiction: the rôle of reward-related learning and memory. Annu Rev Neurosci. 2006; 29: 565-598.
[48] Schultz W. Multiple Dopamine Functions at Different Time Courses. Annu Rev Neurosci. 2007; 30: 259-288.
[49] Schultz W. Behavioral dopamine signals. Trends in Neurosciences. 2007; 30: 203-210.
[50] Faure A, Reynolds SM, Richard JM, Berridge KC. Mesolimbic dopamine in desire and dread: enabling motivation to be generated by localized glutamate disruptions in nucleus accumbens. J Neurosci. 2008; 28: 7184-7192.
[51] Thomas MJ, Kalivas P, Shaham Y. Neuroplasticity in the mesolimbic dopamine system and cocaine addiction. Br J Pharmacol. 2008; 154: 327-342.
[52] Berridge KC, Robinson TE, Aldridge JW. Dissecting components of reward: 'liking', 'wanting', and learning. Curr Opin Pharmacol. 2009; 9[1]:65-73.
[53] Ettenberg A, Pettit HO, Bloom FE, Koob GF. Heroin and cocaine intravenous self-administration in rats: Mediation by separate neural systems. Psychopharmacology. 1982; 78: 204-209.
[54] Kelly PH, Roberts DC. Effects of amphetamine and apomorphine on locomotor activity after 6-OHDA and electrolytic lesions of the nucleus accumbens septi. Pharmacol Biochem Behav. 1983; 19: 137-143.
[55] Pettit HO, Ettenberg A, Bloom FE, Koob GF. Destruction of dopamine in the nucleus accumbens selectively attenuates cocaine but not heroin self-administration in rats. Psychopharmacology [Berl]. 1984; 84: 167-173.
[56] Badiani A, Belin D, Epstein D, Calu D, Shaham Y. Opiate versus psychostimulant addiction: the differences do matter. Nat Rev Neurosci. 2011; 12: 685-700.
[57] Robinson T, Kolb B. Persistent structural modifications in nucleus accumbens and prefrontal cortex neurons produced by previous experience with amphetamine. J Neurosci. 1997; 17: 8491-8497.
[58] Robinson T, Kolb B. Morphine alters the structure of neurons in the nucleus accumbens and neocortex of rats. Synapse. 1999; 33: 160-162.
[59] Robinson T, Kolb B. Alterations in the morphology of dendrites and dendritic spines in the nucleus accumbens and prefrontal cortex following repeated treatment with amphetamine or cocaine. Eur J Neurosci. 1999; 11: 1598-1604.
[60] Robinson T, Kolb B. Structural plasticity associated with exposure to drugs of abuse. Neuropharmacology. 2004; 47 Suppl 1: 33-46.
[61] Robinson TE, Leung AN, Northway WH, Blankenberg FG, Bloch DA, Oehlert JW, Al-Dabbagh H, Hubli S, Moss RB. Spirometer-triggered high-resolution computed tomography and pulmonary function measurements during an acute exacerbation in patients with cystic fibrosis. J Pediatr. 2001; 138: 553-559.
[62] Li Y, Kolb B, Robinson T. The location of persistent amphetamine-induced changes in the density of dendritic spines on medium spiny neurons in the nucleus accumbens and caudate-putamen. Neuropsychopharmacology. 2003; 28: 1082-1085.
[63] Wolf ME, Sun X, Mangiavacchi S, Chao SZ. Psychomotor stimulants and neuronal plasticity. Neuropharmacology. 2004; 47 Suppl 1: 61-79.
[64] Schmidt K, Krishnan B, Xia Y, Sun A, Orozco-Cabal L, Pollandt S, Centeno M, Genzer K, Gallagher JP, Shinnick-Gallagher P, Liu J. Cocaine withdrawal enhances long-

term potentiation induced by corticotropin-releasing factor at central amygdala glutamatergic synapses via CRF, NMDA receptors and PKA. Eur J Neurosci. 2006; 24: 1733-1743.

[65] Fu Y, Pollandt S, Liu J, Krishnan B, Genzer K, Orozco-Cabal L, Gallagher JP, Shinnick-Gallagher P Long-term potentiation [LTP] in the central amygdala [CeA] is enhanced after prolonged withdrawal from chronic cocaine and requires CRF1 receptors. J Neurophysiol. 2007; 97: 937-941.

[66] Bonci A, Borgland S. Role of orexin/hypocretin and CRF in the formation of drug-dependent synaptic plasticity in the mesolimbic system. Neuropharmacology. 2009; 56 Suppl 1: 107-111.

[67] Ahmed SH, Lutjens R, van der Stap LD, Lekic D, Romano-Spica V, Morales M, Koob GF, Repunte-Canonigo V, Sanna PP. Gene expression evidence for remodeling of lateral hypothalamic circuitry in cocaine addiction. Proc Natl Acad Sci U S A. 2005; 102: 11533-11538.

[68] Belin D, Deroche-Gamonet V, Jaber M. Cocaine-induced sensitization is associated with altered dynamics of transcriptional responses of the dopamine transporter, tyrosine hydroxylase, and dopamine D2 receptors in C57Bl/6J mice. Psychopharmacology [Berl]. 2007; 193: 567-578.

[69] Nestler EJ. Common molecular and cellular substrates of addiction and memory. Neurobiol Learn Mem. 2002; 78: 637-647.

[70] Koob G. Neuroadaptive mechanisms of addiction: studies on the extended amygdala. European Neuropsychopharmacology. 2003; 13: 442-452.

[71] Befort K, Filliol D, Ghate A, Darcq E, Matifas A, Muller J, Lardenois A, Thibault C, Dembele D, Le Merrer J, Becker JA, Poch O, Kieffer BL. Mu-opioid receptor activation induces transcriptional plasticity in the central extended amygdala. Eur J Neurosci. 2008; 27: 2973-2984.

[72] Feltenstein MW, See RE. The neurocircuitry of addiction: an overview. Br J Pharmacol. 2008; 154: 261-274.

[73] Corominas M, Roncero C, Casas M. Corticotropin releasing factor and neuroplasticity in cocaine addiction. Life Sci. 2009

[74] Marcinkiewcz CA, Prado MM, Isaac SK, Marshall A, Rylkova D, Bruijnzeel AW. Corticotropin-releasing factor within the central nucleus of the amygdala and the nucleus accumbens shell mediates the negative affective state of nicotine withdrawal in rats. Neuropsychopharmacology. 2009; 34: 1743-1752.

[75] Nestler EJ. The neurobiology of cocaine addiction. Sci Pract Perspect. 2005; 3: 4-10.

[76] Nestler EJ. Epigenetic mechanisms in psychiatry. Biol Psychiatry. 2009; 65: 189-190.

[77] Renthal W, Nestler EJ. Epigenetic mechanisms in drug addiction. Trends Mol Med. 2008; 14: 341-350.

[78] Maze I, Covington HE 3rd, Dietz DM, LaPlant Q, Renthal W, Russo SJ, Mechanic M, Mouzon E, Neve RL, Haggarty SJ, Ren Y, Sampath SC, Hurd YL, Greengard P, Tarakhovsky A, Schaefer A, Nestler EJ. Essential role of the histone methyltransferase G9a in cocaine-induced plasticity. Science. 2010; 327: 213-216.

[79] Russo SJ, Dietz DM, Dumitriu D, Morrison JH, Malenka RC, Nestler EJ. The addicted synapse: mechanisms of synaptic and structural plasticity in nucleus accumbens. Trends Neurosci. 2010

[80] Jedynak J, Uslaner J, Esteban J, Robinson T. Methamphetamine-induced structural plasticity in the dorsal striatum. Eur J Neurosci. 2007; 25: 847-853.

[81] Schoenbaum G, Shaham Y. The role of Orbitofrontal Cortex in Drug Addiction: A Review of Preclinical Studies. Biological Psychiatry. 2008; 63: 256-262.

[82] Winstanley CA, Green TA, Theobald DE, Renthal W, LaPlant Q, DiLeone RJ, Chakravarty S, Nestler EJ. DeltaFosB induction in orbitofrontal cortex potentiates locomotor sensitization despite attenuating the cognitive dysfunction caused by cocaine. Pharmacol Biochem Behav. 2008

[83] Kolb B, Gorny G, Li Y, Samaha AN, Robinson T. Amphetamine or cocaine limits the ability of later experience to promote structural plasticity in the neocortex and nucleus accumbens. Proc Natl Acad Sci U S A. 2003; 100: 10523-10528.

[84] Kolb B, Pellis S, Robinson T. Plasticity and functions of the orbital frontal cortex. Brain Cogn. 2004; 55: 104-115.

[85] Crombag H, Gorny G, Li Y, Kolb B, Robinson T. Opposite effects of amphetamine self-administration experience on dendritic spines in the medial and orbital prefrontal cortex. Cereb Cortex. 2005; 15: 341-348.

[86] Koob G, Le Moal M. Drug Abuse: Hedonic Homeostatic Dysregulation. Science. 1997; 278: 52-58.

[87] Koob G, Le Moal M. Drug addiction, dysregulation of reward, and allostasis. Neuropsychopharmacology. 2001; 24: 97-129.

[88] Koob GF, Le Moal M. Review. Neurobiological mechanisms for opponent motivational processes in addiction. Philos Trans R Soc Lond B Biol Sci. 2008; 363: 3113-3123.

[89] Tsankova N, Renthal W, Kumar A, Nestler EJ. Epigenetic regulation in psychiatric disorders. Nat Rev Neurosci. 2007; 8: 355-367.

[90] McClung CA, Nestler EJ. Neuroplasticity mediated by altered gene expression. Neuropsychopharmacology. 2008; 33: 3-17.

[91] Renthal W, Nestler EJ. Chromatin regulation in drug addiction and depression. Dialogues Clin Neurosci. 2009; 11: 257-268.

[92] Renthal W, Nestler EJ. Histone acetylation in drug addiction. Semin Cell Dev Biol. 2009; 20: 387-394.

[93] Ahmed SH. Validation crisis in animal models of drug addiction: beyond non-disordered drug use toward drug addiction. Neurosci Biobehav Rev. 2010; 35: 172-184.

[94] Clark R, Schuster CR, Brady JV. Instrumental conditioning of jugular self-infusion in the rhesus monkey. Science. 1961; 133: 1829-1830.

[95] Wise RA, Bozarth MA. A psychomotor stimulant theory of addiction. Psychol Rev. 1987; 94: 469-492.

[96] Robinson T, Berridge K. The neural basis of drug craving: an incentive-sensitization theory of addiction. Brain Research Reviews. 1993; 18: 247-291.

[97] APA. Diagnostic and Statistical Manual of Mental Disorders fourth edition, Text revision [DSM-IV TR]. Washington DC: American Psychiatric Association; 2000

[98] Shaham Y, Miczek K. Reinstatement?toward a model of relapse. Psychopharmacology. 2003; 168: 1-2.

[99] Shaham Y, Shalev U, Lu L, De Wit H, Stewart J. The reinstatement model of drug relapse: history, methodology and major findings. Psychopharmacology. 2003; 168: 3-20.

[100] Fuchs RA, Branham RK, See RE. Different neural substrates mediate cocaine seeking after abstinence versus extinction training: a critical rôle for the dorsolateral caudate-putamen. J Neurosci. 2006; 26: 3584-3588.

[101] Belin D, Everitt BJ. Cocaine-Seeking Habits Depend upon Dopamine-Dependent Serial Connectivity Linking the Ventral with the Dorsal Striatum. Neuron. 2008; 57: 432-441.

[102] O'Brien CP. A Range of Research-Based Pharmacotherapies for Addiction. Science. 1997; 278: 66-70.

[103] See RE, Elliott JC, Feltenstein MW. The role of dorsal vs ventral striatal pathways in cocaine-seeking behavior after prolonged abstinence in rats. Psychopharmacology [Berl]. 2007; 194: 321-331.

[104] Fuchs R, Tran-Nguyen LT, Specio SE, Groff RS, Neisewander JL. Predictive validity of the extinction/reinstatement model of drug craving. Psychopharmacology [Berl]. 1998; 135: 151-160.

[105] Shalev U, Grimm JW, Shaham Y. Neurobiology of Relapse to Heroin and Cocaine Seeking: A Review. Pharmacological Reviews. 2002; 54: 1-42.

[106] Capriles N, Rodaros D, Sorge RE, Stewart J. A role for the prefrontal cortex in stress- and cocaine-induced reinstatement of cocaine seeking in rats. Psychopharmacology [Berl]. 2003; 168: 66-74.

[107] Fuchs RA, Evans KA, Parker MP, See RE. Differential involvement of orbitofrontal cortex subregions in conditioned cue-induced and cocaine-primed reinstatement of cocaine seeking in rats. J Neurosci. 2004; 24: 6600-6610.

[108] Fuchs RA, Ramirez DR, Bell GH. Nucleus accumbens shell and core involvement in drug context-induced reinstatement of cocaine seeking in rats. Psychopharmacology [Berl]. 2008; 200: 545-556.

[109] Torregrossa MM, Tang XC, Kalivas PW. The glutamatergic projection from the prefrontal cortex to the nucleus accumbens core is required for cocaine-induced decreases in ventral pallidal GABA. Neurosci Lett. 2008; 438: 142-145.

[110] Zhou W, Kalivas P. N-Acetylcysteine Reduces Extinction Responding and Induces Enduring Reductions in Cue- and Heroin-Induced Drug-Seeking. Biological Psychiatry. 2008; 63: 338-340.

[111] Knackstedt LA, Kalivas PW. Glutamate and reinstatement. Curr Opin Pharmacol. 2009; 9: 59-64.

[112] Rocha A, Kalivas PW. role of the prefrontal cortex and nucleus accumbens in reinstating methamphetamine seeking. Eur J Neurosci. 2010; 31: 903-909.

[113] Kalivas P, Mcfarland K. Brain circuitry and the reinstatement of cocaine-seeking behavior. Psychopharmacology [Berl]. 2003; 168: 44-56.

[114] Kalivas P. Glutamate systems in cocaine addiction. Current Opinion in Pharmacology. 2004; 4: 23-29.

[115] LaLumiere RT, Kalivas PW. Glutamate release in the nucleus accumbens core is necessary for heroin seeking. J Neurosci. 2008; 28: 3170-3177.

[116] Kalivas PW. Perspective: the manifest destiny of cocaine research. Neuropsychopharmacology. 2009; 34: 1089-1090.

[117] Grimm JW, Hope BT, Wise RA, Shaham Y. Neuroadaptation. Incubation of cocaine craving after withdrawal. Nature. 2001; 412: 141-142.

[118] Lu L. Incubation of cocaine craving after withdrawal: a review of preclinical data. Neuropharmacology. 2004; 47: 214-226.

[119] Zernig G, Ahmed S, Cardinal R et al. Explaining the Escalation of Drug Use in Substance Dependence: Models and Appropriate Animal Laboratory Tests. Pharmacology. 2007; 80: 65-119.

[120] Ahmed S, Cador M. Dissociation of Psychomotor Sensitization from Compulsive Cocaine Consumption. Neuropsychopharmacology. 2006; 31: 563-571.

[121] Vanderschuren L, Everitt BJ. Drug Seeking Becomes Compulsive After Prolonged Cocaine Self-Administration. Science. 2004; 305: 1017-1019.

[122] McNamara R, Dalley JW, Robbins TW, Everitt BJ, Belin D. Trait-like impulsivity does not predict escalation of heroin self-administration in the rat. Psychopharmacology. 2010; 212: 453-464.

[123] Lenoir M, Ahmed S. Heroin-Induced Reinstatement is Specific to Compulsive Heroin Use and Dissociable from Heroin Reward and Sensitization. Neuropsychopharmacology. 2007; 32: 616-624.

[124] Corbit LH, Balleine B. The role of prelimbic cortex in instrumental conditioning. Behavioural Brain Research. 2003; 146: 145-157.

[125] Olmstead M, Parkinson J, Miles F, Everitt BJ, Dickinson A. Cocaine-seeking by rats: regulation, reinforcement and activation. Psychopharmacology. 2000; 152: 123-131.

[126] Olmstead M, Lafond M, Everitt BJ, Dickinson A. Cocaine seeking by rats is a goal-directed action. Behavioral Neuroscience. 2001; 115: 394-402.

[127] Zapata A, Minney VL, Shippenberg TS. Shift from goal-directed to habitual cocaine seeking after prolonged experience in rats. J Neurosci. 2010; 30: 15457-15463.

[128] Belin-Rauscent A, Everitt BJ, Belin D. Intrastriatal shifts mediate the transition from drug seeking actions to habits. Biological Psychiatry. 2012; In Press

[129] Goldberg SR, Spealman RD, Kelleher RT. Enhancement of drug-seeking behavior by environmental stimuli associated with cocaine or morphine injections. Neuropharmacology. 1979; 18: 1015-1017.

[130] Goldberg SR, Kelleher RT, Goldberg DM. Fixed-ratio responding under second-order schedules of food presentation or cocaine injection. J Pharmacol Exp Ther. 1981; 218: 271-281.

[131] Parkinson JA, Roberts AC, Everitt BJ, Di Ciano P. Acquisition of instrumental conditioned reinforcement is resistant to the devaluation of the unconditioned stimulus. QJExpPsycholB. 2005; 58: 19-30.

[132] Di Ciano P, Benham-Hermetz J, Fogg AP, Osborne GE. role of the prelimbic cortex in the acquisition, re-acquisition or persistence of responding for a drug-paired conditioned reinforcer. Neuroscience. 2007; 150: 291-298.

[133] Arroyo M, Markou A, Robbins TW, Everitt BJ. Acquisition, maintenance and reinstatement of intravenous cocaine self-administration under a second-order schedule of reinforcement in rats: effects of conditioned cues and continuous access to cocaine. Psychopharmacology [Berl]. 1998; 140: 331-344.

[134] Ito R, Dalley J, Robbins TW, Everitt BJ. Dopamine release in the dorsal striatum during cocaine-seeking behavior under the control of a drug-associated cue. J Neurosci. 2002; 22: 6247-6253.

[135] Ito R, Robbins TW, Everitt BJ. Differential control over cocaine-seeking behavior by nucleus accumbens core and shell. Nat Neurosci. 2004; 7: 389-397.

[136] Lee J, Di Ciano P, Thomas K, Everitt BJ. Disrupting Reconsolidation of Drug Memories Reduces Cocaine-Seeking Behavior. Neuron. 2005; 47: 795-801.

[137] Murray J, Belin D, Everitt BJ. Double dissociation of the dorsomedial and dorsolateral striatal control over the acquisition and performance of cocaine seeking. Neuropsychopharmacology. 2012; In Press

[138] Murray JE, Everitt BJ, Belin D. N-Acetylcysteine reduces early- and late-stage cocaine seeking without affecting cocaine taking in rats. Addict Biol. 2012; 17: 437-440.

[139] Di Ciano P, Everitt BJ. Direct Interactions between the Basolateral Amygdala and Nucleus Accumbens Core Underlie Cocaine-Seeking Behavior by Rats. Journal of Neuroscience. 2004; 24: 7167-7173.

[140] Corbit LH, Nie H, Janak PH. Habitual Alcohol Seeking: Time Course and the Contribution of Subregions of the Dorsal Striatum. Biol Psychiatry. 2012

[141] Murray J, Belin D, Everitt BJ. Double dissociation of the dorsomedial and dorsolateral striatal control over the acquisition and performance of cocaine seeking. Neuropsychopharmacology. 2012; In Press

[142] Vollstädt-Klein S, Wichert S, Rabinstein J, Bühler M, Klein O, Ende G, Hermann D, Mann K. Initial, habitual and compulsive alcohol use is characterized by a shift of cue processing from ventral to dorsal striatum. Addiction. 2010; 105: 1741-1749.

[143] Volkow ND, Wang GJ, Telang F, Fowler JS, Logan J, Childress AR, Jayne M, Ma Y, Wong C. Cocaine Cues and Dopamine in Dorsal Striatum: Mechanism of Craving in Cocaine Addiction. Journal of Neuroscience. 2006; 26: 6583-6588.

[144] Goodman WK, Price LH, Rasmussen SA, Mazure C, Fleischmann RL, Hill CL, Heninger GR, Charney DS. The Yale-Brown Obsessive Compulsive Scale. II. Validity. Arch Gen Psychiatry. 1989; 46: 1012-1016.

[145] Goodman WK, Price LH, Rasmussen SA, Mazure C, Fleischmann RL, Hill CL, Heninger GR, Charney DS. The Yale-Brown Obsessive Compulsive Scale. I. Development, use, and reliability. Arch Gen Psychiatry. 1989; 46: 1006-1011.

[146] Anton RF. Obsessive-compulsive aspects of craving: development of the Obsessive Compulsive Drinking Scale. Addiction. 2000; 95 Suppl 2: S211-7.

[147] Waldorf D, Reinarman C, Murphy S. Cocaine Changes: The Experience of Using and Quitting. Temple University Press; 1991

[148] Burman BD. The nonreimbursed patient. Rehab Manag. 1997; 10: 48-51.

[149] Cunningham JA, Lin E, Ross HE, Walsh GW. Factors associated with untreated remissions from alcohol abuse or dependence. Addict Behav. 2000; 25: 317-321.

[150] Dickinson A, Wood N, Smith J. Alcohol seeking by rats: Action or habit? The Quarterly Journal of Experimental Psychology: Section B. 2002; 55: 331-348.

[151] Miles F, Everitt BJ, Dickinson A. Oral cocaine seeking by rats: Action or habit? Behavioral Neuroscience. 2003; 117: 927-938.

[152] Heyne A, Wolffgramm J. The development of addiction to d-amphetamine in an animal model: same principles as for alcohol and opiate. Psychopharmacology [Berl]. 1998; 140: 510-518.

[153] Spanagel R, Holter SM. Long-term alcohol self-administration with repeated alcohol deprivation phases: an animal model of alcoholism? Alcohol Alcohol. 1999; 34: 231-243.

[154] Heyne A, May T, Goll P, Wolffgramm J. Persisting consequences of drug intake: towards a memory of addiction. J Neural Transm. 2000; 107: 613-638.

[155] Pearce JM, Dickinson A. Pavlovian counterconditioning: changing the suppressive properties of shock by association with food. J Exp Psychol Anim Behav Process. 1975; 1: 170-177.

[156] Azrin NH, Holz WC. Punishment. Operant behavior: Areas of research and application. 1966; 380-447.

[157] Cooper A, Barnea-Ygael N, Levy D, Shaham Y, Zangen A. A conflict rat model of cue-induced relapse to cocaine seeking. Psychopharmacology [Berl]. 2007; 194: 117-125.

[158] Smith SG, Davis WM. Punishment of amphetamine and morphine self-administration behavior. Psychol Rec. 1974; 24: 477-480.

[159] Corbit L, Balleine B. Instrumental and Pavlovian incentive processes have dissociable effects on components of a heterogeneous instrumental chain. Journal of Experimental Psychology: Animal Behavior Processes. 2003; 29: 99-106.

[160] Panlilio LV, Thorndike EB, Schindler CW. Reinstatement of punishment-suppressed opioid self-administration in rats: an alternative model of relapse to drug abuse. Psychopharmacology [Berl]. 2003; 168: 229-235.

[161] Robinson T, Berridge K. The psychology and neurobiology of addiction: an incentive-sensitization view. Addiction. 2000; 95: S91-S117.

[162] Robinson TE, Berridge KC. Review. The incentive sensitization theory of addiction: some current issues. Philos Trans R Soc Lond B Biol Sci. 2008; 363: 3137-3146.

[163] Dieckmann U, Doebeli M. On the origin of species by sympatric speciation. Nature. 1999; 400: 354-357.

[164] Hasegawa M, Yahara T, Yasumoto A, Hotta M. Bimodal distribution of flowering time in a natural hybrid population of daylily [Hemerocallis fulva] and nightlily [Hemerocallis citrina]. Journal of Plant Research. 2006; 119: 63-68.

[165] Ellenbroek BA, Cools AR. Apomorphine susceptibility and animal models for psychopathology: genes and environment. Behav Genet. 2002; 32: 349-361.

[166] Nesse RM, Berridge K. Psychoactive Drug Use in Evolutionary Perspective. Science. 1997; 278: 63-66.

[167] Belin D, Economidou D, Pelloux Y, Everitt BJ. Habit Formation and Compulsion. In: Olmstead MC, editor. Animal models of drug addiction. Humana Press; 2010. p. 337-378.

[168] Anthony JC, Warner LA, Kessler RC Comparative epidemiology of dependence on tobacco, alcohol, controlled substances, and inhalants: Basic findings from the National comorbidity Survey. Exp Clin Psychopharmacol. 1994; 2: 244-268.

[169] Kasanetz F, Deroche-Gamonet V, Berson N, Balado E, Lafourcade M, Manzoni O, Piazza PV. Transition to addiction is associated with a persistent impairment in synaptic plasticity. Science. 2010; 328: 1709-1712.

[170] Everitt BJ, Belin D, Economidou D, Pelloux Y, Dalley J, Robbins TW. Neural mechanisms underlying the vulnerability to develop compulsive drug-seeking habits and addiction. Philos Trans R Soc Lond B Biol Sci. 2008; 363: 3125-3135.

[171] Kreek M, Laforge K, Butelman E. Pharmacotherapy of addictions. Nat Rev Drug Discov. 2002; 1: 710-726.

[172] Kreek M, Nielsen D, Butelman E, Laforge K. Genetic influences on impulsivity, risk taking, stress responsivity and vulnerability to drug abuse and addiction. Nat Neurosci. 2005; 8: 1450-1457.

[173] Teichman M, Barnea Z, Rahav G. Sensation seeking, state and trait anxiety, and depressive mood in adolescent substance users. IntJAddict. 1989; 24: 87-99.
[174] Teichman M, Barnea Z, Ravav G. Personality and substance use among adolescents: a longitudinal study. BrJAddict. 1989; 84: 181-190.
[175] Zuckerman M. The sensation seeking motive. Prog Exp Pers Res. 1974; 7: 79-148.
[176] Zuckerman M. Sensation seeking and the endogenous deficit theory of drug abuse. NIDA Res Monogr. 1986; 74: 59-70.
[177] Zuckerman M. Sensation seeking and behavior disorders. Arch Gen Psychiatry. 1988; 45: 502-504.
[178] Kilpatrick DG, Sutker PB, Roitzsch JC, Miller WC. Personality correlates of polydrug abuse. PsycholRep. 1976; 38: 311-317.
[179] Pomerleau CS, Pomerleau OF, Flessland KA, Basson SM. Relationship of Tridimensional Personality Questionnaire scores and smoking variables in female and male smokers. J Subst Abuse. 1992; 4: 143-154.
[180] Schinka JA, Curtiss G, Mulloy JM. Personality variables and self-medication in substance abuse. JpersAssess. 1994; 63: 413-422.
[181] Wills TA, Vaccaro D, McNamara G. Novelty seeking, risk taking, and related constructs as predictors of adolescent substance use: an application of Cloninger's theory. J Subst Abuse. 1994; 6: 1-20.
[182] Wills TA, Windle M, Cleary SD. Temperament and novelty seeking in adolescent substance use: convergence of dimensions of temperament with constructs from Cloninger's theory. J Pers Soc Psychol. 1998; 74: 387-406.
[183] Scourfield J, Stevens DE, Merikangas KR. Substance abuse, comorbidity, and sensation seeking: gender differences. Compr Psychiatry. 1996; 37: 384-392.
[184] Sarramon C, Verdoux H, Schmitt L, Bourgeois M. [Addiction and personality traits: sensation seeking, anhedonia, impulsivity]. Encephale. 1999; 25: 569-575.
[185] Sher KJ, Bartholow BD, Wood MD. Personality and substance use disorders: a prospective study. J Consult Clin Psychol. 2000; 68: 818-829.
[186] Skinstad AH, Swain A. Comorbidity in a clinical sample of substance abusers. Am Jdrug Alcohol Abuse. 2001; 27: 45-64.
[187] Conway K, Swendsen JD, Rounsaville BJ, Merikangas KR. Personality, drug of choice, and comorbid psychopathology among substance abusers. Drug Alcohol Depend. 2002; 65: 225-234.
[188] Moeller FG, Dougherty DM, Barratt ES, Oderinde V, Mathias CW, Harper RA, Swann AC. Increased impulsivity in cocaine dependent subjects independent of antisocial personality disorder and aggression. Drug Alcohol Depend. 2002; 68: 105-111.
[189] Adams JB, Heath AJ, Young SE, Hewitt JK, Corley RP, Stallings MC. Relationships between personality and preferred substance and motivations for use among adolescent substance abusers. Am J Drug Alcohol Abuse. 2003; 29: 691-712.
[190] Conway K. Personality, substance of choice, and polysubstance involvement among substance dependent patients. Drug and Alcohol Dependence. 2003; 71: 65-75.
[191] O'Leary TA, Rohsenow DJ, Martin R, Colby SM, Eaton CA, Monti PM. The relationship between anxiety levels and outcome of cocaine abuse treatment. Am Jdrug Alcohol Abuse. 2000; 26: 179-194.

[192] Roberts A. Psychiatric comorbidity in white and African-American illicit substance abusers: evidence for differential etiology. ClinPsycholRev. 2000; 20: 667-677.

[193] Forsyth JP, Parker JD, Finlay CG. Anxiety sensitivity, controllability, and experiential avoidance and their relation to drug of choice and addiction severity in a residential sample of substance-abusing veterans. Addictive Behaviors. 2003; 28: 851-870.

[194] Zilberman ML, Tavares H, Hodgins DC, el-Guebaly N. The impact of gender, depression, and personality on craving. J Addict Dis. 2007; 26: 79-84.

[195] Petry NM. Discounting of delayed rewards in substance abusers: relationship to antisocial personality disorder. Psychopharmacology [Berl]. 2002; 162: 425-432.

[196] Hanson KL, Luciana M, Sullwold K. Reward-related decision-making deficits and elevated impulsivity among MDMA and other drug users. Drug Alcohol Depend. 2008; 96: 99-110.

[197] Franques P, Auriacombe M, Tignol J. [Addiction and personality]. Encephale. 2000; 26: 68-78.

[198] Zuckerman M, Neeb M. Sensation seeking and psychopathology. Psychiatry Res. 1979; 1: 255-264.

[199] Zuckerman M. The psychophysiology of sensation seeking. J Pers. 1990; 58: 313-345.

[200] Chandra PS, Krishna VA, Benegal V, Ramakrishna J. High-risk sexual behaviour & sensation seeking among heavy alcohol users. Indian J Med Res. 2003; 117: 88-92.

[201] Pellow S, Chopin P, File SE, Briley M. Validation of open: closed arm entries in an elevated plus-maze as a measure of anxiety in the rat. JneurosciMethods. 1985; 14: 149-167.

[202] Pellow S, File SE. Anxiolytic and anxiogenic drug effects on exploratory activity in an elevated plus-maze: a novel test of anxiety in the rat. PharmacolBiochemBehav. 1986; 24: 525-529.

[203] Pelloux Y, Costentin J, Duterte-Boucher D. Anxiety increases the place conditioning induced by cocaine in rats. Behav Brain Res. 2009; 197: 311-316.

[204] Homberg JR, van den Akker M, Raasø HS, Wardeh G, Binnekade R, Schoffelmeer AN, de Vries TJ. Enhanced motivation to self-administer cocaine is predicted by self-grooming behaviour and relates to dopamine release in the rat medial prefrontal cortex and amygdala. Eur J Neurosci. 2002; 15: 1542-1550.

[205] Bush D, Vaccarino F. Individual differences in elevated plus-maze exploration predicted progressive-ratio cocaine self-administration break points in Wistar rats. Psychopharmacology. 2007; 194: 211-219.

[206] Spanagel R, Montkowski A, Allingham K, Stöhr T, Shoaib M, Holsboer F, Landgraf R. Anxiety: a potential predictor of vulnerability to the initiation of ethanol self-administration in rats. Psychopharmacology [Berl]. 1995; 122: 369-373.

[207] Henniger MS, Spanagel R, Wigger A, Landgraf R, Holter SM. Alcohol self-administration in two rat lines selectively bred for extremes in anxiety-related behavior. Neuropsychopharmacology. 2002; 26: 729-736.

[208] Stewart SH, Karp J, Pihl RO, Peterson RA. Anxiety sensitivity and self-reported reasons for drug use. JsubstAbuse. 1997; 9: 223-240.

[209] Chakroun N, Doron J, Swendsen J. [Substance use, affective problems and personality traits: test of two association models.]. Encephale. 2004; 30: 564-569.
[210] Dilleen R, Pelloux Y, Mar AC, Molander A, Robbins TW, Everitt BJ, Dalley JW, Belin D. High anxiety is a predisposing endophenotype for loss of control over cocaine, but not heroin, self-administration in rats. Psychopharmacology [Berl]. 2012
[211] Conrod PJ, Pihl RO, Stewart SH, Dongier M. Validation of a system of classifying female substance abusers on the basis of personality and motivational risk factors for substance abuse. Psychol Addict Behav. 2000; 14: 243-256.
[212] Khantzian EJ. The self-medication hypothesis of substance use disorders: a reconsideration and recent applications. HarvRevPsychiatry. 1997; 4: 231-244.
[213] Paine TA, Jackman SL, Olmstead MC. Cocaine-induced anxiety: alleviation by diazepam, but not buspirone, dimenhydrinate or diphenhydramine. Behav Pharmacol. 2002; 13: 511-523.
[214] Müller CP, Carey RJ, Wilkisz M, Schwenzner S, Jocham G, Huston JP, De Souza Silva MA. Acute anxiolytic effects of cocaine: the rôle of test latency and activity phase. Pharmacol Biochem Behav. 2008; 89: 218-226.
[215] Dellu F, Mayo W, Vallée M, Maccari S, Piazza PV, Le Moal M, Simon H. Behavioral reactivity to novelty during youth as a predictive factor of stress-induced corticosterone secretion in the elderly--a life-span study in rats. Psychoneuroendocrinology. 1996; 21: 441-453.
[216] Blanchard MM, Mendelsohn D, Stamp JA. The HR/LR model: Further evidence as an animal model of sensation seeking. Neurosci Biobehav Rev. 2009; 33: 1145-1154.
[217] Cain M, Saucier D, Bardo M. Novelty seeking and drug use: Contribution of an animal model. Experimental and Clinical Psychopharmacology. 2005; 13: 367-375.
[218] Piazza PV, Deminiere JM, Le Moal M, Simon H. Factors that predict individual vulnerability to amphetamine self-administration. Science. 1989; 245: 1511-1513.
[219] Hooks MS, Jones GH, Smith AD, Neill DB, Justice JB. Individual differences in locomotor activity and sensitization. PharmacolBiochemBehav. 1991; 38: 467-470.
[220] Hooks MS, Jones GH, Smith AD, Neill DB, Justice JB. Response to novelty predicts the locomotor and nucleus accumbens dopamine response to cocaine. Synapse. 1991; 9: 121-128.
[221] Piazza PV, Rouge-Pont F, Deminiere JM, Kharoubi M, Le Moal M, Simon H. Dopaminergic activity is reduced in the prefrontal cortex and increased in the nucleus accumbens of rats predisposed to develop amphetamine self-administration. Brain Res. 1991; 567: 169-174.
[222] Misslin R, Cigrang M. Does neophobia necessarily imply fear or anxiety? Behavioural processes. 1986; 12: 45-50.
[223] Bevins RA, Klebaur JE, Bardo M. Individual differences in response to novelty, amphetamine-induced activity and drug discrimination in rats. Behav Pharmacol. 1997; 8: 113-123.

[224] Cain ME, Smith C, Bardo M. The effect of novelty on amphetamine self-administration in rats classified as high and low responders. Psychopharmacology [Berl]. 2004; 176: 129-138.

[225] Klebaur JE, Bevins RA, Segar TM, Bardo M. Individual differences in behavioral responses to novelty and amphetamine self-administration in male and female rats. Behavioural Pharmacology. 2001

[226] Bardo M, Neisewander JL, Pierce R. Novelty-induced place preference behavior in rats: effects of opiate and dopaminergic drugs. Pharmacol Biochem Behav. 1989; 32: 683-689.

[227] Dellu F, Mayo W, Piazza PV, Le Moal M, Simon H. Individual differences in behavioral responses to novelty in rats. Possible relationship with the sensation-seeking trait in man. Personality and Individual Differences. 1993; 15: 411-411.

[228] Piazza PV, Ferdico M, Russo D, Crescimanno G, Benigno A, Amato G. Circling behavior: ethological analysis and functional considerations. Behav Brain Res. 1989; 31: 267-271.

[229] Klebaur JE, Bardo M. Individual differences in novelty seeking on the playground maze predict amphetamine conditioned place preference. Pharmacol Biochem Behav. 1999; 63: 131-136.

[230] Kabbaj M. The search for the neurobiological basis of vulnerability to drug abuse: using microarrays to investigate the rôle of stress and individual differences. Neuropharmacology. 2004; 47: 111-122.

[231] Beckmann JS, Marusich JA, Gipson CD, Bardo MT. Novelty seeking, incentive salience and acquisition of cocaine self-administration in the rat. Behav Brain Res. 2010

[232] Dellu F, Piazza PV, Mayo W, Le Moal M, Simon H. Novelty-seeking in rats--biobehavioral characteristics and possible relationship with the sensation-seeking trait in man. Neuropsychobiology. 1996; 34: 136-145.

[233] Zuckerman M, Eysenck S, Eysenck HJ. Sensation seeking in England and America: cross-cultural, age, and sex comparisons. J Consult Clin Psychol. 1978; 46: 139-149.

[234] Cloninger CR. A unified biosocial theory of personality and its rôle in the development of anxiety states: a reply to commentaries. Psychiatr Dev. 1988; 6: 83-120.

[235] Arnett J. Sensation seeking: a new conceptualization and a new scale. Personality and Individual Differences. 1994; 16: 289-296.

[236] Wohlwill JF. What are sensation seekers seeking. Behavioral and Brain Sciences. 1984; 7: 453.

[237] Beck LH, Bransome ED, Mirsky AF, Rosvold HE, Sarason I. A continuous performance test of brain damage. J Consult Psychol. 1956; 20: 343-350.

[238] Robbins TW. The 5-choice serial reaction time task: behavioural pharmacology and functional neurochemistry. Psychopharmacology. 2002; 163[3-4]:362-380.

[239] Bari A, Dalley J, Robbins TW. The application of the 5-choice serial reaction time task for the assessment of visual attentional processes and impulse control in rats. Nature Protocol. 2008; 3[5]:759-767.

[240] Dalley J, Cardinal R, Robbins TW. Prefrontal executive and cognitive functions in rodents: neural and neurochemical substrates. Neuroscience & Biobehavioral Reviews. 2004; 28: 771-784.

[241] Dalley J, Mar A, Economidou D, Robbins TW. Neurobehavioral mechanisms of impulsivity: Fronto-striatal systems and functional neurochemistry. Pharmacology Biochemistry and Behavior. 2008; 90: 250-260.

[242] Dalley JW, Fryer TD, Brichard L, Robinson ES, Theobald DE, Lääne K, Peña Y, Murphy ER, Shah Y, Probst K, Abakumova I, Aigbirhio FI, Richards HK, Hong Y, Baron JC, Everitt BJ, Robbins TW. Nucleus Accumbens D2/3 Receptors Predict Trait Impulsivity and Cocaine Reinforcement. Science. 2007; 315: 1267-1270.

[243] Diergaarde L, Pattij T, Poortvliet I, Hogenboom F, de Vries W, Schoffelmeer AN, De Vries TJ. Impulsive Choice and Impulsive Action Predict Vulnerability to Distinct Stages of Nicotine Seeking in Rats. Biological Psychiatry. 2008; 63: 301-308.

[244] Diergaarde L, Pattij T, Nawijn L, Schoffelmeer ANM, De Vries TJ. Trait impulsivity predicts escalation of sucrose seeking and hypersensitivity to sucrose-associated stimuli. Behavioral Neuroscience. 2009; 123: 794-803.

[245] Jentsch JD, Taylor JR. Impulsivity resulting from frontostriatal dysfunction in drug abuse: implications for the control of behavior by reward-related stimuli. Psychopharmacology. 1999; 146: 373-390.

[246] Molander AC, Mar A, Norbury A, Steventon S, Moreno M, Caprioli D, Theobald DE, Belin D, Everitt BJ, Robbins TW, Dalley JW. High impulsivity predicting vulnerability to cocaine addiction in rats: some relationship with novelty preference but not novelty reactivity, anxiety or stress. Psychopharmacology [Berl]. 2011; 215: 721-731.

[247] Evenden J, Meyerson B. The behavior of spontaneously hypertensive and Wistar Kyoto rats under a paced fixed consecutive number schedule of reinforcement. Pharmacol Biochem Behav. 1999; 63: 71-82.

Section 2

Pathophysiology of Addictions

3

Addictive Drugs and Synaptic Plasticity

José Vicente Negrete-Díaz[1], Gonzalo Flores[1],
Talvinder S. Sihra[2] and Antonio Rodríguez-Moreno[3]
[1]*Universidad Autonoma de Puebla, Puebla,*
[2]*University College London, London,*
[3]*Universidad Pablo de Olavide, Sevilla,*
[1]*México*
[2]*UK*
[3]*Spain*

1. Introduction

The term addiction, derived from a Latin word meaning "bound to" or "enslaved by," was initially not linked to substance use. However, over the past several hundred years, addiction became associated with excessive alcohol and then drug use, such that by the late 1980s it was largely synonymous with compulsive drug use (O'Brien et al., 2006). The core features of addiction are manifest in the continued performance of the behavior despite adverse consequences, compulsive engagement or diminished control over the behavior, and an appetitive urge or craving state prior to the behavioral engagement representing core elements (Holden, 2010).

Addiction is a state of compulsive drug use; despite treatment and other attempts to control drug taking, addiction tends to persist. Hyman (2005) has summarized several studies where the authors have suggested that if the neurobiology is ultimately to contribute to the development of successful treatments for drug addiction, researchers must elucidate the molecular mechanisms by which drug-seeking behaviors are consolidated into compulsive use. Evidence at different levels of analysis suggest that addiction represents a pathological state of the neural mechanisms of learning and memory that, under normal circumstances, serve to shape survival behaviors related to the pursuit of rewards and the cues that predict them (Shultz et el., 1997; Montague et al., 2004; see Badiani et al., 2011 for review). The major substrates of persistent compulsive drug use are hypothesized to be molecular and cellular mechanisms that underlie long-term associative memories in several forebrain circuits (involving the ventral and dorsal striatum and prefrontal cortex) which receive inputs from midbrain dopamine neurons (see Hyman et al., 2006, for review). Also, the basolateral amygdala and nucleus accumbens core are key structures within limbic cortical-striatal circuitry where reconsolidation of a cue-drug memory occurs (Théberge et al., 2010). Vulnerability to stimulant addiction may depend on an impulsivity endophenotype. Impulsivity is the tendency to act prematurely without foresight, and is commonly associated with addiction to drugs, though its causal role in human addiction is unclear. Different groups (Dalley et al., 2007; Bezze et al., 2007 and Dalley et al., 2011) have characterized, in neurobehavioral and neurochemical terms, a rodent model of impulsivity based on premature responses in an attentional task. Evidence suggests that high impulsivity on this task precedes the subsequent escalation of cocaine self-administration behavior (Dalley et al., 2007, and also a tendency towards compulsive cocaine-seeking (Belin et al., 2008) and to relapse (Economidou et al., 2009). On the other hand, excessive consumption of palatable food can trigger neuroadaptive responses in brain reward circuitries similar to those produced by drugs of abuse. Thus, congruent genetic vulnerabilities in brain reward systems can increase predisposition to drug addiction and obesity. Kenny (2011) has recently advanced our understanding of the brain circuitries that regulate hedonic aspects of feeding behavior, with evidence suggesting that obesity and drug addiction may share common mechanisms.

Individuals take addictive drugs to elevate mood, but after repeated use these drugs produce serious unwanted effects, which include: tolerance to some drug effects, sensitization to others, and an adapted state-dependence, these setting the stage for withdrawal symptoms when drug use stops. The most serious consequence of repetitive drug taking is however addiction: a persistent state in which compulsive drug use escapes control, even when serious negative consequences ensue. Addiction is characterized by a long-lasting risk of relapse, which is often initiated by exposure to drug-related cues. Substantial progress has been made in understanding the molecular and cellular mechanisms of tolerance, dependence and withdrawal but, as yet, we understand little of the neural substrates of compulsive drug use and its remarkable persistence. Evidence exists for the possibility that compulsion and its persistence are based on a pathological usurpation of molecular mechanisms that are normally involved in memory (see Hyman and Malenka 2001 for review).

Genetic studies to date have been most successful at identifying factors that influence the transition from regular use to dependence. Numerous and large twin studies have indicated a significant genetic contribution to the process of conversion from eventual use to established use before development of dependence. The availability of large cohort samples for nicotine and alcohol dependence has resulted in significant progress being made in understanding at least some of the genetic contributions to these addictions (Tsuang et al., 1998, Kendler et al., 2003). Fewer studies have replicated specific genetic contributions to illicit drug use. Substance dependence can be thought of as a pharmacogenetic illness and, most likely, hundreds and more probably thousands of genetic variants will be required to fully explain the genetic input to this disease (see Bierut, 211 for review).

1.1 Neurobiology of addiction

Addictive drugs have in common the property that they are voluntarily self-administered by laboratory animals (usually avidly) (Di Chiara et al., 2004), and that they enhance the functioning of the reward circuitry of the brain (producing the 'high' that the drug user seeks). The core reward circuitry consists of an 'in-series' circuit linking the ventral tegmental area (VTA), nucleus accumbens (NAc) and ventral pallidum via the medial forebrain bundle. All addictive drugs have in common that they enhance (directly or indirectly or even transsynaptically) dopaminergic synaptic function in the NAc (Di Chiara et al., 2004), which is implicated in the reward process. Drug self-administration is regulated by NAc dopamine (DA) levels, which are retained within a specific elevated range (to maintain a desired hedonic level). The three classical sets of craving and relapse triggers are (a) reexposure to addictive drugs, (b) stress, and (c) reexposure to environmental cues (people, places, things) previously associated with drug-taking behavior. Knowledge of the neuroanatomy, neurophysiology, neurochemistry and neuropharmacology of addictive drug action in the brain is currently producing a variety of strategies for pharmacotherapeutic treatment of drug addiction, some of which appear promising (Gardner, 2011). Addictive drugs target the mesocorticolimbic dopamine (DA) system. This system originates in the VTA and projects mainly to the NAc and prefrontal cortex (PFC), affecting glutamatergic and GABAergic synaptic transmission in all three brain areas. These changes are refered to as drug-evoked synaptic plasticity, which outlasts the presence of the drug in the brain and contributes to the reorganization of neural circuits. While in most cases these early changes are not sufficient to induce the disease, with repetitive drug exposure, they may add up and contribute to addictive behavior (see Lüscher and Malenka, 2011 for review).

1.2 Learning and memory in addictive behavior

Two forms of cellular and synaptic plasticity, long-term potentiation (LTP) and long-term depression (LTD) remain the most extensively studied. They are considered the cellular and molecular basis of learning and memory (Kandel, 2004; Negrete-Díaz et al., 2007; Adermark et al., 2009; Abusch and Akirav, 2010; Collingridge et al., 2010; Huang et al., 2011, Figure 1).

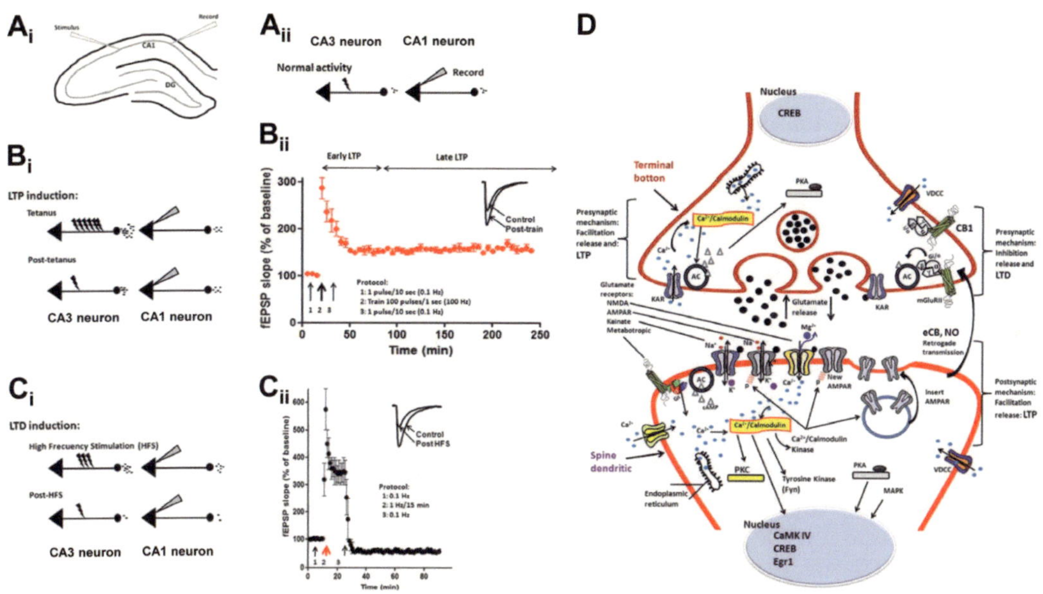

Fig. 1. LTP and LTD. Induction protocols and cellular mechanisms. A_i transverse hippocampal slice and estándar positioning of stimulating and recording electrodes. Hippocampus is the structure in which plasticity mechanisms have been more extensively estudied. A_{ii}, representation of presynaptic and postsynaptic neurons at synapse between CA3 and CA1 pyramidal cells. B_i, LTP protocol, tetanic (100 Hz, 1s) stimulation of presynaptic neurons induce and increase of the amplitude of excitatory postsynaptic potencial EPSP (B_{ii}) recorded from postsynaptic neurons. C_i, LTD protocol, stimulation at 1 Hz during 15 minutes induce a decrease of the amplitude of the EPSP (C_{ii}) recorded from postsynaptic neurons. D, schematic description of intracellular mechanisms involved in LTP and LTD

In addition, they can be used to demonstrate the repertoire of enduring modifications of individual synapses, circuits or neural networks. A classic triad arrangement of DA terminal varicosities, dendritic spines, and cortical inputs allows dopamine to enhance spike-time-dependent plasticity (STDP) at active cortico-striatal and cortico-cortical synapses. The induced LTP and LTD are candidate mechanisms for phasic DA signal to mediate behavioral learning. Thus, by affecting striatal and cortical plasticity, addictive drugs could lead to long-lasting changes of the motor, reward, and cognitive functions of these structures, striatum and PFC (Schultz, 2011). Conditioned stimuli (CSs) by Pavlovian association with reinforcing drugs (unconditioned stimuli; US) are thought to play an important role in the acquisition, maintenance and relapse of drug dependence. Bassareo et al. (2007) using microdialysis investigated the impact of pavlovian drug CSs on behaviour and on basal and drug-stimulated transmitter levels in three terminal DA areas: NAc shell and core, and the PFC. Drug CSs elicited incentive reactions and released DA; pre-exposure to CSs potentiated DA release to drug (Schultz, 2011). Théberge et al. (2010) demonstrated that the basolateral amygdala (BLA) and the NAc core are two structures importantly involved in the reconsolidation of a cocaine–CS memory. They show that, depending on the psychological processes involved, different neural substrates within limbic cortical-ventral striatal circuitry are required for the reconsolidation of a Pavlovian memory. Milton and Everitt, 2010, have shown with more detail the memory reconsolidation mechanisms underlying conditioned reinforcement and its relationship to drug addiction and the subsequent translation to the clinic of preclinical works.

1.3 Dopamine in addiction

DA's contribution appears to chiefly cause 'wanting' for hedonic rewards, more than 'liking' of or learning of those rewards (Schultz, 2011). However, the debate continues over the precise causal contribution made by mesolimbic DA systems to reward. Recent evidence indicates that DA is neither necessary nor sufficient to mediate changes in hedonic 'liking' for sensory pleasures. Other recent evidence indicates that DA is not needed for new learning, and not sufficient to directly mediate learning by causing teaching or prediction signals. Drugs of abuse promote DA signals, short circuit and sensitize dynamic mesolimbic mechanisms that evolved to attribute incentive salience to rewards (Berridge, 2007). The potential use of drugs to enhance cognition, emotion, and executive function has engendered controversy despite the fact that few such agents exist today. Hyman (2011) provided a context for discussions based on medical, regulatory, and ethical concerns that have been raised by the possibility that enhancers will emerge from current efforts to discover drugs for neuropsychiatric disorders. Addiction coopts the brain's neuronal circuits necessary for insight, reward, motivation, and social behaviors. This functional overlap results in addicted individuals making poor choices despite awareness of the negative consequences (Volkow et al., 2011). This explains why previously rewarding life situations and the threat of judicial punishment cannot stop drug taking and why a medical rather than a retributional approach is more effective in curtailing addiction.

We describe in this chapter the effects of cannabinoids, cocaine and amphetamines on the nervous system with particular emphasis on the effects of these compounds in plasticity processes. As the DA transporter is central to the effects of these drugs, we dedicate some special attention to the physiology of this type of transporter.

2. Cannabinoids (Table 1)

The use of marijuana for recreational and medicinal purposes has resulted in a large prevalence of chronic marijuana users (WHO, 2012). In the present decade, cannabis abuse has grown more rapidly than cocaine and opiate abuse. About 147 million people, 2.5% of the world population, consume cannabis (annual prevalence) compared with 0.2% consuming cocaine and 0.6% consuming amphetamine (WHO, 2012). The most rapid growth in cannabis abuse since the 1960s has been in developed countries in North America, Western Europe and Australia (WHO, 2012). Consequences of chronic cannabinoid administration include profound behavioral tolerance and withdrawal symptoms upon drug cessation. A marijuana withdrawal syndrome is only recently gaining acceptance as being clinically significant. Similarly, laboratory animals exhibit both tolerance and dependence following chronic administration of cannabinoids. These animal models are being used to evaluate the high degree of plasticity that occurs at the molecular level in various brain regions following chronic cannabinoid exposure (Lichtman and Martin, 2005).

2.1 The endocannabinoid (eCB) signaling system

The isolation and identification, in 1964 (Gaoni and Mechoulam, 1964), of delta-9-tetrahydrocannabinol (Δ9-THC), the primary psychoactive compound in cannabis, opened the door to a whole new field of medical research. The exploration of the therapeutic potential of THC and other natural and synthetic cannabinoid compounds was paralleled by the discovery of the endocannabinoid system, comprising cannabinoid receptors and their endogenous ligands, which offered exciting new insights into brain function (see Isbell et al., 1967 for review). Besides its well-known involvement in specific brain functions, such as control of movement (Di Marzo et al., 2000; Keeney et al., 2008; Fuss and Gass, 2010), memory (Deadwyler et al., 2007; Deadwyler and Hampson, 2008) and emotions (Paule et al., 2005; Tan et al., 2010), the endocannabinoid system plays an important role in fundamental developmental processes such as cell proliferation, migration and differentiation (Trezza et al., 2008, 2012). For this reason, changes in its activity during stages of high neuronal plasticity, such as the perinatal and the adolescent period, can have long-lasting neurobehavioral consequences (see Trezza et al., 2008 for review). Two subtypes of cannabinoid receptors (CBRs) have been identified to date, the CB1 receptor, essentially located in the CNS, but also in peripheral tissues, and the CB2 receptor, found only at the periphery. Many of the effects of cannabinoids, such as delta (9)-THC (Δ9-THC), the psychoactive principle of *cannabis sativa*, and endocannabinoids (eCBs) are mediated by these two metabotropic receptors, although additional receptors may be implicated. Both CB1 and CB2 are G-protein-coupled receptors (GPCRs), primarily operating through inhibitory G proteins, and are subject to the same pharmacological influences of other GPCRs (Chaperon and Thiébot, 1999; Basavarajappa et al., 2009). Freund et al. (2003) described a fine-grain anatomical distribution of the neuronal cannabinoid receptor CB1 in brain areas, emphasizing its general presynaptic localization and role in controlling neurotransmitter release, synaptic plasticity and network activity patterns. The eCBs as ligands for these CB1 and CB2 receptors are a family of lipidic mediators that signal through the same cell surface receptors that are targeted by Δ9-THC. Unlike neurotransmitter molecules that are typically held in vesicles before synaptic release, eCBs are liberated directly after synthesis and, once released, travel in a retrograde direction to suppress presynaptic neurotransmitter release through activation of CBRs (Basavarajappa, 2007).

Drug	Effect on brain plasticity and behaviour	Structures	Autor
Marijuana or CBR1 pharmacological manipulation	Presence of an 'amotivational' syndrome	Limbic system	Paule, 2005
	Regulation of ion channels, neurotransmitter release and synaptic plasticity	Multiples brain regions	Fisar, 2009
	Profound behavioral tolerance and withdrawal symptoms	Limbic system	Lichtman & Martin, 2005
	Activity of central reward pathways alterated	VTA	Lupica et al., 2004
	↑ Risk of developing psychotic disorders in adolescence Disturbs in glutamate and GABA release	PFC	Bossong & Niesink, 2010
	↑ Density of cannabinoid CB1R binding	Corticolimbic regions	Fernandez-Espejo et al., 2009
	↓ Hippocampal encoding and the ability to encode information into short-term memory	Hippocampus	Deadwyler et al., 2007; Deadwyler and Hampson, 2008.
	Impaired LTP Facilitated LTD	Schaffer collateral-CA1 projection	Abush & Akirav, 2010
	LTD blocked with CB1R antagonist	Glutamatergic and GABAergic synapses in the striatum	Adermark et al., 2009
	Impaired LTP Decrease in LTP prevented by pharmacological inhibition or deletion of the CB1R	Hippocampus	Fan et al., 2010
	Metaplastic effects on brain cortex	Motor cortex	Koch et al., 2009
	↑Response of mPFC neurons Modulate emotional memory formation	mPFC, BLA	Laviolette & Grace, 2006
	↓ Gray matter	Cerebral cortex	Stone et al., 2011
	Blocked LTP and acquisition of conditioned fear memories by CB1R antagonist	BLA-PLC pathway	Tan et al., 2010
	Changes in cell proliferation, migration and differentiation	Central nervous system, eCB system	Trezza et al., 2008

Table 1. Plastic changes on brain regions by chronic use of marijuana, Δ9-THC administration or CB1R pharmacological manipulation.

(Abbreviations: BLA: basolateral amygdale; CB1R: type 1 cannabinoid receptor; eCB: endocannabinoid; GABA: gamma aminobutyric acid; LTP: long-term potentiation; LTD: long-term depression; mPFC: medial prefrontal cortex; PLC: prelimbic cortex; PFC: prefrontal cortex).

Recent results have suggested that the eCB system may play an important role in early neuronal development having been detected from the earliest stages of embryogenesis and throughout pre- and postnatal development. Additionally, the eCB signaling system is being found to be involved in an increasing number of neuropathological conditions, with widespread roles being invoked in neurodegenerative disorders. The fact that eCB signaling is mostly inhibitory, imparts eCBs with the ability to modulate synaptic efficacy with a wide range of functional consequences and provides unique therapeutic possibilities in central nervous system (CNS) diseases, including alcoholism, Alzheimer's disease, Parkinson's disease, Huntington's disease, and multiple sclerosis (see Basavarajappa, 2007; Basavarajappa et al., 2009 for reviews).

Although CB1 receptors are distributed throughout the brain, they are found at very high levels in the cerebellum. Edwards and Skosnik (2007) have integrated two separate literatures. The first literature demonstrates that the eCB system mediates synaptic plasticity, specifically LTD of parallel fibers at the parallel fiber-Purkinje junction in the cerebellar cortex. The second literature suggests that LTD at this junction is necessary for the acquisition of the primary dependent variable in delay eyeblink conditioning. Also, they discuss recent evidence from CB1 knockout mice, human cannabis users, and schizophrenia patients, with the expectation that translational research on the cannabinoid system will be advanced. Wiskerke et al. (2008) summarize studies in which have been used CB1R knockout mice as well as CB1 antagonists to elucidate the role of this neurotransmitter system in psychostimulant addiction. CB1 receptors appear not to be involved in psychostimulant reward, nor in the development of dependence to such substances. In contrast, the eCB system appears to play a role in the persistence of psychostimulant addiction (see Wiskerke et al., 2008 for review). Interactions of the eCB system with afferent glutamatergic and possibly dopaminergic projections to the nucleus accumbens are most likely involved and CB1 receptors seem to modulate drug-related memories, in line with the hypothesized role of the eCB system in memory-related plasticity. Together, these findings suggest that modulators of the eCB system represent a promising novel type of therapy to treat drug addiction.

2.2 The reward system

The reward circuitry of the brain consists of neurons that synaptically connect a wide variety of nuclei. Of these brain regions, the VTA and the NAc play key roles in the processing of rewarding environmental stimuli and in drug addiction. The psychoactive properties of marijuana are produced by Δ9-THC, interacting primarily with CB1 receptors in a large number of brain areas. However, it is the activation of CB1 receptors located in reward circuits that is thought to be instrumental in sustaining the self-administration of marijuana in humans, and in mediating the anxiolytic and pleasurable effects of the drug. It has been suggested that, whereas Δ9-THC alters the activity of central reward pathways in a manner that is consistent with other abused drugs, the cellular mechanism through which this occurs is likely different, relying upon the combined regulation of several afferent pathways to the VTA (see Lupica et al., 2004 for review).

2.3 Cannabis, cannabinoids and neuronal plasticity

Changes in synaptic efficacy are thought to be crucial to experience-dependent modifications of neural function. eCB-mediated plasticity encompasses many forms of transient and long-lasting synaptic depression and is found at both excitatory and inhibitory synapses. Thus, the eCB system is emerging as a major player in synaptic plasticity and, given the wide distribution of CB1 receptors in the CNS, the list of brain structures and synapses expressing eCB-mediated plasticity is likely to expand (see Chevaleyre et al., 2006 for review). Glutamate is the principal excitatory neurotransmitter in CNS and altered glutamatergic transmission during critical periods (such as first postnatal weeks) may disturb circuitry in specific brain areas (including cortex and hippocampus), particularly in experience-dependent maturation. Recent hypotheses regarding disturbances in strengthening and pruning of synaptic connections in the PFC, and the link with latent psychotic disorders suggest that cannabis-induced schizophrenia is due to a distortion of normal late postnatal brain maturation (see Bossong and Niesink, 2010 for review). In this respect, cannabis use during adolescence increases the risk of developing psychotic disorders later in life. In animals, Bossong and Niesink (2010) postulated that adolescent exposure to Δ9-THC transiently disturbs physiological control of the eCB system over glutamate and GABA release. As a result, Δ9-THC may adversely affect adolescent experience-dependent maturation of neural circuitries within prefrontal cortical areas. Depending on dose, exact time window and duration of exposure, this may ultimately lead to the development of psychoses like schizophrenia.

There is substantial evidence that cannabis abuse is a risk factor for psychosis in genetically predisposed people, may lead to a worse outcome of the disease, or it can affect normal brain development during adolescence, increasing the risk for schizophrenia in adulthood. On the other hand, the eCB system is altered in schizophrenia (increased density of CB1 receptors binding in corticolimbic regions). Dysregulation of this system can interact with neurotransmitter systems in such a way that a "cannabinoid hypothesis" can be integrated in the neurobiological hypotheses of schizophrenia. Also, there is evidence that some genetic alterations of the CNR1 gene can act as a protectant factor against schizophrenia or can induce a better pharmacological response to atypical antipsychotics (see Fernandez-Espejo et al., 2009 for review). Awareness of cannabis dependence as a clinically relevant issue has grown in recent years. Clinical and laboratory studies demonstrate that chronic marijuana smokers can experience withdrawal symptoms upon cessation of marijuana smoking and have difficulty abstaining from marijuana use. The behavioral effects that directly contribute to the maintenance of chronic marijuana smoking are reward, subjective effects, and the positive and negative reinforcing effects of marijuana, Δ9-THC or synthetic cannabinoids (Cooper and Haney, 2008).

Studies using population codes derived from ensembles of hippocampal neurons have been assessed to determine whether eCBs were active when rats performed a short-term memory task in presence or absence of CB1 receptor antagonists or agonists. Results show that eCBs, like marijuana, reduced hippocampal encoding necessary to perform long-delay trials (Deadwyler et al., 2007). Also, CB1 receptor antagonism blocked an inherent hippocampal memory encoding bias used by all animals. These findings suggest a direct relationship between the actions of cannabinoids on hippocampal processes and the ability to encode information into short-term memory Deadwyler and Hampson, 2008. Considerable evidence demonstrates that cannabinoid receptor agonists impair, whereas cannabinoid receptor antagonists improve, memory and plasticity (Ademark et al., 2009; Fan et al., 2010). However, recent studies suggest that the effects of cannabinoids on learning do not necessarily follow these simple patterns, particularly when emotional memory processes are involved. Abush and Akirav (2010) have investigated the involvement of the CB system in hippocampal learning and plasticity using behavioral task and cellular models of learning and memory (LTP and LTD). They found that i.p. agonist administration impaired LTP in the Schaffer collateral-CA1 projection, whereas an inhibitor of eCB reuptake facilitated LTD. These findings suggest that the diverse effects of the cannabinoid system on CA1 memory and plasticity cannot be categorized simply into an impairing or an enhancing effect of cannabinoid activation and deactivation, respectively. Previous studies have indicated that eCB mobilization at excitatory synapses might be regulated by afferent activation. LTD at striatal synapses is mediated by postsynaptic eCB release and presynaptic CB1 receptor activation. Adermark et al. (2009) have examined changes in synaptic strength induced by activation of L-type calcium channels at glutamatergic and gamma-aminobutyric acid (GABA)ergic synapses in the striatum. They found that the basic mechanisms for eCB signaling are the same at glutamatergic and GABAergic synapses. LTD was blocked in slices treated with AM251, a CB1 receptor antagonist, but established depression was not reversed at either glutamatergic and GABAergic synapses. It is suggested that the level of neuronal firing regulates eCB signaling by modulating release from the postsynaptic cell, as well as interacting with presynaptic mechanisms to induce LTD at both glutamatergic and GABAergic synapses in the striatum.

Chronic use of marijuana impairs synaptic plasticity and cognitive function. Fan et al. (2010) found that repeated *in vivo* exposures to Δ9-THC for 7 consecutive days significantly impaired hippocampal LTP of excitatory glutamatergic synaptic transmission, and this decrease in LTP was prevented by pharmacological inhibition or deletion of the CB1 receptor. They showed that reduced expression and function of the GluR subunits and phosphorylation of cAMP response element-binding (CREB) may underlie the impaired long-term synaptic plasticity induced by repeated *in vivo* exposure to Δ9-THC. In animal models, the CB system has been convincingly implicated in the regulation of long-lasting synaptic plasticity. Both LTP and LTD can be induced in the human motor cortex by transcranial magnetic theta burst stimulation (TBS). Koch et al. (2009) explored the potential involvement of the CB system in TBS-induced synaptic plasticity in humans with multiple sclerosis. Continuous TBS induced the expected inhibition of motor-evoked potentials (MEPs) before cannabis-based preparation exposure (Sativex), whereas it caused a persisting enhancement of MEP amplitude 4 weeks after. The LTP-like phenomenon induced by intermittent TBS was conversely unaffected by preparation exposure. These results indicate that cannabis ingredients have metaplastic effects on the motor cortex. Laviolette and Grace (2006), using *in vivo* single-unit recordings in rats, found that a CB1 receptor agonist potentiated the response of medial prefrontal cortical (mPFC) neurons to olfactory cues paired previously with a footshock, whereas this associative responding was prevented by a CB1 receptor antagonist, providing the first demonstration that CB signaling in the mPFC can modulate the magnitude of neuronal emotional learning plasticity and memory formation through functional inputs from the basolateral amygdala (BLA, Laviolette and Grace, 2006).

Individuals with an "at risk mental state" (ARMS) are greatly more susceptible to developing a psychotic illness. There has been considerable interest in the interaction between psychosis risk and substance use. Cannabis at low to moderate intake may be associated with lower gray matter in both ARMS subjects and healthy volunteers, possibly representing low-level cortical damage or change in neural plasticity (Stone et al., 2011). The CB1 receptor system is functionally involved in the processing and encoding of emotionally salient sensory information, learning and memory. The CB1 receptor is found in high concentrations in brain structures that are critical for emotional processing, including the BLA and the mPFC. Synaptic plasticity in the form of LTP within the BLA-mPFC pathway is an established correlate of exposure to emotionally salient events (Laviolette and Grace, 2006). *In vivo* LTP studies showed that systemic pretreatment with AM-251, dose-dependently block LTP along the BLA-PLC pathway, and also the behavioral acquisition of conditioned fear memories (Tan et al., 2010). Experiments show that when CB1 receptor transmission within the BLA-PFC circuit was pharmacologically blocked, this prevented the acquisition of emotionally salient associative memory. These results indicate that coordinated CB1 receptor transmission within the BLA-PFC pathway is critically involved in the encoding of emotional fear memories and modulates neural plasticity related to the encoding of emotionally salient associative learning (Tan et al., 2010).

3. Cocaine (Table 2)

Behavioral sensitization is the augmented motor-stimulant response that occurs with repeated, intermittent exposure to most drugs of abuse, including cocaine. Sensitization, which is a long-lasting phenomenon, is thought to underlie drug craving and relapse to drug use (Steketee et al., 2003). The neural mechanisms of sensitization have focused on the NAc and VTA that comprise a part of the mesolimbic DA system. Cocaine sensitization results from a decrease in inhibitory modulation of excitatory transmission from the mPFC

Drug	Effect on brain plasticity and behaviour	Structures	Autor
Cocaine	Induced behavioural sensitization	mPFC, NAc, VTA	Steketee, 2003; 2005
	Induced conditioned place preference	mPFC, NAc shell, VTA	McBride et al., 1999
	↑ BDNF, ↓ mGluR5, LTD impared	NAc shell	Huang et al., 2011
	↑ DA transmission and induce CTA	NAc shell	Di Chiara et al., 2004
	Behavioral deficits at birth and/or during adulthood	Limbic system	Lidow, 2003
	Behavioral rigidity or lack of plasticity	PFC, limbic system	Paule, 2005
	Changes in Fos expression	Lateral hipotalamus	Aston-Jones et al., 2009
	Shift from impulsivity to compulsivity during the development of addictive behavior	PFC, ventral and dorsal striatum	Belin et al., 2008
	Increased MeCP2 expression and microRNA	Dorsal striatum	Welberg, 2010

Table 2. Plastic changes on brain regions by chronic use of cocaine.
(Abbreviations: BDNF: brain-derived neurotrophic factor; CTA: conditioned taste avoidance; DA: dopamine; LTD: long-term depression; MeCP2: methyl CpG binding protein 2; mGluR5: type 5 metabotropic glutamate receptor; mPFC: medial prefrontal cortex; NAc: nucleus accumbens; VTA: ventral tegmental area).

to the VTA and NAc. Repeated cocaine exposure alters DA, gamma-aminobutyric acid (GABA), and glutamate regulation of pyramidal cell activity (Di Chiara et al., 2004; Huang et al., 2011), with cocaine-induced alterations in cortical transmission occuring in two phases. During early withdrawal from repeated cocaine exposure, changes in neurotransmitter release are thought to underlie the decreased inhibitory modulation of pyramidal projection neurons. Following more prolonged withdrawal, the attenuation in inhibitory transmission appears to occur at the receptor level (Steketee, 2005).

3.1 Cocaine and dopaminergic system

Neuroadaptation in the NAc, a central component of the mesolimbic DA system, has been implicated in the development of cocaine-induced psychomotor sensitization and relapse to cocaine seeking (Zhang et al., 2001; Anderson et al., 2003; see Steketee, 2005 for review). Recent results suggest that withdrawal from repeated cocaine exposure may result in increased brain-derived neurotrophic factor (BDNF) levels in the NAc shell, which leads to a selective downregulation of mGluR5 and thereby impairs the induction of mGluR-dependent LTD (Huang et al., 2011). The effects of BDNF on cocaine-seeking are brain region-specific. Infusion of BDNF into subcortical structures, like the NAc and VTA, enhances cocaine-induced behavioral sensitization and cocaine-seeking. Conversely, repeated administration of BDNF antiserum into the NAc during chronic cocaine self-administration attenuates cocaine-induced reinstatement. Three weeks after BDNF antiserum infusion in animals with a cocaine self-administration history, suppressed basal levels of glutamate are normalized, and a cocaine prime-induced increase in extracellular glutamate levels in the NAc is prevented (McGinty et al., 2010). Although the development of behavioral sensitization to psychostimulants such as cocaine and amphetamine is confined mainly to one nucleus in the brain, the VTA, this process is nonetheless complex, involving an interplay between neurotransmitters, neuropeptides and trophic factors. Calcium-stimulated signalling molecules, including the calcium/calmodulin-dependent protein kinases, and the Ras/mitogen-activated protein kinases, represent the major biochemical pathways whereby converging extracellular signals are integrated and amplified, resulting in the biochemical and molecular changes in DA neurons in the VTA that represent the critical neuronal correlates of the development of behavioral sensitization to psychostimulants (see Licata and Pierce, 2003 for review).

Using a mouse model of behavioral sensitization, Huang et al. (2011) showed that animals withdrawn from repeated cocaine exposure have a selective deficit in the ability to elicit metabotropic glutamate receptor (mGluR)-dependent LTD in the shell of the NAc in response to bath application of the group I mGluR agonist DHPG. Experiments demonstrated that the impaired DHPG-LTD is likely attributable to a loss of mGluR5 function. Quantitative real-time reverse transcriptase-PCR and Western blot analysis revealed significant downregulation of mGluR5, but not mGluR1, mRNA or protein levels in the NAc shell. The inhibitory effect of repeated cocaine exposure on DHPG-LTD was selectively prevented when cocaine was coadministered with a selective D1 receptor antagonist. Furthermore, the levels of BDNF protein in the NAc shell increased progressively after cocaine withdrawal, and crucially, the impairment of DHPG-LTD in the NAc shell was not found in slices from BDNF-knock-out mice after cocaine withdrawal. Recent evidence suggests that CB1Rs may represent effective targets for therapeutic agents used to treat cocaine relapse. Li et al. (2008) determinated whether CBRs play a similar role in relapse to ketamine abuse. To establish a ketamine reinstatement model in the conditioned place preference paradigm, rats were trained to develop place preference conditioned by ketamine, which was subsequently extinguished through daily exposure to the test chambers in the absence of ketamine. The effects of rimonabant, a CB1Rs antagonist, were investigated on reinstatement of ketamine-induced place preference. While ketamine priming injections reinstated extinguished place preference, rimonabant administration significantly attenuated the reinstatement of ketamine-induced place preference in a dose-dependent manner. Importantly, rimonabant itself did not produce conditioned place preference or place aversion. Since the reinstatement effects of ketamine administration were inhibited by rimonabant, these findings suggest that a CB1 receptor antagonist may be useful in preventing relapse to ketamine abuse. VTA DA neurons play a pivotal role in processing reward-related information and are involved in drug addiction and mental illness in humans (Wise, 2004). Information is conveyed to the VTA in the large part by glutamatergic afferents that arise in various brain nuclei, including the pedunculopontine nucleus (PPN).

In rat brain slice preparations, Good and Lupica (2010) found that PPN stimulation activates afferents targeting GluR2-containing AMPA receptors (AMPAR) on VTA DA neurons, and these afferents did not exhibit long-term depression (LTD). In contrast, activation of glutamate afferents onto the same DA neurons via stimulation within the VTA evoked both, excitatory postsynaptic currents EPSCs mediated by GluR2-lacking AMPARs which showed LTD, and EPSCs mediated by GluR2-containing AMPA receptors that did not express LTD. Single cocaine injections increase GluR2-lacking AMPA receptors at all glutamate synapses on VTA dopamine neurons (and this permitted LTD expression in both pathways), whereas Δ9-THC selectively increased GluR2-lacking AMPA receptors at subcortical PPN synapses (and permitted LTD in the PPN pathway only), suggesting that different drugs of abuse may exert influence over distinct sets of glutamatergic afferents to VTA DA neurons, which may thereby be associated with different reinforcing or addictive properties of these drugs. Microdialysis studies in animals have shown that addictive drugs preferentially increase extracellular DA levels in the NAc rather than in the core. However, by acting directly on the brain, drugs bypass the adaptive mechanisms (habituation) that constrain the responsiveness of accumbens shell DA to food reward, abnormally facilitating Pavlovian incentive learning and promoting the acquisition of abnormal DA-releasing properties by drug conditioned stimuli (See Di Chiara & Bassareo, 2007 for review). Thus, whereas Pavlovian food conditioned stimuli release core but not shell DA, drug conditioned stimuli do the opposite, releasing shell but not core DA. This process, which results in the acquisition of excessive incentive-motivational properties by drug conditioned stimuli has been suggested to contribute to the initiation of the drug addiction process (Imperato and Di Chiara, 1986; Di Chiara and Bassareo, 2007).

Brain imaging studies, while extending these finding to humans, have shown a correlation between psychostimulant-induced increase of extracellular DA in the striatum and self-reported measures of liking and euphoria (Volkow et al., 2002a; 2002b). Although a correlate of drug reward, independent from associative learning and performance is difficult to obtain in animals, conditioned taste avoidance (CTA) might meet these requirements. Addictive drugs induce CTA to saccharin most likely as a result of anticipatory contrast of saccharin over drug reward. Consistently with a role of DA in drug reward, D2 or combined D1/D2 receptor blockade abolishes cocaine, amphetamine and nicotine CTA. Intracranial self-administration studies with mixtures of D1 and D2 receptor agonists point to the NAc shell as the critical site of DA reward (Di Chiara et al., 2004; Bassareo et al., 2007). NAc shell DA acting on D1 receptors is also involved in Pavlovian learning through pre-trial and post-trial consolidation mechanisms and in the utilization of spatial short-term memory for goal-directed behaviour (Volkow et al., 2011). Stimulation of NAc shell DA transmission by addictive drugs is shared by a natural reward like food, but lacks its adaptive properties (habituation and inhibition by predictive stimuli). These peculiarities of drug-induced stimulation of DA transmission in the NAc shell result in striking differences in the impact of drug-conditioned stimuli on DA transmission. It is speculated that drug addiction results from the impact exerted on behavior by the abnormal DA stimulant properties acquired by drug-conditioned stimuli as a result of their association with addictive drugs (Di Chiara et al., 2004; Everitt & Robbins, 2005). Di Chiara and Bassareo (2007) have summarized that addictive drugs share with palatable food, the property of increasing extracellular DA, preferentially in the NAc shell rather than in the core. However, by acting directly on the brain, drugs bypass the adaptive mechanisms (habituation) that constrain the responsiveness of NAc shell DA to food reward, abnormally facilitating Pavlovian incentive learning and promoting the acquisition of abnormal DA-releasing properties by drug conditioned stimuli. Thus, whereas Pavlovian foods conditioned stimuli release core but not NAc shell DA, drug conditioned stimuli do the opposite, releasing shell but not NAc core DA. Neuroadaptive processes related to the chronic influence of drugs on subcortical DA might secondarily impair the function of prefronto-striatal loops, resulting in impairments in impulse control and decision making that form the basis for the compulsive feature of drug seeking and its relapsing character (Belin and Everitt, 2010).

3.2 Prenatal cocaine exposure

The extent to which cocaine abuse by pregnant women can affect development of their offspring remains a matter of significant debate. In large part, this is due to difficulties in accurate determination of the type, dose, and pattern of cocaine administration by drug abusing women as well as to difficulties in controlling for a wide range of potentially confounding variables, such as other drugs used, race, socioeconomic status, and level of prenatal care. Examination of the effects of prenatal cocaine exposure in highly controlled nonhuman primate models represents an important complement to the human research. Data obtained in several different rhesus monkey models of cocaine exposure *in utero*, has demonstrated the potential of prenatal cocaine exposure to interfere with structural and biochemical development of the brain leading to behavioral deficits at birth and/or during adulthood. The differences in the outcomes between individual models also suggest that the specific types and severity of cocaine effects are likely dependent on the route, dose, gestational period, and daily pattern of administration (see Lidow, 2003 for review). Nonhuman primates (rhesus monkeys, Macaca mulatta) have been used to study the effects of chronic drug exposures on brain function during different stages of development. In the case of the marijuana studies, exposures occurred during the adolescent period; for the cocaine studies, exposures occurred *in utero*. A battery of behavioral tasks, designed to assess aspects of motivation, visual discrimination, time perception, short-term memory, and learning, was used to monitor treatment effects. Chronic marijuana smoke exposure resulted in an 'amotivational' syndrome. *In utero* cocaine exposure was shown to cause behavioral rigidity or lack of plasticity as evidenced by the difficulty of subjects to adjust to rules changes for some tasks. These effects were seen in adult subjects suggesting that the effects of gestational cocaine exposure are long-term or permanent (see Paul, 2005 for review).

3.3 Orexins in drug-seeking

Orexins (also known as hypocretins) are recently discovered neuropeptides, synthetised exclusively in hypothalamic neurons, which have been shown to be important in narcolepsy/cataplexy and arousal (Zhou et al., 2008). Aston-Jones et al. (2009) conducted behavioral, anatomical and neurophysiological studies that show that a subset of these cells, located specifically in lateral hypothalamus (LH), are involved in reward processing and addictive behaviors. They found that Fos expression in LH orexin neurons varied in proportion to preference for cocaine or food. Recently, using a self-administration paradigm, it was discovered that the Ox1 orexin receptor antagonist, SB-334867 (SB), blocks cocaine-seeking induced by discrete or contextual cues, but not by a priming injection of cocaine. Neurophysiological studies revealed that locally applied orexin often augmented responses of VTA DA neurons to activation of the mPFC, consistent with the view that orexin facilitates activation of VTA DA neurons by stimulus-reward associations. These findings are consistent with results from others showing that orexins facilitate glutamate-mediated responses, and are necessary for glutamate-dependent long-term potentiation, in VTA DA neurons (Anston-Jones et al., 2010). Boutrel et al., (2005) show that intracerebroventricular infusions of hypocretin-1 lead to a dose-related reinstatement of cocaine seeking without altering cocaine intake in rats and elevates intracranial self-stimulation threshold. The effect was prevented by blockade of noradrenergic and corticotrophin releasing factor systems, suggesting that hypocretin-1 reinstated drug seeking through induction of a stress-like state.

3.4 Regulation of cocaine intake

Recent studies have started to reveal the contribution of epigenetic regulation to addiction-related behaviours and neuroadaptation. Two studies focused on the role of the X-linked transcriptional repressor methyl CpG-binding protein 2 (MeCP2), wich contributes to the development and function of CNS synapses. They showed that drugs of abuse regulate the expression and/or activity of MeCP2 and that this contributes to behavioural and neural responses to the drug. MeCP2, known for its role in the neurodevelopmental disorder Rett syndrome, is emerging as an important regulator of neuroplasticity in postmitotic neurons.

Cocaine addiction is commonly viewed as a disorder of neuroplasticity (White, 1996; Everitt et al., 1999; Di Chiara, 1999). Heh-In et al. (2010) identified a key role for MeCP2 in the dorsal striatum in the escalating cocaine intake seen in rats with extended access to the drug, a process that resembles in some rats subjected to extended daily access to the drug, the increasingly uncontrolled cocaine use seen in addicted humans (See Badiani et al., 2011 for review). MeCP2 regulates cocaine intake through homeostatic interactions with microRNA-212 (miR-212) to control the effects of cocaine on striatal BDNF levels. They suggest that homeostatic interactions between MeCP2 and miR-212 in dorsal striatum may be important in regulating vulnerability to cocaine addiction. Deng et al. (2010) have shown that acute viral manipulation of MeCP2 expression in the NAc bidirectionally modulates amphetamine (AMPH)-induced conditioned place preference. *Mecp2* hypomorphic mutant mice have more NAc GABAergic synapses and show deficient AMPH-induced structural plasticity of NAc dendritic spines. Furthermore, these mice show deficient plasticity of striatal immediate early gene inducibility after repeated AMPH administration. Notably, psychostimulants induce phosphorylation of MeCP2 at Ser421, a site that regulates MeCP2's function as a repressor. Phosphorylation is selectively induced in GABAergic interneurons of the NAc, and its extent strongly predicts the degree of behavioral sensitization. These data reveal new roles for MeCP2, both, in mesolimbocortical circuit development, and in the regulation of psychostimulant-induced behaviors. Also, Im et al (2010) reported increased MeCP2 expression and miR-212 (as well as miR-132) levels in the dorsal striatum in rats that had extended access to cocaine. Knocking down striatal MeCP2 expression using small hairpin RNA (shRNA) promoted the cocaine-induced increase in miR-212 expression. It also prevented the escalation of cocaine intake that normally occurs with prolonged cocaine access, an effect that could be blocked by disruption of miR-212 signalling using an antisense oligonucleotide. Furthermore, overexpressing miR-212 in the dorsal striatum, a neurobiological locus of control of habitual (Belin and Everitt 2008; Belin et al., 2009, 2010, Zapata et al., 2010, Murray et al., 2012) and compulsive (Jonkman et al., 2012) cocaine seeking, using a lentiviral vector reduced MeCP2 levels and decreased cocaine intake in rats with extended access to the drug (Im et al., 2010). These findings indicate that miR-212 and MeCP2 homeostatically regulate one another in the dorsal striatum and suggest that this interaction has a role in controlling compulsive cocaine intake. Taken together, these results suggest a role for MeCP2 in the behavioural response to psychostimulant drugs, although many questions remain regarding the undoubtedly complex mechanisms involved in its interactions with microRNAs and its modulation of synaptic plasticity (Welberg, 2010).

4. Amphetamine (Table 3)

4.1 Dopaminergic system

The fundamental principle that unites addictive drugs appears to be that each enhances synaptic DA by means that dissociate it from normal behavioral control, so that they act to reinforce their own acquisition. This occurs via the modulation of synaptic mechanisms that can be involved in learning, including enhanced excitation or disinhibition of DA neuron activity, blockade of DA reuptake, and altering the state of the presynaptic terminal to enhance evoked over basal transmission. Amphetamines offer an exception to such modulation in that they combine multiple effects to produce nonexocytotic, stimulation-independent release of neurotransmitter, via reverse-transport, independent from normal presynaptic function (Sulzer, 2011). In addition, behavioral sensitization is accompanied by an increase in postsynaptic DA receptors; an increase in DA synthesis; an increase in DA utilization and/or release (Kalivas and Stewart, 1991; Flores et al., 2011). There is strong evidence to support the notion that behavioral sensitization is due to enhanced mesotelencephalic DA release, especially upon re-exposure to the drug (Robinson and Becker, 1986). The mesocorticolimbic dopamine system, which arises in the VTA and innervates the NAc, among numerous other regions, has been implicated in processes associated with drug addiction, including behavioral sensitization. The mPFC, defined as the cortical region that has a reciprocal innervation with the mediodorsal nucleus of the thalamus, is also a terminal region of the mesocorticolimbic DA system. The mPFC contains pyramidal glutamatergic neurons that serve as the primary output of this region and mPFC transmitter systems are involved in the development of behavioral sensitization to cocaine and amphetamine (Steketee, 2003).

Drug	Effect on brain plasticity and behaviour	Structures	Autor
Amphetamine	Behavioural sensitization	VTA	Licata & Pierce, 2003; Robinson & Becker, 1986
	↑ DA transmission and induce CTA	NAc shell	Di Chiara et al., 2004
	Induced conditioned place preference Enhancement of hippocampal CaMKII activity Alterated structural plasticity of dendritic spines	Hippocampus, NAc	Tan, 2008; Deng et al., 2010
	↑ postsynaptic DAR ↑ DA synthesis ↑DA utilization and/or release Release of neurotransmitter via reverse transport	Mesotelencephalic system	Robinson & Becker, 1986
	Deficits in the passive avoidance and Y-maze tests LTP alterated Pleiotrophin expression regulated	Hippocampus Limbic system	del Olmo et al., 2009; Gramage et al., 2011
	↑ Learning of environmental stimuli ↑ mGluR-dependent facilitation ↑ Susceptible to LTP induction	VTA	Ahn et al., 2010
	↑ NMDA-dependent, AMPA-mediated LTP ↓ LTD	Dopamine neurons	Schultz, 2011
	↓ PFC thickness in control females ↑ Posterior striatum thickness in control males	PFC, Striatum	Muhammad et al., 2011a
	↑ Spine density in NAc and mPFC ↓ Spine density in the OFC	NAc, mPFC, OFC	Muhammad & Kolb, 2011b; 2011c
	Psychosis, similar to paranoid schizophrenia	Limbic system	Robinson & Becker, 1986
	↑ DAT at postpubertal age by prenatal exposure	NAc	Flores et al., 2011

Table 3. Plastic changes on brain regions by chronic use of amphetamine.

(Abbreviations: AMPA: α-amino-3-hydroxy-5-methyl-4-isoxazolepropionic acid; CaMKII: Ca2+/calmodulin-dependent protein kinase II CTA: conditioned taste avoidance; DA: dopamine; DAR: dopamine receptor eCB: endocannabinoid; LTP: long-term potentiation; LTD: long-term depression; mGluR: metabotropic glutamate receptor; mPFC: medial prefrontal cortex; NAc: nucleus accumbens; NMDA: N-Methyl-D-aspartic acid; OFC: orbital frontal cortex; PFC: prefrontal cortex; VTA: ventral tegmental area).

Intracranial self-administration (ICSA) and intracranial place conditioning (ICPC) methodologies have been mainly used to study drug reward mechanisms, but they have also been applied toward examining brain reward mechanisms (McBride et al., 1999; Di Chiara et al., 2004). ICSA studies in rodents have established that the VTA is a site supporting reinforcement. The NAc also appears to have a major role in brain reward mechanisms. Rodents will self-infuse a variety of drugs of abuse (amphetamine and cocaine) into the NAc, and this occurs primarily in the shell region. ICPC studies also indicate that injection of amphetamine into the shell portion of the NAc produces conditioned place preference (CPP). Activation of the DA system within the shell subregion of the NAc appears to play a key role in brain reward mechanisms. The PFC supports the ICSA of cocaine and phencyclidine. The DA system also seems to play a role in this behavior since cocaine self-infusion into the PFC can be blocked by co-infusing a D2 antagonist. Among other regions, ICPC findings suggest that cocaine and amphetamine are rewarding in the rostral ventral pallidum (VP). Finally, substance P-mediated systems within the caudal VP (nucleus basalis magnocellularis) and serotonin systems of the dorsal and median raphe nuclei may also be important anatomical components involved in brain reward mechanisms. Overall, the ICSA and ICPC studies indicate that there are a number discrete CNS sites involved in brain reward mechanisms (McBride et al., 1999).

4.2 Amphetamine alters learning, LTP and LTD

Recent studies suggest LTP expression in locally activated glutamate synapses onto DA neurons (local Glu-DA synapses) of the midbrain VTA following a single or chronic exposure to many drugs of abuse, whereas a single exposure to cannabinoid did not significantly affect synaptic plasticity at these synapses. It is unknown whether chronic exposure of cannabis (marijuana or cannabinoids), the most commonly used illicit drug worldwide, induce LTP or LTD at these synapses. Pleiotrophin (PTN) is a cytokine with important roles in the modulation of synaptic plasticity, which levels of expression are significantly regulated by amphetamine administration. Gramage et al. (2011), have reported that amphetamine during adolescence causes long-term cognitive deficits in rats. Periadolescent amphetamine treatment daily during 10 days in normal and in PTN genetically deficient mice result in significant deficits in the passive avoidance and Y-maze tests (two tasks related to learning and memory abilities), only observed in amphetamine-pretreated PTN mutant mice. However, 13 and 26 days after the last administration, they did not find significant differences in Y-maze between amphetamine- and saline-pretreated PTN-/- mice. A significantly enhanced LTP in CA1 hippocampal slices from saline-pretreated PTN-/- mice compared with saline-pretreated PTN+/+ mice was observed. Interestingly, amphetamine pre-treatment during adolescence significantly enhanced LTP in adult PTN+/+ mice but did not cause any effect in PTN-/- mice, suggesting LTP mechanisms saturation in naïve PTN-/- mice. The data demonstrate that periadolescent amphetamine treatment causes transient cognitive deficits and long-term alterations of hippocampal LTP depending on the endogenous expression of PTN. Pleiotrophin (PTN) is a growth factor that has been shown to be involved in hippocampal synaptic plasticity and learning. Del Olmo et al. (2009), using *in vitro* electrophysiological recordings in PTN-stimulated CA1 from rat hippocampal slices, found that PTN inhibited hippocampal LTP induced by high-frequency stimulation (HFS). Also, they observed significant differences in recognition memory between PTN genetically deficient (PTN-/-) mice and wild type (WT) mice using the Y-maze test, whereas WT mice showed disruption of recognition memory,

PTN -/- mice maintained the recognition memory. The data demonstrate that PTN inhibits hippocampal LTP *in vitro* and might play a role in memory processes *in vivo*.

Synaptic plasticity in the mesolimbic DA system is critically involved in reward-based conditioning and the development of drug addiction (Schultz et al., 1998; Wise, 2004). Ca^{2+} signals triggered by postsynaptic action potentials (APs) drive the induction of synaptic plasticity in the CNS. Ahn et al. (2010) have recently proposed that enhancement of mGluR-dependent n-methyl-d-aspartate receptor (NMDAR) plasticity in the VTA may promote the learning of environmental stimuli repeatedly associated with amphetamine experience. In this study, using brain slices prepared from male rats, it was shown that repeated *in vivo* exposure to the psychostimulant amphetamine upregulates mGluR-dependent facilitation of burst-evoked Ca^{2+} signals in DA neurons of the VTA. Protein kinase A (PKA)-induced sensitization of IP_3 receptors mediates this upregulation of mGluR action. As a consequence, NMDAR-mediated transmission becomes more susceptible to LTP induction after repeated amphetamine exposure. It was also found that the magnitude of amphetamine-conditioned place preference (CPP) in behaving rats correlates with the magnitude of mGluR-dependent Ca^{2+} signal facilitation measured in VTA slices prepared from these rats.

Major drugs of abuse such as cocaine, amphetamine, morphine, heroine, nicotine, and ethanol act on glutamatergic synapses on midbrain DA neurons and lead to NMDA-dependent, AMPA-mediated long-term potentiation in DA neurons. Thus, excitatory influences on these neurons become enhanced; in particular NMDA-dependent burst firing. Amphetamine also leads to reduction of LTD in DA neurons (Swope et al., 1999; Ahn et al., 2010; Liu et al., 2010, Good and Lupica, 2010). Thus, subthreshold fluctuations of excitatory inputs to DA neurons would increase or even generate action potentials in the absence of reward, generating a false reward signal (Schultz, 2011). There are glutamatergic projections from the hippocampus to the NAc, which regulate DA transmission in this structure. Ventral hippocampal (VH) glutamatergic neurons project to the NAc shell region, whereas the dorsal hippocampus (DH) sends glutamatergic projections to the NAc core region. Tan (2008) investigated the roles of hippocampal NMDA receptors and NAc D1 receptor in AMPH-produced conditioned place preference (AMPH-CPP) in rats. It was shown that AMPH-CPP results in the enhancement of hippocampal CaMKII activity which can be impaired by NMDA antagonist (AP5). Inactivation of hippocampal area (dorsal hippocampus or ventral hippocampus) impaired AMPH-CPP, but its effect was diminished by the activation of D1 receptors in NAc core or NAc shell. It was concluded that if the deterioration of AMPH-CPP expression resembles the formation of new learning, then this active process might have been facilitated by the hippocampal NMDA receptor activations during testing.

4.3 Amphetamine sensitization

Muhammad et al. (2011a) studied the effect of postnatal tactile stimulation (TS) on juvenile behavior, adult amphetamine (AMPH) sensitization, and the interaction of TS and AMPH on prefrontal cortical (PFC) thickness and striatum size. AMPH administration resulted in gradual increase in behavioral sensitization that persisted at least for 2 weeks. However, TS rats exhibited attenuated AMPH sensitization compared to sex-matched controls. Neuroanatomically, AMPH reduced the PFC thickness in control females but enlarged the posterior striatum in control males. It was suggested that TS during development modulated the response to novel objects and altered social behaviors and attenuated AMPH-induced behavioral sensitization by preventing drug-induced structural alteration in the PFC and the striatum, brain regions implicated in drug abuse. Subsequently, these same investigators studied the effect of prenatal stress (PS) on juvenile behavior and adult AMPH sensitization, as well as the effect of the interaction between experience and drug on cortical thickness and neuronal morphology in corticolimbic regions in rats. PS did not influence AMPH-induced behavioral sensitization in either male or female rats. Moreover, PS increased the spine density in the NAc and decreased it in the mPFC without any alteration in the orbital frontal cortex (OFC). Similarly, AMPH administration increased spine density in the NAc and mPFC, whereas a decrease was observed in the OFC. However, PS prevented the drug-induced alterations in the spine density observed in controls. In sum, PS modulated juvenile behavior and altered brain morphology without influencing AMPH-induced behavioral sensitization substantially (Muhammad and Kolb, 2011b). Also, more recently Muhammad and Kolb (2011c) studied the long-term influence of maternal separation (MS) on periadolescent behavior, adult amphetamine (AMPH) sensitization, and structural plasticity in the corticolimbic regions in rats. Male and female pups, separated daily for 3h from the dam during postnatal day 3-21, were tested for periadolescent exploratory, emotional, cognitive, and social behaviors. The results showed that MS enhanced anxiety-like behavior in males. Repeated AMPH administration increased the spine density in the NAc and the mPFC, and decreased it in the OFC. MS blocked the drug-induced alteration in these regions. MS during development influenced periadolescent behavior in males, and structurally reorganized cortical and subcortical brain regions without affecting AMPH-induced behavioral sensitization.

4.4 Amphetamine and mental disorders

Individuals who repeatedly use stimulant drugs, such as AMPH, develop an AMPH-induced psychosis that is similar to paranoid schizophrenia. There has been, therefore, considerable interest in characterizing the effects of chronic stimulant drug treatment on brain and behavior in non-human animals (Robinson and Becker, 1986).

5. Dopamine transporter and neural plasticity

Dopamine (DA) is one of the most important neurotransmitters affecting fine brain processes. Dysfunction of dopaminergic neurotransmission precipitates diseases such as Parkinson's disease (PD), schizophrenia, attention-deficit hyperactivity disorder (ADHD), and drug addiction (see Zhang et al., 2010 for review). DA synthesis occurs within the DA neurons. Tyrosine is transported into the cell via amino acid carriers in the blood–brain barrier and cell membranes. Once in the intracellular space, tyrosine is hydroxylated to L-3,4-dihydroxyphenylalanine (L-DOPA) by tyrosine hydroxylase (TH). L-DOPA is then decarboxylated by aromatic acid decarboxylase (AADC) to DA (for review see Miyake et al., 2011). Extracellular DA concentration and lifetime after release is regulated by diffusion, dilution as well as reuptake (for review see Rice and Cragge, 2008). Reuptake of synaptic DA by the dopamine transporter (DAT) is the principal mechanism regulating dopamine neurotransmission, and is often used as a marker for presynaptic DA function (for review see Zhang et al., 2010). In addition DA itself can regulate DAT via its interaction with the transporter or presynaptic autoreceptors (Williams and Galli, 2006). Interestingly, a recent report has found that unmedicated bipolar disorder (BPD) subjects had significantly lower DAT availability relative to healthy controls in bilateral dorsal caudate (Anand et al., 2011), thus the authors suggest that DAT availability may be related to the neuropathology of BPD.

The DAT is a target for the development of pharmacotherapies for a number of central disorders including PD, Alzheimer's disease, schizophrenia, Tourette's syndrome, Lesch-Nyhan disease, ADHD, obesity, depression, and stimulant abuse, as well as normal aging (for review see Runyon and Carroll, 2006). DAT is located on the presynaptic membrane of DA terminals and regulates phasic DA transmission at the synapse by rapidly removing DA from the synaptic cleft through reuptake (for review see Rice and Cragge, 2008). Interestingly, this protein is expressed exclusively by DA neurons and is found extrasynaptically on DA axons in CPu and NAc (for review see Rice and Cragge, 2008). In addition, DA receptors are also predominantly extrasynaptic (Sesack et al., 1994; Yung et al., 1995; Hersch et al., 1995; Khan et al., 1998). Interestingly, several recent reports suggest that synuclein proteins have a critical role in monoamine neurotransmitter homeostasis. In addition, the physical interactions between synuclein proteins and monoamine transporters (DA, serotonin (5HT) and norepinephrine (NE) transporters) indicate an important role for the synucleins in regulating transporter function, trafficking and distribution at the DA, 5HT and NE synapses (for review see Oaks and Sidhu, 2011).

The synuclein family of proteins includes α-synuclein (α-Syn), β-synuclein (β-Syn), and γ-synuclein (γ-Syn). The genes cloned from multiple species demonstrate that synucleins, a group of prevalent pre-synaptic proteins, are highly conserved, but unique to vertebrate organisms (Surguchov, 2008). In addition, these proteins participate in numerous interactions with other proteins, lipid membranes, and nucleic acids, suggesting a possible role in the chaperoning or trafficking of biomolecules (Surguchov, 2008). Two-hybrid and immunoprecipitation experiments have identified a physical interaction between α-Syn and the carboxy terminal of DAT (Lee et al., 2001). In addition, release of DA synthesized by DA neurons in the brain requires packaging of the neurotransmitter into vesicles by the vesicular monoamine transporter 2 (VMAT2). VMAT2 co-localizes with α-Syn in the Lewy bodies of PD (Yamamoto, 2006), and overexpression of α-Syn can disrupt VMAT2 function (Surguchov, 2008). However, the influence of β-Syn and γ-Syn upon VMAT2 expression and activity are not known. Recent reports suggest that psychostimulants such as amphetamines and cocaine induced overexpression of α-synuclein (Fornai et al., 2005; Mauceli et al., 2006; Ajjimaporn et al., 2007; Klongpanichapak et al., 2008; Mukda et al., 2011, Sae-Ung et al., 2011). Interestingly, recent reports suggest that low levels of the γ-synuclein in the NAc results to an increased self-administration of cocaine in the rat (Boyer et al., 2011). In addition, cocaine induced a 1.9-fold increase in locomotor activity after overexpression of α-synuclein in the NAc (Boyer and Dreyer, 2007). It is noteworthy that the neurotoxicity induced by the psychostimulants such as amphetamine are mediated by enhanced oxidative stress and these effects are abolished by melatonin (Govitrapong et al., 2010), a main secretory product of pineal gland. Interestingly, a recent report suggested that this melatonin effect is mediated by the reduction of the overexpression of α-synuclein induced by amphetamine (Sae-Ung et al., 2011).

Amphetamines and cocaine are psychostimulants with a target in the monoaminergic system. These drugs reverse the action of monoamine transporters and enhance the release of DA as well as norepinephrine and 5-hydroxytriptamine (5-HT, serotonin) into the synaptic cleft, increasing their availability to act upon post-synaptic receptors. Reuptake blocking and decreased degradation of these neurotransmitters increases their concentrations in the synaptic cleft.

Locomotor activity induced by psychostimulants such as amphetamine is the result of increases in synaptic DA, by blocking or reversing the direction of DAT (Sulzer et al., 1995; Sulzer et al., 2005), which in turn acts on postsynaptic receptors. Interestingly, mice lacking DAT exhibit spontaneous hyperlocomotion and are unresponsive to amphetamine (Giros et al., 1996). Recent reports suggest that DAT, but not the serotonin transport (SERT), is critical in mediating the reinforcing effects of cocaine. In addition, mice lacking DAT generally failed to acquire and maintain cocaine self-administration (Thompson et al., 2009) compared to wild-type or SERT-/- mice. Therefore, DAT may play a role in mediating the long-lasting neural changes associated with drug addiction (Martin et al., 2011; Schmitt and Reith 2010).

Drug addiction involves several molecules such as CART (Cocaine-and amphetamine-regulated transcript) peptide. This peptide is a neurotransmitter believed to play a homeostatic role in psychostimulant reward and reinforcement, as well as in other processes (Jaworski and Jones, 2006; Rogge et al., 2008). CART has also been proved to attenuate locomotion induced by direct intraaccumbal injections of DA (Jaworski et al., 2003). Recently, it has been documented that the role of CART peptide in the NAc is to homeostatically regulate the activity of the DA system (Rogge et al., 2008). Moreover CART mRNA and CART peptide are found abundantly in the NAc (Douglass et al., 1995; Koylu et al., 1998). CART peptide (CART55-1029) has been shown to have minor psychostimulant-like properties when injected into the VTA, inducing locomotor activity and producing a slightly conditioned place preference (Kimmel et al., 2000, 2002). In this sense, a new study supports the idea that CART peptide reduces the effects of psychostimulants by modulating the simultaneous activation of both D1 and D2 receptors, rather than by affecting the action of any individual DA receptor (Moffett et al., 2011). In addition, our recent report suggests that prenatal amphetamine exposure produced, at postpubertal age, an enhanced DAT in the NAc (Flores et al., 2011, Figures 2, 3, 4) and children with prenatal psychostimulant exposure have greater risk of addictions (McKenna, 2011).

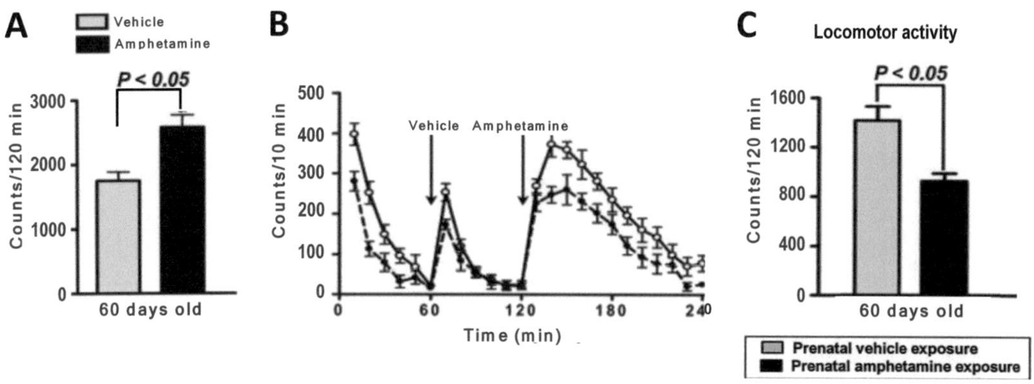

Fig. 2. Effect of amphetamine on locomotor behavior in a novel environment. A) Analysis of total activity scores revealed that the rats at PD60 were more active after amphetamine injection than their corresponding control group. B) Temporal profile of locomotor activity at PD60. C) Rats with prenatal amphetamine exposure were less active than control animals. Modified from Flores et al., 2011.

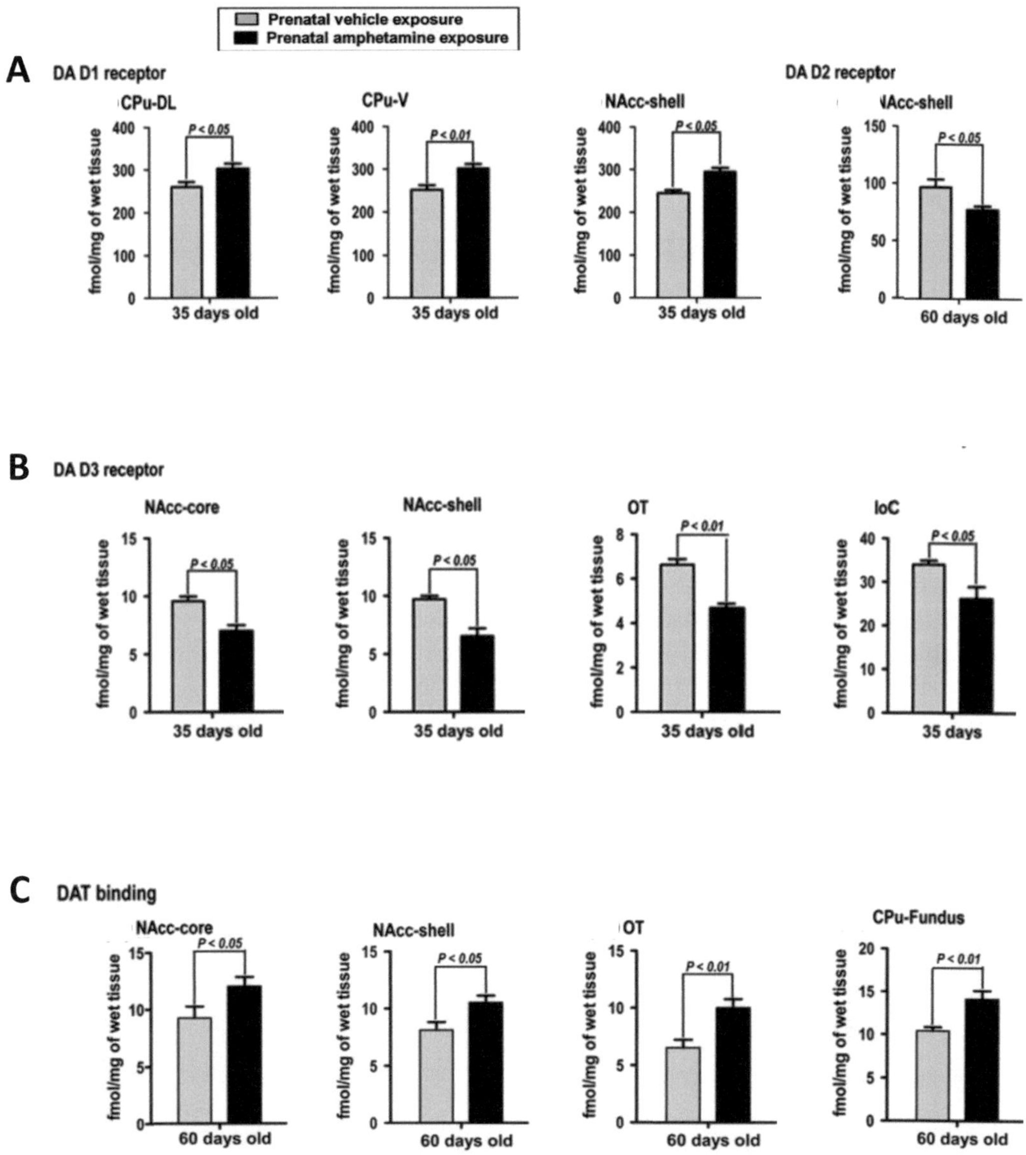

Fig. 3. Quantitative autoradiographic analysis of [3H]- SCH-23390/dopamine D1-like receptor binding, [3H]-spiperone/dopamine D2-like receptor binding, [3H]7-OHDPAT/dopamine D3 receptor binding and [3H] WIN-35428/dopamine transporter binding in prenatal amphetamine exposure (PAE)- and prenatal vehicle exposure (PVE)-rats Dopamine (DA), Postnatal (PD), nucleus accumbens (NAcc), caudate–putamen (CPu), olfactory tubercle (OT) and the island of Calleja. (Modified from Flores et al., 2011).

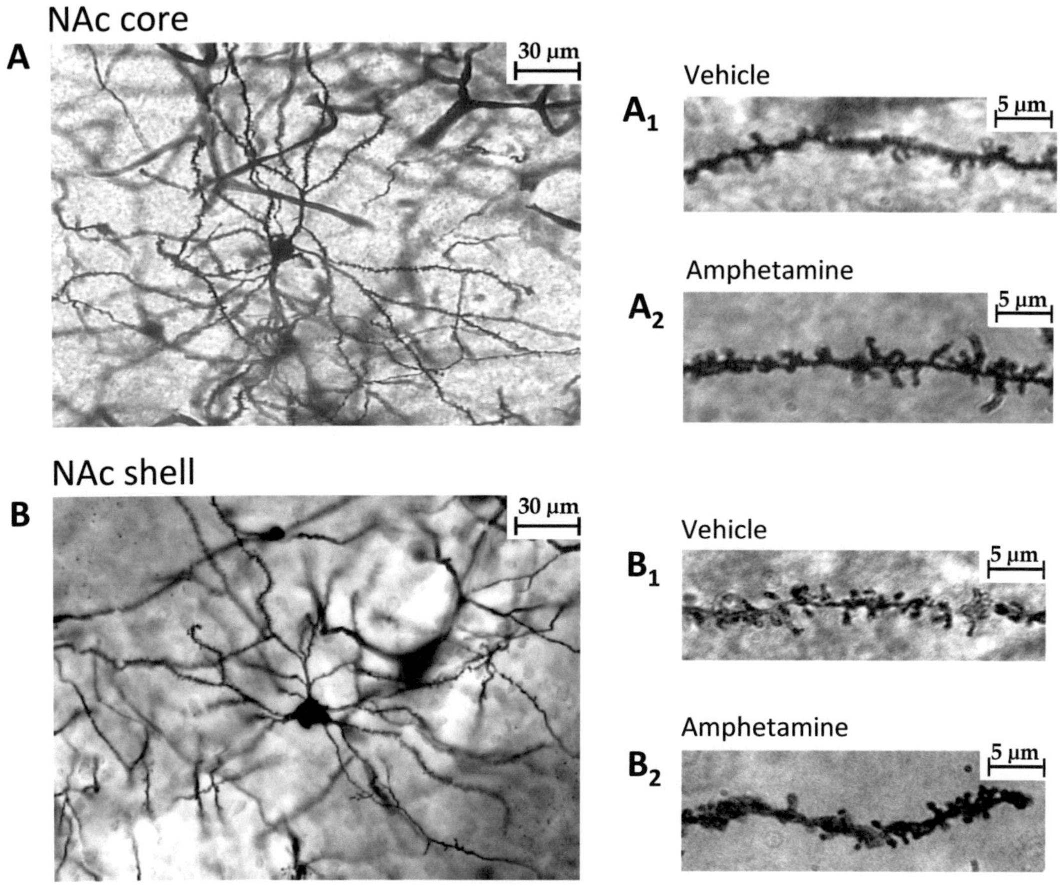

Fig. 4. Photomicrograph showing representative Golgi-Cox-impregnated medium spiny neurons and spines dendritic from the nucleus accumbens. Neurons in the nucleus accumbens core (A) and shell (B). The spine density is higher at PD60 in the dendritic segments from the core (A2) and shell (B2) subregions of the NAc of rats prenatally exposed to amphetamine compared to their corresponding vehicle group.

Cocaine and amphetamine may induce neural changes, including an increase in the density of spines on neuron dendrites in the NAc and PFC (Robinson and Kolb, 2004) associated with locomotor sensitization (Manev and Uz, 2009). More recently it has been suggested that cocaine-induced dendritic spine changes are correlated with the presence of DAT, because mice lacking DAT did not show an increase in dendritic spine density in the NAc (Martin et al., 211). In addition, the stereotypy induced by cocaine is also absent in this transgenic mice (Tilley and Gu, 2008). However, amphetamine and cocaine, although similar in many respects, do not produce identical patterns of structural plasticity when given to rats at different ages. In adult rats, several reports have demonstrated that cocaine increases spine density on the basilar dendrites of pyramidal neurons in the PFC, while amphetamine has either no effect or a weak effect on these dendrites. In contrast, in juvenile (P22–P34) rats, amphetamine increases spine density on the basilar dendrites of PFC (for review see Robinson and Kolb, 2011).

In conclusion, DAT is one of the principal mechanisms regulating DA neurotransmission via reuptake of synaptic DA. The psychostimulants amphetamine and cocaine alter DAT function and alter the lifetime of the DA after release. Exposure to amphetamine or cocaine produced persistent changes in the structure of dendrites and dendritic spines in brain regions such as the NAc and PFC, limbic structures related with the addictions. This structural plasticity associated with the use of the drugs of abuse results in a reorganization of synaptic connectivity in these neural systems, which may associate with addiction symptoms. Several reports suggest that cocaine abusers have an increase in DAT levels with a decrease in gray and white matter density (Gould et al., 2011), however, abstainers have significantly higher gray matter density and lower DAT levels than current cocaine users (Hanlon et al., 2011; Gould et al., 2011). Therefore, both, DAT levels and gray matter density in cocaine users reverse after prolonged abstinence (Volkow et al., 2001; Beverigde et al., 2009; Hanlon et al., 2011). Interestingly, cocaine abstainers perform better cognitive test compared to current cocaine users (Hanlon et al., 2011).

6. Treatment of addiction

Despite intensive research and significant advances, drug addictions remain a substantial public health problem. Drug addictions have a high economical cost annually and impact not only the addicted individuals, but also their spouses, children, employers, and others. Thus, the development of improved prevention and treatment strategies is of importance (Potenza et al., 2011). Learning processes have been shown to play a major role in the maintenance of addictive behaviour (Everitt et al., 1999; Robbins & Everitt, 2002; Everitt & Robbins, 2005; Moreira & Lutz, 2008; Liu et al., 2010). Humans and animals rapidly learn cues and contexts that predict the availability of addictive drugs. Once learned, these cues and contexts initiate drug seeking, craving and relapse in both animal models and clinical studies (Von der Goltz & Kiefer, 2009; De Vries & Schoffelmeer, 2005; Micale et al., 2007). Evidence suggests that several types of neuroadaptation occur, including synapse-specific adaptations of the type thought to underlie specific long-term associative memory. Thus, understanding learning and memory processes in the addicted is an important key for understanding the persistence of addiction, and it is reasonable to hypothesize that the disruption of drug-related memories may help to prevent relapses (von der Goltz & Kiefer, 2009). The study of structure-activity relationships of molecules which influence the cannabinoid system in the brain and body is crucial in the search of medical preparations with the therapeutic effects of the phytocannabinoids without the negative effects on cognitive function attributed to cannabis (see Fisar, 2009 for review).

As discussed before, cannabinoid CB1Rs are novel targets for a new class of therapeutic agents used to treat drug addiction. Blockade of the CB1 receptor is particularly effective in reducing cue-induced reinstatement of drug seeking, an animal analogue of cue-induced relapse in human addicts (See Gardner, 2002, 2005, 2011 for review). These relapse-preventing properties are observed with different classes of abused drug (i.e. psychostimulants, opiates, nicotine and alcohol). In addition, recent evidence indicates a more general role of CB1 receptors in reward-related memories, which is consistent with the proposed role of endocannabinoids in memory-related plasticity. Relapse-preventing actions and inhibitory effects on weight gain were confirmed recently in clinical trials with the CB1 antagonist rimonabant (De Vries and Schoffelmeer, 2005). Preclinical results provide support for the suggestion that targeting the endocannabinoid system may aid in the treatment of disorders associated with impaired extinction-like processes, such as post-traumatic stress disorder (Abush and Akirav, 2010). Liu et al. (2010) provided evidence that NMDA receptor-dependent synaptic depression at VTA dopamine circuitry requires GluR2 endocytosis, also suggest an essential contribution of such synaptic depression to cannabinoid-associated addictive learning, in addition to pointing to novel pharmacological strategies for the treatment of cannabis addiction. They found in rats that chronic cannabinoid exposure activates VTA CB1 receptors to induce transient neurotransmission depression at VTA local Glu-DA synapses through activation of NMDA receptors and subsequent endocytosis of AMPA receptor GluR2 subunits. A GluR2-derived peptide blocks cannabinoid-induced VTA synaptic depression and conditioned place preference, i.e., learning to associate drug exposure with environmental cues.

6.1 Pharmacological treatments and targets

Multiple pharmacological targets have been identified for the treatment of addictive disorders. "Classic" approaches tend to target the drug "reward" system, such as normalization of function through agonist approaches and negative reinforcement strategies. Agonist medications have their main impact on the same types of neurotransmitter receptors as those stimulated by abused substances. Most notably, dextroamphetamine has reduced drug use in short-term clinical trials in cocaine and methamphetamine users. The long-term safety and abuse liability of amphetamines as a treatment for cocaine addiction remains to be determined. Another example of an agonist approach for cocaine dependence is modafinil, a weak DAT inhibitor and increases synaptic DA levels, which has stimulant-like effects. On other hand, antagonists block the effects of drugs by either pharmacological or pharmacokinetic mechanisms. More recently, immunotherapies have been developed for the treatment of cocaine and methamphetamine addictions. The antibodies produced by immunotherapies sequester the drug in the circulation and reduce the amount of drug and the speed at which it reaches the brain. A potentially promising target for agonist and antagonist treatment of cocaine addiction is the D3 dopamine receptor. D3 partial agonists can act like agonists and stimulate DA receptors when endogenous levels of dopamine are low, as in cocaine withdrawal. An important limitation of vaccines is that the antibodies produced are specific for a given drug of abuse, a characteristic that will limit their clinical efficacy in polydrug abusers.

Drug addiction is associated with adaptive changes in multiple neurotransmitter systems in the brain. These adaptive changes are thought to underlie the negative reinforcing effects of abstinence from drug use that are clinically observed as withdrawal symptoms, craving for drug use, and negative mood states like anhedonia and anxiety (Hasin et al., 2007; Treadway and Zald, 2011). Examples of medications targeting negative reinforcement of drugs include methadone or buprenorphine, drugs that relieve opioid withdrawal symptoms. Cocaine users with more severe withdrawal symptoms respond more favorably to propranolol, a beta-adrenergic antagonist (Kampman et al., 2006). Several agents targeting glutamate system are also under investigation as potential treatment medications. Memantine, a noncompetitive NMDA glutamate receptor antagonist, may be efficacious and operate by reducing cognitive measures of compulsivity (Grant et al., 2010). However, clinical trials with an NMDA receptor antagonist have demonstrated negative findings for cocaine dependence (Bisaga et al., 2010).

Activation of cannabinoid receptors on synaptic terminals results in regulation of ion channels, neurotransmitter release and synaptic plasticity. Neuromodulation of synapses by the cannabinoids is proving to have a wide range of functional effects, making them potential targets as medical preparations in a variety of illnesses, including some mental disorders and neurodegenerative illnesses (see Fisar, 2009 for review).

In conclusion, the review of existing evidences indicates that addictive drugs induce synaptic plasticity at DA system and produce changes in DA at different target structures of the brain, affecting glutamateric, GABAergic transmission and LTP and LTD processes (Figure 5). New research will without doubt shed light onto the mechanisms of addiction induction and better design of drug-addiction treatments.

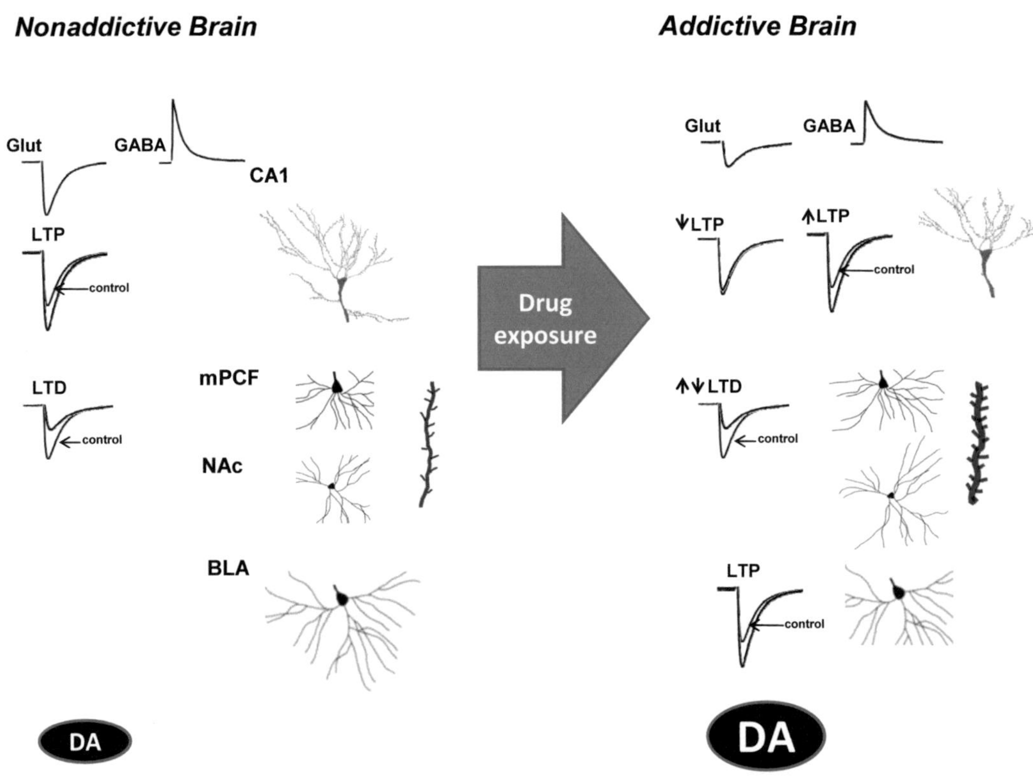

Fig. 5. Addictive drug affects DA levels, glutamatergic and GABAergic transmission and LTP and LTD processes at different brain structures. DA: dopamine; CA1: CA1 region of the hippocampus; PFC, prefrontal cortex; NAc: accumbens nucleus; BLA: basolateral amygdala.

7. References

Abush, H. & Akirav, I. (2010). Cannabinoids modulate hippocampal memory and plasticity. *Hippocampus*, Vol.20, No.10, pp. 1126-1138.

Adermark, L.; Talani, G. & Lovinger, D.M. (2009). Endocannabinoid-dependent plasticity at GABAergic and glutamatergic synapses in the striatum is regulated by synaptic activity. *Eur J Neurosci.*, Vol.29, No.1, pp. 32-41.

Ahn K.C.; Bernier, B.E.; Harnett, M.T. & Morikawa, H. (2010). IP3 receptor sensitization during in vivo amphetamine experience enhances NMDA receptor plasticity in dopamine neurons of the ventral tegmental area. *J Neurosci.*, Vol.30, No.19, pp. 6689-6699.

Ajjimaporn, A.; Phansuwan-Pujito, P.; Ebadi M. & Govitrapong, P. (2007). Zinc protects SK-N-SH cells from methamphetamine-induced alpha-synuclein expression. *Neurosci Lett.*, No.419, pp. 59-63.

Anand, A.; Barkay, G.; Dzemidzic, M.; Albrecht, D.; Karne, H.; Zheng, Q.H,; Hutchins, G.D.; Normandin, M.D. & Yoder, K.K. (2011). Striatal dopamine transporter availability in unmedicated bipolar disorder. *Bipolar Disord.*, No.13, pp. 406-413.

Anderson, S.M.; Bari, A.A. & Pierce, R.C. (2003). Administration of the D1-like dopamine receptor antagonist SCH-23390 into the medial nucleus accumbens shell attenuates cocaine priming-induced reinstatement of drug-seeking behavior in rats. *Psychopharmacology*, No. 168, pp.132–138.

Aston-Jones, G.; Smith, R.J.; Moorman, D.E. & Richardson, K.A. (2009). Role of lateral hypothalamic orexin neurons in reward processing and addiction. *Neuropharmacol.*, No.56, Suppl 1, pp. 112-121.

Aston-Jones, G.; Smith, R.J.; Sartor, G.C.; Moorman, D.E.; Massi, L.; Tahsili-Fahadan, P. & Richardson, K.A. (2010). Lateral hypothalamic orexin/hypocretin neurons: A role in reward-seeking and addiction. *Brain Res.*, Vol.16, No.1314, pp. 74-90.

Badiani, A.; Belin, D. ; Epstein, D. ; Calu, D. & Shaham, Y. (2011). Opiate versus psychostimulant addiction: the differences do matter. Nat Rev Neurosci., Vol. 12, No. 11, pp. 685-70.

Basavarajappa, B.S. (2007). Neuropharmacology of the endocannabinoid signaling system-molecular mechanisms, biological actions and synaptic plasticity. *Curr Neuropharmacol.*, Vol.5, No.2, pp. 81-97.

Basavarajappa, B.S.; Nixon, R.A. & Arancio, O. (2009). Endocannabinoid system: emerging role from neurodevelopment to neurodegeneration. *Mini Rev Med Chem.*, Vol.9, No.4, pp. 448-462.

Bassareo, V.; De Luca, M.A. & Di Chiara, G. (2007). Differential impact of pavlovian drug conditioned stimuli on in vivo dopamine transmission in the rat accumbens shell and core and in the prefrontal cortex. *Psychopharmacol. (Berl)*, Vol.191, No.3, pp. 689-703.

Belin, D.; Mar, A.C.; Dalley, J.W.; Robbins, T.W. & Everitt, B.J. (2008). High impulsivity predicts the switch to compulsive cocaine-taking. Science. Vol. 320, No. 5881, pp. 1352-5.

Belin, D.; Jonkman, S.; Dickinson, A., Robbins, T. & Everitt, B. (2009) Parallel and interactive learning processes within the basal ganglia: Relevance for the understanding of addiction. *Behav. Brain Res.* No. 199, Vol. 11, pp. 89–102.

Belin, D. & Everitt, B.J. (2010). Drug Addiction: The Neural and Psychological Basis of a Compulsive Incentive Habit. In: *Handbook of Basal ganglia. Structure and Function.* Steiner, H. & Tseng, K. Eds. Academic Press.

Berridge, K.C. (2007). The debate over dopamine's role in reward: the case for incentive salience. *Psychopharmacol. (Berl)*, Vol.191, No.3, pp. 391-431.

Beveridge, T.J.; Smith, H.R.; Nader, M.A. & Porrino, L.J. (2009). Abstinence from chronic cocaine self-administration alters striatal dopamine systems in rhesus monkeys. Neuropsychopharmacol., Vol. 34, No. 5, pp. 1162-1171.

Bierut, L.J. (2011). Genetic Vulnerability and Susceptibility to Substance Dependence. *Neuron*, Vol.69, No.4, pp. 618-627.

Bossong, M.G. & Niesink, R.J. (2010). Adolescent brain maturation, the endogenous cannabinoid system and the neurobiology of cannabis-induced schizophrenia. *Prog Neurobiol.*, Vol.92, No.3, pp. 370-385.

Boutrel B, Kenny PJ, Specio SE, Martin-Fardon R, Markou A, Koob GF, de Lecea L. (2005). Role for hypocretin in mediating stress-induced reinstatement of cocaine-seeking behavior. *Proc Natl Acad Sci.*, No. 102, Vol. 52, pp. 19168-19173.

Boyer, F.; Balado, E.; Piazza, P.V.; Dreyer, J.L. & Deroche-Gamonet, V. (2011). A decrease in gamma-synuclein expression within the nucleus accumbens increases cocaine intravenous self-administration in the rat. *Addict Biol.*, No.16, pp. 120-123.

Boyer, F. & Dreyer, J.L. (2007). Alpha-synuclein in the nucleus accumbens induces changes in cocaine behaviour in rats. *Eur J Neurosci.*, No.26, pp. 2764-2776.

Chaperon, F. & Thiébot, M.H. (1999). Behavioral effects of cannabinoid agents in animals. *Crit Rev Neurobiol.*, Vol.13, No.3, pp. 243-281.

Chevaleyre, V.; Takahashi, K.A. & Castillo, P.E. (2006). Endocannabinoid-mediated synaptic plasticity in the CNS. *Annu Rev Neurosci.*, No.29, pp. 37-76.

Cooper, Z.D. & Haney, M. (2008). Cannabis reinforcement and dependence: role of the cannabinoid CB1 receptor. *Addict Biol.*, Vol.13, No.2, pp. 188-195.

Dalley, J.W.; Fryer, T.D.; Brichard, L.; Robinson, E.S.; Theobald, D.E.; Lääne, K.; Peña, Y.; Murphy, E.R.; Shah, Y.; Probst, K.; Abakumova, I.; Aigbirhio, F.I.; Richards, H.K.; Hong, Y.; Baron, J.C.; Everitt, B.J. & Robbins, T.W. (2007). Nucleus accumbens D2/3 receptors predict trait impulsivity and cocaine reinforcement. *Science*, Vol. 15, No. 5816, pp. 1267-70.

Dalley, J.W.; Everitt, B.J. & Robbins, T.W. (2011). Impulsivity, Compulsivity, and Top-Down Cognitive Control. *Neuron* Vol.69, No.4, pp. 680-694.

Deadwyler, S.A.; Goonawardena, A.V. & Hampson, R.E. (2007). Short-term memory is modulated by the spontaneous release of endocannabinoids: evidence from hippocampal population codes. *Behav Pharmacol.*, Vol.18, No.5-6, pp. 571-80.

Deadwyler, S.A. & Hampson, R.E. (2008). Endocannabinoids modulate encoding of sequential memory in the rat hippocampus. *Psychopharmacol (Berl).*, Vol.198, No.4, pp. 577-586.

Del Olmo, N.; Gramage, E.; Alguacil, L.F.; Pérez-Pinera, P.; Deuel, T.F. & Herradón, G. (2009). Pleiotrophin inhibits hippocampal long-term potentiation: a role of pleiotrophin in learning and memory. *Growth Factors*, Vol.27, No.3, pp. 189-194.

Deng, J.V.; Rodriguiz, R.M.; Hutchinson, A.N.; Kim, I.K.; Wetsel, W.C. & West, A.E. (2010). MeCP2 in the nucleus accumbens contributes to neural and behavioral responses to psychostimulants. *Nature Neurosci.*, No.13, pp, 1128–1136.

De Vries, T.J. & Schoffelmeer, A.N. (2005). Cannabinoid CB1 receptors control conditioned drug seeking. *Trends Pharmacol Sci.*, Vol.26, No.8, pp. 420-426.

Di Chiara, G. (1999). Drug addiction as dopamine-dependent associative learning disorder. *Eur J Pharmacol.*, No. 375, pp. 13–30.

Di Chiara, G.; Bassareo, V.; Fenu, S.; De Luca, M.A.; Spina, L.; Cadoni, C.; Acquas, E.; Carboni, E.; Valentini, V. & Lecca, D. (2004). Dopamine and drug addiction: the nucleus accumbens shell connection. *Neuropharmacol.*, No.47, Suppl 1, pp. 227-241.

Di Chiara, G. & Bassareo, V. (2007). Reward system and addiction: what dopamine does and doesn't do. *Curr Opin Pharmacol.*, Vol.7, No.1, pp. 69-76.

Di Marzo, V.; Hill M.P.; Bisogno, T.; Crossman, A.R. & Brotchie, J.M. (2000). Enhanced levels of endogenous cannabinoids in the globus pallidus are associated with a reduction in movement in an animal model of Parkinson's disease. *FASEB J.*, Vol. 14, No. 10, pp.1432-1438.

Economidou, D.; Pelloux, Y., Robbins, T.W.; Dalley, J.W. & Everitt, B.J. (2009) High impulsivity predicts relapse to cocaine-seeking after punishment-induced abstinence. Biol Psychiatry. Vol. 65, No. 10, pp. 851-6.

Edwards, C.R. & Skosnik, P.D. (2007). Cerebellar-dependent learning as a neurobehavioral index of the cannabinoid system. *Crit Rev Neurobiol.*, Vol.19, No.1, pp. 29-57.

Everitt, B. J.; Parkinson, J.A.; Olmstead, M.C.; Arroyo, M.; Robledo, P. & Robbins, T.W. (1999). Associative processes in addiction and reward. The role of amygdala–ventral striatal subsystems. *Ann. NY Acad. Sci.*, No. 877, pp. 412–438.

Everit, B.J. & Robbins, T.W. (2005). Neural systems of reinforcement for drug addiction: from actions to habits to compulsion. Nat Neurosci., Vol. 7, No. 8, pp.1481-1489.

Fan, N.; Yang, H.; Zhang, J. & Chen, C. (2010). Reduced expression of glutamate receptors and phosphorylation of CREB are responsible for in vivo Delta9-THC exposure-impaired hippocampal synaptic plasticity. *J Neurochem.*, Vol.112, No.3, pp. 691-702.

Fernandez-Espejo, E.; Viveros, M.P.; Núñez, L.; Ellenbroek, B.A. & Rodriguez de Fonseca, F. (2009). Role of cannabis and endocannabinoids in the genesis of schizophrenia. *Psychopharmacol (Berl).*, Vol.206, No.4, pp. 531-549.

Fisar, Z. (2009). Phytocannabinoids and endocannabinoids. *Curr Drug Abuse Rev.*, Vol.2, No.1, pp. 51-75.

Flores, G.; de Jesús, Gómez-Villalobos M. & Rodríguez-Sosa, L. (2011). Prenatal amphetamine exposure effects on dopaminergic receptors and transporter in postnatal rats. *Neurochem Res.*, No.36, pp. 1740-1749.

Fornai, F.; Lenzi, P.; Ferrucci, M.; Lazzeri, G.; di Poggio, A.B.; Natale, G.; Busceti, C.L.; Biagioni, F.; Giusiani, M.; Ruggieri, S. & Paparelli, A. (2005). Occurrence of neuronal inclusions combined with increased nigral expression of alpha-synuclein within dopaminergic neurons following treatment with amphetamine derivatives in mice. *Brain Res Bull.*, No.65, pp. 405-413.

Freund, T.F.; Katona, I. & Piomelli, D. (2003). Role of endogenous cannabinoids in synaptic signaling. *Physiol Rev.*, Vol.83, No.3, pp. 1017-1066.

Fuss, J. & Gass, P. (2010). Endocannabinoids and voluntary activity in mice: runner's high and long-term consequences in emotional behaviors. *Exp Neurol.* Vol. 224, No. 1, pp. 103-105.

Gaoni, Y. & Mechoulam, R. (1964). Isolation, structure and partial synthesis of an active constituent of hashish. J Am Chem Soc., No. 86, p.1646.

Gardner, E.L. (2002). Addictive potential of cannabinoids: the underlying neurobiology. *Chem Phys Lipids.*, Vol. 121, No. 1-2, pp. 267-290.

Gardner, E.L. (2005). Endocannabinoid signaling system and brain reward: emphasis on dopamine. *Pharmacol Biochem Behav.*, Vol. 81, No. 2, pp. 263-284.

Gardner, E.L. (2011). Addiction and brain reward and antireward pathways. *Adv Psychosom Med.*, No.30, pp. 22-60.

Giros, B.; Jaber, M.; Jones, S.R.; Wightman, R.M. & Caron, M.G. (1996). Hyperlocomotion and indifference to cocaine and amphetamine in mice lacking the dopamine transporter. *Nature*, No.379, pp. 606-612.

Govitrapong, P.; Boontem, P.; Kooncumchoo, P.; Pinweha, S.; Namyen, J.; Sanvarinda, Y. & Vatanatunyakum, S. (2010). Increased blood oxidative stress in amphetamine users. *Addict Biol.*, Vol.15, No.1, pp. 100-102.

Good, CH. & Lupica, C.R. (2010). Afferent-specific AMPA receptor subunit composition and regulation of synaptic plasticity in midbrain dopamine neurons by abused drugs. *J Neurosci.*, Vol.30, No.23, pp. 7900-7909.

Gould, R.W.; Porrino, L.J. & Nader, M.A. (2011). Nonhuman Primate Models of Addiction and PET Imaging: Dopamine System Dysregulation. Curr Top Behav Neurosci. DIO: 10.1007/7854.

Gramage, E.; Del Olmo, N.; Fole, A.; Martín, Y.B. & Herradón, G. (2011). Periadolescent amphetamine treatment causes transient cognitive disruptions and long-term changes in hippocampal LTP depending on the endogenous expression of pleiotrophin. *Addict Biol.* 2011, August 4, doi: 10.1111/j.1369-1600.2011.00362.x.

Hasin, D.S.; Stinson, F.S.; Ogburn, E. & Grant, B.F. (2007). Prevalence, correlates, disability, and comorbidity of DSM-IV alcohol abuse and dependence in the United States: Results from the National Epidemiologic Survey on Alcohol and Related Conditions. *Arch. Gen. Psychiatry*, No. 64, pp. 830–842.

Hersch, S.M.; Ciliax, B.J.; Gutekunst, C.A.; Rees, H.D.; Heilman, C.J.; Yung, K.K.; Bolam, J.P.; Ince, E.; Yi, H. & Levey, A.I. (2005). Electron microscopic analysis of D1 and D2 dopamine receptor proteins in the dorsal striatum and their synaptic relationships with motor corticostriatal afferents. *J Neurosci.*, No.15, pp. 5222-5237.

Huang, C.C.; Yeh, C.M.; Wu, M.Y.; Chang, A.Y.; Chan, J.Y.; Chan, S.H. & Hsu, K.S. (2011). Cocaine withdrawal impairs metabotropic glutamate receptor-dependent long-term depression in the nucleus accumbens. *J Neurosci.*, Vol.31, No.11, pp. 4194-4203.

Hyman, S.E. & Malenka, R.C. (2001). Addiction and the brain: the neurobiology of compulsion and its persistence. *Nat Rev Neurosci.*, Vol.2, No.10, pp. 695-703.

Hyman, S.E. (2005). Addiction: A Disease of Learning and Memory. *Am J Psychiatry*, No.162, pp. 1414-1422.

Hyman, S.E.; Malenka, R.C. & Nestler, E.J. (2006). Neural mechanisms of addiction: the role of reward-related learning and memory. *Annu Rev Neurosci.*, No.29, pp. 565-598.

Hyman, S.E. (2011). Cognitive enhancement: promises and perils. *Neuron*, Vol.69, No.4, pp. 595-598.

Holden, C. (2010). Psychiatry. Behavioral addictions debut in proposed DSM-V. *Science* , No. 327, pp. 935.

Im, H.I.; Hollander, J.A.; Bali, P. & Kenny, P.J. (2010). MeCP2 controls BDNF expression and cocaine intake through homeostatic interactions with microRNA-212. *Nature Neurosci.* No.13, pp. 1120–1127.

Imperato, A. & Di Chiara, G. (1986). Preferential stimulation of dopamine release in the nucleus accumbens of freely moving rats by ethanol. *J Pharmacol Exp Ther.*, No. 239, pp. 219–228.

Isbell, H.; Gorodetzsky, C.W.; Jasinski, D., Claussen, U.; Spulak, F.V. & Korte, F. (1967). Effects of (-)Delta (9)-Trans-Tetrahydrocannabinol in Man. *Psychopharmacologia (Berl.),* No. 11, pp. 184-188.

Jaworski, J.N.; Kozel, M.A.; Philpot, K.B. & Kuhar, M.J. (2003). Intra-accumbal injection of CART (cocaine-amphetamine regulated transcript) peptide reduces cocaine-induced locomotor activity. *J Pharmacol Exp Ther.*, No.307, pp. 1038-1044.

Jaworski, J.N. & Jones, D.C. (2004). The role of CART in the reward/reinforcing properties of psychostimulants. *Peptides*, No.27, pp. 1993-2004.

Jonkman, S.; Pelloux, Y. & Everitt, B.J. (2012) Differential roles of the dorsolateral and midlateral striatum in punished cocaine seeking. *J Neurosci.*, No. 32, pp. 4645–4650.

Kalivas, P.W. & Stewart, J. (1991) Dopamine transmission in the initiation and expression of drug- and stress-induced sensitization of motor activity. *Brain Res Rev.*, No. 16, pp. 223–244.

Kandel, E.R. (2004). The Molecular Biology of Memory Storage: A Dialogue Between Genes and Synapses. *Science*, No. 294, pp. 1030-1038.

Kendler, K.S., Prescott C.A., J. Myers, J. & Neale, M.C. (2003). The structure of genetic and environmental risk factors for common psychiatric and substance use disorders in men and women. *Arch. Gen. Psychiatry*, 60, pp. 929–937.

Keeney, B.K.; Raichlen, D.A.; Meek, T.H.; Wijeratne, R.S.; Middleton, K.M.; Gerdeman, G.L. & Garland, T. Jr. (2008). Differential response to a selective cannabinoid receptor antagonist (SR141716: rimonabant) in female mice from lines selectively bred for high voluntary wheel-running behaviour. *Behav Pharmacol.,* Vol. 19, No. 8, pp. 812-20.

Kenny, P.J. (2011). Reward Mechanisms in Obesity: New Insights and Future Directions. *Neuron*, Vol.69, No.4, pp. 664-679.

Khan, Z.U.; Gutiérrez, A.; Martín, R.; Peñafiel, A.; Rivera, A. & De La Calle, A. (1998). Differential regional and cellular distribution of dopamine D2-like receptors: an immunocytochemical study of subtype-specific antibodies in rat and human brain. *J Comp Neurol.*, No.402, pp. 353-371.

Kimmel, H.L.; Gong, W.; Vechia, S.D.; Hunter, R.G. & Kuhar, M.J. (2000). Intra-ventral tegmental area injection of rat cocaine and amphetamine-regulated transcript peptide 55-102 induces locomotor activity and promotes conditioned place preference. *J Pharmacol Exp Ther.*, No.294, pp. 784-792.

Kimmel, H.L.; Thim, L. & Kuhar, M.J. (2002). Activity of various CART peptides in changing locomotor activity in the rat. *Neuropeptides*, No.36, pp. 9-12.

Klongpanichapak, S.; Phansuwan-Pujito, P.; Ebadi, M. & Govitrapong, P. (2011). Melatonin inhibits amphetamine-induced increase in alpha-synuclein and decrease in phosphorylated tyrosine hydroxylase in SK-N-SH cells. *Neurosci Lett.*, No. 436, pp. 309-313.

Koch, G.; Mori, F.; Codecà, C.; Kusayanagi, H.; Monteleone, F.; Buttari, F.; Fiore, S.; Bernardi, G. & Centonze, D. (2009). Cannabis-based treatment induces polarity-reversing plasticity assessed by theta burst stimulation in humans. *Brain Stimul.*, Vol.2, No.4, pp. 229-233.

Laviolette, S.R. & Grace, A.A. (2006). Cannabinoids Potentiate Emotional Learning Plasticity in Neurons of the Medial Prefrontal Cortex through Basolateral Amygdala Inputs. *J Neurosci.*, Vol.26, No.24, pp. 6458-6468.

Lee, F.J.; Liu, F.; Pristupa, Z.B. & Niznik, H.B. (2001). Direct binding and functional coupling of alpha-synuclein to the dopamine transporters accelerate dopamine-induced apoptosis. *FASEB J.*, No.15, pp. 916-926.

Licata, S.C. & Pierce, R.C. (2003). The roles of calcium/calmodulin-dependent and Ras/mitogen-activated protein kinases in the development of psychostimulant-induced behavioral sensitization. *J Neurochem.*, Vol.85, No.1, pp. 14-22.

Lichtman, A.H. & Martin, B.R. (2005). Cannabinoid tolerance and dependence. *Handb Exp Pharmacol.*, No.168, pp. 691-717.

Lidow, M.S. (2003). Consequences of prenatal cocaine exposure in nonhuman primates. *Brain Res Dev Brain Res.*, Vol.147, No.1-2, pp. 23-36.

Li, F; Fang, Q.; Liu, Y.; Zhao, M.; Li, D.; Wang, J. & Lu, L. (2008). Cannabinoid CB(1) receptor antagonist rimonabant attenuates reinstatement of ketamine conditioned place preference in rats. *Eur J Pharmacol.*, Vol.589, No.1-3:122-126.

Liu, Z.; Han, J.; Jia, L.; Maillet, J.C.; Bai, G.; Xu, L.; Jia, Z.; Zheng, Q.; Zhang, W.; Monette, R.; Merali, Z.; Zhu, Z.; Wang, W.; Ren, W. & Zhang, X. (2010). Synaptic neurotransmission depression in ventral tegmental dopamine neurons and cannabinoid-associated addictive learning. *PLoS One*, Vol.5, No.12, e15634.

Lupica, C.R.; Riegel, A.C. & Hoffman, A.F. (2004). Marijuana and cannabinoid regulation of brain reward circuits. *Br J Pharmacol.*, Vol.143, No.2, pp. 227-234.

Lüscher, C. & Malenka, R.C. (2011). Drug-Evoked Synaptic Plasticity in Addiction: From Molecular Changes to Circuit Remodeling. *Neuron*, Vol.69, No.4, pp. 650-663.

Manev, H. & Uz, T. (2009). Dosing time-dependent actions of psychostimulants. *Int Rev Neurobiol.*, No.88, pp. 25-41.

Martin, B.J.; Naughton, B.J.; Thirtamara-Rajamani, K.; Yoon, D.J.; Han, D.D.; Devries, A.C. & Gu, H.H. (2011). Dopamine transporter inhibition is necessary for cocaine-induced increases in dendritic spine density in the nucleus accumbens. *Synapse*, No.65, pp. 490-496.

Mauceli, G.; Busceti, C.I.; Pellegrini, A.; Soldani, P.; Lenzi, P.; Paparelli, A. & Fornai, F. (2006). Overexpression of alpha-synuclein following methamphetamine: is it good or bad? *Ann N Y Acad Sci.*, No.1074, pp. 191-197.

McBride, W.J.; Murphy, J.M. & Ikemoto, S. (1999). Localization of brain reinforcement mechanisms: intracranial self-administration and intracranial place-conditioning studies. *Behav Brain Res.*, Vol.101, No.2, 129-152.

McGinty, J.F.; Whitfield, T.W. Jr & Berglind, W.J. (2010). Brain-derived neurotrophic factor and cocaine addiction. *Brain Res.*, No.1314, pp. 183-93.

McKenna, S.A. (2011). Reproducing Hegemony: The Culture of Enhancement and Discourses on Amphetamines in Popular Fiction. *Cult Med Psychiatry*, Vol. 35, No.1, pp. 90-97.

Micale, V.; Mazzola, C. & Drago, F. (2007). Endocannabinoids and neurodegenerative diseases. *Pharmacol Res.*, Vol. 56, No. 5, pp. 382-392.

Milton, A.L. & Everitt, B.J. (2010). The psychological and neurochemical mechanisms of drug memory reconsolidation: implications for the treatment of addiction. *Eur J Neurosci.* Vol. 31, No.12, pp. 2308-19.

Miyake, N.; Thompson, J.; Skinbjerg, M. & Abi-Dargham, A. (2011). Presynaptic dopamine in schizophrenia. *CNS Neurosci Ther.*, No.17, pp. 104-109.

Moffett, M.C.; Song, J. & Kuhar, M.J. (2011). CART peptide inhibits locomotor activity induced by simultaneous stimulation of D1 and D2 receptors, but not by stimulation of individual dopamine receptors. *Synapse*, No.65, pp. 1-7.

Montague, P.R.; Hyman, S.E. & Cohen J.D. (2004). Computational roles for dopamine in behavioural control. *Nature*, No. 431, pp. 760-767.

Moreira, F.A. & Lutz, B. (2008). The endocannabinoid system: emotion, learning and addiction. *Addict Biol.*, Vol.13, No. 2, pp.196-212.

Muhammad, A.; Hossain, S.; Pellis, S.M. & Kolb, B. (2011a). Tactile stimulation during development attenuates amphetamine sensitization and structurally reorganizes prefrontal cortex and striatum in a sex-dependent manner. *Behav Neurosci*, Vol.125, No.2, pp. 161-74.

Muhammad, A. & Kolb, B. (2011b). Mild Prenatal Stress-Modulated Behavior and Neuronal Spine Density without Affecting Amphetamine Sensitization. *Dev Neurosci.* 2011, May 12, (DOI: 10.1159/000324744), [Epub ahead of print].

Muhammad, A. & Kolb, B. (2011c). Maternal separation altered behavior and neuronal spine density without influencing amphetamine sensitization. *Behav Brain Res.*, Vol.223, No.1, pp. 7-16.

Mukda, S.; Vimolratana, O. & Govitrapong, P. (2011). Melatonin attenuates the amphetamine-induced decrease in vesicular monoamine transporter-2 expression in postnatal rat striatum. *Neurosci Lett.*, No.488, pp. 154-157.

Murray, J.; Belin, D. & Everitt, B.J. (2012) Double dissociation of the dorsomedial and dorsolateral striatum control over the acquisition and performance of cocaine seeking. *Neuropsychopharmacology*, In Press.

Oaks, A.W. & Sidhu, A. (2011). Synuclein modulation of monoamine transporters. *FEBS Lett.*, No.585, pp. 1001-1006.

O'Brien, C.P.; Volkow, N. & Li, T.K. (2006). What's in a word? Addiction versus dependence in DSM-V. *Am J Psychiatry*, No. 163, pp. 764–765.

Paule, M.G. (2005). Chronic drug exposures during development in nonhuman primates: models of brain dysfunction in humans. *Front Biosci.*, No.10, pp. 2240-2249.

Pezze, M.A.; Dalley, J.W. & Robbins, T.W. (2007). Differential roles of dopamine D1 and D2 receptors in the nucleus accumbens in attentional performance on the five-choice serial reaction time task. *Neuropsychopharmacol.* Vol. 32, No.2, pp. 273-83.

Potenza, M.N.; Sofuoglu, M.; Carroll, K.M. & Rounsaville, B.J. (2011). Neuroscience of Behavioral and Pharmacological Treatments for Addictions. *Neuron*, Vol.69, No.4, pp. 695-712.

Rice, M.E. & Cragg, S.J. (2008). Dopamine spillover after quantal release: rethinking dopamine transmission in the nigrostriatal pathway. *Brain Res Rev.*, No.58, pp. 303-313.

Robbins, T.W. & Everitt, B.J. (2002). Limbic-striatal memory systems and drug addiction. *Neurobiol Learn Mem.*, Vol.78, No.3, pp. 625-636.

Robinson, T.E. & Becker, J.B. (1986). Enduring changes in brain and behavior produced by chronic amphetamine administration: a review and evaluation of animal models of amphetamine psychosis. *Brain Res.*, Vol.396, No.2, pp. 157-198.

Robinson, T.E. & Kolb, B. (2004). Structural plasticity associated with exposure to drugs of abuse. *Neuropharmacology*, No.47, pp. 33-46.

Robinson, T.E. & Kolb, B. (2011). Structural plasticity associated with exposure to drugs of abuse. *Neuropharmacology* 2004, No.47, Suppl 1, pp. 33-46.

Rogge, G.; Jones, D.; Hubert, G.W.; Lin, Y. & Kuhar, M.J. (2008). CART peptides: regulators of body weight, reward and other functions. *Nat Rev Neurosci.*, No.9, pp. 747-758.

Runyon, S.P. & Carroll, F.I. (2006). Dopamine transporter ligands: recent developments and therapeutic potential. *Curr Top Med Chem.*, No.6, pp. 1825-1843.

Sae-Ung, K.; Uéda, K.; Govitrapong, P. & Phansuwan-Pujito, P. (2012). Melatonin reduces the expression of alpha-synuclein in the dopamine containing neuronal regions of amphetamine-treated postnatal rats. *J Pineal Res.*, Vol. 52, No. 1, pp. 128-137.

Schmitt, K.C. & Reith, M.E. (2010). Regulation of the dopamine transporter: aspects relevant to psychostimulant drugs of abuse. *Ann N Y Acad Sci.*, No.1187, pp. 316-340.

Schultz, W.; Dayan, P. & Montague, P.R. (1997). A neural substrate of prediction and reward. *Science*, No. 275, pp. 1593-1599.

Schultz, W. (1998). Predictive reward signal of dopamine neurons. *J Neurophysiol.*, No. 80, pp.1–27.

Schultz, W. (2011). Potential vulnerabilities of neuronal reward, risk, and decision mechanisms to addictive drugs. *Neuron*, Vol.69, No.4, pp. 603-617.

Sesack, S.R.; Aoki, C. & Pickel, V.M. (1994). Ultrastructural localization of D2 receptor-like immunoreactivity in midbrain dopamine neurons and their striatal targets. *J Neurosci.*, No.14, pp. 88-106.

Steketee, J.D. (2003). Neurotransmitter systems of the medial prefrontal cortex: potential role in sensitization to psychostimulants. *Brain Res Brain Res Rev.*, Vol.41, No.2-3, pp. 203-228.

Steketee, J.D. (2005). Cortical mechanisms of cocaine sensitization. *Crit Rev Neurobiol.*, Vol.17, No.2, pp. 69-86.

Sulzer, D.; Chen, T.K. ; Lau, Y.Y.; Kristensen, H.; Rayport, S. & Ewing, A. (1995). Amphetamine redistributes dopamine from synaptic vesicles to the cytosol and promotes reverse transport. *J Neurosci.*, No.15, pp. 4102-4108.

Sulzer, D.; Sonders, M.S.; Poulsen, N.W. & Galli, A. (2005). Mechanisms of neurotransmitter release by amphetamines: a review. *Prog Neurobiol.*, No.75, pp. 406-433.

Sulzer, D. (2011). How Addictive Drugs Disrupt Presynaptic Dopamine Neurotransmission. *Neuron*, Vol.69, No.4, pp. 628-649.

Surguchov, A. (2008). Molecular and cellular biology of synucleins. *Int. Rev. Cell Mol. Biol.*, No.270, pp. 225–317.

Stone, J.M.; Bhattacharyya, S.; Barker, G.J. & McGuire, P.K. (2011). Substance use and regional gray matter volume in individuals at high risk of psychosis. *Eur Neuropsychopharmacol.* Vol. 22, No. 2, pp. 114-122.

Swope, S.L.; Moss, S.J.; Raymond, L.A. & Huganir, R.L. (1999). Regulation of ligand-gated ion channels by protein phosphorylation. *Adv Second Messenger Phosphoprotein Res.* No. 33, pp. 49-78.

Tan, H.; Lauzon, N.M.; Bishop, S.F.; Bechard, M.A. & Laviolette, S.R. (2010). Integrated cannabinoid CB1 receptor transmission within the amygdala-prefrontal cortical pathway modulates neuronal plasticity and emotional memory encoding. *Cereb Cortex*, Vol.20, No.6, pp. 1486-1496.

Tan, S.E. (2008). Roles of hippocampal NMDA receptors and nucleus accumbens D1 receptors in the amphetamine-produced conditioned place preference in rats. *Brain Res Bull.*, Vol.77, No.6, pp. 412-419.

Théberge, F.R.; Milton, A.L.; Belin, D.; Lee J.L. & Everitt B.J. (2010). The basolateral amygdala and nucleus accumbens core mediate dissociable aspects of drug memory reconsolidation. *Learn Mem.* Vol. 17, No.9, pp. 444-53.

Thompson, B.L.; Levitt, P. & Stanwood, G.D. (2009). Prenatal exposure to drugs: effects on brain development and implications for policy and education. *Nat Rev Neurosci.*, No.10, pp. 303-312.

Tilley, M.R. & Gu, H.H. (2008). Dopamine transporter inhibition is required for cocaine-induced stereotypy. *Neuroreport*, No.19, pp. 1137-1140.

Tsuang, M.T., Lyons, M.J., Meyer, J.M., Doyle, T., Eisen, S.A, Goldberg, J., True, W., Lin, N., Toomey, R. & Eaves, L. (1998). Co-occurrence of abuse of different drugs in men: The role of drug-specific and shared vulnerabilities. *Arch. Gen. Psychiatry,* 55, pp. 967–972.

Treadway, M.T. and Zald, D.H. (2011). Reconsidering anhedonia in depression: Lessons from translational neuroscience. *Neurosci Biobehav Rev.*, No. 35, pp. 537–555.

Trezza, V.; Cuomo, V. & Vanderschuren, L.J. (2008). Cannabis and the developing brain: insights from behavior. *Eur J Pharmacol.*, Vol.585, No.2-3, pp. 441-452.

Trezza, V.; Campolongo, P.; Manduca, A.; Morena, M.; Palmery, M.; Vanderschuren, L.J. & Cuomo V. (2012). Altering endocannabinoid neurotransmission at critical developmental ages: impact on rodent emotionality and cognitive performance. *Front Behav Neurosci.*, Vol. 6, No. 2, pp. 1-12.

White, N. M. (1996). Addictive drugs as reinforcers: multiple partial actions on memory systems. *Addiction Vol.* 91, No. 7, pp. 921–949.

Volkow, N.D.; Fowler, J.S. & Wang, G.J. (2002a). Role of dopamine in drug reinforcement and addiction in humans:results from imaging studies. *Behav Pharmacol.* No. 13, pp. 355–366.

Volkow, N.D; Wang, G.J.; Fowler, J.S.; Thanos, P.P.; Logan, J.; Gatley, S.J.; Gifford, A.; Ding, Y.S.; Wong, C.; Pappas, N. & Thanos, P. (2002b). Brain DA D2 receptors predict reinforcing effects of stimulants in humans:replication study. *Synapse,* No. 46, pp. 79–82.

Volkow, N.D.; Baler, R.D. & Goldstein, R.Z. (2011). Addiction: pulling at the neural threads of social behaviors. *Neuron*, Vol.69, No.4, pp. 599-602.

Von der Goltz, C. & Kiefer, F. (2009). Learning and memory in the aetiopathogenesis of addiction: future implications for therapy? *Eur Arch Psychiatry Clin Neurosci.*, No.259, Suppl 2, pp. S183-S187.

Welberg, L. (2010). Addiction: Cracking the code of addiction. *Nat Rev Neurosci.*, Vol.11, No.10, p. 668.

WHO (2012). Cannabis. In "*Management of substance abuse*". January 6, 2012. Available from: http://www.who.int/substance_abuse/facts/cannabis/en/

Wise, R.A. (2004). Dopamine, learning and motivation. *Nat Rev Neurosci.*, Vol.5, No. 6, pp.483–494.

Wiskerke, J.; Pattij, T.; Schoffelmeer, A.N. & De Vries T.J. (2008). The role of CB1 receptors in psychostimulant addiction. *Addict Biol.*, Vol.13, No.2, pp. 225-238.

Williams, J.M. & Galli, A. (2006). The dopamine transporter: a vigilant border control for psychostimulant action. *Handb Exp Pharmacol.*, No.175, pp. 215-232.

Yamamoto, S.; Fukae, J.; Mori, H.; Mizuno, Y. & Hattori, N. (2006). Positive immunoreactivity for vesicular monoamine transporter 2 in Lewy bodies and Lewy neurites in substantia nigra. *Neurosci. Lett.*, Vol.396, No.3, pp. 187–191.

Yung, K.K.; Bolam, J.P.; Smith, A.D.; Hersch, S.M.; Ciliax, B.J. & Levey, A.I. (1995). Immunocytochemical localization of D1 and D2 dopamine receptors in the basal ganglia of the rat: light and electron microscopy. *Neuroscience*, No.65, pp. 709-730.

Zapata, A.; Minney, V.L. & Shippenberg, T.S. (2010). Shift from goal-directed to habitual cocaine seeking after prolonged experience in rats. *J Neurosci.*, No. 30, pp.15457–15463.

Zhang, J.; Liu, X.; Lei, X.; Wang, L.; Guo, L.; Zhao, G. & Lin, G. (2010). Discovery and synthesis of novel luteolin derivatives as DAT agonists. Bioorg Med Chem., No.18, pp. 7842-7848.

Zhou, Y.; Cui, C.L.; Schlussman, S.D.; Choi, J.C.; Ho, A.; Han, J.S. & Kreek, M.J. (2008). Effects of cocaine place conditioning, chronic escalating-dose "binge" pattern cocaine administration and acute withdrawal on orexin/hypocretin and preprodynorphin gene expressions in lateral hypothalamus of Fischer and Sprague-Dawley rats. *Neuroscience*, Vol. 153, No. 4, pp.1225-1234.

4

Cocaine Addiction: Changes in Excitatory and Inhibitory Neurotransmission

Edgar Antonio Reyes-Montaño and Edwin Alfredo Reyes-Guzmán
Protein Research Group (Grupo de Investigación en Proteínas, GRIP)
Universidad Nacional de Colombia, Sede Bogotá
Colombia

1. Introduction

The principal routes of cocaine administration are oral, intranasal, intravenous, and inhalation. The slang terms for these routes are, respectively, "chewing," "snorting," "mainlining," "injecting," and "smoking" (including freebase and crack cocaine). Cocaine use ranges from occasional use to repeated or compulsive use, with a variety of patterns between these extremes. There is no safe way to use cocaine. Any route of administration can lead to absorption of toxic amounts of cocaine, allowing to acute cardiovascular or cerebrovascular emergencies that could result in sudden death. Repeated cocaine use by any route of administration can produce addiction and other adverse health consequences. Those who snort or sniff cocaine through their noses suffer damage to their nasal and sinus passages. These include nasal crusting, nosebleeds, nasal congestion, irritation, facial pain caused by sinusitis and hoarseness.

Cocaine addiction changes the responsiveness of the brain to various neurotransmitters or chemicals. The development of drug addiction involves persistent cellular and molecular changes in the Central Nervious System. The brain dopamine, GABA and glutamate systems play key roles in mediating drug-induced neuroadaptation. We show some physiological changes that can occur in some key pathways in which glutamate, dopamine and GABA receptors are involved. These chemical changes cause different effects in users, including: anxiety, confusion, dizziness, psychosis, headaches and nausea.

Cocaine use and addiction affects the sympathetic nervous system (which controls automatic functions such as breathing, heartbeat, etc.). This system secretes adrenaline which raises ones heart rate, narrows blood vessels and significantly increases blood pressure. Chest pain, heart attacks and strokes are common side effects of cocaine use.

The most widely studied neurobiological characteristic of cocaine addiction is the role played by dopamine transmission. It is clear that enhanced dopamine transmission in neurons projecting from the ventral mesencephalon to the limbic forebrain, including the medial prefrontal cortex (mPFC) and nucleus accumbens (NAc), is the pharmacological target for cocaine-induced reinforcement and locomotor stimulation (O' Brien., 2001) However, persistence of the behavioral characteristics of cocaine addiction, such as paranoia (sensitization) and the propensity to relapse years after the acute rewarding effects of the drug have disappeared, indicates that there must also be neuronal substrates undergoing long-term neuroplastic changes. Although studies have endeavored to identify enduring changes in dopamine transmission that might underlie behavioral sensitization and the reinstatement of drug-seeking (relapse), the results have not been entirely consistent with an obligatory role for dopamine.

Addiction can be viewed as a form of drug-induced neural plasticity. One of the best-established molecular mechanisms of addiction is up-regulation of the cAMP second messenger pathway, which occurs in many neuronal cell types in response to chronic administration of opiates or other drugs of abuse. This up-regulation and the resulting activation of the transcription factor CREB appear to mediate aspects of tolerance and dependence. In contrast, induction of another transcription factor, termed 1FosB, exerts the opposite effect and may contribute to sensitized responses to drug exposure. Knowledge of these mechanisms could lead to more effective treatments for addictive disorders.

2. The neurobiology of cocaine addiction

Dopamine acts as a modulator for many nerve cells throughout the brain. Dopamine is responsible for keeping those cells operating at the appropriate levels of activity to accomplish our needs and aims (Nestler., 2005). Whenever we need to mobilize our muscles or mind to work harder or faster, dopamine drives some of the involved brain cells to step up to the challenge (Nestler., 2005). The targets in brain and other organs are shown in figure 1.

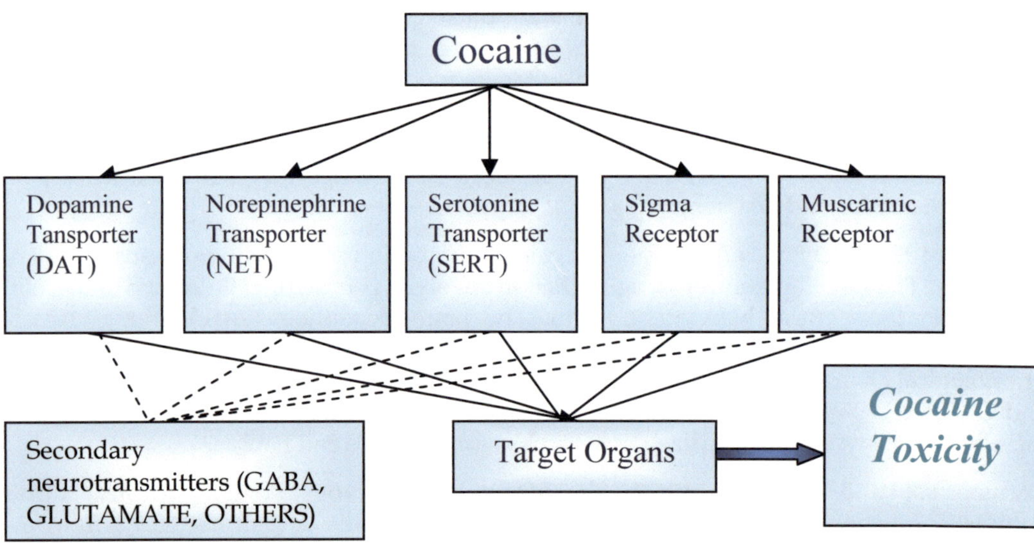

Fig. 1. Cocaine and receptors associated with its toxicity. Continuous lines show the main target organs affected; dashed lines represent the secondary neurotransmitters associated. (Adapted from Nestler., 2005)

Dopamine is originated in dopaminergic neurons and launch them into their surroundings. Some of the free-floating dopamine molecules latch onto receptor proteins on neighboring cells. Once attached, dopamine stimulates the receptors to alter electrical impulses in the receiving cells and thereby alter the cells' function. To keep the receiving cells in each brain region functioning at appropriate intensities for current demands the dopaminergic cells continually increase and decrease the number of dopamine molecules they launch. They further regulate the amount of dopamine available to stimulate the receptors by pulling some previously released dopamine molecules back into themselves (Nestler., 2005).

One of the most addictive drugs is cocaine. Cocaine can act mainly on the mesoaccumbens dopamine (DA) pathway of the midbrain, extending from the ventral tegumental area (VTA) to the nucleus accumbens (NAc). This pathway is also known as the reward pathway as it is the area of the brain that is activated when someone has a pleasurable experience such as eating, sex, or receiving praise. Cocaine interferes with the dopamine control mechanism: It ties up the dopamine transporter. As a result, with cocaine on board, dopamine molecules that otherwise would be picked up remain in action. Dopamine builds up and overactivates the receiving cells. However, DA is not the only system affected by cocaine. Glutamate and neurotransmission mediated for this aminoacid is also modified and has an importantt role in the mechanism of this drug addiction.

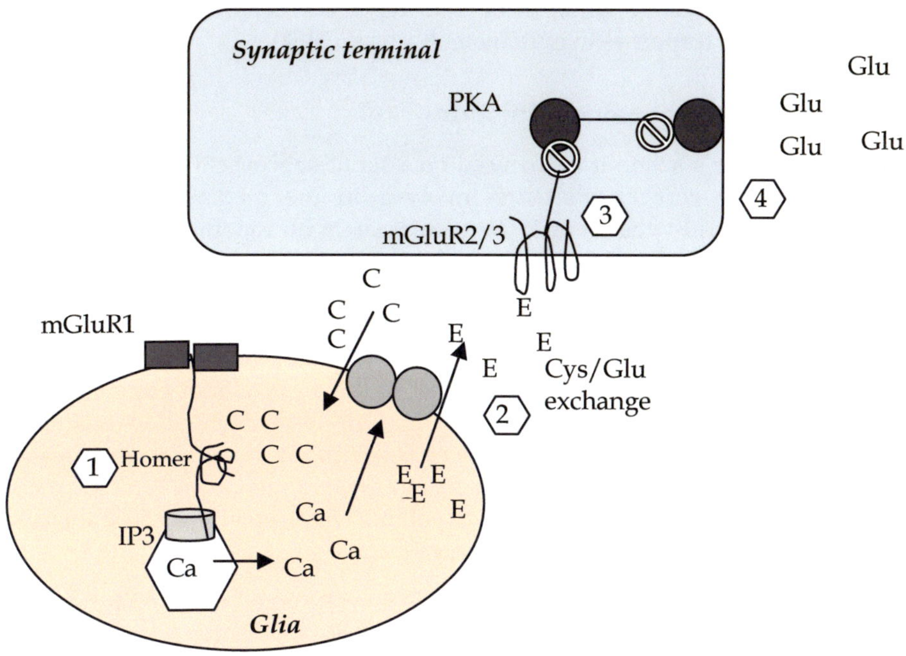

Fig. 2. The potential mechanisms regulating glutamatergic transmission in the NAc that are involved in the reinstatement of drug-seeking behavior. The cocaine-induced changes in extrasynaptic glutamate release outlined below are postulated to increase the signal-to-noise ratio of synaptically released glutamate, thereby facilitating drug-seeking. 1. Homer protein is reduced in the nucleus accumbens, causing a reduction in signaling via mGluR1 receptors through inositol trisphosphate (IP3) receptor regulation of internal calcium (Ca) stores. 2. Because glutamate release stimulated by mGluR1 receptors results from activation of the cystine/glutamate exchanger, it is proposed that down regulated mGluR1 signaling may mediate the reduced activity of the cystine/glutamate exchanger produced by chronic cocaine administration. 3. The reduced heteroexchange of extracellular cystine (C) for intracellular glutamate (E) in glia results in reduced basal extracellular glutamate and reduced tone on mGluR2/3 presynaptic autoreceptors. 4. This reduced tone, accompanied by mGluR2/3 residing in a more phosphorylated (desensitized) state, results in reduced inhibitory regulation of synaptically released glutamate (Glu) (Adapted from Kalivas., 2004)

The way in which this sequence of adaptations could synergize to dysregulate presynaptic glutamate transmission in cocaine addiction is illustrated in Figure 2. This hypothetical model describes how reduced Homer1bc could account for reduced activity of the cystine-glutamate exchanger and the accompanying reduced basal levels of extracellular glutamate. The reduced levels of glutamate, combined with desensitization of the mGluR2/3 receptor, results in a loss of regulatory feedback on synaptic glutamate release. Thus, lower basal levels of glutamate, combined with increased release of synaptic glutamate in response to activation of prefrontal cortical afferents to the NAc, results in an amplified signal and behavioral drive to engage drug seeking (e.g. to relapse). In addition to adaptations in presynaptic and possibly glial release of glutamate that regulate the expression of sensitization and/or reinstatement a variety of changes in postsynaptic glutamate transmission have been documented in the NAc. Interestingly, although presynaptic release of glutamate was augmented by withdrawal from repeated cocaine, most data indicate a reduction in postsynaptic responses to glutamate (Kalivas., 2004).

3. Brain changes during cocaine addiction

Animal studies of cocaine´s action have focused on a set of subcortical gray matter of some structures as paralimbic cortices, that are involved in the mediation of reward and reinforcement, most notably the ventral tegmental area of the midbrain, the nucleus accumbens, the amygdala, and regions of the prefrontal cortex (Makris et al., 2004). Existing studies of brain structure in cocaine users have reported abnormalities only in brain regions connected to the amygdala, such as the orbitofrontal and anterior cingulate cortex (Franklin et al., 2002; Matochik et al., 2003). Markis et al., (2004) sought to evaluate the hypothesis that topological and volumetric abnormalities may exist in the amygdala of cocaine-dependent subjects that may represent a predisposition to cocaine addiction, or an adaptation to protracted exposure to the drug. Amygdala volume and topology were assessed by segmentation-based morphometric analysis, and absolute quantitative volumetric measures were performed. It was observed that amygdala volume of cocaine-dependent subjects was significantly smaller than the one of matched controls.

The amygdala volumes of cocaine-dependent subjects were similar for each hemisphere, whereas those of their matched controls had clear laterality differences. In addition, amygdala volume in addicts did not correlate with (1) measures of anxiety or depression, (2) any measure of the amount of cocaine use, or (3) age at which cocaine use began (Makris et al., 2004)

Barrós-Loscertales et al., (2011) reported reduced gray matter (GM) volume in the striatum and in the supramarginal gyrus. Likewise, another set of cortical and subcortical structures, such as the amygdala, the insula and dorsolateral prefrontal cortex, were seen to have volume reductions related to years of cocaine exposure (Barrós-Loscertales et al., 2011). All these structural changes associated with cocaine addiction seem to merge in the striato-cortico-limbic circuitry linked not only to addiction, but also to the wider set of disinhibitory disorders (Barrós-Loscertales et al., 2011). Although causal relationships are very difficult to determine in human studies, the significant relationship between years of use and reduced GM volumes are consistent with these volumetric effects arising from the cumulative exposure to cocaine or the concomitant lifestyle (e.g., stress) that accompanies prolonged drug use (Yücel et al., 2008).

In other aspects, Ersche et al., (2011) found some differences between healthy and cocaine users, specially in the gray matter abundance in some regions of the brain. There was widespread significant loss of grey matter in orbitofrontal cortex bilaterally in the cocaine user group. Grey matter volume was also abnormally reduced in the insula, the medial frontal and anterior cingulate cortex, temporoparietal cortex and the cerebellum. In contrast to this extensive system of decreased cortical grey matter volume, cocaine users also showed a significant increase of grey matter volume mainly localized to basal ganglia structures (including putamen, caudate nucleus and pallidum), and cerebellum (figure 3).

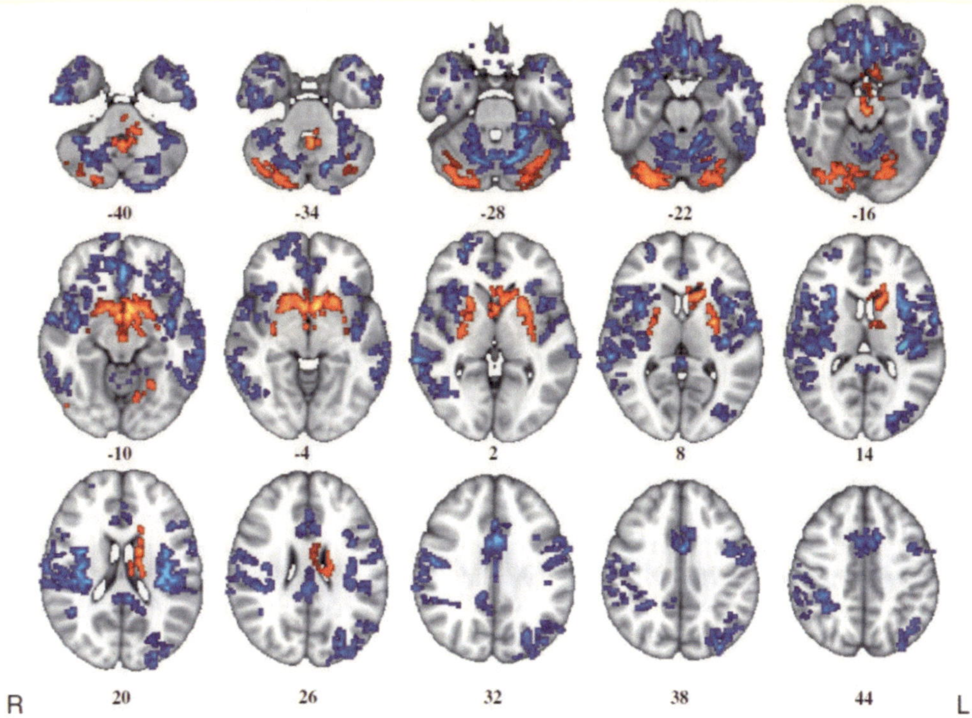

Fig. 3. Whole-brain maps of significant differences in grey matter volume between healthy volunteers and cocaine users. Voxels coloured blue indicate brain areas in which cocaine users have reduced grey matter volume compared with healthy volunteers, and voxels coloured red indicate brain areas in which cocaine users have abnormally increased grey matter volume. These results were generated by permutation testing of voxel cluster statistics with cluster-wise P50.001, at which level we expect less than one false positive cluster per map. The statistical results are overlaid on the FSL MNI152 standard T1 image and the numbers beneath each section of the image refer to its position (mm) relative to the intercommissural plane in standard stereotactic space. L = left; R = right. (Ersche et al., 2011)

In addition, it has been found that the caudate enlargement in cocaine users was associated with significant attentional impairments, whereas the reduction in grey matter in the orbitofrontal cortex was associated with cocaine-related compulsivity. The abnormal changes in grey matter in the striatum and in the orbitofrontal cortex were both related to the duration of cocaine abuse (Ersche et al., 2011).

In another interesting description, Ersche et al., (2011) showed some maps of brain regions demonstrating significant association between grey matter volume and measures of duration of cocaine use, compulsivity and impulsivity in the group of cocaine users (figure 4). This study allow see that is possible find some positive and negative correlations between grey matter and duration of cocaine use, or compulsive cocaine taking or impulsivity in cocaine users.

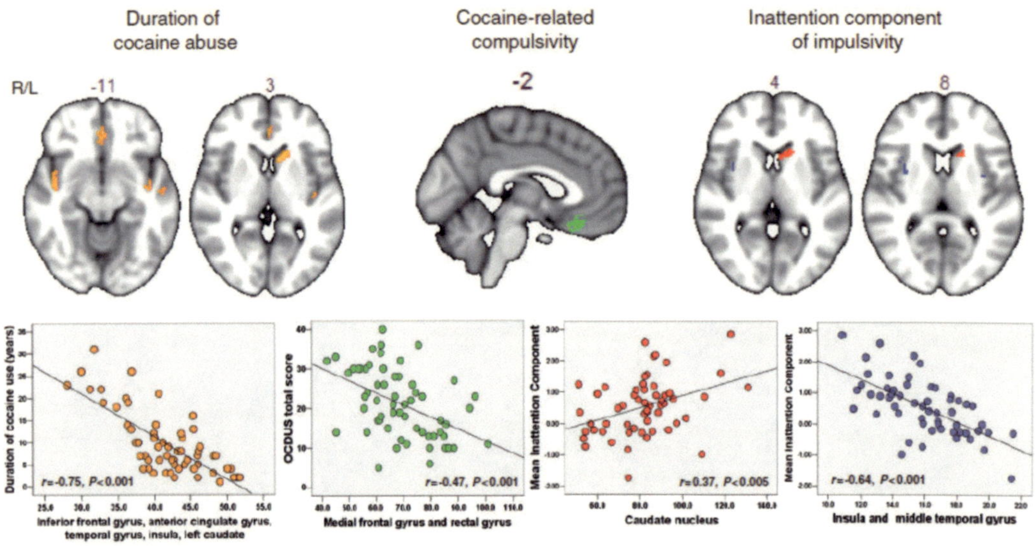

Fig. 4. Maps of brain regions. Regions where grey matter volume correlated significantly with the duration of cocaine use in drug users are indicated in orange. Regions that correlated significantly with compulsive cocaine-taking are coloured in green. Regions where grey matter volume correlated significantly with the inattention component of impulsivity in cocaine users are indicated in red (if the correlation was positive) and blue (if the correlation was negative). The scatter plots beneath each section of the brain image show the correlation between these measures and the total grey matter volume for each drug user. The numbers above each section of the image refer to its plane position (mm) relative to the origin in MNI stereotactic space. L = left; R = right (Ersche et al., 2011).

In addition, there are differences between the cocaine-dependent and healthy groups. For example, the cocaine users had higher depressive scores than the healthy people, and fewer years in formal education (11.5 compared to 12.3 years). Most of the cocaine users also had nicotine dependence (83%), some also had alcohol dependence (27%), cannabis dependence (18%) and heroin dependence (7%). These factors may also have been related to the brain differences seen, rather than just the cocaine use. Morever, Ersche et al., (2011), noted that impulsivity is a complex trait and that the measures they used would not have captured all aspects of it.

4. The signaling pathways involved in cocaine addiction

The drugs of abuse differ greatly in their chemical structure, they act on their own unique target that are mostly proteins involved in synaptic transmission, although different drugs affect different neurotransmitter systems (Nestler, E., 2004).

All addictive drugs facilitate dopamine transmission. The dopamine projection to the prefrontal cortex (PFC), nucleus accumbens (NAc) and amygdala is a primary site of pharmacological action by cocaine, as well as a site where addictive behaviors such as relapse and sensitization can be initiated (Berridge and Robinson., 1998). The regions of the prefrontal cortex most clearly tied to addiction in both neuroimaging studies in addicts and lesion/pharmacological studies in animal models of addiction (rats) are the anterior cingulate/prelimbic cortex and the ventral orbital cortex (Neisewander et al., 2000; Goldstein and Volkow., 2002; Kalivas., 2004).

The NAc is composed of two compartments termed the core and the shell (Zahm and Brog., 1992) and, although the shell is more clearly associated with dopamine-dependent reward, the core has been linked to the enduring cellular changes elicited by repeated use of addictive drugs (Di Ciano and Everitt., 2001; Kalivas and McFarland., 2003). The projections from the amygdala and prefrontal cortex to the nucleus accumbens are glutamatergic, as are the reciprocal connections between the basolateral amygdala and prefrontal cortex (figure 5). The prefrontal cortex also sends glutamatergic efferents to the dopamine cell body region in the ventral tegmental area (VTA). This circuit has primary output through co-localized γ-amino butyric acid (GABA)ergic and peptidergic neurons in the NAc that project to the ventral pallidum (PV) and ventral tegmental area (Kalivas., 2004).

The changes in the NAc, influenced by activation of dopamine receptors, are critically involved in behavioral adaptations (Marinelli and White., 2000). Natural rewards, but also drugs of abuse, increase VTA release of dopamine in downstream structures such as the NAc (Di Chiara, 2002; Schultz., 2002). However, an essential difference between natural rewards and drugs of abuse is that, over time, the dopamine response to the natural rewards, but not drugs of abuse, diminishes (Kalivas and O'Brien., 2008). Additionally, the amount of dopamine released following administration of a drug of abuse, particularly cocaine, typically exceeds what occurs following exposure to a natural reward. Thus, the repeated large release of dopamine is believed to be critical in the development of addiction, as it alters and modifies structures and their connections (Uys and LaLumiere,. 2008).

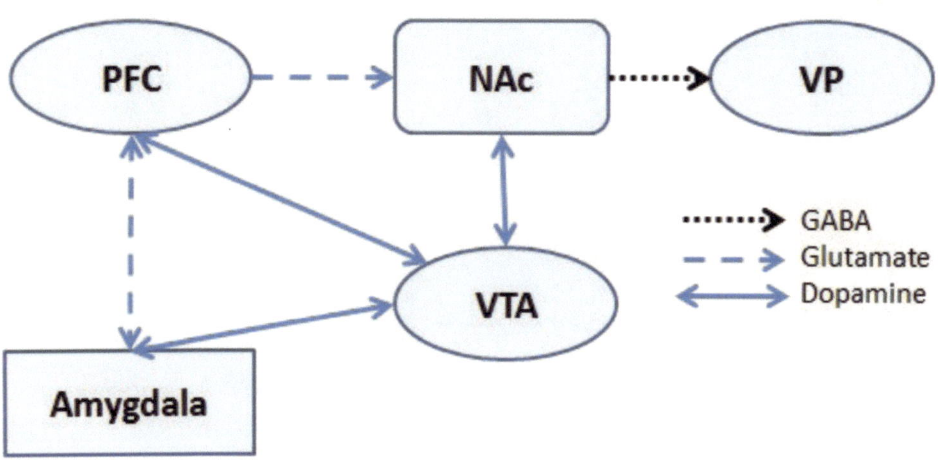

Fig. 5. The schematic diagram identify the critical structures involved in drug reward and relapse to cocaine seeking. VTA, Ventral tegmental area; PFC, Prefrontal cortex; NAc, Nucleus accumbens; VP, Ventral pallidum.

The VTA–NAc, so called mesolimbic, pathway seems to be a site where virtually all drugs of abuse converge to produce their acute reward signals. Two major mechanisms are involved: first, all drugs of abuse increase dopamine-mediated transmission in the NAc, although by very different mechanisms; second, some drugs also act directly on NAc neurons by dopamine-independent mechanisms (Everitt and Wolf., 2002).

An interesting point is the intracellular event precipitated by stimulation of dopamine receptors as a result of repeated use of cocaine. In dopamine D1 receptor stimulation of cAMP-dependent protein kinase (or PKA) and subsequent changes in protein function and gene expression in the NAc and VTA appear critical to establishing sensitization (Nestler., 2001). The most well-characterized effect of increased cAMP-dependent protein kinase activity is the induction of cAMP response element and the subsequent change in ΔFosB and cyclin-dependent kinase 5 (Nestler et al., 2001; Lu et al., 2003). In addition to the immediate consequences of dopamine receptor signaling, calcium/calmodulin and ras/mitogen-activated protein kinase activity in the ventral tegmental area are critical for the development of sensitization (figure 6). The dopamine D1 receptor stimulation–dependent activation of L-type Ca^{2+} channels and CaMKII facilitates the reinstatement of cocaine seeking by promoting the transport of GluA1-containing AMPA receptors in the NAc shell to the plasma membrane. The CaMKII activity in the NAc shell may be an essential link between dopamine and glutamate systems involved in the neuronal plasticity underlying cocaine craving and relapse (figure 6). (Wolf et al., 2004; Boehm and Malinow., 2005; Schmidt and Pierce., 2010).

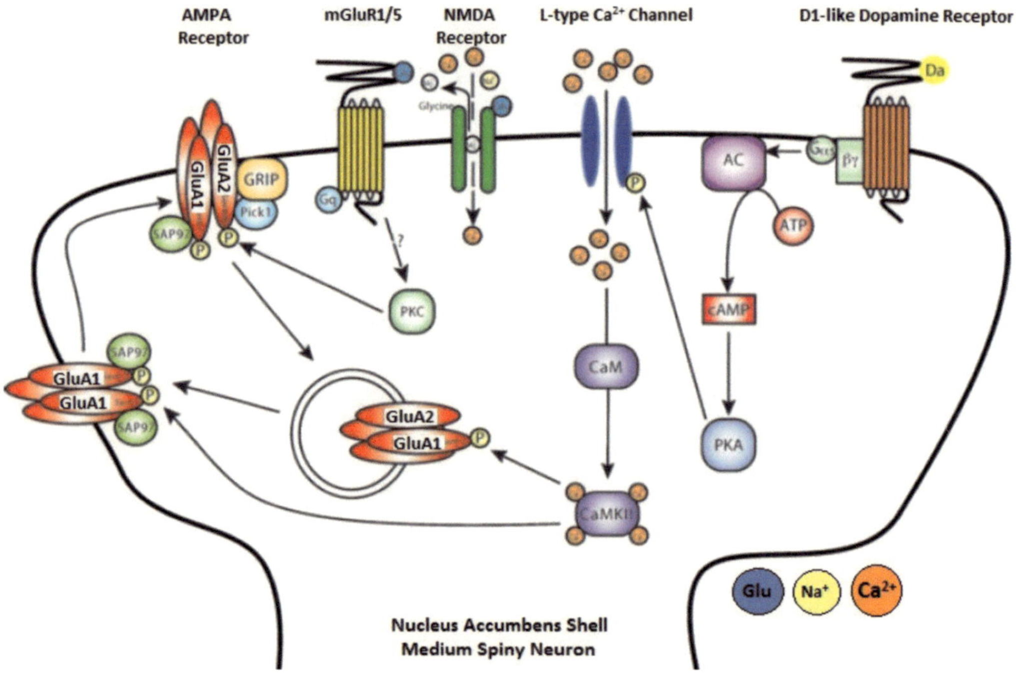

Fig. 6. Pathway between NAc shell dopamine and glutamate systems, via L-type Ca^{2+} channels and Ca^{2+}/calmodulin kinase II (CaMKII), which is proposed to underlie the reinstatement of cocaine seeking. (Adapted from Schmidt and Pierce., 2010).

In contrast to dopamine, glutamate transmission appears to be a primary contributor in the majority of examples of enduring neuroplasticity in the brain, and the development and expression of cocaine addiction is no exception (Winder et al., 2002). The activation of glutamatergic efferents from the amygdala and prefrontal cortex is critical in the expression of addictive behaviors.

Cocaine indirectly influences glutamate transmission in the limbic system, including the NAc, producing persistent changes in neuronal function that can alter the behavioral effects that generate this drug. (Gass and Olive., 2008; Uys and LaLumiere., 2008; Thomas et al., 2008). Thus, maladaptive forms of neuroplasticity in the NAc contribute to cocaine-seeking behavior, and reversing these cocaine-induced neuroadaptations in glutamatergic transmission may prevent relapse of cocaine taking.

The interaction between glutamate and dopamine in VTA and NAc is rather complex, but in simplified terms, glutamatergic input to the VTA increases the activity of dopaminergic cells and enhances dopamine release in the NAc (Tzschentke., 2001). At the level of the NAc, glutamate also facilitates dopaminergic transmission, presumably by presynaptically influencing dopamine release (Floresco et al., 1998; Tzschentke and Schmidt., 2003).

5. The role of glutamate, and GABA receptors in cocaine addiction

The glutamate as neurotransmitter interacts with specific ionotropic glutamate receptors (iGluR) or metabotropic glutamate receptors (mGluR) (Dingledine et al., 1999; Cull-Candy et al., 2001). The ionotropic family of glutamate receptors consists of three subfamilies of tetrameric receptors; *N*-methyl-D-aspartate (NMDA) receptors, α-amino-3-hydroxy-5-methylisoxazole-4-propionic acid receptors (AMPAR), and kainate receptors. Agonist binding induces a conformation change in NMDA, AMPA, and kainate receptors that increases the probability of channel opening. Different subunit compositions of ionotropic glutamate receptors produce functionally diverse NMDA, AMPA, and kainate receptors that are expressed differently throughout the brain (Dingledine et al., 1999).

The latter are the G protein-coupled receptor. Through various G proteins, they connect to multiple second messenger systems. There are three functional groups of mGluRs (group I–III) classified from eight subtypes (mGluR1–8) (Conn and Pin., 1997). Group I mGluRs (mGluR1/5 subtypes) are positively coupled to phospholipase Cβ1 through Gαq proteins. Activation of mGluR1/5 increases phosphoinositol hydrolysis, resulting in intracellular Ca^{2+} release and protein kinase C (PKC) activation (Conn and Pin, 1997). Both group II (mGluR2/3) and group III (mGluR4/6/7/8) receptors are negatively coupled to adenylyl cyclase through Gαi/o proteins. Their activation reduces cAMP formation and inhibits protein kinase A (PKA).

Group I mGlu receptors can also couple Homer proteins through a Homer-phosphatidyl-inositol 3-kinase enhancer (PIKE) adaptor complex (Szumlinski et al., 2008). This is particularly important for mGlu receptor trafficking into and out of the synapse and also to functionally connect mGlu to iGlu receptors.

5.1 Ionotropic receptors and cocaine

The glutamate neurotransmission in the NAc core is necessary for cocaine-induced behaviors, which are regulated by AMPA receptors (Pierce et al., 1996). In addition, chronic cocaine treatment changes iGluR's in both the PFC and NAc. In cocaine sensitized rats, there is an increase in GluN2B receptors in the NAc shell and decreased Tyr1472 phosphorylation in the NAc core with an increase in GluA1 Ser845 phosphorylation in the PFC, NAc shell and core (Zhang et al., 2007). Interestingly, glutamate receptor trafficking may be highly relevant for cocaine-induced neuroplasticity (Lau and Zukin., 2007).

Dopamine D1 receptor stimulation of rat PFC cortical neurons increases surface expression of GluA1-containing AMPA receptors through a protein kinase A-dependent mechanism (Sun et al., 2005). Cocaine self-administration increases synaptic GluA2-lacking AMPA receptors in the NAc after withdrawal (Conrad et al., 2008). Likewise when sensitized animals are re-exposed to cocaine after 10–14 days of withdrawal, both AMPAR surface expression and AMPA/NMDA ratio were shown to be decreased 24 h later (Boudreau et al., 2007; Ferrario et al., 2010; Kourrich et al., 2007; Thomas et al., 2001). GluA2-lacking AMPA receptors may therefore be a novel target for treating cocaine addiction.

The effect of repeated cocaine exposure on the cellular distribution of AMPARs is of functional significance because it has been shown that drug seeking requires AMPAR transmission in the NAc (Cornish and Kalivas, 2000; Di Ciano and Everitt, 2001) and that enhanced AMPAR transmission in the NAc is associated with enhanced drug seeking (Anderson et al., 2008; Conrad et al., 2008; Suto et al., 2004; Wolf and Ferrario, 2010).

Carrie et al., (2011) showed effects of a single cocaine exposure in rats and the difference from those previously reported after repeated cocaine administration. They further suggested that cocaine exerts these effects by influencing neuronal circuits rather than simply stimulating NAc DA transmission.

Cocaine injection administered to rats pretreated with repeated cocaine injections results in increased glutamate release in the NAc core (McFarland et al., 2003; Pierce et al., 1996; Hotsenpiller et al., 2001). There are different neuroadaptations in the accumbens core and the accumbens shell. When cocaine is injected during withdrawal from repeated cocaine exposure, occurs that cocaine decreased presynaptic glutamate immunoreactivity in the accumbens core, but not the accumbens shell (Kozell et al., 2003, 2004). Similarly, cocaine-induced reinstatement of drug seeking was associated with increased glutamate release in the core of the nucleus accumbens, an effect that is attenuated by pharmacological inactivation of the medial prefrontal cortex (mPFC) (McFarland et al., 2003). Then, the administration of an AMPA receptor antagonist into the NAc blocked the reinstatement of cocaine seeking induced by administration of cocaine directly into the mPFC (Park et al., 2002). The activation of the glutamatergic projection from the mPFC to the NAc promotes cocaine seeking (Park et al., 2002)., a finding supported by brain imaging studies of human cocaine addicts, which demonstrate that cocaine craving is associated with metabolic activation of the mPFC (Volkow et al., 2005). These findings also demonstrate that stimulation of AMPA glutamate receptors in the NAc plays a critical role in cocaine seeking (Schmidt and Pierce., 2010).

Has been established an association (correlation) between AMPAR phosphorylation and enduring behavioral plasticity (behavioral sensitization and more significantly drug-seeking behavior), although a causal link between them remains to be proven experimentally (Mao et al., 2011). S845/S831 phosphorylation is likely to be up-regulated to increase surface AMPAR expression thereby enhancing AMPAR transmission related to behavioral plasticity (Boudreau and Wolf, 2005; Conrad et al., 2008). However, self-administration of cocaine induced lesser S845 phosphorylation in the striatum as compared to acute cocaine injection, establishing a tolerance of S845 phosphorylation in response to chronic cocaine (Edwards et al., 2007). This tolerance may reflect a down-regulated GluA1 function in accumbens neurons and may contribute to cocaine sensitization and cocaine-seeking behavior (Sutton et al., 2003; Bachtell et al., 2008). These imply a phosphorylation-dependent mechanism for AMPAR plasticity and drug-seeking (Mao et al., 2011).

In terms of NMDA receptors there is evidence that links post-translational modifications of glutamate receptors to excitatory synaptic plasticity and drug-seeking behavior (Di Ciano, Everitt, 2001). Generally, modification processes of striatal glutamate receptors are sensitive to addictive drugs such as cocaine.

Dopamine D2 receptors are involved in the regulation of NMDA receptor phosphorylation (Liu et al., 2006). A single dose of cocaine induced a heteroreceptor complex formation between D2 receptors and GluN2B-containing NMDA receptor in D2 receptor-bearing striatopallidal neurons. The interaction of D2 receptors with GluN2B disrupted the association of CaMKII with GluN2B, thereby reducing phosphorylation at the CaMKII-sensitive site S1303 and inhibiting NMDA receptor currents. Behaviorally, this phosphorylation, involving D2–GluN2B interaction, suppressed the inhibitory indirect pathway to promote a full motor response to cocaine. Chronic cocaine reduced GluN1 S896 phosphorylation in the rat frontal cortex at 24 h, although not 14 days after of withdrawal (Loftis and Janowsky, 2002). However, acute, repeated, and self-administration of cocaine increased GluN1 S897 phosphorylation in the rat striatum (Edwards et al., 2007). Then the fact that S897 is a sensitive site modified by cocaine can show the importance of post-translational modifications in NMDA receptor plasticity and drug craving (Mao et al., 2011; Hemby et al., 2005).

5.2 Metabotropic receptors and cocaine

An acute injection of cocaine did not alter the total accumbal expression of mGluR5 protein but was enough to reduce surface expression of mGluR5 in the nucleus accumbens, suggesting that trafficking of mGluRs plays a critical role in cocaine-induced synaptic plasticity (Fourgeaud et al., 2004). There is evidence that indicates that mGluR2/3 and mGluR5 proteins are redistributed to the synaptosomal membrane fraction after a period of extended, but not acute, forced abstinence (Ghasemzadeh et al., 2009).

In fact, mGluR2/3s have already been demonstrated to play a key role in the excessive glutamate release believed to promote drug-seeking (Kalivas, 2004). Acute and chronic cocaine treatment alter the normal function, expression or traficking of group I metabotropic receptors in the NAc of rats (Mitrano et al., 2008). A single injection of cocaine decreases the proportion of plasma membrane-bound mGluR1a in the NAc shell dendrites 45 minutes after the injection, while chronic cocaine treatment decreased mGluR1a in the NAc core dendrites. This is in contrast to acute and chronic cocaine treatment having no effect on the localization of mGluR5 receptors (Mitrano et al., 2008). Another study found a decrease in mGluR1a in the NAc shell of chronic cocaine treated rats (Ary and Szumlinski., 2007; Uys and LaLumiere., 2008). Mice lacking mGluR5 receptors do not self-administer cocaine or show an increase in locomotor activity after cocaine treatment, despite having a similar increase in dopamine levels in the NAc as compared to wild-type mice (Chiamulera et al., 2001). Activation of the perisynaptic group II mGluR receptors, mGluR2/3, decreases presynaptic glutamate release in the NAc (Xi et al., 2002; Moran et al., 2005)

Likewise the cocaine-induced plasticity in excitatory synapses within the NAc initiates adaptive changes in neuronal ensembles that lead to drug-seeking behavior and alters subsequent physiological responses to cocaine, including increased trafficking and surface expression of AMPA receptors, during protracted withdrawal (Schmidt and Pierce., 2010).

Glutamate receptors antagonists produce undesirable side effects on neurological functions. Therefore, modulation, rather than blockade, of glutamatergic transmission would be more advantageous. Accordingly, glutamate transmission-modulating agents have emerged as possible therapeutic compounds in preclinical and clinical studies (Kalivas, 2004).

5.3 GABA in cocaine addiction

GABA is an inhibitory neurotransmitter that is found primarily in the brain. As mentioned previously, the VTA plays a role in the reinforcing effects of most drugs of abuse, including cocaine, and consists of both dopaminergic and GABAergic cell bodies along with afferent terminals containing a variety of neurotransmitters. Then GABA acts as the primary inhibitory neurotransmitter in the VTA, and the GABAergic environment in the VTA has been understudied in the realm of cocaine abuse. High GABA levels result in low levels of dopamine. However cocaine diminishes transmission through of type a GABA-A receptor on dopaminergic cells in the VTA, and stimulation of other GABA-B receptor, instead, can counteract the reinforcing properties of cocaine.

The activation of GABA-A and GABA-B receptors inhibit VTA neurons, reduce dopamine release, and reduce cocaine-induced increases in extracellular dopamine (Klitenick et al., 1992; Fadda et al., 2003). GABA-A receptors are also located on GABAergic interneurons presynaptic to dopaminergic VTA neurons, and activation of these receptors would be predicted to inhibit GABAergic interneurons, disinhibit VTA neurons, enhance dopamine release, and enhance cocaine-induced increases in extracellular dopamine (Klitenick et al., 1992; Xi and Stein, 1998). Now, given the interactions between GABA and dopaminergic systems, GABAergic ligands may be useful for modifying some of the abuse-related effects of cocaine. Then the use of an among mechanistically diverse GABA agonists, high-efficacy GABA-A modulators may be the most effective for modifying the abuse-related effects of cocaine (Barrett et al., 2005).

On the other hand, acute cocaine toxicity is frequently associated with seizures. The mechanisms underlying the convulsant effect of cocaine are not well understood. Previously, studies have shown that cocaine depresses whole-cell current evoked by gamma-aminobutyric acid (GABA) in hippocampal neurons freshly isolated from rats. Cocaine's effect was voltage-independent and concentration-dependent. Ye and Ren, (2006), suggest that cocaine induces an increase from intracellular calcium [Ca]i, which stimulates phosphatase activity and thus leads to dephosphorylation of GABA receptors. This dephosphorylation-mediated disinhibitory action may play a role in cocaine-induced convulsant states.

6. Therapeutical targets for cocaine addiction

Studying the pathways involved in cocaine addiction, it is possible to know that pharmaceutical industries are hardly working on pharmacotherapies to treat this addiction and that must be directed toward the molecular transductors of abnormalities found in cocaine users. In the present section, we´ll show some of the most used pharmacotherapies and the usual targets that are regulated for them. In general, we can say that most of those therapies have been used firstly in other pathologies and assayed in cocaine addiction according to their action mode or target.

Topiramate: is a sulphamatefructopyranose derivative, thought to antagonize a drug's rewarding effects by inhibiting mesocorticolimbic dopamine release via the gamma aminobutyric acid (GABA) activity and inhibition of glutamate function after drug intake. Through this activity, topiramate may decrease extracellular release of dopamine in the VTA projecting to the nucleus accumbens. This action may mediate drug-seeking behaviors and craving by reducing the rewarding effects associated with drug use (Johnson et al., 2004).

Disulfiram: inhibits plasma and microsomal carboxylesterases and plasma cholinesterase that inactivate cocaine systemically thereby increasing blood levels of cocaine without any cardiovascular toxicity. Another important role is that disulfiram chelates copper, and since copper is essential in the function of the dopamine beta-hydroxylase enzyme, disulfiram inhibits the conversion of dopamine to norepinephrine. Dopamine betahydroxylase inhibition by disulfiram leads to decreases in peripheral and central norepinephrine and increases in dopamine levels. This effect is believed to contribute to disulfiram's efficacy in treating cocaine addiction (McCance-Katz et al., 1998)

Ondansetron: Post-synaptic 5-HT3 receptors are located densely on the terminals of corticomesolimbic dopamine containing neurons, where they promote DA release. A primary effect of ondansetron a 5-HT3 antagonist is to decrease dopamine release, especially under suprabasal conditions in these regions (Haile et al., 2009)

Baclofen: is a GABA B receptor agonist used to reduce muscle spasticity in different neurological diseases. It is believed to modulate cocaine-induced dopamine release in the nucleus accumbens. In animal studies baclofen was found to reduce cocaine self-administration, reinstatement, and cocaine seeking behaviors in rats suggesting its potential utility as a medication for treatment of cocaine addiction. In humans, an open label study found that baclofen 20 taken three times daily significantly reduced cocaine craving in cocaine-dependent subjects. However, this trial had a sample size of 10 and did not have a placebo arm. An analysis of the same data found that baclofen significantly reduced cocaine use in the subgroup of patients with the heaviest cocaine use only (Fadda et al., 2003)

Modafinil: a functional stimulant, is FDA approved for the treatment of narcolepsy and idiopathic hypersomnia. The mechanisms underlying modafinil's therapeutic actions remain unknown. It is believed to occupy both the dopamine and norepinephrine transporters consistent with a stimulant like effect. In addition, modafinil appears to increase release of the excitatory neurotransmitter glutamate, and decrease the inhibitory neurotransmitter GABA. Modafinil is usually well tolerated, although up to 3% of patients on modafinil experienced cardiovascular side-effects such as hypertension, tachycardia, and palpitations. Because of its stimulant-like activity, modafinil was suggested and later tested as a treatment for cocaine dependence. It was believed to diminish not only the symptoms of cocaine withdrawal, but also act as a "substitution treatment" for cocaine (Ballon and Feifel., 2006).

Naltrexone: (NTX) has long been available as an orally available antagonist at opioid receptors, with a relative selectivity for the μ-opioid receptor at lower doses. It was originally studied as a potential treatment for opiate dependence, where it seems to be effective in special cases, but not across the broad range of patients. NTX taps into known EtOH actions in a seemingly logical manner. EtOH administration leads to release of endogenous opioid peptides, and one of the downstream effects of this is to activate mesolimbic dopamine (DA) release. This in turn contributes to acute positive reinforcing properties of drugs of abuse (Kreek et al., 2002). Consistant with this chain of events, μ-receptor null-mutant mice do not self-administer EtOH (Roberts et al., 2000; Heilis and Egli., 2006).

Other medications that interact with GABA- or glutamate-mediated neuronal systems have been tried as potential treatment for cocaine dependence. While there is preclinical evidence that acamprosate can inhibit conditioned place preference to cocaine and attenuates both drug and cue-induced reinstatement of cocaine-seeking behavior there is to date, no clinical trial testing its utility in treating humans with cocaine dependence. Gabapentin is another gabanergic drug used to treat both epilepsy and neuropathic pain. Its exact pharmacological mechanism remains unclear. Gabapentin has showed some promising results in an open-label study and case series suggesting that it might have utility in the treatment of cocaine dependence. There are encouraging preclinical data that support the utility of vigabatrin as a treatment agent for cocaine dependence. Vigabatrin is another anticonvulsant that increases GABA neurotransmission but this time by inhibiting GABA transaminase. It is a drug with great potentials but needs to be tested in adequately powered placebo controlled randomized studies. Tiagabine is yet another anticonvulsant that increases GABA neurotransmission by blocking the presynaptic reuptake of GABA. In 2 randomized clinical trials involving cocaine dependent patients who were maintained on methadone, tiagabine (12-24 mg/day) was found to decrease cocaine use compared with placebo (Bowers et al., 2007; Gonzalez et al., 2003) .

Finally, the use of stimulants has been tried for the treatment of cocaine dependence under the premise of a drug substitution for a drug with slower onset formulation and less abuse liability. Methylphenidate, a dopamine and nerepinephrine reuptake inhibitor used to treat attention deficit hyperactivity disorders (ADHD) was found to be no better than placebo in the treatment of cocaine dependent patients without comorbid ADHD. However when used in a population with dual diagnosis of cocaine dependence and ADHD, results from clinical trials were mixed. While a controlled clinical trial using immediate release methylphenidate (90 mg/day) found no difference between the active drug and placebo groups, another trial using sustained release methylphenidate (60 mg/day), found significant improvement in ADHAD symptoms that were associated with decrease in cocaine use compared with placebo. Though medications such as those that facilitate gabaergic function, modulate dopaminergic function or act as an agonist replacement therapy show promise in treating cocaine dependence, there are certain drawbacks (Levin et al., 2007).

Other authors (Heilis and Egli., 2006) have organized medication used in cocaine addiction in three different groups. The medications described in past paragraphs are classified in the "first wave: currently available treatments" and "second wave: the near future". Those medications have been used in mixes between them and have shown interesting results.

Table 1 summarizes some aspects related to treatment and targets of first, and second wave medications.

Medication	Group (wave)	Target, mechanism	References
Disulfiram	First	Blocking aldehyde dehydrogenase (alcohol treatment), and dopamine beta-hydroxylase (cocaine dependence)	Carroll et al., 2004
Naltrexone (NTX)	First	Antagonist at opioid receptors	Kirchmayer et al., 2000
Acamprosate (ACM)	First	Glutamate antagonist, attenuates NMDA signaling through spermidine site and actions at metabotropic glutamate receptors	Spanagel & Zieglgansberger, 1997; Harris et al., 2002.
NTX and ACM mixed	First	Opioid receptors, NMDA receptors and metabotropic receptors	Rist et al., 2005; Spanagel & Mann, 2005.
Ondansetron	Second	Serotonin receptors	Higgins et al., 1992; Meert, 1993; Tomkins et al., 1995.
Baclofen	Second	Agonist at GABA-B receptor. Treatment when in detected additional alcohol dependence	Stromberg, 2004.
Topiramate	Second	Proposed effects: blockade of voltage dependent sodium channels, antagonism of kainite receptors and potentiation of GABA signaling through increased GABA availability	Zona et al., 1997; Gryder & Rogawski, 2003; Kaminski et al., 2004, White et al.,1997

Table 1. Medications used in cocaine dependence, showing its classification and possible mechanism (or target) of action. The main use of those medications is in alcohol dependence treatment but they have shown good results in other dependences as cocaine addiction (adapted from Heilis and Egli., 2006)

The third wave medications in cocaine addiction have been used with promising results. The development of pharmacotherapy for cocaine addiction is based on previous strategies designed to alleviate other chemical dependencies such as alcoholism and opiate addiction, focusing on the neurobiological and the behavioral bases of addiction. To date, however, no pharmacotherapy has been approved by the U.S. Food and Drug Administration for cocaine dependence, but two major classes of medications have been investigated: (1) dopaminergic agents and (2) antidepressants. Studies have been relatively brief for both types of agents and have focused on abstinence initiation rather than on relapse prevention. In addition to dopaminergic agents and antidepressants, other compounds such as calcium channel blockers, have been examined as potential treatments of cocaine dependence (figure 7) (Carrera et al., 2004)

In the first group, some dopaminergic agents have been used based on the theory that chronic cocaine use reduces the efficiency of central DA neurotransmission, several dopaminergic compounds, including amantadine, bromocriptine, mazindol, and methylphenidate, have been examined as treatments for cocaine abuse. Investigators hoped that these dopaminergic agents, which have a fast onset of action, would correct the DA dysregulation and alleviate the withdrawal symptoms that often follow cessation of stimulant use.

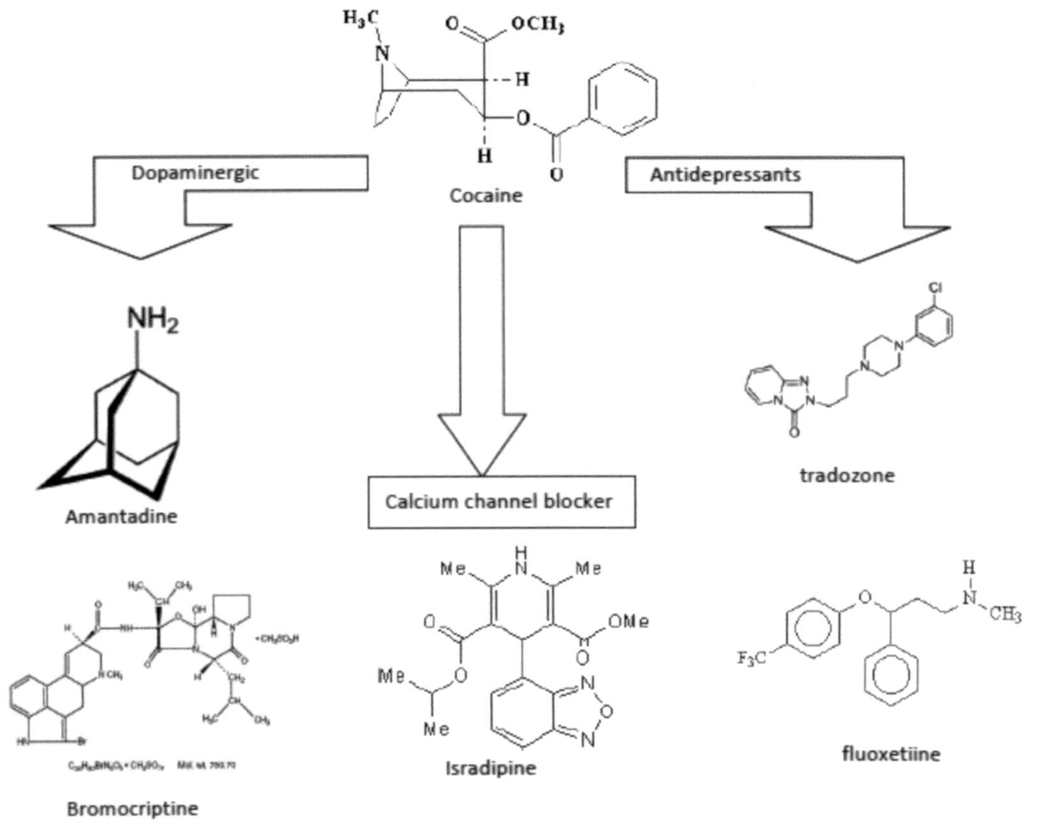

Fig. 7. Classification of medications used for cocaine addiction, based on target and mechanism of action (based on Carrera et al., 2004).

Large array of cocaine analogues and other dopamine uptake inhibitors (see Table 2) including analogues of WIN-35,065, GBR-12909, nomifensine, and benztropine have been developed in the last years. The largest class of compound studies is the class of 3-phenyltropane analogues, of which many hundreds have been made and tested. The analogues RTI-112 and PTT are in preclinical evaluation. Like cocaine, RTI-112 and PTT both have good affinity for all three monoamine transporters, but in contrast to cocaine they enter the brain slowly and are long-lasting. A number of other 3-phenyltropanes are potent and selective for the dopamine transporter relative to inhibition of serotonin and norepinephrine transporters, are long-lasting, and also enter the brain more slowly than cocaine, for example, RTI-113 and RTI-177 (Carrera et al., 2004).

The effect of inhibiting neurotransmitter uptake is to stimulate neurotransmitter receptors; thus the use of direct receptor agonists as substitute agonist medications also has been suggested. Data on dopamine receptor agonists have been extensively reviewed. Animal studies indicate that dopamine receptor agonists such as apomorphine and bromocriptine maintain self-administration in rodents.

Compound	CNS target
RTI-113, RTI-177, GBR-12909	DA uptake inhibitors (selective for DAT)
Mazindol, methyl phenidate, nomifensine, benztropine	DA uptake inhibitors (not selective)
Apomorphine, bromocriptine, SKF38393, quinpirole	DA receptor agonists and partial agonist
Desipramine	Antagonist of cocaine binding that spare DA uptake
Fluoxetine, alaproclate	5HT uptake inhibitors
Quipazine	5HT receptor agonist
Ketanserin, ritanserin, ondansetron	Calcium channel blockers

Table 2. List of some compounds that have been used as pharmacotherapy in cocaine addiction and target identified in Central Nervous System (adapted from Carrera et al., 2004)

The second class of medications used to treat cocaine dependence, antidepressants, are thought to down regulate synaptic catecholamine receptors, and this action is opposite to the presynaptic up-regulation caused by chronic stimulant use. Although antidepressants have a relatively benign side-effect profile, good patient compliance rates, and lack of abuse liability, they have a delayed onset of action ranging from 10 to 20 days. Therefore, the physician may consider beginning antidepressant treatment during early withdrawal and continuing for weeks or longer as clinically indicated. The tricyclic antidepressant desipramine has been studied most extensively as a treatment of cocaine dependence. Early studies of desipramine to treat cocaine dependence showed positive results but placebo-controlled trials have not produced impressive findings. A meta-analysis of placebo-controlled studies by Levin and Lehman showed that although desipramine did not improve retention in treatment, it did produce greater cocaine abstinence relative to placebo. However, treatment with desipramine has induced "early tricyclic jitteriness syndrome" and cocaine craving, as well as relapse to cocaine use in some patients. Therefore, desipramine as pharmacotherapy would hold serious clinical caveats. Additional studies have focused on the involvement of the 5HT3 receptor subtype in the neuropharmacology of cocaine, but the results obtained are somewhat inconsistent. Several 5HT3-selective antagonists, including MDL-72222 and ondansetron were reported to attenuate cocaine-induced locomotor activityin rodents. However, ondansetron failed to block the reinforcing or discriminative-stimulus effects of cocaine in rodents. Several other antidepressants, including fluoxetine, sertraline, and trazodone, that work predominantly through serotonergic mechanisms also have been used as pharmacotherapy for cocaine dependence. Although some reports indicated that treatment with fluoxetine reduced cocaine craving and use in cocaine-abusing heroin addicts, other investigators have not found fluoxetine to be effective in attenuating cocaine use and withdrawal symptoms. Bupropion, a "second-generation" antidepressant, has been studied as pharmacotherapy for cocaine dependence (Heilis and Egli., 2006; Carrera et al., 2004)

Various studies suggest that L-type calcium channel blockers potentially reduce the rewarding effects of cocaine. One such compound, the L-type calcium channel blocker isradipine (Fig. 7), attenuated the cocaine induced dopamine release in the striatum of rats. Another report described isradipine-induced attenuation of condition place preference and the discriminative stimulus properties of cocaine. Also, pretreatment with isradipine resulted in a dose-dependent decrease in intravenous cocaine self-administration. Because of the antihypertensive quality of calcium channel blockers, the potential increase in cardiac output in patients with normal ventricular function could complicate their use as pharmacotherapies for cocaine abuse (Carrera et al., 2004)

Notwithstanding the impressive amount of research effort in this area, a large number of studies using dopaminergic drugs have failed to yield encouraging results. To date, no pharmacotherapeutic agent of this type used on an experimental basis has been shown effectiveness that would merit medical implementation.

7. Perspectives

The fact that GABA and glutamate are so widely present makes it likely that they will be altered during drug addiction. This fact also makes it difficult to treat addiction with drug therapy. Say that a drug affects GABA and glutamate in way that relieves craving. Because GABA and glutamate are so widely present, these drugs could produce a mess of side effects as well. If we had drugs that could selectively stimulate or block certain receptors, then we could treat addiction and avoid doing people more harm than good.

Treatment studies should continue the present emphases on (1) identifying and systematically testing pharmacological agents that may be useful in achieving abstinence from cocaine and reducing the likelihood of relapse; (2) characterizing and understanding the processes and outcomes of existing treatments by using field studies with outcomes studied over a 1-year post treatment period and longer; and (3) testing the efficacy of specific psychosocial interventions such as psychotherapies, behavioral treatments, and relapse prevention strategies. The need for theory-based treatment approaches should be recognized. Promising pharmacotherapies also should be field tested in clinical programs to understand issues related to compliance with medication regimens.

Recent efforts to discover new pharmacs have been oriented to get a vaccine for cocaine addiction. However, to improve existing treatment, there should be a systematic effort to integrate research and treatment. Research should develop and test criteria for client-treatment matching so that the most cost-effective treatments can be provided for cocaine dependent users. Additional research should focus on better understanding motivation as a factor for increasing the retention of cocaine users in treatment. This focus would include use of motivational incentives to enter and remaining treatment. There is a need to better understand the role of self-help in treating cocaine users.

Additional studies for the current cocaine vaccine are planned to confirm and extend the discussed outpatient studies, and there are ongoing developmental studies of alternative adjuvants and vaccine constructs which will likely improve the quantity and quality of antibodies produced, as well as the proportion of high response subjects. Such results would lead to clinical application of these vaccines for in the treatment of cocaine abusers. Better vaccines or newer methods will not be the end of the game for treating substance abuse, however. The motivated cocaine addict will need other interventions such as therapy and rehabilitation programs in order to overcome this seductive addiction. Anti-drug programs in schools should be strengthened, as cocaine addiction often starts before age 20. The criminal justice system should reconsider the wholesale incarceration of cocaine users, and offer help rather than punishment. Let us hope that in the years ahead anti-cocaine vaccination will be one of numerous arrows in our therapeutic quiver to combat drug addiction (Kinsey et al., 2010).

Incorporation of technology into treatment methods is also being explored. Computer-assisted therapies may offer more consistent and convenient delivery of instruction and reinforcement in conjunction with CBT. An additional and innovative approach, to be used with a structured treatment program, is the administration of a therapeutic cocaine vaccine. The vaccine is shown to inhibit the cocaine 'high' through antibodies binding to cocaine in the circulation and inhibiting entry to the brain. However, it does not stop drug cravings. In addition, recent findings suggest that only those subjects who attain high (> 43 ug/L) IgG anticocaine antibody levels benefited from significantly reduced cocaine use. Unfortunately, only 38% of the vaccinated subjects achieved such high IgG levels. Psychosocial therapy is still essential in medication and vaccine studies because the underlying issues of the dependence and use behavior must be addressed or individuals may relapse or resort to misusing another drug. The intent of the vaccine is to immunize motivated patients as part of a comprehensive recovery program and to inhibit the reinforcing activity of cocaine and decrease the likelihood of relapse (Penberthy et al., 2010).

8. Acknowledgements

Authors want to express a special thanks to people who have worked so hard in developing science in our country, Colombia, and specially to three people who now are making amazing science in the kingdom of God, Leonardo Lareo, Gerardo Pérez and Luis Osses. In memoriam of Leonardo, Gerardo and Luis, Professors and friends.

9. References

Anderson, SM, Famous, KR, Sadri-Vakili, G, Kumaresan, V, Schmidt HD, Bass CE, Terwilliger EF, Cha JH, Pierce RC. (2008). CaMKII: A biochemical bridge linking accumbens dopamine and glutamate systems in cocaine seeking. *Nat Neurosci* 11,3 (March 2008), pp. 344-53, ISSN 1097-6256

Ary, A.W.; Szumlinski, K.K. (2007). Regional differences in the effects of withdrawal from repeated cocaine upon Homer and glutamate receptor expression: a two-species comparison. *Brain Res,* 12,1184 (December 2007), pp. 295-305, ISSN 0006-8993

Bachtell, RK, Choi, KH, Simmons, DL, Falcon, E, Monteggia, LM, Neve, RL, Self, DW.(2008). Role of GluR1 expression in nucleus accumbens neurons in cocaine sensitization and cocaine-seeking behavior.*Eur J Neurosci,* 27, 9 (May 2008), pp. 2229-40 ISSN 1460-9568

Ballon J, Feifel D. (2006). A systematic review of modafinil: potential clinical uses and mechanisms of action. J Clin Psychiatry, 67, 4 (april 2006), pp. 554-66. ISSN 0160-6689

Barrett, A. C., Negus, S. S, Mello, N. K., and Caine, S. B. (2005). Effect of GABA Agonists and GABA-A Receptor Modulators on Cocaine- and Food-Maintained Responding and Cocaine Discrimination in Rats. *JPET,* 315, 2 (November 2005), pp. 858-871, ISSN 0022-3565

Barrós-Loscertales, A; Garavan, H; Bustamante, J; Ventura-Campos, N; Llopis, J; Belloch, V; Parcet, M; Ávila, C. (2011). Reduced striatal volume in cocaine-dependent patients.*Neuroimage* 56, 3 (june 2011), pp. 1021-1026. ISSN 1053-8119.

Berridge, K, Robinson T. (1998). What is the role of dopamine in reward: hedonic impact, reward learning, or incentive salience? *Brain Res Rev,* 28 (December 1998), pp. 309-369, ISSN 0165-0173

Boehm, J. and Malinow, R. (2005).AMPA receptor phosphorylation during synaptic plasticity.*Biochem. Soc. Trans.* 33, pt 6 (December 2005), pp. 1354–1356, ISSN 0300-5127

Boudreau, A.C, and Wolf, M.E. (2005). Behavioral sensitization to cocaine is associated with increased AMPA receptor surface expression in the nucleus accumbens. *J Neurosci ,* 25, 40 (October 2005), pp. 9144-9151, ISSN 0270-6474

Boudreau, AC, Reimers, JM, Milovanovic, M, Wolf ME. (2007). Surface AMPA receptors in the rat nucleus accumbens increase during cocaine withdrawal but internalize after cocaine challenge in association with altered activity of mitogen-activated protein kinases. *J Neurosci,* 27,39 (September 2007), pp. 10621–10635, ISSN 0270-6474

Bowers, M.; Chen, B.; Chou, J.; Osborne, M.; Gass, J.; See, R.; Bonci, A.; Janak, P.; Olive, M. (2007). Acamprosate attenuates cocaine- and cue-induced reinstatement of cocaine-seeking behavior in rats. *Psychopharmacology,* 195, 3 (December 2007), pp. 397-406. ISSN 0033-3158Carrera, M; Meijler, M; Janda, K. (2004).Cocaine pharmacology and current pharmacotherapies for its abuse.*Bioorganic & Medicinal Chemistry,*12 (October 2004)pp. 5019–5030. ISSN 0968-0896

Carroll, K. M., Fenton, L. R., Ball, S. A., Nich, C., Frankforter, T. L., Shi, J., Rounsaville, B. (2004). Efficacy of disulfiram and cognitive behavior therapy in cocaine dependent outpatients: a randomized placebo-controlled trial. *Arch Gen Psychiatry,* 61, 3, (march 2004) pp. 264−272. ISSN 0003-990x

Chiamulera, C.; Epping-Jordan, M.P.; Zocchi, A.; Marcon, C.; Cottiny, C.; Tacconi, S.; Corsi, M.; Orzi, F.; Conquet, F. (2001).Reinforcing and locomotor stimulant effects of cocaine are absent in mGluR5 null mutant mice. *Nat. Neurosci,* 4,9 (September 2001), pp. 873-4, ISSN 1097-6256

Conn, P. J., and Pin, J. P. (1997).Pharmacology and functions of metabotropic glutamate receptors.*Annu. Rev. Pharmacol. Toxicol.*37 (1997), pp. 205–237. ISSN 0362-1642

Conrad, KL, Tseng, KY, Uejima JL, Reimers JM, Heng LJ, Shaham Y, Marinelli M, Wolf ME. (2008). Formation of accumbens GluR2-lacking AMPA receptors mediates incubation of cocaine craving. *Nature* 454, (July 2008), pp. 118-121. ISSN0028-0836

Cornish, JL, Kalivas, PW. (2000). Glutamate transmission in the nucleus accumbens mediates relapse in cocaine addiction. *J Neurosci* 20 (May 2000), pp. RC89, ISSN 0270-6474

Cull-Candy, S., Brickley, S., and Farrant, M. (2001). NMDA receptor subunits: diversity, development and disease. *Curr.Opin.Neurobiol,* 11(2001), pp. 327–335,ISSN 0959-4388

Di Chiara, G. (2002). Nucleus accumbens shell and core dopamine: differential role in behavior and addiction. *Behav Brain Res,* 137 (December 2002), pp. 75-114. ISSN 0166-4328

Di Ciano, P, Everitt, BJ. (2001). Dissociable effects of antagonism of NMDA and AMPA/KA receptors in the nucleus accumbens core and shell on cocaine-seeking behavior.*Neuropsychopharmacology,* 25, 3 (September 2001), pp. 341-360, ISSN 1461-1457

Dingledine, R., Borges, K., Bowie, D., and Traynelis, S. F. (1999).The glutamate receptor ion channels.*Pharmacol. Rev.* 51,1 (March 1999), pp. 7–61, ISSN 0031-6997

Edwards, S., Graham, D. L., Bachtell, R. K., and Self, D. W. (2007).Region-specific tolerance to cocaine-regulated cAMP-dependent protein phosphorylation following chronic self-administration.*Eur. J. Neurosci,* 25 (April 2007), pp. 2201–2213,ISSN 1460-9568

Ersche, K; Barnes, A; Jones, S; Morein-Zamir, S; Robbins, T; Bullmore, E. (2011). Abnormal structure of frontostriatal brain systems is associated with aspects of impulsivity and compulsivity in cocaine dependence. *Brain.*134, 7, (july 2011) pp. 2013-2024. ISSN 0006-8950.

Everitt, B.J. and Wolf, M.E. (2002) Psychomotor stimulant addiction: a neural systems perspective. *J. Neurosci,* 22 (May 2002), pp. 3312–3320, ISSN 0270-6474

Fadda P, Scherma M, Fresu A, Collu M, Fratta W. (2003). Baclofen antagonizes nicotine-, cocaine-, and morphine-induced dopamine release in the nucleus accumbens of rat. Synapse. 50, 1 (October 2003), pp. 1-6. ISSN 0887-4776

Ferrario, CR, Li X, Wang, X, Reimers, JM, Uejima, JL, Wolf ME. (2010). The role of glutamate receptor redistribution in locomotor sensitization to cocaine. *Neuropsychopharmacology*35 (February 2010), pp. 818–833,ISSN 1461-1457

Floresco, SB, Yang, CR, Phillips, AG, Blaha, CD. (1998). Basolateral amygdala stimulation evokes glutamate receptor-dependent dopamine efflux in the nucleus accumbens of the anesthetised rat. *Eur J Neurosci* 10,4 (April 1998), pp. 1241–1251, ISSN 1460-9568

Fourgeaud, L. Mato Susana, Bouchet, Delphine, Hémar, Agnès, Worley, Paul F, and Manzoni, Olivier J. (2004). A single in vivo exposure to cocaine abolishes endocannabinoid-mediated longterm depression in the nucleus accumbens. *J. Neurosci.* 24, 31 (August 2004), pp. 6939–6945,ISSN 0270-6474

Franklin, T.R., Acton, P.D., Maldjian, J.A., Gray, J.D., Croft, J.R., Dackis, C.A., O'Brien, C.P., and Childress, A.R. (2002). Decreased gray matter concentration in the insular, orbitofrontal, cingulate, and temporal cortices of cocaine patients.*Biol. Psychiatry,51,* 2 (january 2002), pp. 134–142, ISSN 0006-3223

Gass, J.T. and M.F. Olive.(2008). Glutamatergic substrates of drug addiction and alcoholism.*Biochem.Pharmacol.* 75,1 (January 2008), pp. 218–265, ISSN 0006-2952

Ghasemzadeh, M.B., C. Mueller and P. Vasudevan. (2009). Behavioral sensitization to cocaine is associated with increased glutamate receptor trafficking to the postsynaptic density after extended withdrawal period. *Neuroscience* 159 (March 2009), pp. 414–426, ISSN 0306-4522

Goldstein, RA, Volkow, ND. (2002). Drug addiction and its underlying neurobiological basis: neuroimaging evidence for the involvement of the frontal cortex. *Am J Psychiatry*, 159,10 (2002), pp. 1642-1652. ISSN 0002-953X

Gonzalez, G.; Sevarino, K.; Sofuoglu, M.; Poling, J.; Oliveto, A.; Gonsai, K.; George, T.; Kosten, T. (2003). Tiagabine increases cocaine-free urines in cocaine-dependent methadone-treated patients: results of a randomized pilot study. *Addiction*, 98, 11 (November 2003), pp. 1625-32. ISSN 0965-2140.

Gryder, D. S., &Rogawski, M. A. (2003).Selective antagonism of GluR5 kainate-receptor-mediated synaptic currents by topiramate in rat basolateral amygdala neurons.*J Neurosci*, 23, 18 (August 2003) pp. 7069–7074. ISSN 0270-6474

Haile CN, Kosten TR, Kosten TA. (2009). Pharmacogenetic treatments for drug addiction: cocaine, amphetamine and methamphetamine. *Am J Drug Alcohol Abuse.* 35, 3 (June 2009), pp. 161-77. ISSN 0095-2790.

Harris, B. R., Prendergast, M. A., Gibson, D. A., Rogers, D. T., Blanchard, J. A., Holley, R. C.,Fu, M., Hart, S., Pedigo, N., Littleton, J. (2002). Acamprosate inhibits the binding and neurotoxic effects of trans-ACPD, suggesting a novel site of action at metabotropic glutamate receptors. *Alcohol: ClinExp Res* 26, 12, (December 2002), pp. 1779–1793. ISSN 1530-0277

Heilig, M., Egli, M. (2006) Pharmacological treatment of alcohol dependence: Target symptoms and target mechanisms.*Pharmacology & Therapeutics* 111, 3, (September 2006), pp. 855–876. ISSN 0163-7258

Higgins, G. A., Tomkins, D. M., Fletcher, P. J., & Sellers, E. M. (1992). Effect of drugs influencing 5-HT function on ethanol drinking and feeding behavior in rats: studies using a drinkometer system. *NeurosciBiobehav Rev*, 16, 4 (winter 1992) pp. 535–552. ISSN 0147-7634

Hotsenpiller,G., M. Giorgetti and M.E.Wolf. (2001). Alterations in behaviour and glutamate transmission following presentation of stimuli previously associated with cocaine exposure. *Eur. J. Neurosci.* 14, 11 (December 2001), pp. 1843–1855, ISSN 1460-9568

Kalivas, P.W and McFarland, K. (2003).Brain circuitry and the reinstatement of cocaine-seeking behavior.*Psychopharmacology* (Berl), 168 (July 2003), pp. 168:44-56, ISSN 0033-3158

Kalivas, P. W. (2004). Glutamate systems in cocaine addiction.*Current Opinion in Pharmacology*, 4 (February 2004), pp. 23–29, ISSN1471-4892

Kalivas, P.W and O'Brien C. (2008). Drug addiction as a pathology of staged neuroplasticity. *Neuropsychopharmacology*, 33,1 (January 2008), pp. 166–180, ISSN 1461-1457

Kaminski, R. M., Banerjee, M., &Rogawski, M. A. (2004).Topiramate selectively protects against seizures induced by ATPA, a GluR5 kainate receptor agonist. *Neuropharmacology*, 46, 8 (june 2004) pp. 1097–1104. ISSN 0028-3908

Kantak, KM, Black Y, Valencia, E, Green-Jordan, K, Eichembaum, HB. (2002). Dissociable effects of lidocaine inactivation of the rostral and caudal basolateral amygdala on the maintenance and reinstatement of cocaine-seeking behavior in rats.*J Neurosci*, 22, 3 (February 2002), pp. 1126-1136, ISSN 0270-6474

Kinsey, B; Kosten, T; Orson, F. (2010).Anti-cocaine vaccine development.*Expert Rev Vaccines.* 9, 9 (September 2010), pp. 1109–1114. ISSN 1476-0584.

Kirchmayer, U., Davoli, M., &Verster, A. (2003).Naltrexone maintenance treatment for opioid dependence. (Cochrane Review) *In the cochraneLybrary*. 1 (January 2003). ISSN 1464-780X

Klitenick, M. A., DeWitte, P. and Kalivas, P. W. (1992). Regulation of somatodendritic dopamine release in the ventral tegmental area by opioids and GABA: an in vivo microdialysis study. *J. Neurosci*, 12,7 (July 1992), pp. 2623–2632, ISSN 0270-6474

Kourrich, S, Rothwell, PE, Klug, JR, Thomas, MJ. (2007). Cocaine experience controls bidirectional synaptic plasticity in the nucleus accumbens. *J Neurosci*, 27, 30 (July 2007), pp. 7921–7928,ISSN 0270-6474

Kozell, L.B. & C.K. Meshul.(2004). Nerve terminal glutamate immunoreactivity in the rat nucleus accumbens and ventral tegmental area after a short withdrawal from cocaine.*Synapse* 51, 4 (March 2004), pp. 224–232, ISSN 0887-4476

Kozell,B. and K.Meshul. (2003). Alterations in nerve terminal glutamate immunoreactivity in the nucleus accumbens and ventral tegmental area following single and repeated doses of cocaine.*Psychopharmacology* (Berl) 165, 4 (February 2003), pp. 337–345, ISSN 0033-3158

Kreek, M. J., LaForge, K. S., &Butelman, E. (2002).Pharmacotherapy of addictions.*Nat Rev Drug Discov*, 1, 9, (September 2002), pp. 710−726.ISSN 1474-1776.

Johnson B. (2004). An overview of the development of medications including novel anticonvulsants for the treatment of alcohol dependence.*Expert OpinPharmacother*, 5, 9 (September 2004), pp. 1943-55. ISSN 1465-6566

Lau, C.G. and Zukin, R.S. (2007).NMDA receptor trafficking in synaptic plasticity and neuropsychiatric disorders.*Nat. Rev. Neurosci.* 8 (June 2007), pp. 413-426 ISSN 1471-0048

Levin, F.; Lehman, A. F.(1991).Meta-Analysis of Desipramine as an Adjunct in the: Treatment of Cocaine Addiction. J. Clin. Psychopharmacol.11,6 (December 1991), pp. 374-378. ISSN 0271-0479.

Levin FR, Evans SM, Brooks DJ, Garawi F. (2007). Treatment of cocaine dependent treatment seekers with adult ADHD: double-blind comparison of methylphenidate and placebo. Drug *Alcohol Dependence*, 87, 1 (February 2007), pp. 20-29. ISSN 0376-8716

Liu, XY, Chu, XP, Mao, LM, Wang, M, Lan, HX, Li, MH, *et al.* (2006). Modulation of D2R-NR2B interactions in response to cocaine.*Neuron*, 52, 5 (December 2006), pp. 897-909, ISSN 0896-6273

Loftis, J. M., and Janowsky, A. (2002). Cocaine treatment- and withdrawal- induced alterations in the expression and serine phosphorylation of the NR1 NMDA receptor subunit. *Psychopharmacology*, 164 (2002), pp. 349–359, ISSN 0033-3158

Lu, L, Grimm, JW, Shaham, Y, Hope, BT. (2003). Molecular neuroadaptations in the accumbens and ventral tegmental area during the first 90 days of forced abstinence from cocaine self-administration in rats. *J Neurochem* 85, 6 (June 2003), pp. 1604-1613, ISSN 0022-3042

Makris N., Gasic GP, Seidman LJ, Goldstein JM, Gastfriend DR, Elman I, Albaugh DM, Hodge SM, Ziegler DA, Sheahan F, Caviness VS Jr., Tsuang MT, Kennedy DN, Hyman SE, Rosen BR, Breiter HC. (2004). Decreased Absolute Amygdala Volume in Cocaine Addicts. *Neuron*, 44 (November 2004), pp. 729–740, ISSN 0896-6273

Mao, Li-Min, Guo, Ming-Lei, Jin, Dao-Zhong, Fibuch, Eugene E., Choe, Eun Sang, and Wang John Q. (2011). Post-translational modification biology of glutamate receptors and drug addiction.*Frontiers in neuroanatomy*, 5, 19 (March 2011), pp. 1-11, ISSN 1662-5129

Marinelli M, White FJ (2000) Enhanced vulnerability to cocaine self-administration is associated with elevated impulse activity of midbrain dopamine neurons. J Neurosci 20:8876–8885

Matochik, J.A., London, E.D., Eldreth, D.A., Cadet, J.L., and Bolla, K.I. (2003). Frontal cortical tissue composition in abstinent cocaine abusers: a magnetic resonance imaging study. *Neuroimage19*, 3 (july 2003), pp. 1095–1102. ISSN 1053-8119

McCance-Katz E, Kosten T, Jatlow P. (1998).Disulfiram effects on acute cocaine administration. *Drug Alcohol Depend.* 52. 1 (september 1998), pp. 27-39. ISSN 0376-8716

McFarland, K., C.C. Lapish and P.W. Kalivas.(2003). Prefrontal glutamate release into the core of the nucleus accumbensmediates cocaine-induced reinstatement of drug-seeking behavior.*J. Neurosci.* 23 (April 2003), pp. 3531–3537, ISSN 0270-6474

Mitrano, D.A, Arnold, C, Smith, Y. (2008). Subcellular and subsynaptic localization of group I metabotropic glutamate receptors in the nucleus accumbens of cocaine-treated rats.*Neuroscience,* 154, 2 (June 2008), pp. 653-66 ISSN 0306-4522

Meert, T. F. (1993). Effects of various serotonergic agents on alcohol intake and alcohol preference in Wistar rats selected at two different levels of alcohol preference. *Alcohol Alcohol,* 28, 2 (march 1993) pp. 157−170. ISSN 0735-0414

Moran, M.M, McFarland, K, Melendez, R.I, Kalivas, P.W, Seamans, J.K. J. (2005).Cystine/Glutamate Exchange Regulates Metabotropic Glutamate Receptor Presynaptic Inhibition of Excitatory Transmission and Vulnerability to Cocaine Seeking. *J. Neurosci,* 25,27 (July 2005), pp. 6389-6393 ISSN 0270-6474

Neisewander, JL, Baker, DA, Fuchs, RA, Tran-Nguyen, LTL, Palme,r A, Marshall, JF. (2000). Fos protein expression and cocaine seeking behavior in rats after exposure to a cocaine self-administration environment. *J Neurosci,* 20 (January 2000), pp. 798-805 ISSN 0270-6474

Nestler, E. J. (2001).Molecular basis of long-term plasticity underlying addiction. Nature Rev Neurosci, 2, 2 (February 2001), pp. 119-128, ISSN 1471-003X

Nestler, EJ, Barrot, M, Self, DW. (2001). DeltaFosB: a sustained molecular switch for addiction. ProcNatlAcadSci USA 98, 20 (September 2001), pp. 11042-11046 ISSN 0027-8424

Nestler, E. J. (2004).Molecular and cellular mechanisms of opiate and cocaine addiction.*Trends in Pharmacological Sciences,* 25, 4 (April 2004), pp. 210-218, ISSN 0165-6147

Nestler, E. (2005).Neurobiology of drug addiction.*Science & practice perspectives,* 3, 4 (December 2005), pp. 6-10, ISSN 1930-4307

Nestler, E.J. 2005. The Neurobiology of Cocaine Addiction. Sci Pract Perspect. December; 3(1): 4–10.

O'Brien, C. 2001. Drug addiction and drug abuse. In The Pharmacological Basis of Therapeutics. Edited by Hardman J, n Limbird L, Gilman AG. New York: McGraw-Hill; 2001:621-642.

Park, W.K, Bari, A.A, Jey, A. R, Anderson, S. M, Spealman, R. D, Rowlett, J. K, Pierce, R. C. (2002). Cocaine administered into the medial prefrontal cortex reinstates cocaine-seeking behavior by increasing AMPA receptor-mediated glutamate transmission in the nucleus accumbens. *J. Neurosci.* 22,7 (April 2002), pp. 2916–2925, ISSN 0270-6474

Penberthy, J; Ait-Daoud, N; Vaughan, M; Fanning, T. (2010) Review of Treatment for Cocaine Dependence.*Current Drug Abuse Reviews, 3,(march 2010), pp.* 49-62. ISSN 1874-4737.

Pierce, R.C, Bell, R.C, Duffy, K, Kalivas, P.W. (1996). Repeated cocaine augments excitatory amino acid transmission in the nucleus accumbens only in rats having developed behavioral sensitization. *J. Neurosci.* 16 (February 1996), pp. 1550–1560, ISSN 0270-6474

Rist, F., Randall, C. L., Heather, N., & Mann, K. (2005). New developments in alcoholism treatment research in europe. *Alcohol: ClinExp Res.* 29,6 (june 2005) pp. 1127−1132. ISSN 1530-0277

Schmidt, H. D. and Pierce, R. C. (2010).Cocaine-induced neuroadaptations in glutamate transmission Potential therapeutic targets for craving and addiction.*Ann. N.Y. Acad. Sci.* 1187 (January 2010), pp. 35–75, ISNN 0077-8923

Schultz, W. (2002).Getting formal with dopamine and reward.*Neuron,* 36, 2 (October 2002), pp. 241-63, ISSN 0896-6273

Spanagel, R., &Zieglgansberger, W. (1997). Anti-craving compounds for ethanol: new pharmacological tools to study addictive processes. *Trends PharmacolSci,* 18, 2 (February 2007), pp. 54−59. ISSN 0165-6147

Spanagel, R., Pendyala, G., Abarca, C., Zghoul, T., Sanchis-Segura, C., Magnone, M. C., Lascorz, J., Depner, M., Holzberg, D., Soyka, M., Schreiber, S., Matsuda, F., Lathrop, M., Schumann, G., Albrecht, U. (2005). The clock gene Per2 influences the glutamatergic system and modulates alcohol consumption. *Nat Med* 11, 1 (January 2005). Pp. 35−42. ISSN 1078-8956

Stromberg, M. F. (2004). The effect of baclofen alone and in combination with naltrexone on ethanol consumption in the rat.*PharmacolBiochemBehav,* 78, 4 (august 2004) pp. 743−750. ISSN 0091-3057

Sun, X, Zhao, Y, Wolf, M.E. (2005). Dopamine receptor stimulation modulates AMPA receptor synaptic insertion in prefrontal cortex neurons. *J Neurosci,* 25, 32 (August 2005), pp. 7342-7351, ISSN 0270-6474

Suto, N, Tanabe, LM, Austin, JD, Creekmore, E, Pham, CT, Vezina, P. (2004). Previous exposure to psychostimulants enhances the reinstatement of cocaine seeking by nucleus accumbens AMPA. *Neuropsychopharmacology*29 (December 2004), pp. 2149–2159, ISSN 1461-1457

Sutton, M.A., Schmidt, E.F., Choi, K.-H., Schad, C.A., Whisler, K., Simmons, D., *et al.* (2003). Extinction-induced up-regulation in AMPA receptors reduces cocaine-seeking behaviour. Nature, 421 (January 2003), pp, 70–75, ISSN 0028-0836

Szumlinski, K.K, Ary, A.W, Lominac, K.D. (2008). Homers regulate drug-induced neuroplasticity: implications for addiction. Biochem.Pharmacol, 75(January 2008), pp. 112-33, ISSN 0006-2952

Thomas, M.J., P.W. Kalivas and Y. Shaham.(2008). Neuroplasticity in the mesolimbic dopamine system and cocaine addiction.*Br. J. Pharmacol,* 154 (May 2008), pp. 327–342, ISSN 0007-1188

Thomas, MJ, Beurrier, C, Bonci, A, Malenka, RC. (2001). Long-term depression in the nucleus accumbens: A neural correlate of behavioral sensitization to cocaine. *Nat Neurosci,* 4 (December 2001), pp. 1217–1223, ISSN ISSN 1097-6256

Tomkins, D. M., Le, A. D., & Sellers, E. M. (1995).Effect of the 5-HT3 antagonist ondansetron on voluntary ethanol intake in rats and mice maintained on a limited access procedure.*Psychopharmacology*, 117, 4 (February 1995) pp. 479–485. ISSN 0033-3158

Tzschentke, TM and Schmidt, WJ. (2003). Glutamatergic mechanisms in addiction.*Molecular Psychiatry*, 8 (September 2003), pp. 373–382, ISSN 1476-5578

Tzschentke, TM. (2001). Pharmacology and behavioural pharmacology of the mesocortical dopamine system.*ProgNeurobiol*, 63, 3 (February 2001), pp. 241–320, ISSN 0555-4047

Uys, J. D. and LaLumiere, R. T. (2008). Glutamate: The New Frontier in Pharmacotherapy for Cocaine Addiction. *CNS & Neurological Disorders - Drug Targets*, 7, 5 (November 2008), pp. 482-491, ISSN 1871-5273

Volkow, N.D, Wang, G-J, Ma, Y, Fowler, J.S, Wong, C, Ding, Y-S, Hitzemann, R, Swanson, J, and Kalivas, P. (2005). Activation of orbital and medial prefrontal cortex by methylphenidate in cocaineaddicted subjects but not in controls: relevance to addiction. *J. Neurosci*, 25, 15 (April 2005), pp. 3932–3939, ISSN 0270-6474

Winder, D.G, Egli, R.E, Schramm, N.L, Matthews, R.T. (2002).Synaptic plasticity in drug reward circuitry.*CurrMol Med*, 2, 7 (November 2002), pp. 667-676, ISSN 1566-5240

White, H. S., Brown, S. D., Woodhead, J. H., Skeen, G. A., & Wolf, H. H. (1997). Topiramate enhances GABA-mediated chloride flux and GABAevoked chloride currents in murine brain neurons and increases seizure threshold. *Epilepsy Res*, 28, 3 (October 2008) pp. 167–179. ISSN 0920-1211

Wolf, M.E, Ferrario, C.R. (2010). AMPA receptor plasticity in the nucleus accumbens after repeated exposure to cocaine.*NeurosciBiobehav Rev*, 35 (January 2010), pp. 185–211, ISSN 0149-7634

Wolf, M.E, Sun, X, Mangiavacchi, S, Chao, SZ. (2004). Psychomotor stimulants and neuronal plasticity.*Neuropharmacology*, 47, suppl 1 (September 2004), pp. 61–79, ISSN 0028-3908

Xi, Z.X, Ramamoorthy, S, Baker, D.A, Shen, H, Samuvel, D.J, Kalivas, P. (2002), Modulation of group II metabotropic glutamate receptor signaling by chronic cocaine. *J. Pharmacol. Exp. Ther*, 303, 2 (November 2002), pp., 608-15, ISSN 0022-3565

Xi, Z.X. and Stein, E.A. (1998). Nucleus accumbens dopamine release modulation by mesolimbic GABAA receptors-an in vivo electrochemical study. *Brain Res*, 798 (1998), pp. 156-165 ISSN 0006-8993

Ye, J.H and Ren, J. (2006). Cocaine inhibition of GABA(A) current: role of dephosphorylation. *Crit Rev Neurobiol*, 18, 1-2 (2006), pp. 85-94, ISSN 0892-0915

Yücel, M; Solowij, N; Respondek, C; Whittle, S; Fornito, A; Pantelis, C; Lubman, D. (2008). Regional Brain Abnormalities Associated With Long-term Heavy Cannabis Use. *Arch Gen Psychiatry*, 65, 6 (June 2008) pp. 694-701.ISSN 0003-990x.

Zahm DS, Brog JS. 1992. On the significance of subterritories in the "accumbens" part of the rat ventral striatum. Neuroscience 50:751–767

Zhang, X, Lee, T.H, Davidson, C, Lazarus, C, Wetsel, W.C, Ellinwood, E.H. (2007).Reversal of cocaine-induced behavioral sensitization and associated phosphorylation of the NR2B and GluR1 subunits of the NMDA and AMPA receptors. *Neuropsychopharmacology*, 32, 2 (February 2007), pp. 377-387, ISSN 0893-133X

Zona, C., Ciotti, M. T., &Avoli, M. (1997).Topiramate attenuates voltage-gated sodium currents in rat cerebellar granule cells. *NeurosciLett*, 231, 3 (august 1997) pp 123–126. ISSN 0304-3940

5

Role of Prefrontal Cortex Dopamine and Noradrenaline Circuitry in Addiction

Ezio Carboni*, Roberto Cadeddu and Anna Rosa Carta
Dept. of Biomedical Sciences,
University of Cagliari, Cagliari,
Italy

1. Introduction

Understanding the mechanisms of drug dependence has been the goal of a large number of neuroscientists, pharmacologists and clinicians who carried out research with the hope of individuating and proposing an efficacious therapy for this disorder (Sofuoglu, 2010; Kalivas and Volkow, 2011). Unfortunately, although huge efforts, drug dependence is still a relevant health, social and economical problem (Popova et al., 2012; Hiscock et al., 2011; Shorter and Kosten, 2011). Treatments for drug abuse are for the most part ineffective because the molecular and cellular mechanisms through which drugs of abuse alter neuronal circuitry are still unexplained and above all, because drugs of abuse determine a global alteration of cerebral functions that govern behaviour through decision formation, making therefore unfocused the identification of a pharmacological target (Volkow et al., 2011; Schultz 2011). One of the first strategies pursued in drug dependence therapy was directed to removal of pleasure associated with drug taking, but the compliance with the treatment has been always limited, although it could improve when it was supported by psychology based motivational therapy as in alcohol dependence (Krampe and Ehrenreich, 2010; Simkin and Grenoble, 2010). On the other hand it is not infrequent that heavy smokers or heavy drinkers stop suddenly dependence just because their will overcome year-long habits. Decision making is a process based on the interaction between prefrontal cortex (PFC) and subcortical regions involved in reward and motivation, therefore it is likely that failure in self-regulatory behavior, that is common in addicted subjects, could be dependent upon the alteration of interactions between the prefrontal cortex and subcortical regions (Heatherton and Wagner, 2011). In this chapter we will review the role of PFC in addiction with particular attention to dopamine and norepinephrine transmission.

2. Brief overview on the prefrontal cortex

The PFC has a prominent role in governing behavior. This function is achieved through a complex interaction of many different areas within the PFC which cooperate with subcortical areas integrating cognitive and executive functions to produce the "optimal choice". The result of this interaction can be also a deleterious one, as observed in drug

* Corresponding Author

addicted subjects. This interaction has been elegantly discussed by Kennerley and Walton (2011) by comparing the functional correspondence between neurophysiological and neuropsychological studies to help define the roles of different PFC areas in supporting optimal decision making. The following brief overview on PFC is not intended to be exhaustive, as far as regards discussion of cognitive and executive functions of sub areas of PFC, but it will address specific features of PFC areas in which catecholamine transmission plays relevant role in drug addiction.

Dopamine transmission in PFC is directly involved in cognitive processes (Seamans and Yang, 2004), in the regulation of emotions (Sullivan, 2004), in working memory (Khan and Muly 2011), as well as in executive functions such as motor planning, inhibitory response control and sustained attention (Fibiger and Phillips, 1988; Granon et al., 2000; Robbins, 2002). The association of PFC functions with impulse control is supported by the evidence that damage to the ventromedial PFC causes persistent motivational impulsivity associated with affective instability, reduced capability for decision making, poor executive planning and general apathy towards social life (Damasio et al., 1994). In general damage of PFC function in humans can therefore affect one or more of the above functions producing personal and social difficulties as observed in disorders such as Alzheimer's disease (Melrose et al., 2011), schizophrenia (Arnsten, 2011), and Parkinson's disease (Luft and Schwarz, 2009). Loss of PFC function can be also generated by traumas (Bechara and Van Der Linden, 2005), or can result from drug addiction (Koob and Volkow, 2010; Van den Oever et al., 2010). Moreover, PFC functional or anatomical abnormalities are frequently found in individuals with drug abuse disorders (Liu et al., 1998a and 1998b; Franklin et al., 2002) and at the same time PFC is thought to have an important role in the onset and in the progression of psychiatric disorders associated with poor decision making such as schizophrenia (Arnsten, 2004), attention deficit/hyperactivity disorder (ADHD) (Sullivan and Brake, 2003) and depression (Davidson et al., 2002). Also, clinical studies report that when traumatic brain injury damages the PFC it often facilitate the emergence of drug use disorders (Ommaya et al., 1996, Delmonico et al., 1998).

The knowledge on PFC functions in mammals has been accumulated through research on different species but anatomy differences between primates and rodents is object of discussion when comparing experimental evidence on PFC function. In particular the dorsolateral PFC of mammals is thought to be involved in working memory, in attention processes, in reasoning-based decision making and in the timing of behavioural organization (Curtis and Lee, 2010; Arnsten, 2011). The prominent role of PFC catecholamine transmission in motivation is also supported by its anatomical and functional connection with other important areas of the brain, such as the nucleus accumbens (NAcc) (Di Chiara et al., 2011), and the ventral tegmental area (Omelchenko and Sesack, 2007) (Fig. 1). Chambers et al. (2003) provided an interesting definition for the role of the PFC: - It plays a determining role in the representation, execution and inhibition of motivational drives by influencing patterns of neural ensemble firing in the NAcc and poor PFC function could increase the probability of performing inappropriate motivated drives viewed clinically as impulsive. This view may acquire increasing relevance by integrating it in a scenario in which neural transmission in the NAcc is considered a common molecular pathway for addiction (Nestler, 2005; Di Chiara et al., 2004). Furthermore, one of the primary outputs of the accumbens is the gabaergic innervation (Fig. 2) directed to the ventral pallidum that in turn innervate the mediodorsal thalamic nucleus by GABA neurons. Mediodorsal thalamus in turn sends and excitatory output to the prelimbic and infralimbic PFC (O'Donnel et al., 1997). The PFC in primates receives the projection from the medio-dorsal nucleus of the thalamus that innervates the dorsolateral, medial and orbital cortices (Vertes, 2006) but in general, the thalamic innervation of PFC is a part of a loop which includes cortical thalamic glutamatergic excitatory projection that has a role in working memory (Watanabe and Funahashi, 2012) and is involved in the reward circuit (Haber and Knutoson, 2010).

Recent reviews suggest that the medial PFC in rat is functionally equivalent to the medial PFC of primates (Brown and Bowman 2002; Wilson et al. 2010). It has also been suggested that the rat PFC is not differentiated and therefore can subserve cognitive function localized in the dorsolateral PFC of primates as discussed elegantly by Brown and Bowman, (2002). These authors recognised that behavioural deficits following PFC damage in rats could reflect impaired behavioural flexibility similar to that reported in primates (De Bruin et al., 1994; Joel et al., 2005) and although the ability of shifting attention from one complex stimulus to another can be characterized by different abstraction level among different species, mammals could share executive processing mechanisms [selective attention, working memory, updating (manipulating the contents of working memory)] and rerouting attention (Shimamura, 2000; Brown and Bowman 2002). Due to the complexity of reciprocal neurotransmitter relationship in PFC, this chapter will mainly consider the role of dopamine and norepinephine in the PFC and their relationship with the effects of drugs of abuse and therapy of addiction. This choice is based on the important role of dopaminergic transmission in the effects of drugs of abuse and on the modulation of cognitive control (van Schouwenburg et al., 2010).

3. Dopamine in the prefrontal cortex: innervation, receptors and functions

The PFC receives multiple ascending innervations (Fig. 1 and Fig. 2). Whereas Acetylcholine (Ach) and serotonin (5-HT), contact widely all the subregions of PFC, dopamine innervations are more localized (e.g., prelimbic and infralimbic cortex) although they have a discrete grade of overlapping with norepinephrine innervation (Del Campo et al., 2011). The PFC is reciprocally connected with the VTA by dopaminergic afferents and glutamatergic efferents. Dopaminergic innervation of the PFC is predominantly provided by VTA dopamine cells sublocated in the parabrachialis pigmentosus nucleus which projects to cortical deep layers that contain the highest density of dopamine D1 and D2 receptors (Oades and Halliday, 1987). The main target of these innervations are the dendritic spines of pyramidal cells that project to GABA neurons of the NAcc which in turn complete a circuit by projecting back to VTA cells (Omelchenko and Sesack, 2007). A small population of PFC neurons that project to the VTA form synaptic contact with dopamine neurons that project onto the PFC, and a second population synapse onto GABA neurons that project to the nucleus accumbens, however no synaptic contact was found between PFC neurons and dopamine neurons that project to the NAcc (Carr and Sesack, 2000b). Lastly, to emphasize the complexity of the circuits in which the PFC is involved, it is important to underline that the majority of PFC terminals within the VTA area appear to target dopamine and GABA neurons that project onto target sites different from PFC and NAcc (Carr and Sesack, 2000a). Among them, some innervate ventral pallidum (Papp et al., 2012) and others, such as the putative gabaergic cells of the rostral linear nucleus that innervate the mediodorsal thalamic nucleus may have relevance in reward mechanism (Del Fava et al., 2007). Efferent projections from VTA to hippocampus influence spatial working memory performance (Martig and Mizumori, 2011). Dopamine innervation of PFC is functionally inhibitory either by direct action on pyramidal cells or via GABA interneurons (Grobin, and Deutch, 1998) reducing glutamatergic excitatory output to NAcc and VTA. Therefore, an increase in dopamine stimulation of PFC conversely attenuates dopamine activity in striatal and limbic terminal regions (Karreman and Moghaddam, 1996) and attenuates the motor stimulatory effects of systemically administered stimulants such as amphetamine and cocaine (Karler et al., 1998).

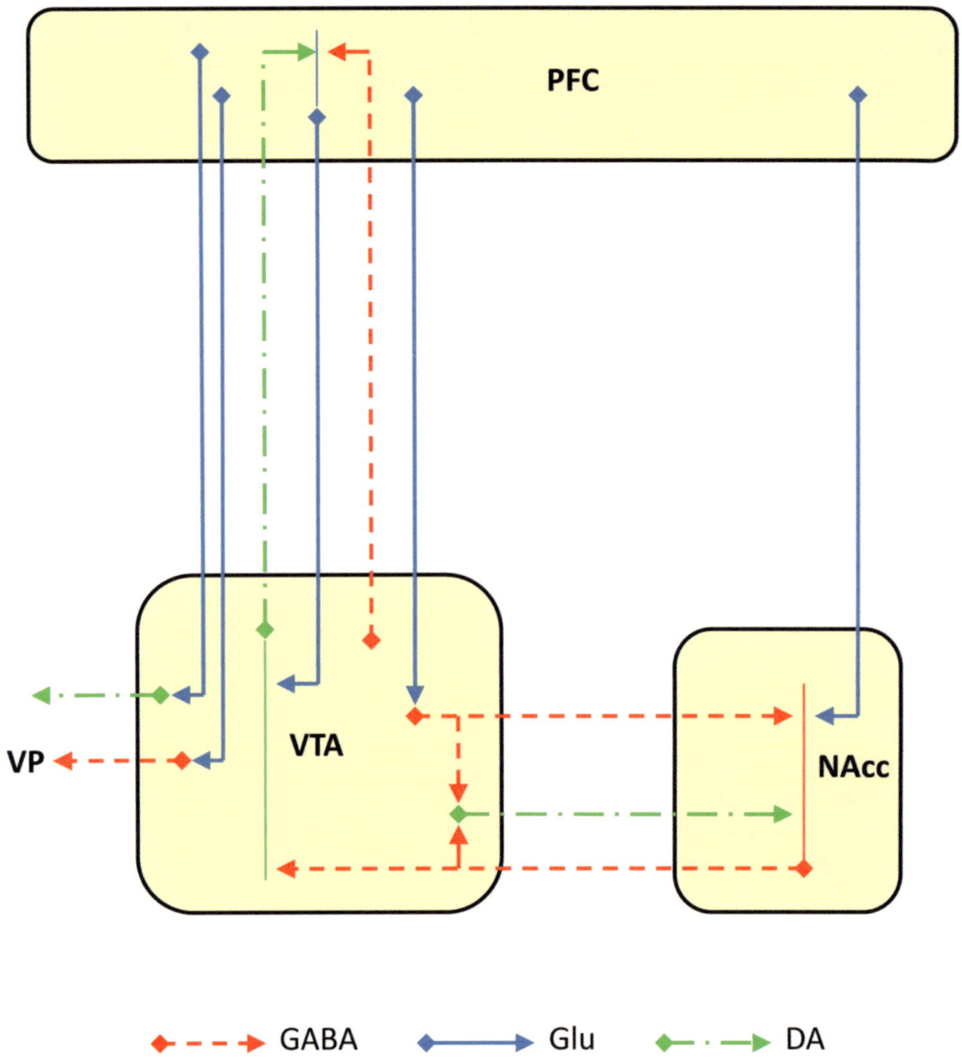

Fig. 1. Schematic representation of few major sites of interaction between prefrontal cortex (PFC) glutamate neurons, ventral tegmental area (VTA) dopamine and GABA neurons, and nucleus accumbens (NAcc) GABA neurons. Dendrites are occasionally represented for drawing clarity.

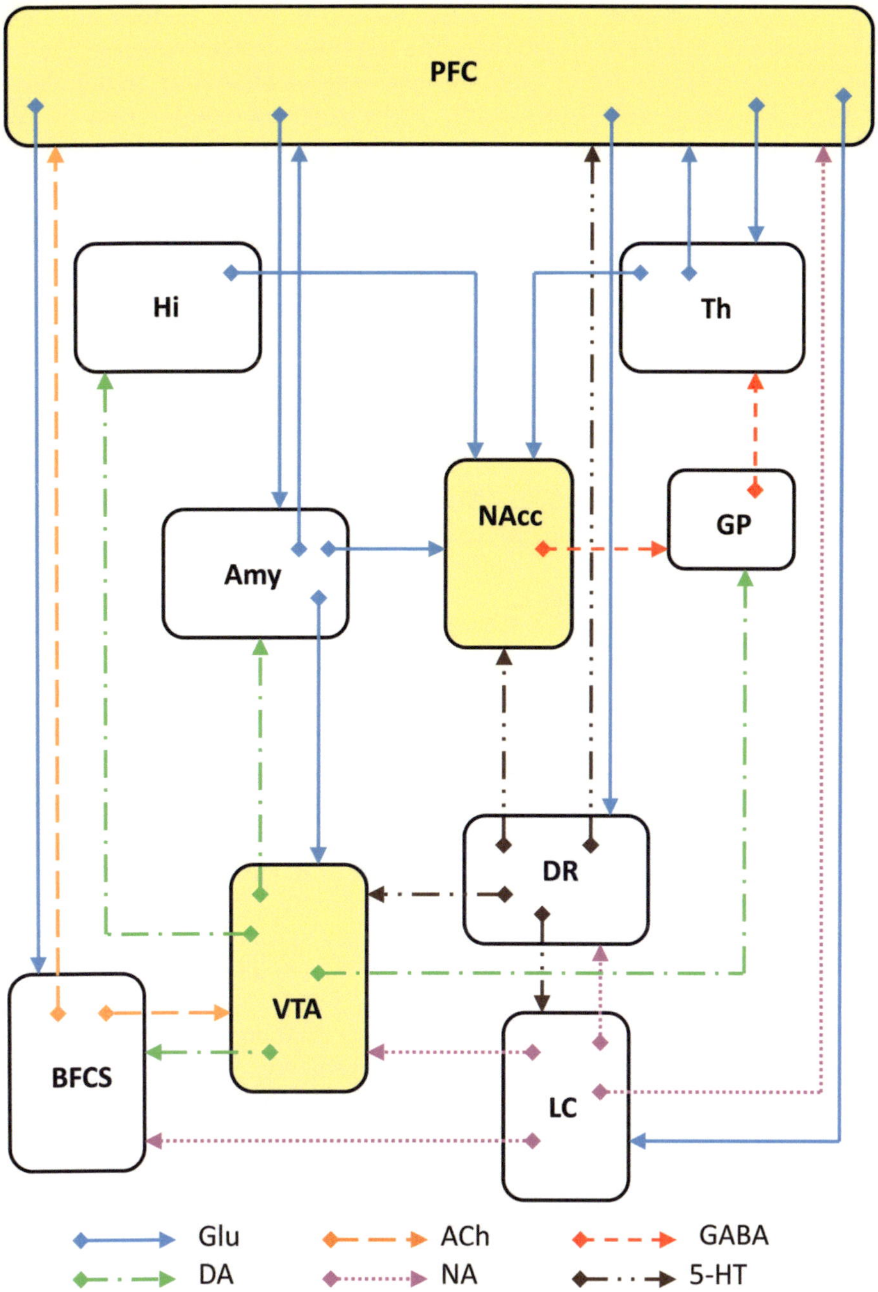

Fig. 2. Schematic representation of several major sites of interaction between prefrontal cortex (PFC) and thalamus (Th), hippocampus (Hi), amygdala (Amy), ventral tegmental area (VTA), dorsal raphe (DR), basal forebrain cholinergic system (BFCS), locus coeruleus (LC) globus pallidus (GP). Glutamate (Glu), Dopamine (DA), GABA, Acetylcholine (Ach), Norepinephrine (NA), and Serotonin (5-HT) neurons and axons are represented. The detailed connection represented in Fig. 1 have been omitted for drawing clarity.

Dopamine is a model of slow synaptic transmission; therefore it does not mediate fast synaptic transmission but instead modulates the response of other systems. The majority of D1 and D2 type receptors in the medial PFC appear to be located on pyramidal cells with the density of D2, apparently considerably lower than that of D1 (see the review by Tzschentke, 2001). Although both receptors are also present in GABAergic interneurons, the D4 subtype in particular (Ariano et al., 1997; Defagot et al., 1997a and 1997b) appears to be located on GABAergic interneurons rather than on pyramidal cells (Mrzljak et al., 1996). It is interesting to note that in the same postsynaptic pyramidal cell of the mPFC, dopaminergic terminals are localized in close opposition to each other with glutamatergic terminal originating in both the mediodorsal thalamus and the controlateral medial PFC. The former is not affected by VTA activation which instead inhibits the excitation of pyramidal cells generated by the input from recurrent collaterals of efferent glutamatergic output (Tzschentke, 2001). By acting on D1 receptors and through cAMP for the activation of cAMP sensitive protein kinase, dopamine determines an increase in the phosphorylation of DARP-32 and an inhibition of phosphatase 1 modulating mechanisms that involve ion channel and transcription factors (Greengard, 2001). D1 receptor optimal stimulation is essential to working memory process (Williams and Goldman-Rakic, 1995) and therefore either an increase or a decrease of the transmission leads to an inverted U response (Desimone, 1995). The involvement of dopamine activity through D1 receptor in cognitive function has a strong impact in schizophrenia research because of the importance of cognitive impairment in this disorder (Barch and Ceaser, 2012).

Although the result of dopamine interaction on pyramidal cells is complex and is influenced by a number of factors (e.g. dopamine concentration, receptor interaction, direct or indirect effect, depolarization status of the cells), dopamine generally, as also described in the previous paragraph, inhibits the activity of pyramidal cells in the medial PFC (see Tzschentke, 2001 for a review). The direct dopamine action on pyramidal cells (Geijo-Barrietos and Pastore, 1995; Gulledge and Jaffe, 1998) or the indirect action by a stimulation of the GABA interneurons may in turn inhibit pyramidal cells (Mercuri et al., 1985; Penit-Soria et al., 1987; Pirot et al., 1992). This latter action appears to be mediated through D2 receptors (Retaux et al., 1991; Grobin and Deutch, 1998). On the other hand, pyramidal cells respond more to NMDA stimulation through D1 receptors in the presence of a low concentration of dopamine, whereas a high concentration would instead reduce this response (Zheng et al., 1999) by acting through D2 receptors. The role of D1/5 receptor is also crucial in suppressing the sustained neuronal firing that takes place during working memory activity (Vijayraghavan et al., 2007). This property is displayed by D1/5 dopamine receptor agonists, which have been found to cause a decrease in extracellular glutamate in PFC in vivo (Abekawa et al. 2000; Harte and O'Connor 2004). Interestingly D1/5 dopamine receptor agonists are also effective in normalizing aberrant network activity induced by both hallucinogens and minimal GABAA antagonism, although clinical efficacy remains to be determined (Aghajanan, 2009). The close relationship between dopamine and glutamate is functionally expressed at NAcc level where medial PFC efferents terminate in close opposition to dopamine terminals originating in the VTA, often in the same spine of GABAergic accumbal cells (Bouyer et al, 1984; Sesack and Pickel, 1992). It is interesting to note that only about 30-40 % of the VTA projection to PFC is dopaminergic, while the rest is likely to be an inhibitory GABAergic innervation (Carr and Sesack 2000a). Of further relevance is that PFC glutamate innervations of the NAcc is part of the motivational circuit completed by accumbal GABA neurons projecting onto the ventral globus pallidus, by pallidal GABA neurons that project to the thalamus and lastly by thalamic glutamate neurons that project back to the PFC (see Chambers et al., 2003, for a review). Hence, PFC and NAcc work together to produce a behavioral output resulting from brain activity that processes input information concerning the internal status of the individual and the external environment (Dorman and Gaudiano, 1998). Considering that firing patterns in both the NAcc and PFC are influenced by glutamatergic input from the hippocampus and amygdala (Aggleton, 2011; Miller et al., 2010), it may be suggested that abnormalities in these distal structures may produce both psychiatric disorders as well as higher vulnerability to drug addiction (Chambers et al., 2001). As far as regards dopamine transmission in the PFC it is necessary to remind that dopamine could be captured by norepinephrine reuptake system (Carboni et al., 1990; Carboni et al., 2006)

4. Noradrenaline in the prefrontal cortex: Innervation, receptors and interactions

The long established observation that catecholamine depletion in PFC can be considered as destructive as tissue ablation (Brozoski et al., 1979) confirms the prominent role of catecholamine innervation in the PFC. The noradrenergic system that originates in the locus coeruleus and in other small nuclei in the medulla and the pons has the peculiar feature of projecting onto the entire neuraxis, although it originates in a relatively small group of cells. This extensive, irradiating anatomical arrangement allows the noradrenergic system to potentially influence all brain activity. In particular, noradrenaline innervations of PFC depend on neurons located in the locus coeruleus (Foote et al., 1983; Bjorklund and Lindvall, 1986) that project to dendrites of both pyramidal cells and interneurons. An interesting feature of locus coeruleus noradrenergic innervation of the cerebral cortex is that individual locus coeruleus neurons simultaneously innervate functionally and cyto-architectonically distinct cortical regions. In fact, locus coeruleus neurons arborize more extensively in the anterior-to-posterior axis of the cortex and exhibit relatively minimal medial-to-lateral collateralization (Swanson, 1976; Aoki et al., 1998). Individual locus coeruleus cells were also shown to innervate both superficial and deep layers of a cortical region (Loughlin et al., 1982). Furthermore, the PFC projects back to the locus coeruleus thereby completing a circuitry which plays a role in relevant brain activity, i.e. maintaining vigilance (reviewed by Aston Jones, 1985) or modulating the behavioural response to stress (Morilak et. al., 2005). Functionally, the noradrenergic system can be viewed as a modulatory system because it can increase the "signal to noise ratio" of responses evoked by other neurotransmitters that excite or inhibit target cells (Woodward et al., 1991). Modulatory actions of this type can be mediated through either α or β noradrenergic receptors (Waterhouse et al., 1991; Woodward et al., 1991). This modulatory type action is also supported by the fact that in the monkey PFC noradrenaline produces its effects predominantly through α2A adrenoceptors that occur in spines, localized discretely over postsynaptic membranes that are most likely PFC pyramidal cells (Aoki et al., 1998). Yet α2A receptors are most prevalent along axons, and are found also in dendritic shafts and astrocytic processes that lack evident synaptic junction. This suggests that these receptors are activated by volume transmission (Aoki et al., 1998). In particular, axonal α2A adrenoceptors have a pre-terminal location; by closing voltage dependent Ca^{++} channels, they are probably able to reduce neurotransmitter release such as serotonin as well as noradrenaline release (Frankhuyzen and Mulder, 1980; Maura et al., 1982).

Moreover, it appears that noradrenaline receptors with different affinities may mediate responses triggered by different extracellular concentrations of this transmitter. As reviewed by Arnsten (2007), moderate levels of noradrenaline released during waking act on high affinity α2A adrenoceptors coupled with Gi proteins to inhibit cAMP signalling, whereas higher levels released during stress not only activate lower affinity β1 coupled to phosphatidyl inositol signalling but also low affinity β1 adrenoceptors coupled to Gs, to increase cAMP signalling (Arnsten, 2000). In general, the role of noradrenaline in the PFC can be seen as being an inhibitory action with a long onset and protracted effect, and can be defined as being neuromodulatory. By inhibiting ongoing background discharge, noradrenaline produces an increase in the signal–to-noise ratio that helps to filter irrelevant stimuli while enhancing behaviorally significant stimuli (Bjorklund and Lindvall, 1986). According to this view NA is crucial for many PFC functions mediated by α2A post synaptic adrenoceptors, such as working memory, attention regulation, planning and behavioural inhibition as suggested by experimental research on various mammals (Arnsten, 2006 and 2009).

Catecholamine transmission in PFC is also dependent on the location of receptors in the dendritic tree of pyramidal cells and may occur through both α2A adrenoceptors increasing delay-related firing for the preferred spatial direction or through D1 receptor decreasing delay-related firing for the nonpreferred direction (Vijayraghavan et al., 2007). Catecholamine transmission is thus essential for reducing the effect of distracting stimulus, or "noise" (Miller et al., 1996) and inhibiting inappropriate behaviours (Funahashi et al., 1993 Arnsten, 2007). More recent data have indicated that both D1 and α2A adrenoceptors can either stimulate or reduce cAMP production respectively, i.e. may increase or reduce the probability of hyperpolarization-activated cyclic nucleotide gated cation channels opening (HCN) (Arnsten, 2007). Moreover, dopamine and NA can inhibit GABA interneurons in the PFC via D4 receptors for which noradrenaline has a high affinity (Wang et al., 2002).

5. Addiction and prefrontal cortex function: Similarities and differences between humans and other mammals

Addiction is the result of numerous factors and the PFC circuitry contributes to the expression of several behaviours that are associated with addiction (Goldstein and Volkow, 2011; Heatherton and Wagner, 2011, George and Koob, 2010). A large majority of addicted subjects do not seek treatment, likely because they do not even recognize their condition as a disease that requires a therapeutic intervention (Goldstein et al. 2009). This condition is probably generated by viewing the abused substance as an essential ingredient of their life, regardless of the consequences of its use. The knowledge of mPFC role in drug dependence can be improved comparing the results of studies performed in animals with those performed in humans although the complexity of addiction behaviour suggests attention in comparing directly specific components of drug dependence (i.e. chronic drug exposure, drug abstinence, drug seeking, cue or drug induced relapse and stress induced relapse). Indeed, if drug addiction in humans can be considered a disorder of self-control because the reinforcing properties of drugs of abuse prevail on the conscious awareness of the negative consequences of addiction behaviour (Heatherton and Wagner, 2011), in animals drug self-administration is supported mostly by the direct rewarding property of the drug (see O'Connor et al. 2011 for a critical evaluation). Therefore, if a man is conscious of the risk associated with drug taking either as far as regards legal or health or social consequences, the same cannot apply to monkeys or rats.

A second important difference among humans and animals deals with the beginning of drug taking. In man it is often the consequence of a complex psychological motivation in which expectations is a strong component (Berridge et al., 2009) while it is often a passive outcome in animals. Moreover, the consequences of drug taking may vary substantially depending on the age of the first experience. In fact drug taking can be started in adolescence, or at adult age and the consequences can be very different because the incomplete brain maturation at adolescence age can offer a fertile ground to the strong reinforcing properties of drugs of abuse (Casey and Jones, 2010). On the other hand, at adult age drug taking can be started to react to a stressful situation and although it may have multiple origin, it may offer again a common fertile ground because the altered status of brain circuitry. Now, if drug taking produces relevant changes in the mPFC of humans and animals, those changes are produced upon a rather different brain circuitry status and therefore the intrinsic rewarding effects in humans can be basically different from those produced in other mammals. When a drug of abuse is administered to animals, the effects observed are those produced on a brain circuitry ensemble that is in a balanced basal condition (unless specific treatments have been applied previously), therefore a great caution should be taken comparing those results to men.

6. Drugs of abuse: Acute effects on prefrontal cortex dopamine and noradrenaline transmission

Substantial evidence confirms the direct involvement of mPFC in addiction. Firing of mPFC neurons is strictly related to i.v. injections of cocaine and heroin (Chang et al., 1998), whereas 6-OH dopamine lesions of mPFC enhance cocaine self-administration (Schenk et al., 1991) and excitotoxic lesions of mPFC determine facilitation of cocaine self-administration (Weissenborn et al., 1997). In particular mPFC has a critical role in drug seeking, craving and relapse either triggered by drugs or by stress or cues associated with drug taking either in humans or in animals (Kalivas et al, 2005; Kalivas and Volkow, 2005). Moreover image studies allowed to observe a reduction in blood flow and cellular metabolism in dorsal PFC of individuals who abused psychostimulants and opioids (Daglish et al., 2001; Bolla et al., 2003; Adinoff et al., 2012). On the contrary an increase has been observed when addicts are exposed to drug-associated cues (Goldstein and Volkow, 2002; Langleben et al., 2008). Nevertheless a reduction in blood flow and cellular metabolism in ventral PFC has been observed in cocaine abusers upon exposition to cocaine related cues (Bonson et al., 2002). Taken together these data support the view that drug addiction increases the motivational value of drug-associated cues while, most likely, negatively affects the function of mPFC in reducing the value of natural reinforcers (see Van den Oever et al., 2010).

Nevertheless, although the dorsal mPFC is critically involved in reinstatement of drug seeking behaviour after abstinence (Berglind et al., 2007) pharmacological inactivation of the dorsal mPFC had no effect on cocaine seeking induced by cocaine cues (Koya et al., 2009). Psychostimulants and other drugs that block dopamine or noradrenaline carrier increase directly extracellular concentration of these catecholamine in all brain areas innervated by dopamine and noradrenaline neurons (Carboni et al., 1989; Tanda et al., 1997; Carboni et al.,

1990; Carboni et al., 2006) including the PFC. The increase in dopamine extracellular concentration can determine the inhibition of the firing of dopamine neurons through an action on D2 auto-receptors and in turn increase K^+ conductance at cell body level (Mercuri et al., 1992). The simultaneous reduction of firing and increase of transmitter extracellular concentration at terminal level produced by psychostimulants and cocaine on catecholamine transmission in the mPFC cortex and other brain areas determines a complex effect on cognition, attention and learning circuitry. Indeed either an increase or a decrease in dopamine transmission in the mPFC may lead to dysfunctions in the ability to inhibit inappropriate actions or thoughts (Arnsten and Li, 2005).

Investigations on the effects of non-psychostimulants substances of abuse on dopamine and norepinephrine transmission in the rat PFC have produced disaccording results. Devoto et al., (2002) have found that acute morphine reduced extracellular norepinephrine, and failed to modify extracellular dopamine level in the mPFC whereas the administration of naloxone, in morphine dependent rats, precipitated a typical abstinence syndrome associated with a concomitant dramatic increase of extracellular dopamine and noreadrenaline (by about 200 and 100%, respectively) in the PFC. The direct role of norepinephrine transmission in the effects of morphine was demonstrated by the alpha(2)-adrenoceptor agonist clonidine that suppressed naloxone-precipitated abstinence symptoms and brought both noradrenaline and dopamine output in PFC to less than 50 % of basal levels (Devoto et al., 2002). In contrast it has been reported that morphine enhances norepinephrine and dopamine release in the mPFC and that norepinephrine transmission is necessary for morphine rewarding effects, reinstatement and mesoaccumbens dopamine release (Ventura et al., 2005). More recently it was found that the released levels of dopamine and its major metabolites in the anterior cingulate cortex were increased by either the electrical stimulation of VTA neurons or by microinjection of a selective μ-opioid receptor agonist, (D-Ala^2,N-$MePhe^4$,Gly^5-ol) enkephalin (DAMGO), into the VTA (Narita et al., 2010).

The ability of nicotine to stimulate dopamine and norepinephrine release in the mPFC has been also investigated to assess the involvement of PFC circuitry in the addiction mechanism of nicotine and to explore the potential of modulation of this transmission for cognition enhancement. At this regard Livingstone et al., (2010) reported that a selective alpha7 nicotinic acetylcholine receptors (nAChRs) agonist evoked dopamine overflow in the prefrontal cortex in vivo, and this effect was potentiated by PNU-120596, an allosteric modulator of alpha7 nACh receptor. Moreover, antagonists of NMDA and AMPA receptors blocked [^{3}H]dopamine release from tissue prisms in vitro. On these bases the authors proposed that alpha7 nAChRs were present on glutamate terminals and could increase glutamate release that in turn coordinately could enhances dopamine release from neighboring buttons.

The effect of other drugs of abuse such ethanol and cannabinoids on dopamine and noradrenaline transmission in the PFC received less attention although the effects of these drugs on cognition and mental health are well known. It has been found that posterior VTA dopamine neurons projecting to the ventral pallidum and mPFC are stimulated by local administration of ethanol and that these stimulating effects are mediated, at least in part, by 5-HT(3)receptors (Ding et al., 2011). The presence of cannabinoid receptors in the PFC has been shown by neuroanatomical data suggesting that cortical norepinephrine release may be modulated, in part, by CB1 receptors that are presynaptically distributed on noradrenergic axon terminals (Oropeza et al., 2006). Moreover, repeated treatment with delta-9-tetrahydrocannabinol (THC), the major psychoactive constituent of marijuana, or WIN 55,212-2 (WIN), a synthetic cannabinoid receptor agonist caused a persistent and selective reduction in mPFC dopamine turnover (Verrico et al., 2003). Thereby these evidences suggest that dopamine and norepinephrine transmission in the PFC are involved in the effects of many drugs of abuse, although their precise role is far to be clarified.

7. Abstinence, dopamine and noradrenaline transmission in the PFC

Although the intrinsic meaning of abstinence, as far as regards drug addiction, is referred to a drug free condition, the status of PFC during abstinence may vary depending on the time interval elapsed from the interruption of drug use. Abrupt drug removal can produce a rather similar abstinence syndrome as both men and rats will experience a neuro-physiological adaptation to drug absence. This effect cannot be trivial considering the strong impact of drug effects on brain. Nevertheless once the acute abstinence has been overtaken, strong differences may be found between men and other mammals, in particular when abstinence is generated by a gradual quitting process in humans or extinction process in animals as in self-administration experiments. For instance, in these experiments, upon removal of the reinforcing drug, rats will soon experience the absence of drug effect. This condition will initially generate an enhanced activity at the operant administration mechanism (e.g. lever pressing, nose poke etc.) that will be followed by a reduction because operant activity becomes emptied of pleasurable consequences. This condition will activate a parsimonious process that drives rat behaviour to ignore the ineffective lever pressing with a come back to the routine cage activity. Thus, drug disappearance can be view as an uncontrollable variable and it is likely that rats will not go through the experience of choosing whether or not going back to the drug. Therefore, although it is hard to appraise in rats the role of memories associated with drug administration, we can suggest that medial PFC circuitry will respond to drug removal through adapting progressive changes, thus generating the relative abstinence condition.

On the other hand in man, abstinence is a multiple component condition in which the lack drug effects is strictly associated with an internal struggle between the desire of the reward associated with drug taking and the evaluation of the consequences of that behaviour in terms of money, social life and health involvement (e.g. smoking, cocaine use). It is therefore likely that mPFC circuitry response to abstinence in man will be unique, although it is obviously dependent on the abused drug and on plenty of other environmental factors such as recreational habits, family or economic problems or other stress related conditions. Therefore, craving for drugs is characterized in animals by an initial stereotyped search for drug, that ends relatively quickly with the reaching of a relatively stable brain circuitry equilibrium. Instead in man, mPFC brain circuitry reaches only a pseudo-equilibrium to which contribute the lack of drug effects and its desire (in common with animals), together with of the effort of self-controlling environmental stimuli that often were those that generated drug addiction. In this scenario the result of the exposition to cues associated with drug taking can trigger relapse either in animals or humans, but again involvement of mPFC circuitry can be completely different. The role of PFC in extinction has been recently investigated in humans and animals though the circuitry involved is poorly understood (See the recent review by Millan et al., 2011).

Here we will briefly discuss mPFC changes related to immediate abstinence generated from drug withdrawal. For instance interruption of nicotine exposure in humans, determines a rather fast appearance of withdrawal syndrome that is characterized by depressed mood, irritability, mild cognitive deficits accompanied by other peripheral physiological symptoms (Shiffman et al., 2004). We observed that either mecamylamine or naloxone determine the precipitation of an abstinence syndrome in rats carrying an osmotic minipump that continuously delivers nicotine (Carboni et al., 2000). This syndrome was characterized by physical abstinence signs appearing to be dissociated from dopamine extracellular concentration. Mecamylamine decreased dopamine in the NAcc while increasing it the mPFC whereas naloxone did not (Carboni et al., 2000). Interestingly withdrawal from a schedule of increasing doses of morphine or the administration of naloxone determined an increase in the extracellular concentration of dopamine mPFC (Bassareo et al., 1995). Preclinical research in animal models have also shown that early nicotine withdrawal is characterized by decreased function of presynaptic inhibitory metabotropic glutamate 2/3 receptors (Markou, 2008). At the same time it has been observed an increased expression of postsynaptic glutamate receptor subunits in limbic and frontal brain sites. This increase may explain why a protracted abstinence may be associated with increased glutamate response to stimuli associated with nicotine administration (as reviewed by Markou, 2008).

As far as regards cocaine addiction it has been reported (Kalivas et al., 2005) that enhanced D1 activity would lead to an increased inhibitory state of the PFC during withdrawal, so that only particularly strong stimuli, such as those associated with drug consumption, would be able to activate and guide behaviour. Moreover repeated cocaine administration change functional properties of the D1 receptors in the PFC through an enhancement of the activity of the G protein signalling 3 (AGS3), coupled to D1 receptors, whereas the G protein activity coupled to D2 was reduced following cocaine withdrawal (Bowers et al., 2004). These alterations in the mPFC may determine alteration of prefrontal glutamatergic innervation of the accumbens promoting the compulsive character of drug seeking in addicts by decreasing the value of natural rewards, diminishing cognitive control (choice), and enhancing glutamatergic drive in response to drug-associated stimuli.

8. Relapse, dopamine and noradrenaline transmission in the prefrontal cortex

The relapse to drug use is a major problem in drug addiction therapy. Essentially, relapse can be categorized in three major types: drug induced relapse, reinstatement of self-administration behaviour upon exposition to drug related cues and stress induced relapse (Stewart, 2003; Crombag et al., 2008; Van den Oever et al., 2010). Drug-induced relapse could be associated with similar processes in humans and animals and will determine the resumption of drug intake behaviour, whereas cue-induced relapse may engage different brain circuitry depending on the involvement of self-control mechanisms. If a rat will just start pressing a lever, a man, who probably went through a strong involving process to achieve drug taking interruption, will go through a complex decision making process (e.g. a man will evaluate the strong effect of the cue and only when self control processes will be defeated will resume drug taking; alternatively he can resume drug taking without craving, or even he can rationally decide to take the drug because he has the conviction to be able to control drug taking). Thus, it is likely that reinstatement in man involves a more complex mPFC circuitry than in other mammals. Nevertheless one of the major determinants of reinstatement to cocaine use among human addicts is acute re-exposure to the drug, which often precipitates cocaine craving and relapse (Cromabag et al., 2008; Volkow et al., 2010). As far as regards animal studies, it has been reported that the mPFC plays a major role during reinstatement, either because its direct role in cognition or because its connections with subcortical areas (Kalivas et al., 2005; Crombag et al., 2008; Van den Oever et al., 2010). Projections from the mPFC to the NAcc are stratified in a dorso-ventral pattern with the dorsal mPFC projecting predominantly to the NAcc core and the ventral mPFC projecting to the NAcc shell (Heidbreder and Groenewegen, 2003; Voorn et al., 2004). These anatomical features have been used to assume that during reinstatement the increase in extracellular glutamate in the NAcc core is associated with an increased excitatory activity of pyramidal neurons of dorsal mPFC that in turn may drive heroin (LaLumiere and Kalivas, 2008) or cocaine seeking behaviour in rats (Mac Farland et al., 2003).

On the other hand, glutamatergic projections from the ventral mPFC to the NAcc shell have been found to suppress conditioned drug seeking after extinction learning (Peters et al., 2009) whereas interruption of this neuronal link or pharmacological inactivation of the NAcc shell produce resumption of drug craving (Peters et al., 2008; Fuchs et al., 2008). At this regard it has been proposed that the mPFC regulates the expression of both fear and drug memories after extinction, through divergent projections to the amygdala and nucleus accumbens, respectively. Therefore a common neural circuit for extinction of fear and drug memories would suggest shared mechanisms and treatment strategies across both domains (Peters et al., 2009). These experimental evidences support the view of mPFC neurons controlling drug craving whereas its suppression may occur through two separate but balanced pathways by acting directly in the two NAcc sub-regions. This view has been contradicted by numerous studies (for a review see Van den Oever et al., 2010) and therefore it can be suggested that drug dependence in rats cannot be the product of a single neuronal pathway

VTA dopaminergic neurons that innervate the dorsal mPFC have been reported to be involved in the initiation of drug seeking responses (for a review see Crombag et al., 2008 and Van den Over et al., 2010). In particular dopamine administration into the dorsal mPFC has been shown to be sufficient to elicit a reinstatement of self-administration behavior (McFarland and Kalivas, 2001), whereas microinjections of the D1/D2 antagonist fluphenazine into the dorsal PFC but not into the NAcc core or ventral pallidum, prevented cocaine induced reinstatement (McFarland and Kalivas 2001). A role for dopamine transmission in reinstatement is also supported by the findings of Park and coworkers (Park et al., 2002). These authors showed that intra-mPFC administration of the dopamine antagonist flupentixol blocked cocaine reinstatement triggered by systemic cocaine administration in rats that were first trained to self-administer cocaine intravenously and later underwent through extinction by substitution of cocaine (i.v.) with saline (Park et al., 2002). These authors also showed that reinstatement of cocaine seeking behavior could be induced by intra-mPFC cocaine and could be blocked by local administration of the AMPA receptor antagonist CNQX into NAcc shell or the border with the core (Park et al., 2002). Interestingly, it has been recently reported that the infralimbic mPFC, and specifically its glutamatergic and beta-adrenergic systems, regulates the consolidation of extinction of cocaine self-administration. Therefore the transmission at level of infralimbic cortex can be manipulated to influence the retention of extinction (LaLumiere and Kalivas, 2008).

Moreover, a role for dopamine transmission in the mPFC has been also proposed in cue and in stress induced reinstatement of self-administration behavior. In fact intracranial infusion of the dopamine D1 receptor antagonist, SCH 23390 into the prelimbic cortex potently, and dose dependently, attenuated heroin-seeking in response to either cue presentations or a priming dose of heroin, confirming that dopamine D1 receptors regulate prefrontal cortex pathways necessary for the reinstatement of heroin-seeking in rats (See, 2009). In addition systemic blockade of D1 receptors prevents an increase in Fos expression in the dorsal mPFC (Ciccocioppo et al., 2001) suggesting an increase in dopamine transmission in this area during reinstatement. Moreover the role of the mPFC and in particular the involvement of dopamine transmission in stress induced reinstatement of cocaine seeking have been investigated in rats (Capriles et al., 2003). These authors have shown that inactivation of prelimbic cortex by tetrodotoxin blocked reinstatement of cocaine seeking induced by either foot shock or by cocaine priming, whereas the effects of tetrodotoxin injections in the orbitofrontal cortex (OFC) were mixed. Moreover, Capriles and coworkers found that infusion of the D1 dopamine antagonist SCH23390 into either the prelimbic or into the OFC blocked foot-shock induced reinstatement. These results suggest that the prelimbic and the orbitofrontal cortices form part of the circuitry mediating the effects of foot shock stress in reinstatement of drug seeking and that the prelimbic region may be a common pathway for cue, drug and foot-shock stress-induced reinstatement of drug seeking (Capriles et al., 2003). Nevertheless, the dichotomy in mPFC function, attributing to dorsal mPFC (prelimbic, cingulate subregions) promotion of drug seeking and to ventral mPFC (infralimbic) inhibition of drug seeking in cocaine-experienced rats (Peters et al., 2009), has been challenged by studies on heroin self-administration suggesting that heroin seeking is promoted by a minority of selectively activated ventral mPFC neurons (Bossert et al., 2011). These authors thus suggested that different brain mechanisms mediate heroin and cocaine relapse in the rat model.

9. Genetic variation, catecholamine transmission in the prefrontal cortex and predisposition to addictions

Dopamine neurons projecting to the PFC possess an interesting feature as compared with other systems. In fact they have a higher baseline rate firing and a higher rate of dopamine turnover. This feature renders them very sensitive to alteration in dopamine synthesis and metabolism either underlained by gene variation or induced by drugs of abuse (Bannon et al., 1981; Hallman, 1984; Garris et al., 1993; Garris and Wightman, 1994; Cass and Gerhardt, 1995). Improved performances in cognitive tasks requiring working memory and inhibition have been observed in subjects that carry variations in the catechol-O-methyltransferase (COMT) gene (Dumontheil et al., 2011). COMT degrades the catecholamine neurotransmitters dopamine, epinephrine, and norepinephrine. A functional polymorphism in the COMT gene (val^{158}met) accounts for a four-fold variation in enzyme activity (Heinz and Smolka, 2006). The low activity met^{158} allele causes approximately 75 % reduction in dopamine methylation and increased dopamine function. This has been associated with improved working memory, executive functioning, and attention control, but is also linked to a higher risk of anxiety-related behaviours. The latter, in turn, may be related to an excessive activation of the HPA axis and relative responses due to elevated noradrenaline transmission in the PFC (Heinz and Smolka, 2006). On the other hand, limbic and prefrontal activation elicited by unpleasant stimuli in subjects with more met^{158} alleles might contribute to the observed lower emotional resilience against negative mood states (Smolka, et al., 2005). The increase in dopamine function is particularly relevant in areas such as the prefrontal cortex because it contains significantly less dopamine transporter (Sesack et al.,

1998; Lammel et al., 2008), and because dopamine clearance (approx. 60 %) is carried out by the COMT enzyme, unlike in other dopamine areas such as the striatum where dopamine is cleared promptly by the reuptake system (Karoum et al., 1994).

Furthermore, Adele Diamond (2007) makes an interesting observation on the difference found between males and females. COMT activity in females is in fact roughly 30 % lower, due probably to estrogen activity (Cohn and Axelrod, 1971; Boudikova et al., 1990). This gender variation may render females able to better perform cognitive tasks because of the more elevated dopamine function in the PFC whereas they perform worse under even minor stress. On the other hand there is also substantial evidence that males perform better or no worse if slightly stressed (Shors and Miesegaes, 2002; Shors and Leuner, 2003; Shansky et al., 2004). This observation fits well with the above reported characteristics of the PFC dopamine function being highly sensitive to stress (Thierry et al., 1972; Reinhard et al., 1982; Roth et al., 1988; Deutch and Roth, 1990; Arnsten and Goldman-Rakic 1998; Arnsten, 1999 and 2000). Thus, as reported by Diamond (2007), cognitive functioning in men would benefit from the expression of COMT variation with reduced activity whereas females would instead benefit from the expression of a faster-acting valine version of the COMT enzyme that would moderate excess dopamine functioning in the PFC. Altered activity of COMT, which has a primary role in the degradation of dopamine in the frontal cortex (Karoum et al., 1994), might thus also be involved in the magnification of the reinforcing properties of drugs of abuse. Considering that the increase of extracellular dopamine and norepinephrine in PFC is a peculiar effect of drugs such as amphetamine and cocaine one can wonder if subjects that carry variations in the catechol-O-methyltransferase (COMT) gene are predisposed to psychostimulant addiction. Genetic studies suggest that while occasional use of drugs of abuse is predominantly linked to environmental or familiar factors, over 60 % of the cocaine users inherited their vulnerability to heavy use and dependence (Kendler et al., 2000; Kendler and Prescott, 1998).

Nevertheless there are no convincing studies that correlate cocaine addiction with variation of genes related to dopaminergic system such as the genes DRD2, COMT, SLC6A3 (coding for the dopamine transporter DAT) and DBH (coding for the dopamine beta hydroxylase). However an interesting hypothesis (Brousse et al., 2010) suggested that individuals carrying genetic variation of the DBH gene, that has particularly been linked with the psychotic effects caused by cocaine, could be predisposed to cocaine-induced psychosis making the development of cocaine addiction less probable. This can also apply to mutations of the Val158Met of the gene COMT, TaqI A of the gene DRD2 and VNTR 9 repeat of the DAT. On the other hand Hosak et al., (2006) found that consumers of methamphetamine carrying the Met allele of the COMT gene Val158Met polymorphism showed higher novelty seeking scores. This polymorphism is associated with low COMT enzyme activity and high endogenous dopamine synaptic levels in the PFC. According to the authors this leads to a decrease in dopaminergic neurotransmission in the NAcc and a need to stimulate it through novelty seeking behaviour or psychostimulant use.

10. Prefrontal cortex dopamine transmission in adolescence and drug addiction

Adolescence (see chapter XX) is a crucial developmental period of life in which physical and psychological remarkable changes occurring after puberty, model the personality to allow the assumption of adult roles and responsibilities (Dahl, 2004a and 2004b; Steinberg, 2008). In this scenario PFC represents a crucial brain area because its function in expressing a specific behaviour. This may be the outcome of multiple interactions such as those between the hormonal triggered desires, and the representation of increasingly complex and distant social goals. The shaping of this objective in turn will be influenced by the social and family environment. Therefore the maturation of PFC occurring in adolescence may definitively shape the adult personality and at the same time, dysfunctions happening in this process may constitute a milieu necessary and often sufficient for developing psychiatric disorders such as schizophrenia and depression or for predisposing individuals to a high vulnerability to drug addiction (see Davey, et al., 2008).

The PFC has a prominent role in controlling impulsiveness (Fineberg et al., 2010) and in adolescence it is likely that this control is insufficient due to incomplete maturation of cognitive function. Accordingly, working memory, abstract thinking and complex problem solving improve during adolescence to peak at late adolescence (Feinberg, 1983; Woo et al., 1997; Williams et al., 1999). These acquired abilities are supported by distinct developmental changes occurring in the PFC during adolescence and involve changes in densities of dendritic processes and synapses, increased myelination, increased neuronal membrane synthesis and in turn, increase in white matter (Paus et al., 1999; Giedd et al., 1999a, 1999b). Among these changes, synaptic pruning has been considered a way to reduce energy use through a selective reduction of synaptic contacts that are not necessary to sustain a particular ability; in humans PFC synaptic density, after reaching a maximum at the age of 5 years, diminishes by about 35 % by late adolescence (Lewis, 1997). This synapse reduction involves mostly local PFC circuits (Woo et al., 1997) and both excitatory and inhibitory inputs are implicated (Anderson et al., 1995). During the pruning that occurs in adolescence there is a prevalent reduction of the excitatory stimulation that reaches the PFC (Rakic et al., 1994). In particular synapse elimination of presumed glutamatergic inputs occurs in PFC. Binding to NMDA receptors in rat brain peaks at 28 post natal day (PND) whereas a successive reduction leads to a 33 % reduction by the 60 PND (Insel et al., 1990).

On the contrary, dopamine functional activity in the PFC increases in adolescence, peaking to levels much higher than those seen in adulthood (for a review see Lewis et al., 1998). In rats, dopamine innervation is maximum at 35 PND in superficial layers and at 60 PND in deeper layers (Kalsbeek et al., 1988); moreover, the density of DAT, often used as an index of dopamine innervation in the PFC, is about 70 % of adult levels in weaning rats. On the other hand the increase in dopamine fiber density observed in development may be associated to a decline in synthesis and turnover; in fact synthesis peaks at PND 30 and then declines in late adolescence (Andersen, et al., 1997). Adolescence has a peculiar feature from an energetically point of view. In fact cortex energy consumption in humans peaks at 3-4 years and is maintained up to the age of 20, to progressively decline in later life (Chugani et al., 1987). In general synaptic pruning and myelination can be considered parallel processes that apparently have the role of strengthening regularly used innervations rendering them able to fire in a more concerted pattern (Lewis, 1997; Miller, 1996). At the same time infrequently used innervations are eliminated (Rutherford et al., 1998). Furthermore dopamine modulation of fast-spiking interneurons changes dramatically during adolescence (PND 45-50 in rats) with D2 agonists switching from being mildly inhibitory in prepubertal rats to strongly excitatory in young adult rats. In vivo recordings in adult rats reveal that deep-layer pyramidal neurons respond to endogenous DA release with suppression of firing while interneurons are activated (Tseng and O'Donnell, 2007; Gruber et al., 2010). Thus the increase in dopamine functional activity that peaks in adolescence together with the reduction of excitatory innervation are two delicate processes which reduce the activity of pyramidal cells. Therefore either a deficiency in excitatory reduction or a defective increased inhibitory activity may lead to an excessive pyramidal cell activity that in turn may be reflected by the onset of a psychiatric disorder or drug abuse.

Substantial evidence points to the higher risk of drug exposure in adolescence (Barron et al., 2005; Crews and Hodge, 2007; Schramm-Sapyta et al., 2009). In particular alcohol consumption during adolescence causes diffuse brain alterations and greatly increases the likelihood that an alcohol use disorder will develop later in life (Nixon and McClain, 2010). Diffusion tensor imaging studies have shown that adolescent binge drinking damages white matter tracts throughout the brain, including main hippocampus efferent fibers and those interconnecting the PFC (McQueeny et al., 2009; Jacobus et al., 2009). Adolescents respond to the effects of alcohol distinctly from adults in fact they are less sensitive to negative effects of alcohol, they do no perceive cues that may suggest reduction of intake, but are more sensitive to positive effects such as those related to social interaction, which may serve to reinforce or promote excessive intake (Spear et al., 2005). Adolescence is also critical for cannabis abuse, indeed it is widely reported that cannabis use during adolescence increases the risk of developing psychotic disorders later in life (Bossong and Niesink, 2010, Malone et al, 2010). However, although the neurobiological processes underlying this relationship are unknown, alteration of PFC circuitry is more than likely. Very recently it was found that marijuana users had decreased cortical thickness in right caudal middle frontal, bilateral insula and bilateral superior frontal cortices (Lopez-Larson, 2011). These results suggest that age of regular use may be associated with altered PFC gray matter development in adolescents. According to the authors of this study reduced insular cortical thickness may be used as a biological marker for ascertain increased risk of substance dependence (Lopez-Larson, 2011). An interesting comparison in adolescent alcohol and marijuana users has been proposed by evaluating participants who performed a verbal paired associates encoding task during functional magnetic resonance imaging (fMRI) scanning. The results of this study suggested that adolescent substance users demonstrated altered fMRI response relative to non-using controls, yet binge drinking appeared to be associated with more differences in activation than marijuana use (Schweinsburg et al., 2011). Alcohol and marijuana may have interactive effects that alter these differences, particularly in prefrontal brain regions (Schweinsburg et al., 2011).

As far as regards cocaine effects, rats with adolescent-onset cocaine self-administration experience were more impaired in an OFC-related learning task than rats with adult-onset cocaine self-administration experience (Harvey et al., 2009). Treatment with cocaine during adolescence also caused acute alterations in the expression of genes encoding cell adhesion molecules and transcription factors within the PFC. In particular, a decrease in histone methylation was observed and this effect may indicate a role for chromatin remodelling in gene expression patterns. These findings allowed the authors to suggest that exposure to cocaine during adolescence has extensive molecular and behavioural effects in the rat PFC. These consequences develop over time and endure long after drug administration has ceased (Black et al., 2006). Smoking and nicotine exposure during adolescence is a very relevant heath problem because the higher dependence developed in individuals who start smoking early (see O'Dell, 2009 for review). Early tobacco use is facilitated by the legal possibility to purchase tobacco in most of the western countries. Besides other health consequences, tobacco smoking and nicotine exposure during adolescence interfere with PFC development and leads to cognitive impairments in later life with enduring attentional disturbances (Cunotte et al., 2009). Among molecular alteration, early nicotine exposure determines reduced mGluR2 protein and function on presynaptic terminals of PFC glutamatergic synapses. Interestingly restoring mGluR2 activity in vivo by local infusion of a group II mGluR agonist in adult rats that received nicotine as adolescents rescued attentional disturbances (Counotte et al., 2011).

Among others, novelty directed behavior is highly expressed in adolescence. It may represent a strong risk for the use of addictive drugs and consequently for the developing of drug dependence. Novelty directed behavior can be observed in periadolescent rats, in fact they show a strong exploratory behavior in a novel open field. Although it is not clear the role of dopamine and norepinephrine transmission in this behavior, periadolescent rats show hypo-responsivity to dopamine agonists and hypersensitivity to antagonist action suggesting that their dopamine transmission is hyperactive as compared with adult rats (Spear and Brake, 1983). Moreover the response of adolescent animals to amphetamine (an indirect dopamine and noradrenaline agonist) supports the peculiarity of catecholamine transmission in adolescence (Mathews and McCormick, 2011). Paradoxically amphetamine reduces novelty preference when adolescent mice are paired with a novel environment while it increases novelty preference when this test is performed in normal adult mice (Adriani et al., 1998). Thus we can hypothesize that typical adolescent behaviors such as novelty seeking, impulsivity and risk taking are the result of a natural drive that emerges in adolescence possibly linked to the need of spreading individuals of a species in a territory. It may be likely that this behaviour could be maintained by an overactive excitatory transmission in the prefrontal cortex and in subcortical areas that are balanced by an increasing active inhibitory catecholamine transmission. On the other hand catecholamine innervations reaching their maximal inhibitory activity at the end of adolescence, may have a role in stabilizing those brain processes that have been developed in adolescence and will be then acquired as behaviour reference in adult life.

As far as nicotine effect in adolescents, we observed that nicotine-stimulated dopamine release was higher in the mPFC of adolescent rats as compared with adults (Carboni et al., 2010). These results suggest that the higher response observed in adolescents might be correlated to their higher sensitivity to the effects of nicotine. This trait might have a contributory role in the strong nicotine addiction that is observed in smokers who start nicotine abuse during adolescence (see the review of O'Dell, 2009). In fact, although nicotine abuse has much in common with other drugs of abuse in that it increases dopamine output in the NAcc shell (Di Chiara, 2000) or in other brain areas (Carboni et al., 2000), its ability to determine a higher increase of dopamine in the PFC of adolescents could potentially be correlated to the alteration of the brain maturation process that occurs in adolescent smokers (Carboni et al., 2010). Consequently this feature may alter the PFC's role in the ability to establish a rational evaluation of smoking even during adult age. We also observed that nicotine increased noradrenaline release in the PFC (Carboni et al., 2010) thus suggesting that this increase may have a role in the nicotine enhancement of cognition (see the review of Poorthuis et al., 2009). Furthermore local infusion of nicotine in the prelimbic mPFC can increase mPFC glutamate extracellular concentration supporting the role of nAChRs in modulating thalamocortical input to the PFC (Gioanni et al., 1999). These findings therefore suggest that such a mechanism may be relevant to the cognitive effects of nicotine and nicotinic agonists.

11. Role of stress (prenatal, adolescent and adult) on prefrontal cortex function and drug addiction

Acute stress modulates the neuronal activity of brain regions such as mPFC (Hains and Arnsten, 2008), amygdala (Goldstein et al., 1996), hippocampus (Belujon and Grace 2011) , OFC (Capriles et al., 2003), insula, and striatum (Koob, 2009) that are also areas of the brain involved in regulation of appetitive behaviors, such as feeding and drug taking (Marchant et al., 2012). These areas share common a consistent dopaminergic innervation pointing to a role of dopamine in stress-induced reinstatement of drug taking (Erblich et al., 2004; Shaham and Stewart, 1995; Shaham et al., 2003). The preclinical early work of Piazza and collaborators has shown a clear relationship between drugs of abuse, stress and glucocorticoids levels (Piazza et al., 1996), although most of their work was focused on sub-cortical areas. They have indeed shown that drugs of abuse acutely activate the hypothalamic-pituitary-adrenal (HPA) axis and that drug dependence was characterized by a dysregulation of HPA axis (Piazza and Le Moal, 1996). Moreover they showed that stressors facilitate the acquisition of cocaine and amphetamine self-administration (Piazza and Le Moal, 1998). Stress plays and important role in drug addiction either by triggering relapse in abstinent addicts, or by altering PFC function thus predisposing for drug use and abuse (Stewart, 2003; George and Koob, 2010; Van den Oever et al., 2010). Human studies suggested that the incapacity to resist to drug cues, such as the sight of drug, can also be amplified by stress (Swan et al., 1988; Breese et al., 2011; Potenza et al., 2012). Although moderate stress can have a positive value on cognition, strong or repeated stress will either be deleterious for cognitive functions or may be a determining factor in vulnerability to mental illness and drug addiction, likely through an alteration of catecholamine transmission in the PFC (Holmes and Welman 2009, George and Koob, 2010; Goldstein and Volkow, 2011). Indeed, it has recently been reported (Radley et al., 2008) that selectively ablating noradrenergic input into the rat medial PFC attenuates the effects of stress in the paraventricular hypothalamic nucleus, as well as the HPA axis secretory responses, while stress-induced Fos expression in dorsal medial PFC was enhanced and was negatively correlated with stress-induced paraventricular hypothalamic nucleus activation. These observations identify the locus coeruleus as an upstream component of a circuitry providing for dorsal medial PFC modulation of emotional stress-induced HPA activation. Since noradrenergic projection, and its innervations of the prefrontal cortex play an important role in the modulation of working memory and attention, it may be likely that noradrenaline release in the medial PFC could modulate stress response, depending on the evaluation and comparison of environmental stimuli with past experience in mounting adequate behaviourally adaptive responses to emotional stress and environmental challenge in general.

Further, the artificial activation of catecholamine transmission in the PFC, such as that produced by amphetamine administration, similarly to stress, can have beneficial or a deleterious effects on cognition depending on the dose and on basal dopamine and noradrenaline transmission. The ability of stress to alter neuronal function has been investigated in 15 smokers undergoing functional magnetic resonance imaging who were exposed to a psychosocial stressor, followed by smoking drug cues (Dagher et al., 2009). The results allowed to observe a significant change in neural activity during stress with an increased neural response to drug cues in the medial prefrontal cortex, posterior cingulate cortex, dorsomedial thalamus, medial temporal lobe, caudate nucleus, and primary and association visual areas. A stress-induced limbic deactivation that predicted subsequent neural cue-reactivity was also observed. The authors thus suggested that stress increases the incentive salience of drug cues (Dagher et al., 2009). The role of mPFC in the ability of stress to enhance the reinforcing properties of morphine has been recently investigated (Rozeske et al., 2009). The results obtained show that escapable stress activates the ventral regions of the mPFC while inescapable stress does not. On the other hand inescapable stress potentiates morphine-conditioned place preference while escapable stress does not. Moreover these effects are modulated by intra-mPFCv microinjection of the GABAA agonist muscimol 1 h before stress session (Rozeske et al., 2009).

It was early reported that the adult offspring of stressed pregnant rats exhibited higher locomotor response to novelty and to an injection of amphetamine but also a higher level of amphetamine self-administration, suggesting that prenatal stress (PNS) could determine an individual predisposition to drug self-administration (Deminiére et al., 1992). The effect of PNS was also observed to elevate active lever responding in rats either during extinction or in cocaine-primed reinstatement, but not during self-administration or in conditioned-cued reinstatement, thus suggesting that early environmental factors contribute to an individual's initial responsiveness to cocaine and propensity to relapse to cocaine-seeking (Kipping et al., 2008). We recently investigated in rats the effect of PNS on dopamine and noradrenaline transmission in the mPFC (Carboni et al., 2010) and in the NAcc shell (Silvagni et al., 2008). We observed that PNS did not change dopamine but decreased noradrenaline basal output in the PFC of both adolescents and adult rats (Carboni et al, 2010). Moreover we observed that PNS decreased amphetamine stimulated dopamine output and increased amphetamine-stimulated noradrenaline output. PNS decreased nicotine-stimulated noradrenaline (but not dopamine output) in adults, though not in adolescents (Carboni et al., 2010). These data support a contributing role of PNS in the development of psychiatric disorders and that its effect may augment drug addiction vulnerability.

12. Areas of prefrontal cortex, decision making and drug addiction.

Preclinical and human studies have provided unequivocal evidence that drug addiction involves many subregions of the PFC. Nevertheless the correspondence between these subregions among rodents and primates has been long debated (Brown and Bowman, 2002). Moreover it is claimed that PFC function is more than the sum of the functions of individual PFC sub-regions (Wilson et al., 2010). An exhaustive review of PFC dysfunction in addiction has been recently provided (Goldstein and Volkow, 2011). In this section we will briefly consider some preclinical and human studies on the involvement of the OFC in addiction because this PFC sub region has recently received much attention in drug addiction (Shoenbaum et al., 2006). The orbitofrontal area is interconnected in both rat and primates with mediodorsal talamus, the basolateral amigdala and NAcc, and has been proposed to use associative information handled by this circuitry to guide behaviour on the basis of the expected outcome of a specific action (See the review of Shoenbaum et al., 2006 for specific anatomical location and relationship with other brain areas). In particular this area is activated in humans during anticipation of expected outcomes and therefore can allow prediction of reward or punishment using this information to guide decisions (Arana et al., 2003). Rats with OFC lesions fail to behave correctly in reinforcing devaluation tasks where they have to make decisions on the basis of outcome expectancies (Gallagher et al., 1999). As far as regards addicted they may suffer of OFC circuitry alteration because, often under the control of drug-associated cues, they are unable to control drug-seeking behaviour despite they are aware of adverse consequences associated with their compulsive and impulsive behaviour and despite a stated desire to stop. The alteration of OFC have been detected by imaging studies of addicts and in particular it has been observed a reduction in OFC activation during acute withdrawal whereas an over-activation of OFC associated with high level of craving has been observed in addicts exposed to drug-related cues (see the review of Dom et al., 2005). Furthermore, in addicts are observed impairments of OFC-dependent behaviours that strongly parallel those that are observed in individuals carrying OFC damage (Grant et al., 2000).

Nevertheless in humans it is difficult to state that functional deficits at the level of OFC are due to drug exposure because it could be attributable to pre-existing condition. At this regard Volkow and collaborators proposed an interesting hypothesis (Volkow et al., 2009). They suggested an association between an impairment of the OFC and other PFC areas involved in addiction, and a decrease of striatal dopamine D2 receptors availability. This condition would render subjects more vulnerable to drug addiction (Volkow et al., 2009). Further, a study done in subjects who have a high risk for alcoholism but were not alcoholics showed higher than normal striatal D2 receptor levels and a normal metabolism in OFC, anterior cingulate cortex and dorsolateral PFC (Volkow et al., 2006). On this basis the authors proposed that normal PFC function may have protected these subjects from alcohol abuse. A further recent evolution of this hypothesis suggested that OFC and cingulate function are involved in individual positive emotionality which in turn is a defence against drug of abuse vulnerability (Volkow et al., 2011). Nevertheless these stimulating hypotheses have to be evaluated taking into account that dopoamine D2 availability does not distinguish between an increase in the released dopamine or in a decrease of receptors. On the other hand rats trained to self-administer amphetamine show a long term (one month) reduction of dendritic spine density specifically in the OFC whereas spine density was increased in the medium spiny neurons of the NAcc and in pyramidal neurons of the mPFC (Crombag et al., 2005). Moreover others have reported an increase of dendritic spine density in the medial PFC and in the NAcc after treatment with psychostimulant (Robinson and Kolb, 1999). It has been reported that chronic cocaine use causes long lasting impairment in OFC function as established by studies on reversal learning in animals, thus suggesting that this damage is expressed by the inability of using the value of predicted outcome to guide behavior (Shoenbaum et al., 2004, 2006 and 2009). The results of these experiments allowed Shoenbaum et al. (2006) to claim that "cocaine use can drive to the loss of outcome expectancies making addicts to continue to seek drugs despite the almost inevitable negative consequences of such behaviour concluding that changes in the OFC-dependent signal would by themselves contribute powerfully to a transition from normal goal-directed behaviour to compulsive habitual responding".

Moreover a dysregulation of the ventral, dorsomedial and dorsolateral striatal systems has been hypothesized to play a fundamental role in the transition from voluntary drug use to more habitual and compulsive drug use (Everitt and Robbins, 2005; Belin and Everitt, 2008). These sub cortical areas are strictly connected with PFC regions and in particular the NAcc shell receives glutamatergic inputs from the ventromedial PFC and insular cortex, the NAcc core receives glutamatergic inputs from the dorsomedial PFC, insular cortex and OFC whereas the dorsomedial and the dorsolateral striatum receive glutamatergic inputs from the OFC, the anterior cingulate cortex and the sensory and motor cortices (Reynolds and Zahm, 2005; Gabbott et al., 2005). Therefore it is objectively possible that the dysfunction in the cortical areas observed after chronic cocaine use (Shoenbaum et al., 2006 and 2009) are a consequence of a complex neural adaptative response that occurs during the transition from voluntary drug use to a more habitual and compulsive drug use. This transition has been hypothesized to be mediated at neural level through a shift from PFC to striatal control over drug seeking and drug taking (Everitt and Robbins, 2005). Nevertheless a recent review of neuroimaging studies have revealed a generalized PFC dysfunction in drug addicted individuals and although the activity of PFC regions is highly integrated and plastic, pre-existing dysfunction of specific PFC regions may confer individual vulnerability to drug addiction (Goldstein and Volkow, 2011).

13. Addiction a disorder of awareness, motivation, or self-control

Addiction may be considered the product of an imbalance between two separate, but interacting, neural systems: an immediate one that generates decision making, based on the impulsivity-related amygdala system for signalling pain or pleasure of immediate prospects and a reflective one, based on PFC circuitry for elaborating the value of signalling pain or pleasure of future prospects (Bechara, 2005). The capacity of controlling behavior is challenged by the ability of cues associated with reinforcing activities (food, sex, drugs of abuse, pleasure) of activating circuitry in which dopamine release in the NAcc has a fundamental value (Schultz, 2010). On the other hand self-control efforts involve increased activity in regions of the PFC regulating emotions and cognition (i.e. dorsolateral and ventrolateral PFC) and a reduced activity in regions associated with reward processing and craving. These brain areas include the ventral striatum, subgenual cingulate, amygdala, ventral tegmental area and OFC as observed in neuroimaging studies in cocaine users (Volkow et al., 2010) or smokers (Kober et al., 2010) when they are required to inhibit craving. In smokers a decrease in craving correlated with a decrease in ventral striatum activity and an increase in dorsolateral prefrontal cortex activity, with ventral striatal activity fully mediating the relationship between lateral prefrontal cortex and reported craving (Kober et al., 2010).

Interestingly, the activation of similar regions was seen in healthy volunteers who were requested to control response to cues associated with monetary rewards (Delgado et al., 2008). Therefore, emotional and cognitive processes that influence decision-making and which may also lead to impulsive behavior or motivational disturbances such as food abuse, drug addiction, excessive spending, risky sexual behavior, may be indicative of an abnormal functioning of PFC or subcortical ventral striatal regions as observed in neuroimaging studies (Breiter et al., 2001). A further feature of PFC role in cognition deals with the overlapping dopamine and ACh innervations in the PFC. It suggests that all the cognitive processes in which are involved these two transmitters may occur involving local mechanisms (Briand et al., 2007). In particular it is of relevance that dopamine agonists increase Ach release and social cognition in rats (Di Cara et al., 2006). Several authors suggested that dopaminergic modulation of PFC cholinergic output is mediated primarily through activation of D1 and D5 type receptors (see Briand et al., 2007 for a review).

Moreover the importance of PFC in expressing self-control is supported by the fact that failure occurs when frontal executive control is compromised such as following alcohol consumption or injury (Crews and Boettinger, 2009) as reported in patients with frontal lobe damage (Sellito et al., 2010) and in subjects who were subjected to transient disruption of functions in the lateral PFC by repetitive transcranial magnetic stimulation in lateral PFC (Figner et al., 2010). The lateral PFC is considered the area which activity allows self-control as proposed by the top-down model although two types of subcortical activities could be distinguished: one related to drug addiction that involves primarily the control of PFC over NAcc and one related to amygdala that controls the emotions. Therefore PFC could be associated with long term outcomes whereas sub-cortical activity is associated with more immediate outcomes. The prevalence of subcortical areas in managing drug taking is gained progressively during drug taking experience. At this regard Belin and Everett (2010) have proposed the incentive habit hypothesis. According to these authors drug seeking habits progressively dominate goal directed drug seeking behavior that in turn ca be highly influenced by Pavlovian incentive mechanisms. This process in humans may crucially affect the transition from drug use to drug abuse, involves a strong emotional component but the outcome of this process likely depends on the individual resilience of neuronal circuit to resist to the neurochemical insult of the drug abused. In fact drug addiction depending on the situation can involve a strong component of emotion (Burke et al., 2008; Heatherton and Wagner, 2011; Artiges et al., 2009). The similarity between the control over drug addiction and over emotion share many commonalities although reactivity to emotion may involve an immediate response while drug addiction control is the result of a complex outcome of brain elaborating activity. According to a simplified point of view addiction is the result of a hypersensitivity of the brain reward systems that escapes the control from PFC regions (Bechara, 2005; Koob et al. 2008). In fact it has been reported that during alcohol intoxication, together with a shift toward right versus left brain metabolic laterality, can be observed a shift in the predominance of activity from cortical to limbic brain regions (Volkow et al., 2008). The widespread nature of these brain changes may contribute to the marked disruption of behaviour, mood, cognition and motor activity induced by alcohol (Volkow et al., 2008) or other drugs of abuse (Goldstein and Volkow, 2011) and can cause degeneration in cortical areas deputed to controlling impulsivity in case of heavy alcohol use (Crews and Bottinger, 2009).

14. Concluding remarks

In summary it has been proposed that according to the theory of top-down control, the PFC and in particular the lateral PFC is responsible for controlling different domains of behavior (Cohen and Lieberman, 2010) regardless their content that may vary depending on the subcortical area involved. It may range from food intake, to drug addiction behaviour up to control of emotions and may explain why the effect of resource depletion are no tied to any one self-regulatory domain, as discussed by Heatherton and Wagner (2010). Among PFC areas many are definitively involved in drug addiction as well as in self-control and decision making. Nevertheless an interesting observation suggested that the PFC is involved in cognitive functions exceeding the sum of specific functions attributed to its subregions (Wilson et al., 2010). Thus if behaviour and decision making are considered as an overall result of PFC activity it is interesting to investigate the reason why self-control fails in drug addicts. Thus it could be hypothesized as mentioned before, that chronic exposure to a drug of abuse could disrupt the balance between cortical and sub-cortical activities but it is less clear why some people start taking drugs of abuse. Do they miss an unspecified activity in brain (genetic theory) or is the environment (psychological pressure and need to emulate companion behaviour to be accepted in the group), or is the sum of each factor to push to drug use. Fortunately, in the case of prevalence of the second factor drug taking may not necessarily lead to drug abuse. Considering that an optimal therapy for drug addiction is far to be proposed it remains to pursue prevention by involving young subject, and especially those at risk for drug use and abuse with involving activities in order to occupy brain activities in thoughts that are far from drug taking. Nevertheless drug therapy aimed at controlling drug taking impulse could be directed on improving the awareness of the consequences associated with pleasure directed behaviours and the capacity to take decisions directed to break the vicious circle of drug dependence.

Abbreviations

HPA, hypothalamic-pituitary-adrenal; NAcc Nucleus Accumbens; nAChRs, nicotinic acetylcholine receptors; OFC, orbitofrontal cortex; PFC, prefrontal cortex; PND, postnatal day; PNS, prenatal stress; VTA, ventral tegmental area.

Acknowledgements

This work has been supported by the Fondazione Banco di Sardegna, and by RAS Legge Regionale 7, 2007.

This work was supported by grants from Regione Autonoma della Sardegna (RAS: Legge 7 n° 2007) and from Fondazione Banco di Sardegna.

15. References

Abekawa T., Ohmori T., Ito K., Koyama T. (2000). D1 dopamine receptor activation reduces extracellular glutamate and GABA concentrations in the medial prefrontal cortex. *Brain Res.* 867, 250-254.

Adinoff B., Braud J., Devous M.D., Harris T.S. (2012). Caudolateral orbitofrontal regional cerebral blood flow is decreased in abstinent cocaine-addicted subjects in two separate cohorts. Addict Biol. In press

Adriani W., Chiarotti F., Laviola G. (1998). Elevated novelty seeking and peculiar d-amphetamine sensitization in periadolescent mice compared with adult mice. *Behav. Neurosci.*, 112, 152-1166.

Aggleton J.P. (2011). Multiple anatomical systems embedded within the primate medial temporal lobe: Implications for hippocampal function. *Neurosci Biobehav Rev.* in press.

Aghajanian GK. (2009). Modeling "psychosis" in vitro by inducing disordered neuronal network activity in cortical brain slices. *Psychopharmacology (Berl).* 206, 575-585.

Andersen S.L., Dumont N.L., Teicher M.H. (1997). Developmental differences in dopamine synthesis inhibition by (+/-)-7-OH-DPAT. *Naunyn Schmiedebergs Arch. Pharmacol.*, 356, 173-181.

Anderson S.A., Classey J.D., Condé F., Lund J.S., Lewis D.A. (1995). Synchronous development of pyramidal neuron dendritic spines and parvalbumin-immunoreactive chandelier neuron axon terminals in layer III of monkey prefrontal cortex. *Neuroscience, 67,* 7-22.

Aoki C., Venkatesan C., Go C.G., Forman R., Kurose H. (1998). Cellular and subcellular sites for noradrenergic action in the monkey dorsolateral prefrontal cortex as revealed by the immunocytochemical localization of noradrenergic receptors and axons. *Cereb. Cortex,* 8, 269-277.

Arana F.S., Parkinson J.A., Hinton E., Holland A.J., Owen A.M,. Roberts A.C. (2003). Dissociable contributions of the human amygdala and orbitofrontal cortex to incentive motivation and goal selection. *J Neurosci.* 23, 9632-9638.

Ariano M.A., Wang J., Noblett K.L., Larson E.R., Sibley D.R. (1997). Cellular distribution of the rat D4 dopamine receptor protein in the CNS using anti-receptor antisera. *Brain Res.,* 752, 26-34.

Arnsten A.F., Goldman-Rakic P.S. (1998). Noise stress impairs prefrontal cortical cognitive function in monkeys: evidence for a hyperdopaminergic mechanism. *Arch. Gen. Psychiatry,* 55, 362-368.

Arnsten A.F. (1999). Development of the cerebral cortex: XIV. Stress impairs prefrontal cortical function. *J. Am Acad. Child Adolesc. Psychiatry,* 38, 220-222.

Arnsten A.F. (2000). Through the looking glass: differential noradenergic modulation of prefrontal cortical function. *Neural Plast.,* 7, 133-146.

Arnsten A.F. (2004). Adrenergic targets for the treatment of cognitive deficits in schizophrenia. *Psychopharmacology,* 174, 25-31.

Arnsten A.F., Li B.M. (2005). Neurobiology of executive functions: catecholamine influences on prefrontal cortical functions. *Biol Psychiatry.* 57, 1377-1384.

Arnsten A.F. (2006). Fundamentals of attention-deficit/hyperactivity disorder: circuits and pathways. *J. Clin. Psychiatry,* 67, *Suppl.* 8, 7-12.

Arnsten A.F. (2007). Catecholamine and second messenger influences on prefrontal cortical networks of "representational knowledge": a rational bridge between genetics and the symptoms of mental illness. *Cereb. Cortex.,* 17, Suppl *1,* 6-15.

Arnsten A.F. (2009). Toward a new understanding of attention-deficit hyperactivity disorder pathophysiology: an important role for prefrontal cortex dysfunction. *CNS Drugs.* 23 Suppl 1, 33-41.

Arnsten A.F. (2011). Catecholamine Influences on Dorsolateral Prefrontal Cortical Networks. Biol Psychiatry. 69, e89–e99.

Artiges E., Ricalens E., Berthoz S., Krebs M.O., Penttilä J., Trichard C., Martinot J.L. (2009) Exposure to smoking cues during an emotion recognition task can modulate limbic fMRI activation in cigarette smokers. *Addict Biol.* 14, 469-477.

Aston-Jones, G., Foote, S.L., Segal, M. (1985). Impulse conduction properties of noradrenergic locus coeruleus axons projecting to monkey cerebrocortex. *Neuroscience,* 15, 765-777.

Bannon M.J., Bunney E.B., Roth R.H. (1981). Mesocortical dopamine neurons: rapid transmitter turnover compared to other brain catecholamine systems. *Brain Res.,* 218, 376-382.

Barch DM, Ceaser A. (2012). Cognition in schizophrenia: core psychological and neural mechanisms. *Trends Cogn Sci.* 16, 27-34.

Barron S., White A., Swartzwelder H.S., Bell R.L., Rodd Z.A., Slawecki C.J., Ehlers C.L., Levin E.D., Rezvani A.H., Spear L.P. (2005). Adolescent vulnerabilities to chronic alcohol or nicotine exposure: findings from rodent models. *Alcohol Clin Exp Res.* 29, 1720-1725.

Bassareo V, Tanda G, Di Chiara G. (1995). Increase of extracellular dopamine in the medial prefrontal cortex during spontaneous and naloxone-precipitated opiate abstinence. *Psychopharmacology (Berl).* 122, 202-205.

Belujon P., Grace A.A. (2011). Hippocampus, amygdala, and stress: interacting systems that affect susceptibility to addiction. *Ann N Y Acad Sci.* 1216, 114-121.

Bechara A. (2005) Decision makin, impulse control and loss of willpower to resist drugs: a neurocognitive perspective. *Nat Neurosci* 8, 1445-1449.

Bechara A., Van Der Linden M. (2005). Decision-making and impulse control after frontal lobe injuries. *Curr Opin Neurol.* 18, 734-739.

Belin D, Everitt BJ (2008). Cocaine seeking habits depend upon dopamine-dependent serial connectivity linking the ventral with the dorsal striatum. *Neuron,* 57, 432-441.

Belin D, Everitt BJ (2010) The Neural and Psychological Basis of a Compulsive Incentive Habit. In: Handbook of basal ganglia structure and function, 20 (Steiner H, Tseng K, eds), pp 571-592. Elsvier, Academic Press.

Berglind W.J., See R.E., Fuchs R.A., Ghee S.M., Whitfield T.W. Jr., Miller S.W., McGinty J.F. (2007). A BDNF *infusion into the medial prefrontal cortex suppresses cocaine seeking in rats. Eur* J Neurosci. 26, 757-766.

Berridge K.C., Robinson T.E., Aldridge J.W. (2009). Dissecting components of reward: 'liking', 'wanting', and learning. *Curr Opin Pharmacol.* 9, 65-73.

Björklund, A., Lindvall, O. (1986) Catecholaminergic brain stem regulatory systems. In: Handbook of Physiology. The Nervous System IV: Intrinsic Regulatory Systems of the Brain, (pp 677-700). American Physiology Society, Washington.

Black Y.D., Maclaren F.R., Naydenov A.V., Carlezon W.A. Jr., Baxter M.G., Konradi C. (2006). Altered attention and prefrontal cortex gene expression in rats after binge-like exposure to cocaine during adolescence. *J Neurosci.* 26, 9656-965.

Bolla K.I., Eldreth D.A., London E.D., Kiehl K.A., Mouratidis M., Contoreggi C., Matochik J.A., Kurian V., Cadet J.L., Kimes A.S., Funderburk F.R., Ernst M. (2003). Orbitofrontal cortex dysfunction in abstinent cocaine abusers performing a decision-making task. *Neuroimage.* 19, 1085-1094.

Bonson K.R., Grant S.J., Contoreggi C.S., Links J.M., Metcalfe J., Weyl H.L., Kurian V., Ernst M., London E.D. (2002). Neural systems and cue-induced cocaine craving. *Neuropsychopharmacology.* 26, 376-386.

Bossert J.M., Stern A.L., Theberge F.R., Cifani C., Koya E., Hope B.T., Shaham Y. (2011). Ventral medial prefrontal cortex neuronal ensembles mediate context-induced relapse to heroin. *Nat Neurosci.* 14, 420-422.

Bossong M.G., Niesink R.J. (2010). Adolescent brain maturation, the endogenous cannabinoid system and the neurobiology of cannabis-induced schizophrenia. *Prog Neurobiol.* 92, 370-385.

Boudíková B., Szumlanski C., Maidak B., Weinshilboum R. (1990). Human liver catechol-O-methyltransferase pharmacogenetics. *Clin. Pharmacol. Ther.,* 48, 381-389.

Bouyer J.J., Joh T.H., Pickel V.M. (1984). Ultrastructural localization of tyrosine hydroxylase in rat nucleus accumbens. *J. Comp, Neurol.,* 227, 92-103.

Bowers M.S., McFarland K., Lake R.W., Peterson Y.K., Lapish C.C., Gregory M.L., Lanier S.M., Kalivas P.W. (2004). Activator of G protein signaling 3: a gatekeeper of cocaine sensitization and drug seeking. *Neuron.* 42, 269-281.

Breese GR, Sinha R, Heilig M. (2011). Chronic alcohol neuroadaptation and stress contribute to susceptibility for alcohol craving and relapse. *Pharmacol Ther.* 129, 149-171.

Breiter H.C., Aharon I., Kahneman D., Dale A., Shizgal P. (2001). Functional imaging of neural responses to expectancy and experience of monetary gains and losses. *Neuron,* 30, 619-639.

Briand L.A., Gritton H., Howe W.M., Young D.A., Sarter M. (2007). Modulators in concert for cognition: modulator interactions in the prefrontal cortex. *Prog Neurobiol.* 83, 69-91.

Brousse G., Vorspan F., Ksouda K., Bloch V., Peoc'h K., Laplanche J.L., Mouly S., Schmidt J., Llorca P.M., Lepine J.P. (2010). Could the inter-individual variability in cocaine-induced psychotic effects influence the development of cocaine addiction? Towards a new pharmacogenetic approach to addictions. *Med Hypotheses.* 75, 600-604.

Brown V.J., Bowman E.M. (2002). Rodent models of prefrontal cortical function. *Trends Neurosci.* 25, 340-343.

Brozoski T.J., Brown R.M., Rosvold H.E., Goldman P.S. (1979). Cognitive deficit caused by regional depletion of dopamine in prefrontal cortex of rhesus monkey. *Science,* 205, 929-932.

Burke K.A., Franz T.M., Miller D.N., Schoenbaum G. (2008) The role of the orbitofrontal cortex in the pursuit of happiness and more specific rewards. *Nature* 454, 340-344.

Capriles N., Rodaros D., Sorge R.E., Stewart J. (2003). A role for the prefrontal cortex in stress- and cocaine-induced reinstatement of cocaine seeking in rats. *Psychopharmacology (Berl)* 168, 66-74.

Carboni E., Imperato A., Perezzani L., Di Chiara G. (1989). Amphetamine, cocaine, phencyclidine and nomifensine increase extracellular dopamine concentrations preferentially in the nucleus accumbens of freely moving rats. *Neuroscience,* 28, 653-661.

Carboni E., Tanda G.L., Frau R., Di Chiara G. (1990). Blockade of the noradrenaline carrier increases extracellular dopamine concentrations in the prefrontal cortex: evidence that dopamine is taken up in vivo by noradrenergic terminals. *J. Neurochem.,* 55, 1067-1070.

Carboni E., Bortone L., Giua C., Di Chiara G. (2000). Dissociation of physical abstinence signs from changes in extracellular dopamine in the nucleus accumbens and in the prefrontal cortex of nicotine dependent rats. *Drug Alcohol Depend.* 58, 93-102.

Carboni E., Silvagni A., Rolando M.T., Di Chiara G. (2000). Stimulation of in vivo dopamine transmission in the bed nucleus of stria terminalis by reinforcing drugs. *J Neurosci.* 20, RC102.

Carboni E., Silvagni A., Vacca C., Di Chiara G. (2006). Cumulative effect of norepinephrine and dopamine carrier blockade on extracellular dopamine increase in the nucleus accumbens shell, bed nucleus of stria terminalis and prefrontal cortex. *J. Neurochem,* 96, 473-481.

Carboni E., Barros V.G., Ibba M., Silvagni A., Mura C., Antonelli M.C. (2010). Prenatal restraint stress: an in vivo microdialysis study on catecholamine release in the rat prefrontal cortex. *Neuroscience.* 168, 156-66.

Carr D.B., Sesack S.R. (2000a). Projections from the rat prefrontal cortex to the ventral tegmental area: target specificity in the synaptic associations with mesoaccumbens and mesocortical neurons. *J. Neurosci.,* 20, 3864-3873.

Carr D.B., Sesack, S.R. (2000b). GABA-containing neurons in the rat ventral tegmental area project to the prefrontal cortex. *Synapse,* 38, 114-23.

Casey BJ, Jones RM. (2010). Neurobiology of the adolescent brain and behavior: implications for substance use disorders. *J Am Acad Child Adolesc Psychiatry.* 49, 1189-1201;

Cass, W.A., Gerhardt, G.A. (1995). In vivo assessment of dopamine uptake in rat medial prefrontal cortex: comparison with dorsal striatum and nucleus accumbens. *J. Neurochem., 65,* 201-207.

Chambers R.A., Krystal J.H., Self D.W. (2001). A neurobiological basis for substance abuse comorbidity in schizophrenia. *Biol. Psychiatry,* 50, 71-83.

Chambers R.A., Taylor J.R., Potenza M.N. (2003). Developmental neurocircuitry of motivation in adolescence: a critical period of addiction vulnerability. *Am. J. Psychiatry,* 160, 1041-1052.

Chang J.Y., Janak P.H., Woodward D.J. (1998). Comparison of mesocorticolimbic neuronal responses during cocaine and heroin self-administration in freely moving rats. *J. Neurosci.* 18, 3098-3115.

Chugani H.T., Phelps M.E., Mazziotta J.C. (1987). Positron emission tomography study of human brain functional development. *Ann. Neurol.,* 22, 487-497.

Ciccocioppo R., Sanna P.P., Weiss F. (2001). Cocaine-predictive stimulus induces drug-seeking behavior and neural activation in limbic brain regions after multiple months of abstinence: reversal by D(1) antagonists. *Proc Natl Acad Sci U S A.* 98, 1976-1981.

Cohen J.R. and Lieberman M.D. (2010). The common neural basis of exerting self-control in multiple domains. *In Self Control in Society, Mind, and Brain* (Hassin, R. et al., eds), pp. 141–162, Oxford University Press.

Cohn C.K., Axelrod J. (1971). The effect of estradiol on catechol-O-methyltransferase activity in rat liver. *Life Sci.,* 10, 1351-1354.

Counotte D.S., Spijker S., Van de Burgwal L.H., Hogenboom F., Schoffelmeer A.N., De Vries T.J., Smit A.B., Pattij T. (2009). Long-lasting cognitive deficits resulting from adolescent nicotine exposure in rats. *Neuropsychopharmacology.* 34, 299-306.

Counotte D.S., Goriounova N.A., Li K.W., Loos M., van der Schors R.C., Schetters D.,
Schoffelmeer A.N., Smit A.B., Mansvelder H.D., Pattij T., Spijker S. (2011). Lasting synaptic changes underlie attention deficits caused by nicotine exposure during adolescence. *Nat Neurosci.* 14, 417-419.

Crews F., He J., Hodge C. (2007). Adolescent cortical development: a critical period of vulnerability for addiction. Pharmacol Biochem Behav. 86, 189-199.

Crews F.T., Boettiger C.A. (2009). Impulsivity, frontal lobes and risk for addiction. *Pharmacol Biochem Behav.* 93, 237-247.

Crombag H.S., Gorny G., Li Y., Kolb B., Robinson TE. (2005). Opposite effects of amphetamine self-administration experience on dendritic spines in the medial and orbital prefrontal cortex. *Cereb Cortex.* 15, 341-8.

Crombag H.S., Bossert J.M., Koya E., Shaham Y. (2008). Context-induced relapse to drug seeking: a review. *Philos Trans R Soc Lond B Biol Sci.* 363, 3233-3243.

Curtis C.E., Lee D. (2010). Beyond working memory: the role of persistent activity in decision making. *Trends Cogn Sci.* 14, 216-222.

Dagher A., Tannenbaum B., Hayashi T., Pruessner J.C., McBride D. (2009). An acute psychosocial stress enhances the neural response to smoking cues. *Brain Res.* 1293, 40-48.

Daglish M.R., Weinstein A., Malizia A.L., Wilson S., Melichar J.K., Britten S., Brewer C., Lingford-Hughes A., Myles J.S., Grasby P., Nutt D.J. (2001). Changes in regional cerebral blood flow elicited by craving memories in abstinent opiate-dependent subjects. *Am J Psychiatry.* 158, 1680-168.

Dahl R.E. (2004a). Adolescent brain development: a period of vulnerabilities and opportunities. Keynote address. *Ann. N. Y. Acad. Sci.,* 1021, 1-22.

Dahl R.E. (2004b). Adolescent development and the regulation of behavior and emotion: introduction to part VIII. *Ann. N. Y. Acad. Sci.,* 1021, 294-295.

Damasio H., Grabowski T., Frank R., Galaburda A.M., Damasio A.R. (1994). The return of Phineas Gage: clues about the brain from the skull of a famous patient. *Science, 264,* 1102-1105.

Davey C.G., Yücel M., Allen N.B. (2008). The emergence of depression in adolescence: development of the prefrontal cortex and the representation of reward. *Neurosci. Biobehav. Rev.,* 32, 1-19.

Davidson R.J., Pizzagalli D., Nitschke J.B., Putnam K. (2002). Depression: perspectives from affective neuroscience. *Annu. Rev. Psychol.* 53, 545-74.

De Bruin J.P., Sànchez-Santed F., Heinsbroek R.P., Donker A., Postmes P. (1994). A behavioural analysis of rats with damage to the medial prefrontal cortex using the Morris water maze: evidence for behavioural flexibility, but not for impaired spatial navigation. *Brain Res.* 652, 323-333.

Defagot M.C., Antonelli M.C. (1997a). Autoradiographic localization of the putative D4 dopamine receptor in rat brain. *Neurochem. Res.,* 22, 401-407.

Defagot M.C., Malchiodi E.L., Villar M.J., Antonelli M.C. (1997b) Distribution of D4 dopamine receptor in rat brain with sequence-specific antibodies. *Brain Res. Mol. Brain Res.,* 45, 1-12.

Del Campo N., Chamberlain S.R., Sahakian B.J., Robbins T.W. (2011). The roles of dopamine and noradrenaline in the pathophysiology and treatment of attention-deficit/hyperactivity disorder. *Biol Psychiatry.* 69, 145-57.

Del-Fava F., Hasue R.H., Ferreira J.G., Shammah-Lagnado S.J. (2007). Efferent connections of the rostral linear nucleus of the ventral tegmental area in the rat. *Neuroscience.* 145, 1059-1076.

Delgado M.R., Gillis M.M., Phelps E.A. (2008). Regulating the expectation of reward via cognitive strategies. *Nat Neurosci.* 11, 880-881.

Delmonico R.L., Hanley-Peterson P., Englander J. (1998). Group psychotherapy for persons with traumatic brain injury: management of frustration and substance abuse. *J. Head Trauma Rehabil.* 13, 10-22.

Deminière JM, Piazza PV, Guegan G, Abrous N, Maccari S, Le Moal M, Simon H. (1992) Increased locomotor response to novelty and propensity to intravenous amphetamine self-administration in adult offspring of stressed mothers. *Brain Res.* 586, 135-139.

Desimone R. (1995). Neuropsychology. Is dopamine a missing link? *Nature, 376,* 549-550.

Deutch A.Y., Roth R.H. (1990). The determinants of stress-induced activation of the prefrontal cortical dopamine system. *Prog. Brain Res.,* 85, 367-402.

Devoto P., Flore G., Pira L., Diana M., Gessa G.L. (2002). Co-release of noradrenaline and dopamine in the prefrontal cortex after acute morphine and during morphine withdrawal. *Psychopharmacology,* 160, 220-224.

Diamond A. (2007). Consequences of variations in genes that affect dopamine in prefrontal cortex. *Cereb. Cortex,* 17, Suppl 1, i161-i170.

Di Cara B., Panayi F., Gobert A., Dekeyne A., Sicard D., De Groote L., Millan M.J. (2006). Activation of dopamine D1 receptors enhances cholinergic transmission and social cognition: a parallel dialysis and behavioural study in rats. *Int J Neuropsychopharmacol.* 10, 383-399.

Di Chiara G. (2000). Role of dopamine in the behavioural actions of nicotine related to addiction. *Eur J Pharmacol.* 393, 295-314.

Di Chiara G., Bassareo V., Fenu S., De Luca M.A., Spina L., Cadoni C., Acquas E., Carboni E., Valentini V., Lecca D. (2004) Dopamine and drug addiction: the nucleus accumbens shell connection. *Neuropharmacology* 47, Suppl 1, 227-241.

Ding Z.M., Oster S.M., Hall S.R., Engleman E.A., Hauser S.R., McBride W.J., Rodd Z.A. (2011). The stimulating effects of ethanol on ventral tegmental area dopamine neurons projecting to the ventral pallidum and medial prefrontal cortex in female Wistar rats: regional difference and involvement of serotonin-3 receptors. *Psychopharmacology (Berl).* 216, 245-55.

Dom G., Sabbe B., Hulstijn W., van den Brink W. (2005). Substance use disorders and the orbitofrontal cortex: systematic review of behavioural decision-making and neuroimaging studies. *Br. J Psychiatry.* 187, 209-220.

Dorman C., Gaudiano P. (1998). Motivation in: Arbib, M.A. (Ed) The Handbook of Brain Theory and Neuronal Networks. (pp 189-226).Cambridge, Mass. MIT Press.

Dumontheil I, Roggeman C, Ziermans T, Peyrard-Janvid M, Matsson H, Kere J, Klingberg T. (2011). Influence of the COMT genotype on working memory and brain activity changes during development. *Biol Psychiatry.* 70, 222-229.

Erblich J., Lerman C., Self D.W., Diaz G.A., Bovbjerg D.H. (2004). Stress-induced cigarette craving: effects of the DRD2 TaqI RFLP and SLC6A3 VNTR polymorphisms. *Pharmacogenomics J.* 4, 102-109.

Everitt BJ, Robbins TW (2005). Neural systems of reinforcement for drug addiction: from actions to habits to compulsion. *Nat Neurosci,* 8, 1481-1489.

Feinberg I. (1983). Schizophrenia: caused by a fault in programmed synaptic elimination during adolescence? *J. Psychiatr. Res.,* 17, 319-334.

Fibiger H.C. and Phillips A.G. (1988). Mesocorticolimbic dopamine systems and reward. *Ann. N. Y. Acad. Sci. 537,* 206-215.

Figner B., Knoch D., Johnson E.J., Krosch A.R., Lisanby S.H., Fehr E., Weber E.U. (2010). Lateral prefrontal cortex and self-control in intertemporal choice. *Nat Neurosci.* 13, 538-539.

Fineberg N.A., Potenza M.N., Chamberlain S.R., Berlin H.A., Menzies L., Bechara A., Sahakian B.J., Robbins T.W., Bullmore E.T., Hollander E. (2010). Probing compulsive and impulsive behaviors, from animal models to endophenotypes: a narrative review. Neuropsychopharmacology. 35, 591-604.

Foote S.L., Bloom F.E., Aston-Jones G. (1983). Nucleus locus coeruleus: new evidence of anatomical and physiological specificity. *Physiol. Rev.,* 63, 844-914.

Frankhuyzen A.L., Mulder A.H. (1980). Noradrenaline inhibits depolarization-induced 3H-serotonin release from slices of rat hippocampus. *Eur. J. Pharmacol., 63,* 179-182.

Franklin T.R., Acton, P.D., Maldjian, J.A., Gray, J.D., Croft, J.R., Dackis, C.A., O'Brien, C.P., Childress, A.R. (2002). Decreased gray matter concentration in the insular, orbitofrontal, cingulate, and temporal cortices of cocaine patients. *Biol. Psychiatry,* 51, 134-142.

Fuchs R.A., Ramirez D.R., Bell G.H. (2008). Nucleus accumbens shell and core involvement in drug context-induced reinstatement of cocaine seeking in rats. *Psychopharmacology (Berl).* 200, 545-556.

Funahashi S., Inoue M., Kubota K. (1993). Delay-related activity in the primate prefrontal cortex during sequential reaching tasks with delay. *Neurosci. Res.,* 18, 171-175.

Gabbott PL, Warner TA, Jays PR, Salway P, Busby SJ (2005). Prefrontal cortex in the rat: projections to subcortical autonomic, motor, and limbic centers. *J Comp Neurol,* 492, 145-177.

Gallagher M., McMahan R.W., Schoenbaum G. (1999). Orbitofrontal cortex and representation of incentive value in associative learning. *J Neurosci.* 19, 6610-4.

Garris P.A., Collins L.B., Jones S.R., Wightman R.M. (1993). Evoked extracellular dopamine in vivo in the medial prefrontal cortex. *J. Neurochem.,* 61, 637-647.

Garris P.A., Wightman R.M. (1994). Different kinetics govern dopaminergic transmission in the amygdala, prefrontal cortex, and striatum: An in vivo voltammetric study. *J. Neurosci,* 14, 442–450.

Geijo-Barrientos E., Pastore C. (1995). The effects of dopamine on the subthreshold electrophysiological responses of rat prefrontal cortex neurons in vitro. *Eur. J. Neurosci., 7,* 358-366.

George O., Koob G.F. (2010). Individual differences in prefrontal cortex function and the transition from drug use to drug dependence. *Neurosci Biobehav Rev.* 35, 232-247.

Giedd J.N., Jeffries, N.O., Blumenthal J., Castellanos F.X., Vaituzis A.C., Fernandez T., Hamburger S.D., Liu H., Nelson J., Bedwell J., Tran L., Lenane M., Nicolson R., Rapoport J.L. (1999a). Childhood-onset schizophrenia: progressive brain changes during adolescence. *Biol. Psychiatry,* 46, 892-898.

Giedd J.N., Blumenthal J., Jeffries N.O., Castellanos F.X., Liu H., Zijdenbos A., Paus T., Evans A.C., Rapoport J.L. (1999b). Brain development during childhood and adolescence: a longitudinal MRI study. *Nat. Neurosci., 2,* 861-863.

Gioanni Y., Rougeot C., Clarke P.B., Lepousé C., Thierry A.M., Vidal C. (1999). Nicotinic receptors in the rat prefrontal cortex: increase in glutamate release and facilitation of mediodorsal thalamo-cortical transmission. *Eur J Neurosci.* 11, 18-30.

Goldstein L.E., Rasmusson A.M., Bunney B.S., Roth R.H. (1996). Role of the amygdala in the coordination of behavioral, neuroendocrine, and prefrontal cortical monoamine responses to psychological stress in the rat. *J Neurosci.* 16, 4787-4798.

Goldstein RZ, Craig AD, Bechara A, Garavan H, Childress AR, Paulus MP, Volkow ND (2009). The neurocircuitry of impaired insight in drug addiction. *Trends Cogn Sci.* 13, 372-380.

Goldstein R.Z., Volkow N.D. (2002). Drug addiction and its underlying neurobiological basis: neuroimaging evidence for the involvement of the frontal cortex. *Am J Psychiatry.* 159, 1642-52.

Goldstein R.Z., Volkow N.D. (2011). Dysfunction of the prefrontal cortex in addiction: neuroimaging findings and clinical implications. *Nat Rev Neurosci.* 12, 652-669.

Granon S., Passetti F., Thomas K.L., Dalley J.W., Everitt B.J., Robbins T.W. (2000). Enhanced and impaired attentional performance after infusion of D1 dopaminergic receptor agents into rat prefrontal cortex. *J. Neurosci.,* 20, 1208-1215.

Grant S., Contoreggi C., London ED. (2000). Drug abusers show impaired performance in a laboratory test of decision making. *Neuropsychologia.* 38, 1180-1187.

Greengard P. (2001). The neurobiology of slow synaptic transmission. *Science, 294,* 1024-1030.

Grobin A.C., Deutch A.Y. (1998). Dopaminergic regulation of extracellular gamma-aminobutyric acid levels in the prefrontal cortex of the rat. *J. Pharmacol. Exp. Ther.,* 285, 350-357.

Gulledge A.T., Jaffe D.B. (1998). Dopamine decreases the excitability of layer V pyramidal cells in the rat prefrontal cortex. *J. Neurosci.,* 18, 9139-9151.

Haber S.N., Knutson B. (2010). The reward circuit: linking primate anatomy and human imaging. *Neuropsychopharmacology.* 35, 4-26.

Gruber AJ, Calhoon GG, Shusterman I, Schoenbaum G, Roesch MR, O'Donnell P (2010). More is less: a disinhibited prefrontal cortex impairs cognitive flexibility. *J Neurosci.* 30, 17102-17110.

Hains A.B., Arnsten A.F. (2008). Molecular mechanisms of stress-induced prefrontal cortical impairment: implications for mental illness. *Learn Mem.* 15, 551-564.

Hallman H., Jonsson G. (1984). Neurochemical studies on central dopamine neurons--regional characterization of dopamine turnover. *Med. Biol.,* 62, 198-209.

Hamlin A.S., Clemens K.J., McNally G.P. (2008). Renewal of extinguished cocaine-seeking. *Neuroscience.* 151, 659-670.

Harte M., O'Connor W.T. (2004). Evidence for a differential medial prefrontal dopamine D1 and D2 receptor regulation of local and ventral tegmental glutamate and GABA release: a dual probe microdialysis study in the awake rat. *Brain Res.* 1017, 120-9.

Harvey R.C., Dembro K.A., Rajagopalan K., Mutebi M.M., Kantak K.M. (2009). Effects of self-administered cocaine in adolescent and adult male rats on orbitofrontal cortex-related neurocognitive functioning. *Psychopharmacology (Berl).* 206, 61-71

Heatherton T.F., Wagner D.D. (2011). Cognitive neuroscience of self-regulation failure. *Trends Cogn Sci.* 15, 132-139.

Heidbreder C.A., Groenewegen H.J. (2003). The medial prefrontal cortex in the rat: evidence for a dorso-ventral distinction based upon functional and anatomical characteristics. *Neurosci Biobehav Rev.* 27, 555-79.

Heinz A., Smolka,M.N. (2006). The effects of catechol O-methyltransferase genotype on brain activation elicited by affective stimuli and cognitive tasks. *Rev. Neurosci.,* 17, 359-367.

Hiscock R., Bauld L., Amos A., Fidler J.A., Munafò M. (2012). Socioeconomic status and smoking: a review. Ann N Y Acad Sci. 1248, 107-123.

Holmes A, Wellman CL. (2009). Stress-induced prefrontal reorganization and executive dysfunction in rodents. *Neurosci Biobehav Rev. 33,* 773-783.

Hosák L., Libiger J., Cizek J., Beránek M., Cermáková E. (2006). The COMT Val158Met polymorphism is associated with novelty seeking in Czech methamphetamine abusers: preliminary results. *Neuro Endocrinol Lett.* 27, 799-802.

Insel T.R., Miller L.P., Gelhard R.E. (1990). The ontogeny of excitatory amino acid receptors in rat forebrain--I. N-methyl-D-aspartate and quisqualate receptors. *Neuroscience, 35,* 31-43.

Jacobus J., McQueeny T., Bava S., Schweinsburg B.C., Frank L.R., Yang T.T., Tapert S.F. (2009). White matter integrity in adolescents with histories of marijuana use and binge drinking. *Neurotoxicol Teratol.* 31, 349-355.

Joel D., Doljansky J., Schiller D. (2005). 'Compulsive' lever pressing in rats is enhanced following lesions to the orbital cortex, but not to the basolateral nucleus of the amygdala or to the dorsal medial prefrontal cortex. *Eur J Neurosci.* 21, 2252-2262.

Kalivas P.W., Volkow N., Seamans J. (2005). Unmanageable motivation in addiction: a pathology in prefrontal-accumbens glutamate transmission. *Neuron.* 45, 647-650.

Kalivas P.W., Volkow N.D. (2005). The neural basis of addiction: a pathology of motivation and choice. *Am J Psychiatry.* 162, 1403-1413.

Kalivas P.W., Volkow N.D. (2011). New medications for drug addiction hiding in glutamatergic neuroplasticity. *Mol Psychiatry.* 16, 974-86.

Kalsbeek A., Voorn P., Buijs R.M., Pool C.W., Uylings H.B. (1988). Development of the dopaminergic innervation in the prefrontal cortex of the rat. *J. Comp. Neurol.,* 269, 58-72.

Karler R., Calder L.D., Thai D.K., Bedingfield J.B. (1998). The role of dopamine and GABA in the frontal cortex of mice in modulating a motor-stimulant effect of amphetamine and cocaine. *Pharmacol. Biochem. Behav.,* 60, 237-244.

Karoum F., Chrapusta S.J., Egan M.F. (1994). 3-Methoxytyramine is the major metabolite of released dopamine in the rat frontal cortex: reassessment of the effects of antipsychotics on the dynamics of dopamine release and metabolism in the frontal cortex, nucleus accumbens, and striatum by a simple two pool model. *J. Neurochem.,* 63, 972-979.

Karreman M., Moghaddam B. (1996). The prefrontal cortex regulates the basal release of dopamine in the limbic striatum: an effect mediated by ventral tegmental area. *J. Neurochem., 66,* 589-598.

Kendler K.S., Prescott C.A. (1998). Cocaine use, abuse and dependence in a population-based sample of female twins. *Br J Psychiatry.* 173, 345-350.

Kendler K.S., Karkowski L.M., Neale M.C., Prescott C.A. (2000). Illicit psychoactive substance use, heavy use, abuse, and dependence in a US population-based sample of male twins. *Arch Gen Psychiatry.* 57, 261-269.

Kennerley SW, Walton ME. (2011). Decision making and reward in frontal cortex: *Behav Neurosci.* 125, 297-317.

Khan ZU, Muly EC. (2011). Molecular mechanisms of working memory. *Behav Brain Res.* 219, 329-341.

Kippin T.E., Szumlinski K.K., Kapasova Z. Rezner B., See R.E. (2008). Prenatal stress enhances responsiveness to cocaine. *Neuropsychopharmacology.* 33, 769-782.

Kober H., Mende-Siedlecki P., Kross E.F., Weber J., Mischel W., Hart C.L., Ochsner K.N. (2010). Prefrontal-striatal pathway underlies cognitive regulation of craving. *Proc Natl Acad Sci U S A.* 107, 14811-14816.

Koob G.F. (2008). A role for brain stress systems in addiction. *Neuron. 59(1),* 11-34.

Koob G.F., Volkow N.D. (2010). Neurocircuitry of addiction. *Neuropsychopharmacology.* 35, 217-238.

Koya E., Uejima J.L., Wihbey K.A., Bossert J.M., Hope B.T., Shaham Y. (2009). Role of ventral medial prefrontal cortex in incubation of cocaine craving. *Neuropharmacology.* 56 (S 1), 177-185.

Krampe H., Ehrenreich H. (2010). Supervised disulfiram as adjunct to psychotherapy in alcoholism treatment. *Curr Pharm Des.* 16, 2076-2090.

LaLumiere R.T., Kalivas P.W. (2008). Glutamate release in the nucleus accumbens core is necessary for heroin seeking. *J Neurosci.* 28, 3170-3177.

Lammel S., Hetzel A., Häckel O., Jones I., Liss B., Roeper J. (2008). Unique properties of mesoprefrontal neurons within a dual mesocorticolimbic dopamine system. *Neuron*, 57, 760-773.

Langleben D.D., Ruparel K., Elman I., Busch-Winokur S., Pratiwadi R., Loughead J., O'Brien C.P., Childress A.R. (2008). Acute effect of methadone maintenance dose on brain FMRI response to heroin-related cues. *Am J Psychiatry*. 165, 390-394.

Lewis D.A. (1997). Development of the prefrontal cortex during adolescence: insights into vulnerable neural circuits in schizophrenia. *Neuropsychopharmacology, 16*, 385-398.

Lewis D.A., Sesack S.R., Levey A.I., Rosenberg D.R. (1998). Dopamine axons in primate prefrontal cortex: specificity of distribution, synaptic targets, and development. *Adv. Pharmacol.*, 42, 703-706.

Liu X., Vaupel D.B., Grant S., London E.D. (1998a). Effect of cocaine-related environmental stimuli on the spontaneous electroencephalogram in polydrug abusers. *Neuropsychopharmacology*, 19, 10-17.

Liu X., Matochik J.A., Cadet J.L., London E.D. (1998b). Smaller volume of prefrontal lobe in polysubstance abusers: a magnetic resonance imaging study. *Neuropsychopharmacology*, 18, 243-252.

Livingstone P.D., Dickinson J.A., Srinivasan J., Kew J.N., Wonnacott S. (2010). Glutamate-dopamine crosstalk in the rat prefrontal cortex is modulated by Alpha7 nicotinic receptors and potentiated by PNU-120596. *J Mol Neurosci*. 40, 172-176.

Lopez-Larson M.P., Bogorodzki P., Rogowska J., McGlade E., King J.B., Terry J., Yurgelun-Todd D. (2011). Altered prefrontal and insular cortical thickness in adolescent marijuana users. *Behav Brain Res*. 220, 164-172.

Loughlin S.E., Foote S.L., Fallon J.H. (1982). Locus coeruleus projections to cortex: topography, morphology and collateralization. *Brain Res. Bull., 9*, 287-294.

Luft A.R., Schwarz S. (2009). Dopaminergic signals in primary motor cortex. *Int J Dev Neurosci*. 27, 415-421.

Malone D.T., Hill M.N., Rubino T. (2010). Adolescent cannabis use and psychosis: epidemiology and neurodevelopmental models. *Br J Pharmacol*. 160, 511-522.

Marchant N.J., Millan E.Z., McNally G.P. (2012). The hypothalamus and the neurobiology of drug seeking. *Cell Mol Life Sci*. 69, 581-597.

Markou A. (2008). Review. Neurobiology of nicotine dependence. *Philos Trans R Soc Lond B Biol Sci*. 363, 3159-3168.

Markram H., Toledo-Rodriguez M., Wang Y., Gupta A., Silberberg G., Wu C.(2004). Interneurons of the neocortical inhibitory system. *Nat Rev Neurosci*. 5, 793-807.

Martig A.K., Mizumori S.J. (2011). Ventral tegmental area disruption selectively affects CA1/CA2 but not CA3 place fields during a differential reward working memory task. *Hippocampus*. 21, 172-184.

Mathews IZ, McCormick CM. (2011). Role of medial prefrontal cortex dopamine in age differences in response to amphetamine in rats: Locomotor activity after intra-mPFC injections of dopaminergic ligands. *Dev Neurobiol*. In press

Maura G., Gemignani A., Raiteri M. (1982). Noradrenaline inhibits central serotonin release through alpha 2-adrenoceptors located on serotonergic nerve terminals. *Naunyn Schmiedebergs Arch. Pharmacol.*, 320, 272-274.

McFarland K., Kalivas P.W. (2001). The circuitry mediating cocaine-induced reinstatement of drug-seeking behavior. *J Neurosci*. 21, 8655-8663.

McFarland K., Lapish C.C., Kalivas P.W. (2003). Prefrontal glutamate release into the core of the nucleus accumbens mediates cocaine-induced reinstatement of drug-seeking behavior. *J Neurosci.* 23, 3531-3537.

McQueeny T., Schweinsburg B.C., Schweinsburg A.D., Jacobus J., Bava S., Frank L.R., Tapert S.F. (2009). Altered white matter integrity in adolescent binge drinkers. Alcohol *Clin Exp Res.* 33, 1278-1285.

Melrose R.J., Ettenhofer M.L., Harwood D., Achamallah N., Campa O., Mandelkern M., Sultzer DL. (2011). Cerebral metabolism, cognition, and functional abilities in Alzheimer disease. *J Geriatr Psychiatry Neurol.* 24, 127-34.

Mercuri N., Bernardi G., Calabresi P., Cotugno A., Levi G., Stanzione P. (1985). Dopamine decreases cell excitability in rat striatal neurons by pre- and postsynaptic mechanisms. *Brain Res.,* 358, 110-121.

Mercuri N.B., Calabresi P., Bernardi G. (1992). The electrophysiological actions of dopamine and dopaminergic drugs on neurons of the substantia nigra pars compacta and ventral tegmental area. *Life Sci.* 51, 711-718.

Millan E.Z., Marchant N.J., McNally G.P. (2011). Extinction of drug seeking. *Behav Brain Res.* 217, 454-462.

Miller E.K., Erickson C.A., Desimone R. (1996). Neural mechanisms of visual working memory in prefrontal cortex of the macaque. *J. Neurosci.,* 16, 5154-5167.

Miller E.J., Saint Marie L.R., Breier M.R., Swerdlow N.R. (2010). Pathways from the ventral hippocampus and caudal amygdala to forebrain regions that regulate sensorimotor gating in the rat. *Neuroscience.* 165, 601-611.

Morilak D.A., Barrera G., Echevarria D.J., Garcia A.S., Hernandez A., Ma S., Petre C.O. (2005). Role of brain norepinephrine in the behavioral response to stress. *Prog Neuropsychopharmacol Biol. Psychiatry,* 29, 1214-1224.

Mrzljak L., Bergson C., Pappy M., Huff R., Levenson R., Goldman-Rakic PS. (1996) Localization of dopamine D4 receptors in GABAergic neurons of the primate brain. *Nature,* 381, 245-248.

Narita M., Matsushima Y., Niikura K., Narita M., Takagi S., Nakahara K., Kurahashi K., Abe M., Saeki M., Asato M., Imai S., Ikeda K., Kuzumaki N., Suzuki T. (2010). Implication of dopaminergic projection from the ventral tegmental area to the anterior cingulate cortex in μ-opioid-induced place preference. *Addict Biol.* 15, 434-47.

Nestler E.J. (2005) Is there a common molecular pathway for addiction? *Nature Neurosci* 8, 1445-1449.

Nixon K., McClain J.A. (2010). Adolescence as a critical window for developing an alcohol use disorder: current findings in neuroscience. *Curr Opin Psychiatry.* 23, 227-232.

Oades R.D., Halliday G.M. (1987). Ventral tegmental (A10) system: neurobiology. 1. Anatomy and connectivity. *Brain Res.* 434, 117-165.

O'Connor EC, Chapman K, Butler P, Mead AN. (2010). The predictive validity of the rat self-administration model for abuse liability. *Neurosci Biobehav Rev.* 35, 912-938.

O'Dell LE. (2009). A psychobiological framework of the substrates that mediate nicotine use during adolescence. *Neuropharmacology.* 56 Suppl 1, 263-78.

O'Donnell P. (2010). Adolescent maturation of cortical dopamine. *Neurotox Res.* 18, 306-312.

O'Donnell P, Lavín A, Enquist LW, Grace AA, Card JP. (1997). Interconnected parallel circuits between rat nucleus accumbens and thalamus revealed by retrograde transynaptic transport of pseudorabies virus. *J Neurosci.* 17, 2143-2167.

Omelchenko N., Sesack S.R. (2007). Glutamate synaptic inputs to ventral tegmental area neurons in the rat derive primarily from subcortical sources. *Neuroscience,* 146, 1259-1274.

Ommaya A.K., Salazar A.M., Dannenberg A.L., Ommaya A.K., Chervinsky A.B., Schwab K. (1996). Outcome after traumatic brain injury in the U.S. military medical system. *J. Trauma.* 41, 972-975.

Oropeza VC, Mackie K, Van Bockstaele EJ. (2006). Cannabinoid receptors are localized to noradrenergic axon terminals in the rat frontal cortex. *Brain Res.* 1127,36-44.

Papp E., Borhegyi Z., Tomioka R., Rockland K.S., Mody I., Freund T.F. (2012). Glutamatergic input from specific sources influences the nucleus accumbens-ventral pallidum information flow. *Brain Struct Funct.* 217, 37-48.

Park W.K., Bari A.A., Jey A.R., Anderson S.M., Spealman R.D., Rowlett J.K., Pierce R.C. (2002). Cocaine administered into the medial prefrontal cortex reinstates cocaine-seeking behavior by increasing AMPA receptor-mediated glutamate transmission in the nucleus accumbens. *J Neurosci.* 22, 2916-2925.

Paus T., Zijdenbos A., Worsley K., Collins D.L., Blumenthal J., Giedd J.N., Rapoport J.L., Evans A.C. (1999). Structural maturation of neural pathways in children and adolescents: in vivo study. *Science,* 283, 1908-1911.

Penit-Soria J., Audinat E., Crepel F. (1987). Excitation of rat prefrontal cortical neurons by dopamine: an in vitro electrophysiological study. *Brain Res.,* 425, 263-274.

Peters J., LaLumiere R.T., Kalivas P.W. (2008). Infralimbic prefrontal cortex is responsible for inhibiting cocaine seeking in extinguished rats. *J Neurosci. 28 (23),* 6046-53.

Peters J., Kalivas P.W., Quirk G.J. (2009). Extinction circuits for fear and addiction overlap in prefrontal cortex. *Learn Mem.* 16, 279-288.

Piazza PV, Rougé-Pont F, Deroche V, Maccari S, Simon H, Le Moal M. (1996). Glucocorticoids have state-dependent stimulant effects on the mesencephalic dopaminergic transmission. Proc Natl Acad Sci U S A. 93, 8716-8720.

Piazza PV, Le Moal ML. (1998). Pathophysiological basis of vulnerability to drug abuse: role of an interaction between stress, glucocorticoids, and dopaminergic neurons. Annu Rev Pharmacol Toxicol. 36, 359-378.

Pirot S., Godbout R., Mantz J., Tassin J.P., Glowinski J., Thierry A.M. (1992). Inhibitory effects of ventral tegmental area stimulation on the activity of prefrontal cortical neurons: evidence for the involvement of both dopaminergic and GABAergic components. *Neuroscience,* 49, 857-865.

Poorthuis R.B., Goriounova N.A., Couey J.J., Mansvelder H.D. (2009). Nicotinic actions on neuronal networks for cognition: general principles and long-term consequences. *Biochem Pharmacol.* 78, 668-676.

Popova S., Mohapatra S., Patra J., Duhig A., Rehm J. (2011). A literature review of cost-enefit analyses for the treatment of alcohol dependence. *Int J Environ Res Public Health.* 8, 3351-3364.

Potenza MN, Hong KI, Lacadie CM, Fulbright RK, Tuit KL, Sinha R. Neural correlates of stress-induced and cue-induced drug craving: influences of sex and cocaine dependence. *Am J Psychiatry.* 169, 406-414.

Radley J.J., Williams B., Sawchenko P.E. (2008). Noradrenergic innervation of the dorsal medial prefrontal cortex modulates hypothalamo-pituitary-adrenal responses to acute emotional stress. *J. Neurosci.,* 28, 5806-5816.

Rakic P., Bourgeois J.P., Goldman-Rakic P.S. (1994). Synaptic development of the cerebral cortex: implications for learning, memory, and mental illness. *Prog. Brain Res.*, 102, 227-243.

Reinhard J.F. Jr, Bannon M.J., Roth R.H. (1982). Acceleration by stress of dopamine synthesis and metabolism in prefrontal cortex: antagonism by diazepam. *Naunyn Schmiedebergs Arch. Pharmacol.*, 318, 374-377.

Rétaux S., Besson M.J., Penit-Soria J. (1991). Opposing effects of dopamine D2 receptor stimulation on the spontaneous and the electrically evoked release of [3H]GABA on rat prefrontal cortex slices. *Neuroscience*, 42, 61-71.

Reynolds SM, Zahm DS (2005). Specificity in the projections of prefrontal and insular cortex to ventral striatopallidum and the extended amygdala. *J Neurosci.* 14, 25, 11757-11767.

Robbins T.W. (2002). The 5-choice serial reaction time task: behavioural pharmacology and functional neurochemistry. *Psychopharmacology*, 163, 362-380.

Robinson T.E., Kolb B. (1999). Alterations in the morphology of dendrites and dendritic spines in the nucleus accumbens and prefrontal cortex following repeated treatment with amphetamine or cocaine. *Eur J Neurosci.* 11, 1598-1604.

Roth R.H., Tam S.Y., Ida Y., Yang J.X., Deutch A.Y. (1988). Stress and the mesocorticolimbic dopamine systems. *Ann. N. Y. Acad. Sci.*, 537, 138-147.

Rozeske R.R., Der-Avakian A., Bland S.T., Beckley J.T., Watkins L.R., Maier S.F. (2009). The medial prefrontal cortex regulates the differential expression of morphine-conditioned place preference following a single exposure to controllable or uncontrollable stress. *Neuropsychopharmacology.* 34, 834-843.

Rutherford L.C., Nelson S.B., Turrigiano G.G. (1998). BDNF has opposite effects on the quantal amplitude of pyramidal neuron and interneuron excitatory synapses. *Neuron*, 21, 521-530.

Schenk S., Horger B.A., Peltier R., Shelton K. (1991). Supersensitivity to the reinforcing effects of cocaine following 6-hydroxydopamine lesions to the medial prefrontal cortex in rats. *Brain Res.* 543, 227-235.

Schoenbaum G., Saddoris M.P., Ramus S.J., Shaham Y., Setlow B. (2004). Cocaine-experienced rats exhibit learning deficits in a task sensitive to orbitofrontal cortex lesions. *Eur J Neurosci.* 19, 1997-2002.

Schoenbaum G., Roesch M.R., Stalnaker T.A. (2006). Orbitofrontal cortex, decision-making and drug addiction. *Trends Neurosci.* 29, 116-124.

Schoenbaum G., Roesch M.R., Stalnaker T.A., Takahashi Y.K. (2009). A new perspective on the role of the orbitofrontal cortex in adaptive behaviour. Nat *Rev Neurosci.* 10, 885-892.

Schramm-Sapyta N.L., Walker Q.D., Caster J.M., Levin E.D., Kuhn C.M. (2009). Are adolescents more vulnerable to drug addiction than adults? Evidence from animal models. *Psychopharmacology (Berl).* 206, 1-21.

Schultz W. (2010). Multiple functions of dopamine neurons. *F1000 Biol Rep.* 2, pii: 2.

Schultz W. (2011). Potential vulnerabilities of neuronal reward, risk, and decision mechanisms to addictive drugs. *Neuron.* 69, 603-617.

Schulz S. (2011). MDMA & cannabis: a mini-review of cognitive, behavioral, and neurobiological effects of co-consumption. Curr Drug Abuse Rev. 4, 81-86.

Schweinsburg A.D., Schweinsburg B.C,. Nagel B.J., Eyler L.T., Tapert S.F. (2011). Neural correlates of verbal learning in adolescent alcohol and marijuana users. *Addiction.* 106, 564-573

Seamans J.K.and Yang C.R. (2004). The principal features and mechanisms of dopamine modulation in the prefrontal cortex. *Prog. Neurobiol.* 74, 1-58.

See R.E. (2009). Dopamine D1 receptor antagonism in the prelimbic cortex blocks the reinstatement of heroin-seeking in an animal model of relapse. *Int J Neuropsychopharmacol.* 12, 431-436.

Sellitto M., Ciaramelli E., di Pellegrino G. (2010). Myopic discounting of future rewards after medial orbitofrontal damage in humans. *J Neurosci.* 30, 16429-16436.

Sesack S.R., Pickel V.M. (1992). Prefrontal cortical efferents in the rat synapse on unlabeled neuronal targets of catecholamine terminals in the nucleus accumbens septi and on dopamine neurons in the ventral tegmental area. *J. Comp. Neurol.*, 8, 145-160.

Sesack S.R., Hawrylak V.A., Guido M.A., Levey A.I. (1998). Cellular and subcellular localization of the dopamine transporter in rat cortex. *Adv. Pharmacol.*, 42, 171-174.

Shaham Y., Stewart J. (1995). Stress reinstates heroin-seeking in drug-free animals: an effect mimicking heroin, not withdrawal. *Psychopharmacology (Berl).* 119, 334-341.

Shaham Y., Shalev U., Lu L., De Wit H., Stewart J. (2003). The reinstatement model of drug relapse: history, methodology and major findings. *Psychopharmacology (Berl).* 168, 3-20.

Shansky R.M., Glavis-Bloom C., Lerman D., McRae P., Benson C., Miller K., Cosand L., Horvath T.L., Arnsten A.F. (2004). Estrogen mediates sex differences in stress-induced prefrontal cortex dysfunction. *Mol. Psychiatry,* 9, 531-538.

Shiffman S., Waters A., Hickcox M. (2004). The nicotine dependence syndrome scale: a multidimensional measure of nicotine dependence. *Nicotine Tob Res.* 6, 327-348.

Shimamura A.P. (2000). Toward a cognitive neuroscience of metacognition. *Conscious Cogn.* 9(2 Pt 1), 313-323.

Shors T.J., Miesegaes G. (2002). Testosterone in utero and at birth dictates how stressful experience will affect learning in adulthood. *Proc. Natl. Acad. Sci. U S A,* 99, 13955-13960.

Shors T.J., Leuner B. (2003). Estrogen-mediated effects on depression and memory formation in females. *J. Affect. Disord.*, 74, 85-96.

Shorter D., Kosten T.R. (2011). Novel pharmacotherapeutic treatments for cocaine addiction. *BMC Med.* 9, 119.

Silvagni A, Barros VG, Mura C, Antonelli MC, Carboni E (2008). Prenatal restraint stress differentially modifies basal and stimulated dopamine and noradrenaline release in the nucleus accumbens shell: an 'in vivo' microdialysis study in adolescent and young adult rats. *Eur J Neurosci.* 28, 744-758.

Simkin D.R., Grenoble S. (2010). Pharmacotherapies for adolescent substance use disorders. *Child Adolesc Psychiatr Clin N Am.* 19, 591-608.

Smolka M.N., Schumann G., Wrase J., Grüsser S.M., Flor H., Mann K., Braus D.F., Goldman D., Büchel C., Heinz A. (2005). Catechol-O-methyltransferase val158met genotype affects processing of emotional stimuli in the amygdala and prefrontal cortex. *J. Neurosci.*, 25, 836-842.

Sofuoglu M. (2010). Cognitive enhancement as a pharmacotherapy target for stimulant addiction. *Addiction.* 105, 38-48.

Spear L.P., Brake S.C. (1983). Periadolescence: age-dependent behavior and psychopharmacological responsivity in rats. *Dev. Psychobiol.,* 16, 83-109.

Spear L.P., Varlinskaya E.I. (2005). Adolescence. Alcohol sensitivity, tolerance, and intake. *Recent Dev Alcohol.* 17, 143-59.

Steinberg L. (2008). A Neurobehavioral Perspective on Adolescent Risk-Taking. *Dev. Rev.,* 28, 78-106.

Stewart J. (2003). Stress and relapse to drug seeking: studies in laboratory animals shed light on mechanisms and sources of long-term vulnerability. *Am J Addict.* 12, 1-17.

Sullivan R.M., Brake, W.G. (2003). What the rodent prefrontal cortex can teach us about attention-deficit/hyperactivity disorder: the critical role of early developmental events on prefrontal function. *Behav. Brain Res.* 146, 43-55.

Sullivan R.M. (2004) Hemispheric asymmetry in stress processing in rat prefrontal cortex and the role of mesocortical dopamine. *Stress,* 7,131-143.

Sun W., Rebec G.V. (2005). The role of prefrontal cortex D1-like and D2-like receptors in cocaine-seeking behavior in rats. *Psychopharmacology (Berl).* 177, 315-323.

Swanson L.W. (1976). The locus coeruleus: a cytoarchitectonic, Golgi and immunohistochemical study in the albino rat. *Brain Res.,* 110, 39–56.

Swan G.E., Denk C.E., Parker S.D., Carmelli D., Furze C.T., Rosenman R.H. (1988). Risk factors for late relapse in male and female ex-smokers. *Addict Behav.* 13, 253-266.

Tanda G., Pontieri F.E., Frau R., Di Chiara G. (1997). Contribution of blockade of the noradrenaline carrier to the increase of extracellular dopamine in the rat prefrontal cortex by amphetamine and cocaine. *Eur. J. Neurosci.,* 9, 2077-2085.

Thierry A.M. (1972). Effect of stress on various characteristics of norepinephrine metabolism in central noradrenergic neurons. *Adv. Exp. Med. Biol., 33,* 501-508.

Tseng KY, O'Donnell P (2007). D2 dopamine receptors recruit a GABA component for their attenuation of excitatory synaptic transmission in the adult rat prefrontal cortex. *Synapse.* 61, 843-850.

Tzschentke T.M. (2001). Pharmacology and behavioral pharmacology of the mesocortical dopamine system. *Prog. Neurobiol.,* 63, 241-320.

Van den Oever M.C., Spijker S., Smit A.B., De Vries T.J. (2010). Prefrontal cortex plasticity mechanisms in drug seeking and relapse. *Neurosci Biobehav Rev.* 35, 276-284.

Van Schouwenburg M., Aarts E., Cools R. (2010). Dopaminergic modulation of cognitive control: distinct roles for the prefrontal cortex and the basal ganglia. *Curr Pharm Des.* 16, 2026-2032.

Ventura R., Alcaro A., Puglisi-Allegra S. (2005). Prefrontal cortical norepinephrine release is critical for morphine-induced reward, reinstatement and dopamine release in the nucleus accumbens. *Cereb Cortex.* 15, 1877-1886

Verrico C.D., Jentsch J.D., Roth R.H. (2003). Persistent and anatomically selective reduction in prefrontal cortical dopamine metabolism after repeated, intermittent cannabinoid administration to rats. *Synapse.* 49, 61-66.

Vertes R.P. (2006). Interactions among the medial prefrontal cortex, hippocampus and midline thalamus in emotional and cognitive processing in the rat. *Neuroscience.* 142, 1-20.

Vijayraghavan S., Wang M., Birnbaum S.G., Williams G.V., Arnsten A.F. (2007). Inverted-U dopamine D1 receptor actions on prefrontal neurons engaged in working memory. *Nat. Neurosci.,* 10, 376-384.

Volkow ND, Wang GJ, Begleiter H, Porjesz B, Fowler JS, Telang F, Wong C, Ma Y,Logan J, Goldstein R, Alexoff D, Thanos PK. (2006). High levels of dopamine D2 receptors in unaffected members of alcoholic families: possible protective factors. *Arch Gen Psychiatry*. 63, 999-1008.

Volkow N.D., Ma Y., Zhu W., Fowler J.S., Li J., Rao M., Mueller K., Pradhan K., Wong C., Wang GJ. (2008). Moderate doses of alcohol disrupt the functional organization of the human brain. *Psychiatry Res.* 162, 205-213.

Volkow ND, Fowler JS, Wang GJ, Baler R, Telang F. (2009). Imaging dopamine's role in drug abuse and addiction. *Neuropharmacology.* 56 Suppl 1, 3-8.

Volkow N.D., Fowler J.S., Wang G.J., Telang F., Logan J., Jayne M., Ma Y., Pradhan K., Wong C., Swanson J.M. (2010). Cognitive control of drug craving inhibits brain reward regions in cocaine abusers. *Neuroimage.* 49, 2536-2543.

Volkow N.D., Wang G.J., Fowler J.S., Tomasi D., Telang F. (2011). Addiction: beyond dopamine reward circuitry. *Proc Natl Acad Sci U S A.* 108, 15037-15042.

Voorn P., Vanderschuren L.J., Groenewegen H.J., Robbins T.W., Pennartz C.M. (2004). Putting a spin on the dorsal-ventral divide of the striatum. *Trends Neurosci.* 27, 468-474.

Wang X., Zhong P., Yan Z. (2002). Dopamine D4 receptors modulate GABAergic signaling in pyramidal neurons of prefrontal cortex. *J. Neurosci.,* 22, 9185-9193.

Watanabe Y., Funahashi S. (2012). Thalamic mediodorsal nucleus and working memory. *Neurosci Biobehav Rev.* 36, 134-42.

Waterhouse B.D., Sessler F.M., Liu W., Lin C.S. (1991). Second messenger-mediated actions of norepinephrine on target neurons in central circuits: a new perspective on intracellular mechanisms and functional consequences. *Prog. Brain Res.,* 88, 351-362.

Weissenborn R., Robbins T.W., Everitt B.J. (1997). Effects of medial prefrontal or anterior cingulate cortex lesions on responding for cocaine under fixed-ratio and second-order schedules of reinforcement in rats. *Psychopharmacology (Berl)* 134, 242-57.

Williams B.R., Ponesse J.S., Schachar R.J., Logan G.D., Tannock R. (1999). Development of inhibitory control across the life span. *Dev. Psychol.,* 35, 205-213.

Williams G.V., Goldman-Rakic P.S. (1995). Modulation of memory fields by dopamine D1 receptors in prefrontal cortex. *Nature, 376,* 572-575.

Wilson S.J., Sayette M.A., Fiez J.A. (2004) Prefrontal responses to drug cues: a neurocognitive analysis. *Nat Neurosci.* 7, 211-214.

Wilson CR, Gaffan D, Browning PG, Baxter MG (2010). Functional localization within the prefrontal cortex: missing the forest for the trees? *Trends Neurosci.* 33, 533-540.

Woo T.U., Pucak M.L., Kye C.H., Matus C.V., Lewis D.A. (1997). Peripubertal refinement of the intrinsic and associational circuitry in monkey prefrontal cortex. *Neuroscience, 80,* 1149-1158.

Woodward D.J., Moises H.C., Waterhouse B.D., Yeh H.H., Cheun J.E. (1991). Modulatory actions of norepinephrine on neural circuits. *Adv. Exp. Med. Biol., 287,* 193-208.

Zheng P., Zhang X.X., Bunney B.S., Shi W.X. (1999). Opposite modulation of cortical N-methyl-D-aspartate receptor-mediated responses by low and high concentrations of dopamine. Neuroscience, 91, 527-535.

6

A Molecular Mechanism of Ethanol Dependence: The Influence of the Ionotropic Glutamate Receptor Activated by N-Methyl-D-Aspartate

Sonia Luz Albarracín Cordero[1,*], Bernd Robert Stab II[1,*], Felipe Guillen[1,**] and Edgar Antonio Reyes Montano[2,**]

[1]Pontificia Universidad Javeriana, Colombia
[2]Universidad Nacional de Colombia
Colombia

1. Introduction

The World Health Organization (WHO) estimates that there are about 2 billion people world-wide who consume alcoholic beverages (WHO, 2004). Alcohol use is related to a wide range of physical, mental, and social detriments. Additionally, alcohol affects almost every organ in the human body as well as the central nervous system (CNS) (Spanagel, 2009). There are several theories as to how alcohol affects the CNS. They are classified into two main groups depending on the primary target of ethanol. These two groups are lipid and protein theories (Goldstein, 1986). Before the 1990s, different lipid theories postulated that alcohol acted via some perturbation of the membrane lipids in CNS neurons. In particular, the effects on membrane fluidity and the disordering of the bulk lipid phase of membranes were originally attractive hypotheses for alcohol action. However, recently the protein hypothesis has become the predominant theory (Lovinger, 1997). This hypothesis predicts that alcohol acts specifically on membrane proteins such as receptors and ion channels. The main reason for a shift towards the protein theory originates from evidence that alcohol, at concentrations in the 10–20 mM range, directly interferes with the function of several ion channels (K^+, Ca^{2+}) and receptors (Lovinger et al., 1989). These ethanol effects are mediated through a number of neural transmitter systems including γ-aminobutyric acid (GABA) and glutamate (Takadera et al., 2008; Murail et al., 2011).

The GABA receptor is involved in GABA signalling and the ionotropic glutamate receptor complex activated by *N*-methyl-D-aspartate (iGluR-NMDA) is involved in glutamate signalling. The GABA and NMDA receptors have competing roles in neural excitability and transmission. Activation of GABA receptors results in a decrease in neural activity. In contrast, activation of iGluR-NMDA results in an increase in neural activity. Alcohol has been shown to have opposite effects on these two types of receptors. Alcohol administration leads to increases in GABA receptor activity and decreases in iGluR-NMDA activity (Suzdak et al., 1986; Tsai et

* Primary Authors
** Contributing Authors

al., 1995). The GABA receptor is a key inhibitory neurotransmitter receptor in the CNS (Figure 1). There are two types of GABA receptors. The $GABA_A$ receptor is a ligand-gated ion channel receptor and the $GABA_B$ receptor is a G coupled-protein receptor. Both are associated with the influx of chloride ions into the cell upon activation by GABA. Under normal conditions GABA binds to the GABA receptor and the chloride channel opens (Figure 1). This allows negatively charged chloride ions to enter the cell and inhibit neuronal cell activity. The GABA receptor is affected by low concentrations of alcohol (Suzdak et al., 1986). Also, ethanol has been shown to reduce the number of $GABA_A$-receptor sub-units, and GABA receptor polymorphisms have been associated with several alcoholic phenotypes (Mihic et al., 1997; Sander et al., 1999). The effects of alcohol are not limited to the modulation of GABA receptor activity; they also modulate iGluR-NMDA activity.

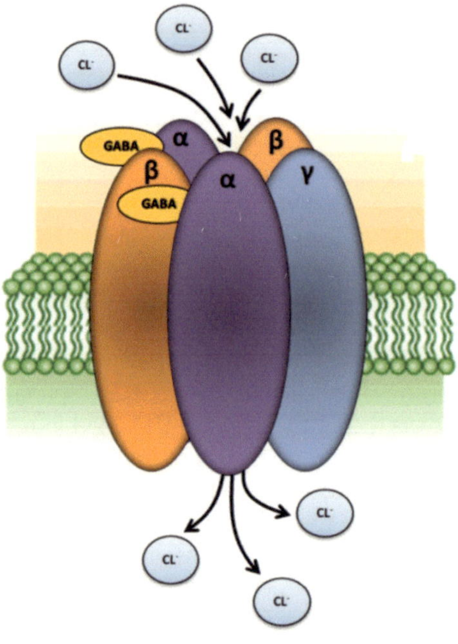

Fig. 1. The GABA receptor composition and potential GABA binding sites. Adapted from Belelli, 2005.

Most GABA receptors are believed to assemble as pentamers with two α subunits, two β subunits, and one γ subunit. The figure shows the influx of Cl^- ions into the cell during GABA activation of the GABA receptor. The GABA molecules bind to interfaces between the α and β subunits.

The iGluR-NMDA is one of the most active molecules in the central nervous system that is involved in learning and memory. It has been extensively studied during the last 30 years. iGluR-NMDA function is inhibited by ethanol in a concentration-dependent manner over the range of 5–50 mM. This is also the concentration range that produces intoxication and that is linearly related to the intoxication potency (Ron, 2004). This suggests that ethanol-induced inhibition of responses to the iGluR-NMDA activation may contribute to the neural and the cognitive impairments associated with alcohol intoxication. However, the mechanism(s) of ethanol interference on NMDA receptor function remains in question.

The iGluR-NMDA is a ligand-gated ion channel with a heteromeric assembly of GluN1, GluN2 (A-D), and GluN3 subunits. The GluN1 and GluN2 subunits contain the co-agonist and agonist binding sites for glycine and glutamate respectively. The GluN3 subunit has some modulatory functions on channel activity especially under pathological conditions (Paoletti, 2011; Traynelis et al., 2010). Electrophysiological studies demonstrated ethanol interactions with domains that influence channel activity. This suggested that residues within the transmembrane (TMD) domains were involved. In the search for these possible binding sites of alcohol in the iGluR-NMDA, several putative binding sites were discovered. Utilizing site-directed mutagenesis, several studies reported putative binding sites in the TM3 and TM4 domains of the GluN1 and GluN2 subunits, respectively. Furthermore, the substitution of an alanine for a phenylalanine residue in the TM3 domain of the GluN1 subunit strongly reduced ethanol sensitivity in recombinant iGluR-NMDAs (Ren et al., 2003, Ren et al., 2008).

The iGluR-NMDA functions as a modulator of synaptic response and a molecular coincidence detector. At resting membrane potentials, iGluR-NMDAs are inactive. This is due to a voltage-dependent block of the channel pore by magnesium ions. This prevents ion flow. For example, the depolarization of the post-synaptic cell occurs through a train of impulses arriving at the pre-synaptic terminal. These impulses sustain the activation of α-amino-3-hydroxy-5-methyl-4-isoxazolepropionic acid (AMPA) receptors. AMPA receptors are a non-NMDA-type ionotropic transmembrane receptor for glutamate. This depolarization caused by the influx of sodium ions into the post-synaptic cell leads to the repulsion of magnesium ions in the iGluR-NMDAs. This repulsion of magnesium ions releases the channel inhibition and allows for iGluR-NMDA activation. However, this is not the only factor necessary for iGluR-NMDA channel function. Other factors include the agonist (glutamate) and the co-agonist (glycine) that allows the channel to open. Unlike GluA2-containing AMPA receptors, NMDA receptors are permeable to calcium ions as well as being permeable to other ions such as sodium and potassium. Therefore, iGluR-NMDA activation leads to a calcium influx into the post-synaptic cell. This event is important in the activation of a number of signaling cascades. Depending on the specific impulse received, the iGluR-NMDA is responsible for a wide range of post-synaptic functions that are involved in physiological processes such as long-term potentiation (LTP) and synaptic plasticity (Van Dongen, 2009). These processes have essential functions in learning and memory (Traynelis et al., 2010). In addition, the iGluR-NMDA is involved in different neurodegenerative diseases such as Alzheimer's, Huntington's, and Parkinson's (Ułas et al., 1994; Hallett et al., 2005; Levine et al., 2010; Saft et al., 2010). It is also involved in psychiatric disorders and pathophysiological conditions such as neuropathic pain (Javitt & Zukin, 1991; Collins et al., 2010). Recently, the iGluR-NMDA has been proposed as an important factor that can be altered in several addictions such as drug and alcohol addiction.

Ethanol inhibits iGluR-NMDA activity at very low concentrations that are typically found during alcohol dependence and abuse (Vengeliene et al., 2005). Several studies have investigated the direct involvement of the N-methyl D-aspartate receptor subtype 2B (NR2B)-containing iGluR-NMDA in ethanol dependence. Narita et al. demonstrated that the protein levels of NR2B subunits in the limbic forebrain but not the cerebral cortex were significantly increased during chronic ethanol dependence in mice. These findings suggest that the up-regulation of NR2B subunits during chronic ethanol exposure may be implicated in the initial development of physical dependence on ethanol (Narita et al., 2007). Sheela et al. reported that NR2B mRNA was significantly elevated in cultured mouse cortical neurons during chronic ethanol exposure (intermittent and non-intermittent) and remained elevated 5 days after withdrawal (Sheela et al., 2006). Studies such as these and others demonstrate that ethanol is a potent inhibitor of the iGluR-NMDA in a number of brain regions (Lovinger, et al., 1989; Lovinger, 1995; Weitlauf & Woodward, 2008). The ability of ethanol to inhibit responses to the iGluR-NMDA is dependent on the subunit combination of the iGluR-NMDA. The N-methyl D-aspartate receptor subtypes 1/2A (NR1/NR2A) and 1/2B (NR1/NR2B) combinations are preferentially sensitive to ethanol inhibition (Otton et al., 2009).

Structural information about the putative alcohol-binding sites on proteins such as the iGluR-NMDA continues to be discovered (Peoples & Weight, 1992; Mirshahi & Woodward, 1995). The functional impact of these binding sites also remains to be elucidated. Substitution studies have shown that a complete substitution for ethanol is exerted by iGluR-NMDA antagonists and certain GABA-mimetic drugs acting through different sites within the $GABA_A$ receptor complex. It has been consistently shown in mice, rats, and monkeys that noncompetitive antagonists of the iGluR-NMDA such as dizocilpine (MK-801), phencyclidine (PCP), ketamine, or memantine (which all act as an ion channel blockers) result in a generalized ethanol response. However, competitive iGluR-NMDA antagonists have often shown only partial substitution for ethanol. Moreover, it has been demonstrated that ketamine produced dose-related ethanol-like subjective effects in detoxified alcoholics. This suggests that NMDA receptors mediate the subjective effects, at least in part, of ethanol in humans (Ren et al., 2003).

In recent years the iGluR-NMDA has emerged as one of the most important and relevant molecules in all neural processes and a key structure in all excitable tissues. The iGluR-NMDA participates in almost all physiological, pathological, and pharmacological processes of the postsynaptic neural membrane. In addition, the iGluR-NMDA is a major target of alcohol (ethanol) in the brain and has been implicated in acute tolerance, long-term facilitation (LTF), sensitization, dependence, withdrawal, and craving (Nagy & László, 2002; Trujillo & Akil, 1995; De Witte, 2004). This chapter's focus is to present in a coherent and comprehensive approach as to why the iGluR-NMDA is one of the most important therapeutic targets in alcohol addiction. It will provide important information for understanding the effects produced by ethanol on the iGluR-NMDA such as the signaling pathways involved and the physiological consequences. It will also summarize information regarding the potential use of different iGluR-NMDA modulators as therapeutic treatments for the adverse effects of alcoholism. In addition, the review will summarize key results obtained from preclinical research such as *in vivo* animal models, *in vitro* cellular models, and *ex vivo* organotypic/acute brain slice models that are currently used to investigate CNS addictions.

2. Structural and functional aspects of the iGluR-NMDA

The iGluR-NMDA is a post-synaptic receptor involved in most neural functions that include fundamental processes such as learning, memory, and possibly consciousness (Lebel et al., 2006; Lareo & Corredor, 2007). The NMDARs are heteromeric complexes composed of three major types of subunits: NR1, with eight isoforms generated by the alternative splicing of the Grin1 gene (Perez-Otano et al., 2001); four NR2 subunits (A–D) generated by the genes

Grin2A–D (Sun et al., 2000); and two NR3 subunits generated by the genes *Grin3A* and *Grin3B* (Andersson et al., 2001). The stoichiometry of the NMDAR remains unknown. It is also not clear whether the NMDAR is a trimeric, tetrameric, or pentameric subunit complex (Ferrer-Montiel & Montal, 1996; Laube et al., 1998; Rosenmund et al., 1998; Hawkins et al., 1999; Nusser, 2000). However, it is known that the various cellular, biophysical, and pharmacological properties of NMDARs are dependent on the splice variants and the composition of these subunits within the receptor complex (Cull-Candy & Leszkiewicz, 2004; Paoletti & Neyton, 2007). The NMDAR is differentially distributed throughout the CNS and has been shown to mediate the fast synaptic action of the major excitatory neurotransmitter L-glutamate (Cochilla & Alfors, 1999; Nusser, 2000). These receptors are multimodulated. Glycine, polyamines (spermine and spermidine), histamine, and cations can act as positive modulators (McBain & Mayer, 1994; Hirai et al., 1996; Kashiwagi et al., 1997; Paoletti et al., 1997). The NMDA receptors are coupled to high conductance cationic channels that are permeable to Ca^{+2}, K^{+}, and Na^{+} ions (Cushing et al., 1999).

NMDAR subunits contain a long extracellular N-terminal domain, three true transmembrane segments, a re-entrant pore loop, and an intracellular C-terminal domain of variable length (Mayer, 2005). The C-terminus of both NR1 and NR2 subunits interact with several intracellular scaffolding proteins and are subject to phosphorylation. As such, they are involved in the regulation of receptor trafficking and function (Salter & Kalia, 2004; Lau & Zukin, 2007). Glutamate, an agonist, binds to the NR2 subunits while the co-agonist glycine binds to the NR1 subunit. The N-terminal domain of the NR2 subunit is subject to allosteric inhibition by compounds such as ifenprodil and zinc (Figure 2) (Perin-Dureau et al., 2002; Hatton & Paoletti, 2005). Synaptic NMDA receptors are localized in the post-synaptic density where they are structurally organized into large macromolecular complexes that interact with signaling molecules such as kinases and phosphatases. They also interact with other transmembrane proteins such as adhesion proteins and metabotropic glutamate receptors (mGluRs) (Husi et al., 2000). Membrane export and synaptic insertion of NMDA receptors involves intrinsic trafficking signals specific for each subunit, splice variant, and complex interaction between NMDA receptors and a variety of interacting proteins. These interacting proteins include the post-synaptic density protein (PSD95), Drosophila disc large tumor suppressor (Dlg1), and zonula occludens-1 protein (zo-1) also known collectively as PDZ-domain proteins. Membrane insertion and regulated endocytosis of NMDA receptors are also tightly controlled by phosphorylation events (Chen & Roche, 2007; Lau & Zukin, 2007). The synaptic activity of NMDARs influence the number and the subunit composition of other synaptic membrane receptors (Zhou & Baudry, 2006; Lau & Zukin, 2007).

The NMDAR requires simultaneous activation by glutamate and glycine for channel opening (Dingledine et al., 1999). Ion passage also requires depolarization because magnesium directly blocks the ion channel in a voltage-dependent manner. Although the physiological significance remains unknown, the receptor is also modulated by polyamines such as spermine and spermidine in a biphasic manner (Figure 2) (Lynch & Guttmann, 2002). At low micromolar concentrations, polyamines promote channel opening by increasing the affinity of the receptor for glycine as well as by removing tonic proton inhibition (Dingledine et al., 1999). In contrast, polyamines at high concentrations that are probably not achievable *in vivo* block the channel in a voltage dependent manner. Three other types of endogenous compounds (zinc, redox modulators, and nitric oxide) also inhibit the NMDA receptor allosterically through different sites (Lynch & Guttmann, 2002). Several compounds such as haloperidol, amitriptyline, and amantidine have been characterized for their ability to inhibit NMDA receptors. These diverse pharmacological antagonists produce different effects when given to animals which suggest that the NMDA receptor population within the brain is heterogeneous.

2.1 NMDA receptor complexes: Structure and function

The NMDA type of glutamate receptor is thought to play a role in long-term potentiation, memory formation, and controlling brain development (MacDonald et al., 2006; Ewald & Cline, 2009; Vastagh et al., 2012). NMDA receptor-mediated neurotoxicity is implicated in neurodegeneration associated with epilepsy, ischemia, Huntington's chorea, Alzheimer's disease, and AIDS encephalopathy (Durand et al., 1993; Reyes et al., 2006).

Three gene families encoding NMDA receptor subunits have been identified in rat brain. One family is composed of the NR1 gene. The NR1 gene encodes RNA that undergoes alternate splicing to yield at least eight receptor variants. These variants arise from the splicing of three alternative exons which have been designated as N1, C1, and C2. Exon N1 encodes 21 amino acids that can be inserted into the N-terminal domain. Exons C1 and C2 are adjacent and encode the last portion of the C-terminal domain. Exon C1 encodes 37 amino acids and exon C2 encodes 38 amino acids before reaching a stop codon followed by an additional 239 nucleotides from the 3′ non-coding region. The splicing out of exon C2 removes the first stop codon. This yields an open reading frame that encodes an unrelated sequence C2′ which consists of 22 amino acids before a second stop codon is reached. The NR1 subunit is essential for channel activity and has glycosylated and de-glycosylated functionally active forms (Reyes et al., 2006).

There are four subtypes (A–D) of the NR2 subunit which bind glutamate (Figure 2). These subunits confer the majority of pharmacological and biophysical properties associated with NMDA receptor (NMDAR) subtypes (Chen & Wyllie, 2006). Since the cloning of NMDAR subunits, the identification of many native NMDARs has been elucidated by comparing the properties of native receptors with those of known recombinant subunit compositions. These studies determined that NR2A and NR2B-containing NMDARs are widely expressed throughout the CNS while NR2C-containing NMDARs are mainly expressed in the cerebellum. Expression levels of NR2D subunits peak around the first week of postnatal development and are thought to be retained in certain neurons that express receptors with properties indistinguishable from recombinant receptors containing only NR1 and NR2D subunits (Monyer et al., 1992; Momiyama et al., 1996; Misra et al., 2000). Activation of NR1/NR2D NMDARs at synaptic sites are thought to produce long lasting synaptic events since recombinant forms deactivate with a time constant of several seconds following rapid synaptic-like glutamate application (Vicini et al., 1998; Wyllie et al., 1998; Wyllie, 2008). The NR2 subunits contain divergent sequences that regulate unique protein-protein interactions and distinct receptor trafficking properties. For example, the NR2A and NR2B intracellular C-terminal domains contain trafficking motifs that regulate NMDAR endocytosis and intracellular trafficking (Tang et al., 2010).

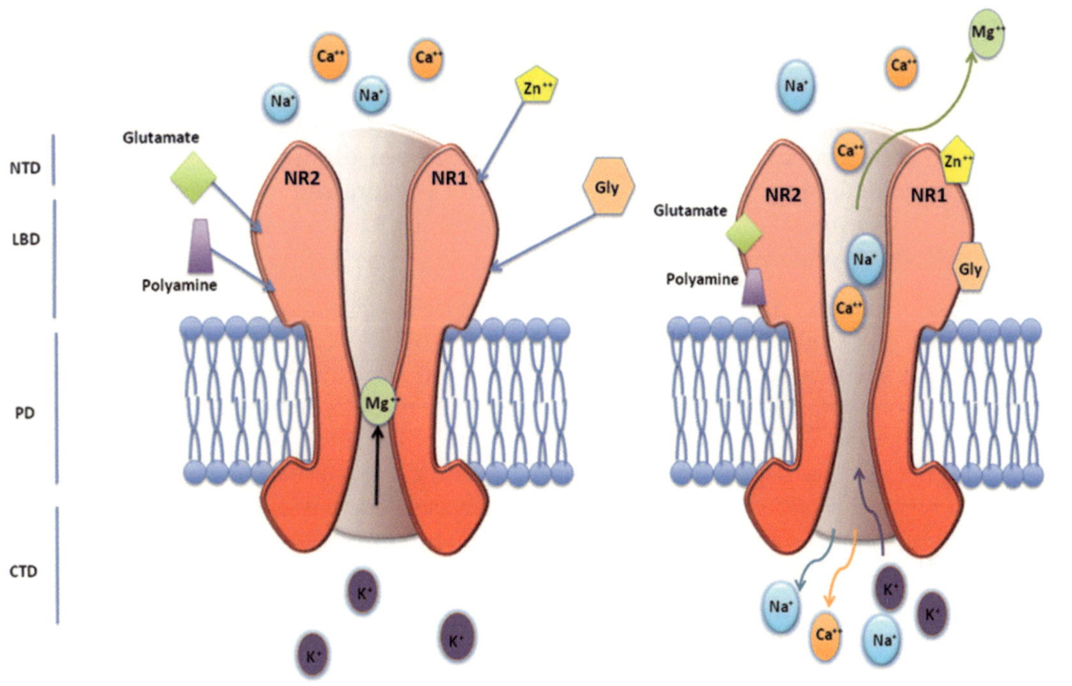

A B

Fig. 2. NMDA receptor composition and potential ligand binding sites.

Most NMDARs are believed to assemble as tetramers that associate two NR1 and two NR2 subunits in a "dimer of dimers" quaternary structure. The diagram shows an assembly with the heterodimer NR1/NR2. For clarity, only one of the two NR1/NR2 heterodimers is shown. The extracellular region is composed of the N-terminal domain (NTD) and ligand binding domain (LBD). Allosteric modulators such as zinc interact with the NTD. Competitive agonists such as glycine, glutamate, and polyamines interact with the LBD. The intermembrane region is composed of the Pore Domain (PD). The Mg^{2+} ion is the endogenous pore blocker of the PD. The intracellular region is composed of the C-terminal domain (CTD). The CTD is involved in receptor trafficking and cell signaling processes.

The successful cloning of NR3, the third subunit of the NMDA receptor, has taken the complexity of NMDA receptors to a new level. NR3 subunits have been identified in rat brains in two variants known as NR3A and NR3B (Méndez et al., 2008; Ciabarra et al., 1995; Sucher et al., 1995). The NR3 subunits have been reported in GenBank as L34938 and U29873, respectively. NR3A has 27% similarity to the other NMDA receptor subunits and 23% similarity to other non-NMDA receptor proteins. Despite this low homology, NR3A was grouped under the NMDA receptor because the CTD and the region upstream of M1 are structurally related to other NMDA receptor subunits (Ciabarra et al., 1995; Moreno et al., 2010; Vargas et al., 2010). The NR3B subunit was initially discovered in 1995. Its complete characterization was published later by other groups (Forcina et al., 1995;

Sevarino et al., 1996; Matsuda et al., 2003; Méndez, 2008). NR3B is also the most similar to NR3A with 47% similarity in amino acid sequence, but it has only 17-21% similarity to NR1 and NR2. There is greater similarity between NR3 and NR1 than with NR2 (Andersson et al., 2001). The mouse homolog of NR3B has 1003 residues whereas the rat homolog is one residue shorter (Chatterton et al., 2002; Nishi et al., 2001; Low & Wee, 2010). NR3 subunits have been reported to be expressed differentially in space and in time. Méndez et al. reported that the NR3A subunit is expressed in different proportions between 1 day postnatal and adult rats, while NR3B has the same expression at both age groups (Méndez et al., 2008).

The "dimer of dimers" quaternary structure of the NMDAR contains at least 2 glutamate binding sites and 2 glycine-binding sites (Figure 2). NMDARs can also assemble with 2 different NR1 splice isoforms and 2 different NR2 subunits. Studies on the AMPA receptor (AMPAR), another member of the ionotropic glutamate receptor family, have given insights into the structure of the NMDA receptor. Crystallographic analyses coupled with electrophysiologic studies indicate a tetrameric structure similar to AMPARs. In the NMDAR, regions of NR2 and NR1 subunits are necessary for transmitting allosteric signals between the glutamate and glycine-binding sites that are analogous to the areas of dimer interactions in AMPARs. This suggests that the NMDARs have similar dimer-dimer interactions. Therefore, collected research suggests that functional NMDAR complexes are tetramers of 2 NR1 and 2 NR2 subunits with an evolutionary link between glutamate receptors and potassium channels (Figure 2). The actual process of assembly of the individual subunits into the functional channel has not been well characterized. However, critical residues in this process are known to be located in the N-terminal domain of the NMDAR (Prybylowski & Wenthold, 2004).

2.2 Stoichiometry

The stoichiometry of NMDA receptors has not been completely established, but the consensus is that they are mostly tetramers composed of two NR1 subunits and two NR2 subunits (Paoletti & Neyton, 2007; Ulbrich & Isacoff, 2008) (Figure 3). NMDARs assemble from two glycine-binding NR1 subunits with two glutamate-binding NR2 subunits to form glutamate-gated excitatory receptors that mediate synaptic transmission and plasticity (Figure 2, 3). The role of glycine-binding NR3 subunits is less clear. In *Xenopus laevis* oocytes, two NR3 subunits co-assemble with two NR1 subunits to form a glycine-gated receptor; such a receptor has yet to be found in mammalian cells. The NR1, NR2, and NR3 appear to co-assemble into tri-heteromeric receptors in neurons, but it is not clear whether this occurs in oocytes (Figure 3). To test the rules that govern subunit assembly in NMDA receptors, Ulbrich and Isacoff developed a single-molecule fluorescence co-localization method. They found that NR1, NR2, and NR3 follow an exclusion rule that yields separate populations of NR1/NR2 and NR1/NR3 receptors on the surface of oocytes. In contrast, co-expression of NR1, NR3A, and NR3B yields tri-heteromeric receptors with a fixed stoichiometry of two NR1 subunits with one NR3A subunit and one NR3B subunit (Figure 3). Therefore, at least part of the regulation of subunit stoichiometry appears to be caused by internal retention. Cell-to-cell differences in these rules may help sculpt distinct physiological properties (Ulbrich & Isacoff, 2008).

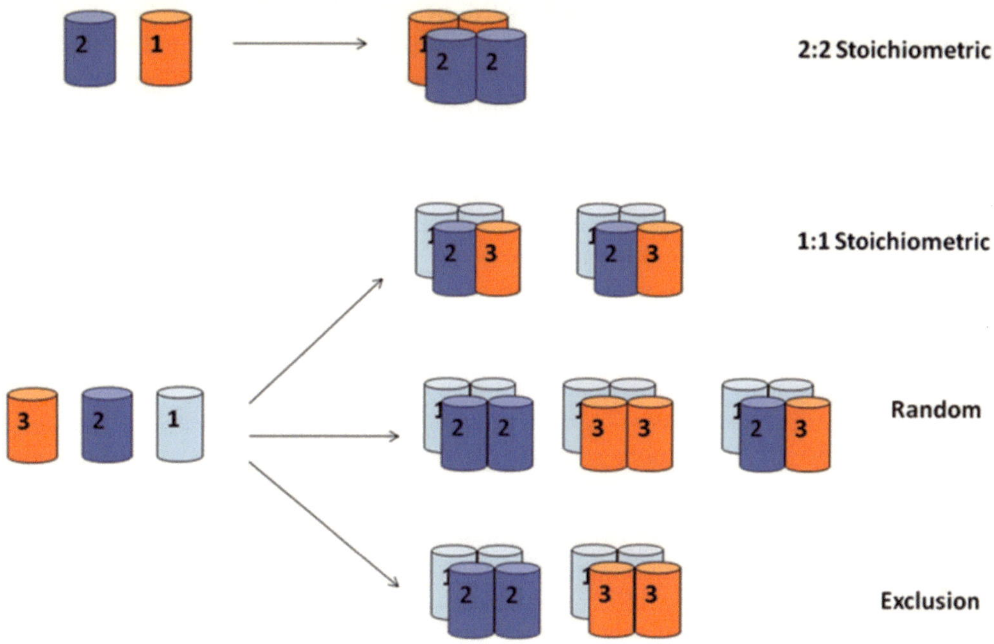

Fig. 3. The different assembly scenarios for NMDA receptors:

Scenario (i) is a 2:2 stoichiometric assembly where two NR1 (orange) and two NR2 (blue) subunits co-assemble. Scenario (ii) is a 1:1 stoichiometric assembly where two NR1 (light blue) subunits assemble with one NR2 (blue) and one NR3 (orange) subunit. Scenario (iii) is a random assembly where two NR1 (light blue) subunits assemble randomly with two NR2 (blue) or two NR3 (orange) subunits, or one NR2 (blue) and one NR3 (orange) subunit. Scenario (iv) is an exclusion rule where two NR1 (light blue) subunits assemble with either two NR2 (blue) or two NR3 (orange) subunits but never form a tri-heteromeric receptor (adapted from Ulbrich & Isacoff, 2008).

3. The impact of alcohol on the NMDA receptor

Alcohol has a complex pharmacology that acts by disrupting distinct receptor or effector proteins via direct or indirect interactions (protein theory). At very high concentrations, it might even change the composition of lipids in the surrounding membrane (lipid theory). At concentrations in the 5–20 mM range, (which constitutes the legal intoxication range for driving in many countries) alcohol directly interferes with and/or influences the function of several membrane receptors. Lovinger et al. showed that NMDA function was inhibited by alcohol in a concentration dependent manner in the range of 5-50 mM. The amplitude of the NMDA-activated current was reduced 61% by 50 mM alcohol (Lovinger et al., 1989). Also, the potency of several alcohols to inhibit the NMDA-activated current is linearly related to their intoxicating potency. This suggests that alcohol-induced inhibition of NMDA receptor activation may contribute to the neural and cognitive impairments associated with intoxication. Several other ionotropic receptors have also been characterized as primary targets of alcohol. These other ionotropic receptors include $GABA_A$ and glycine receptors that have their functions enhanced by alcohol (Mihic, 1999). Alcohol has also been shown to potentiate the function of other non-ionotropic receptors such as neuronal nicotinic ACh receptor (nAChR) and 5-hydroxytryptamine 3 (5-HT3) that is also known as serotonin (Lovinger, 1999; Narahashi et al., 1999).

The influence of alcohol on ionotropic receptors depends on the alcohol concentration and receptor subunit composition. For example, NMDA receptors composed of either NR1/NR2A or NR1/NR2B subunit complexes are more sensitive to alcohol's inhibitory effects than those composed of NR1/NR2C or NR1/NR2D subunit complexes (Kalluri et al., 1998; Allgaier, 2002). Another example is $GABA_A$. $GABA_A$ receptors are composed of α, β, γ, and δ subunits. Most subunit compositions of $GABA_A$ receptors are deficient in δ subunits and only display responses to alcohol at high concentrations (460 mM). However, $GABA_A$ receptors containing δ subunits are affected by very low concentrations (1-3 mM) of alcohol. Also in α4βδ subunit complexes, $GABA_A$ receptors containing the β3 subunit have been found to be almost 10 times more sensitive to alcohol than receptors containing the β2 subunit (Wallner et al., 2003).

In summary, despite the generally held view that alcohol is a non-specific pharmacological compound recent studies demonstrate that it specifically targets certain receptors such as NMDA, GABA, 5-HT3, and nAChRs. Concentrations as low as 1 mM produce alterations in the function of these ionotropic receptors. The complex interaction of alcohol on these receptors is generally characterized by the inhibition of NMDA receptors and by the inhibition of GABA receptors. This complex interaction of alcohol with different receptors is responsible for the psychotropic effects seen with alcohol consumption. These pathways involved in the effects of alcohol on the brain continue to be elucidated.

3.1 The stages of alcohol effects and NMDAR function

The effects of alcohol can be categorized into several stages. These stages are referred to as initiation of alcohol consumption (acute alcohol effects), maintenance of alcohol consumption (chronic alcohol effects and loss of control), craving and alcohol seeking (withdrawal), and relapse to alcohol use (compulsive alcohol consumption) (Wolffgramm et al., 2000; Heyne et al., 1998; Heyne et al., 2000; Ferko, 1994). The glutamatergic system which is a fast-signaling system important for information processing has been shown to play a pivotal role in these stages. The glutamatergic system is composed of at least three major types of glutamate receptors: the AMPA receptor, the NMDA receptor, and the kainate receptor. The NMDA receptor has been demonstrated to have major influence in the first and last stages of alcohol effects and minor or no influence in the middle stages. The AMPA receptor has been shown to have a major influence in the craving and reinstating of alcohol seeking stage (middle stage).

In the initiation of alcohol consumption stage, glutamate has been shown to enhance the central depressant action of alcohol because glutamate can alter the alcohol induced loss of righting reflex (LORR) (Petrakis et al., 2004). NMDARs are associated with decreases in LORR response time and are primary targets of alcohol. This suggests that altered NMDAR function contributes to the initial pathophysiological response during acute alcohol exposure (Ge et al., 2007). Accordingly, NMDAR antagonists are capable of preventing initial alcohol responses. This was shown by the elimination of alcohol-induced conditioned place preference in rats during administration of dizocilpine (a non-competitive NMDAR antagonist). It was also shown by the attenuation of alcohol self-administration in a free-choice operant task with administration of 2-amino-5-phosphopentanoic acid (a competitive NMDAR antagonist) microinjections (Biala & Kotlinska, 1999; Rassnick et al., 1992).

Nitric oxide (NO) production has also been correlated to the initiation of alcohol consumption stage. The glutamatergic/NMDA receptor system is closely linked to NO production. NO is an intracellular and extracellular messenger which is produced by nitric oxide synthase (NOS) (Bredt et al., 1990). The stimulation of NMDARs leads to a calcium influx within the cell and the binding of calcium to calmodulin activates neuronal NOS (nNOS) activity (Spanagel et al., 2002). Other studies have also implicated NOS activity in the modulation of alcohol mediated effects on the CNS (Spanagel et al., 2002; Deng & Deitrich, 2007). Alcohol has been shown to increase inducible NOS (iNOS) activity in glial cells and inhibit nNOS activity in neurons. The link between the NMDA receptor system and NO production implies that both iNOS and nNOS activity within the brain may also be involved in the modulation of acute alcohol effects. NOS activity has also been implicated in the maintenance of alcohol consumption stage (Deng & Deitrich, 2007).

In the maintenance of alcohol consumption stage, adaptive responses occur such as changes in the number and/or affinity of synaptic glutamate receptors or their subunits (Henniger et al., 2003; Vengeliene et al., 2008). These adaptive responses act to counterbalance the acute inhibitory effect of alcohol on iGluR-NMDA function (Nagy et al., 2003; Wu et al., 2010). However, studies suggest that iGluR-NMDA has no influence during this stage. For example, NR2A subunit deletion in mice does not affect voluntary alcohol intake (Boyce-Rustay & Holmes, 2006). Also studies utilizing knockout mice (GluR1 and GluR3 deletions) did not have any effect on either home cage alcohol drinking or operant self-administration (Cowen et al., 2003; Sanchis-Segura & Spanagel, 2006). In contrast, two studies did report that antagonists against the non-ionotropic receptor mGluR5 were capable of reducing alcohol-reinforced responding in mice and alcohol-preferring P/Fawn-Hooded rats (Cowen et al., 2005; Schroeder et al., 2005). This suggests a role for non-ionotropic receptors during this stage of alcohol effects.

In the craving and alcohol seeking stage, adaptive responses in the glutamatergic system cause hyper-excitability in the Central Nervous System (CNS) during withdrawal or conditioned withdrawal. Animal studies have shown that the overactivation of glutamate receptors contributes to the generation of hyper-excitability (Grant et al., 1990; Gulya et al., 1991; Davidson et al., 1995; Grant, 1999). Human studies have supported this hyper-excitability by demonstrating that excitatory neurotransmitters were elevated in the cerebrospinal fluid of alcohol-dependent patients (Tsai & Coyle, 1998). These adaptive responses may represent one mechanism that causes alcohol cravings (Gass & Olive, 2008). Both NMDA receptors and non-NMDA ionotropic glutamate receptors such as AMPA receptors have major roles during this stage (Bachteler et al., 2005; Sanchis-Segura et al., 2006). More specifically, as in the previous stage, mGluRs have also been implicated in this alcohol-craving/seeking behavior. For example, mGluR5 receptor antagonists have been effective in attenuating alcohol cravings (Bäckström et al., 2004). In regards to the NMDA receptor, ethanol withdrawal has been shown to potentiate NMDA-induced damage to the hippocampus by increases in mRNA expression of the NR2 subunit which is correlated with withdrawal seizures (Davidson et al., 1993; Follesa & Ticku, 1996). Also, the competitive

NMDA receptor antagonist, CGP-39551, is a potent inhibitor of withdrawal seizures and hyperexcitability (Liljequist, 1991; Ripley & Little, 1995).

In the last stage, relapse to alcohol use, one major hypothesis proposes that the glutamatergic system is critically involved (Gass & Olive, 2008). Several studies have demonstrated a major role for the NMDA receptors during this stage. For example, the clinical drug acamprosate, known to attenuate hyper-glutamatergic activity, was capable of reducing the alcohol deprivation effect (ADE) in Wistar rats under home cage and operant conditions (Spanagel et al., 1996; Spanagel et al., 2005; Heyser et al., 1998). Furthermore, Hölter et al. demonstrated that chronic treatment with a non-competitive NMDA receptor antagonist selectively abolished the increased alcohol intake during the ADE (Hölter et al., 2000). Similarly, reduction of relapse-like alcohol drinking after a deprivation phase was reported during the administration of competitive and non-competitive antagonists of the NMDA receptor (Vengeliene et al., 2005).

3.2 Acute and chronic alcohol exposure

Acute and chronic effects of alcohol exposure on NMDARs have been observed in hippocampal brain slices in which resistance develops 5-15 min after exposure to ethanol (100 mM) (Miyakawa et al., 1997; Yaka et al., 2003; Nelson et al., 2005). However, the mechanisms of this resistance are not fully understood. Wu et al. proposes that time and dose dependent effects of ethanol produce adaptive changes in the NMDAR which may also occur during exposure to ethanol in *ex vivo* conditions. These changes may be the basis for the functional adaptation of these receptors to alcohol exposure (Wu et al., 2011). It has been shown that changes in the process of adaptation can also occur as a result of NMDAR overexpression, or by other signaling mechanisms that are mediated by selective dephosphorylation of the NMDAR after acute or chronic alcohol exposure (Roberto et al., 2004; Lack et al., 2007; Clapp et al., 2010; Wu et al., 2011).

The NMDAR is considered one of the primary molecular targets of ethanol in the brain. Ethanol inhibits NMDAR function via a non-competitive mechanism and induces the dephosphorylation of NR2 subunits (Wirkner et al., 2000; Suvarna et al., 2005; Wang et al., 2007). For example, NR2A and NR2B in hippocampal and cortical brain slices were characterized after acute ethanol exposure. They exhibited a decrease in tyrosine phosphorylation levels. Both the inhibition of NMDAR function and the decrease in tyrosine phosphorylation of NR2 subunits produced by acute ethanol exposure were blocked by protein tyrosine phosphatases (PTP) inhibitors (Alvestad et al., 2003; Ferrani-Kile et al., 2003). This suggests that ethanol's inhibition of NMDAR function is a result of a decrease in tyrosine phosphorylation of NMDARs by ethanol enhancement of PTP activity (Mahadev & Vemuri, 1999).

NMDARs have also been strongly implicated in synaptic development and cellular models of learning and memory such as long-term potentiation (LTP) and long-term depression (LTD) (Medina et al., 2001; Malenka & Bear, 2004). It has been shown that ethanol inhibits the induction of several forms of neural plasticity such as LTP in the hippocampus, dorsal striatum, and bed nucleus of the stria terminalis while enhancing LTD in the hippocampus (Blitzer et al., 1990; Morrisett et al., 1993; Pyapali et al., 1999; Hendricson et al., 2002; Weitlauf et al., 2004; Hendricson et al., 2007; Yin et al., 2007). Such mechanisms of synaptic plasticity could subsequently lead to the reorganization of neural circuitry by altering gene and protein expression of neuronal receptors such as NMDAR. LTP and LTD have thus become important candidate mechanisms for alcohol induced alterations of neural circuit function in alcohol addiction (Hyman & Malenka, 2001). These studies have proposed the intriguing possibility that disruptions and subsequent adaptive changes in glutamate signaling through NMDARs may contribute to adaptations in brain function. These adaptions in return may produce ethanol tolerance and/or dependence similar to processes involved in experience-dependent plasticity.

The ability of ethanol to inhibit NMDAR function is dependent on various factors including the NR1 splice variant that is co-assembled with NR2 subunits (Jin & Woodward, 2006). While homomeric NR1 subunits form an active ion channel that conducts Na^+ and Ca^{2+} currents, the incorporation of NR2 subunits allows this channel to be modulated by the Src family of kinases (SFKs), phosphatases, and other small molecules such as ethanol. Therefore, NMDAR complexes containing subunits NR1/NR2A or NR1/NR2B are more sensitive to the inhibitory effects of alcohol than complexes that contain the subunits NR1/NR2D or NR1/NR2C. Additionally, given the differential distribution of NMDAR subunits in the brain, alcohol affects certain brain regions more than others. For example, the NR1/NR2B subtype that is mainly expressed in forebrain regions is more sensitive to the inhibitory effects of ethanol (Allgaier, 2002; Smothers et al., 2001; Popp, 1998).

Recently, it has been found that acute ethanol exposure inhibits NMDAR function by modifying STriatal enriched protein tyrosine phosphatase (STEP) activity. STEP is a brain-specific protein that is thought to play a critical role in synaptic plasticity (Fitzpatrick & Lombroso, 2011). The genetic deletion of STEP61, the active form of STEP within the brain, leads to marked attenuation of acute ethanol inhibition of NMDAR currents. Also, STEP61 negatively regulates Fyn and p38 mitogen-activated protein kinase (p38 MAPK). Both of these proteins are members of the NMDAR super molecular complex. The adaptation of NMDAR responses to acute alcohol is associated with 1) a partial inactivation of STEP61, 2) an activation of p38 MAPK, and 3) a requirement for NR2B activity. Together this data indicates that altered STEP61 and p38 MAPK signaling contributes to the modulation of ethanol inhibition of NMDAR activity in brain neurons (Wu et al., 2011).

The functional activity of the NMDAR is increased by SFKs, but its activity is also regulated by protein tyrosine phosphatases (Pelkey et al., 2002; Salter & Kalia, 2004; Snyder et al., 2005; Paul et al., 2007). STEP61 co-immunoprecipitates with NMDARs suggesting a strong physical association between these two molecules as a signaling unit (Pelkey et al., 2002; Braithwaite et al., 2006; Xu et al., 2009). Inhibition of STEP61, the only actively expressed isoform of STEP in the hippocampus, has been shown to enhance NMDAR function and to attenuate ethanol inhibition of the NMDA receptor (Pelkey et al., 2002; Hicklin et al., 2011). Acute ethanol exposure has been shown to decrease phosphorylation at the tyrosine (Y) 1472 phosphorylation site of the NR2B subunit without altering its protein levels (Alvestad et al., 2003; Wu et al., 2010). Y-1472 is a site in the C-terminal tail of the NR2B subunit where STEP61 has been shown to interact. This suggests that acute ethanol treatment activates STEP61 which is involved in the dephosphorylation of the Y-1472 site (Paul et al., 2007; Braithwaite et al., 2006). In accordance, several studies have also shown that the inhibition of NMDAR currents by the action of ethanol requires the participation of STEP61. When STEP61 activity is repressed, ethanol's ability to inhibit NMDAR current is attenuated

(Alvestad et al., 2003; Wu et al., 2010; Hicklin et al., 2011). During the adaptive response increased levels of STEP33 and phospho-p38 mitogen-activate protein kinase (pp38 MAPK) along with decreased levels of STEP61 were correlated with the failure of acute alcohol exposure to inhibit NMDAR currents (Wu et al., 2010; Wu et al., 2011). STEP33 is produced by the cleavage of STEP61. This cleavage process may be one of the mechanisms involved in the partial inhibition of STEP61 during the adaptive phase of alcohol exposure. Studies such as these have suggested that the adaptive resistance of NMDAR currents to acute ethanol inhibition likely involves NR2B subunit activity.

The mechanism of resistance to acute and chronic alcohol exposure during the adaptive response is not well understood. Several studies have reported increases in the expression level of several subunits of the NMDAR such as NR1, NR2A, and NR2B during the adaptive phase under chronic alcohol exposure conditions (Snell et al., 1996; Roberto et al., 2004; Roberto et al., 2006; Lack et al., 2007). Other studies have reported increases in the accumulation of synaptic NMDARs during this phase as well (Carpenter-Hyland et al., 2004; Clapp et al., 2010). For example, hippocampal neurons exposed to ethanol chronically for 7 days demonstrated an increase and accumulation of synaptic NMDARs that was quickly reversed once ethanol exposure ceased (Clapp et al., 2010). This suggests that alcohol inhibition of NMDAR activity regulates the expression and accumulation of NMDARs. In contrast, other studies reported no changes in the expression levels of the NMDAR or its subunits. Instead these studies showed an increased inhibition of NMDAR activity using NR2B antagonists and concluded that resistance may be attributed to increases in NR2B activity (Ferreira et al., 2001; Wu et al., 2010). Even though increases in NR2B activity have not been directly verified, increases in STEP33 and pp38 as mentioned previously are characteristic of excessive NMDAR activation (Floyd et al., 2003; Hardingham, 2009; Xu et al., 2009).

Other mechanisms involved in the adaptive response have been proposed but proven to be untrue. For example, several studies proposed that tolerance could occur in presynaptic neurons, postsynaptic neurons, or both (Wu et al., 2001). Thus, the inhibitory actions of ethanol on postsynaptic glutamate receptors could be counteracted by an increase in presynaptic glutamate release. This hypothesis was tested via a paired pulse facilitation (PPF) experiment. The PPF ratio proves to be inversely proportional to the amount of neurotransmitter release in neurons (Dobrunz & Stevens, 1997; Dittman et al., 2000; Wu et al., 2001). No significant effects of chronic ethanol in the PPF ratio were seen. This suggested that chronic ethanol did not significantly alter the pre-synaptic mechanisms of NMDA neurotransmission. Another group of studies proposed that alterations in the Mg^{2+} blockade were responsible for the alcohol resistance seen during the adaptive phase. However, acute ethanol inhibition of NMDAR currents did not significantly differ in low Mg^{2+} and control Mg^{2+} conditions. This demonstrated that alterations in the Mg^{2+} blockade were unlikely to be responsible for this adaptive response as well (Alvestad et al., 2003; Hicklin et al., 2011; Wu et al., 2011).

Studies in humans have shown that individuals with low initial sensitivity (high resistance) to acute ethanol effects on cognition are at greater risk for becoming alcohol dependent (Schuckit & Smith, 2001). However, other studies have shown that those individuals that develop greater acute ethanol tolerance (low initial resistance) also have a greater risk for alcohol dependence (Newlin & Renton, 2010). Even though the underlying mechanisms for alcohol dependence are not clear, the general consensus is that STEP61 and p38 MAPK activities have critical roles in the modulation of acute and chronic alcohol exposure. These studies also suggest that NR2B subunit antagonists are likely to be effective in regulating the acquisition of functional tolerance to the acute and chronic inhibitory effects of ethanol.

3.3 Mechanisms of alcohol-induced brain damage

The mechanisms of alcohol-induced brain damage and abstinence-induced regeneration are complex (Crews et al., 1998; Farber et al., 2004). The extent of neurodegeneration and potential regeneration varies by brain region and is dependent on many factors including pattern of intake (Crews & Nixon, 2009). Alcoholics display cycles of excessive ethanol intake, abstinence, and relapse behavior. For example, Bell et al showed that high alcohol drinking rats consumed significantly more alcohol upon re-exposure than control rats after a period of alcohol abstinence (Bell et al., 2008). Another studied showed that repeated alcohol deprivation cycles increased the severity of relapse within rats (Rodd et al., 2008). These studies suggest a strong correlation between abstinence and relapse that perpetuate the detrimental cycle of alcohol consumption.

Chronic exposure to ethanol causes an adaptive increase in NMDA receptor sensitivity both *in vivo* and *in vitro*. This leads to an increased vulnerability to the glutamate-induced cytotoxic response (excitotoxicity) (Dodd et al., 2000). This sensitization of neuronal cells is one of the most important factors in the mechanism underlying ethanol-induced brain damage. Increased calcium influx through NMDA receptors, as a result of hyper-sensitivity, is tightly coupled to the increase in calcium influx within the mitochondria. This results in the increased production of reactive oxygen species and oxidative damage that eventually attenuates mitochondrial function. Primary inhibition of the mitochondrial respiratory chain can also indirectly induce further NMDA receptor stimulation and damage (Matsumoto et al., 2001).

Various studies show the effect of alcohol on the induction of brain damage. Cell culture models *in vitro* suggest that chronic ethanol intake inhibits the NMDARs which over time results in a hyper-sensitivity that is alleviated by alcohol withdrawal (Chandler et al., 1993; Chandler et al., 2006, Chandler et al., 1999). These studies suggest that neurotoxicity occurs through NMDARs during withdrawal (Butler et al., 2008; Smith et al., 2008). However, other studies *in vivo* using different NMDAR antagonists such as MK801 (dizocilpine), memantine, and DNQX failed to reduce binge ethanol neurotoxicity. Surprisingly, some doses even increased neurodegeneration (Collins et al., 2010; Corso et al., 1998; Crews et al., 2004; Hamelink et al., 2005). These studies suggest that the mechanism of ethanol-induced brain damage is not glutamate excitotoxicity. Therefore, ethanol-induced brain damage in the binge model occurs during intoxication. Other studies also support the hypothesis that alcohol-induced neurodegeneration occurs primarily during intoxication and is related to increased oxidative stress and pro-inflammatory signaling (Qin et al., 2008). Abstinence after binge ethanol intoxication results in brain cell genesis that could contribute to the return to normal brain function and structure found in abstinent humans (Crews & Nixon, 2009).

Additionally, transcription factors such as the cAMP responsive element-binding protein (CREB) and the nuclear factor κB (NF-κB) regulate the gene expression that increases plasticity and survival of damaged neurons (Walton & Dragunow, 2000; Mabuchi et al.,

2001; Hara et al., 2003). In the presence of ethanol changes can be seen in DNA binding protein activities such as increased DNA binding by NF-κB and reduced DNA binding by CREB. NMDAR activation by synaptic glutamate release is associated with decreased DNA binding by CREB as a result of a decrease in CREB phosphorylation (pCREB) (Papadia & Hardingham, 2007). This decrease in pCREB has also been observed in an *in vivo* model of alcohol consumption where rats were treated with ethanol. Therefore, pCREB is reduced during intoxication (Bison & Crews, 2003). NMDAR inhibition is caused by saturation with ethanol and is expected to enhance neurodegeneration and inhibit neurogenesis. During ethanol withdrawal there is a notable increase in pCREB, 3 days post-withdrawal, which is consistent with the neurogenesis observed (Bison & Crews, 2003). Therefore, it is possible that during abstinence NMDAR activity recovers leading to an increase in the pCREB activated transcription of genes involved in plasticity, cell growth, cell proliferation, and neurogenesis. However, oxidative stress and pro-inflammatory cytokines could attenuate the regeneration process due to imbalances generated by brain cell damage (Collins & Neafsey, 2011; Qin et al., 2008).

3.3.1 Alcoholic neurodegeneration and glial cells

Studies in nonhuman primate adolescents show alcohol-induced changes during neurogenesis in the hippocampus. Alcohol significantly reduced the number of different neural progenitor cell types 1, 2a, and 2b as well as glial progenitor cells (Taffe et al., 2010). This suggests that alcohol interferes with the division and migration of progenitor cells in the hippocampus preneuronal region. Thus, the effect of alcohol decreases neurogenesis and increases degeneration. These results demonstrate that the neurogenic niche of the hippocampus during adolescence is very vulnerable to alcohol. It also demonstrates that alcohol decreases the turnover of neurons in the hippocampus by altering the process of neural development. This effect diminishes slowly and can be seen two months after alcohol abstinence. These findings could explain the deficit in the hippocampus associated with cognitive tasks that may be associated with increased DNA binding of NF-kB and reduced DNA binding of CREB (Fulton et al., 2009, Taffe et al., 2010).

Alcohol-related neuronal loss has been documented in specific regions of the cerebral cortex (superior frontal association cortex), hypothalamus, and cerebellum (Harper et al., 2003; Baker et al., 1999). Glial cells, also contribute to neurodegeneration because astroglial degeneration has been reported during ethanol exposure (Miguel-Hidalgo et al., 2006, Miguel-Hidalgo & Rajkowska, 2003). Glial cells are non-neuronal cells that provide physical and functional support for neurons and are essential for normal neuronal cell function. The loss of glial cells results in a deficiency of metabolic and trophic support for neuronal cells. For example, loss of glial cells leads to the inactivation of neurotransmitters such as glutamate and loss of ionic homeostasis, particularly K^+ (Bezzi & Volterra, 2001; Volterra & Meldolesi, 2005; Obara et al., 2008). This loss directly enhances the deleterious effects of ethanol on neurons. An increase in the glial fibrillary acidic protein (GFAP), a glial-specific cell marker, has been reported after brain injury which suggests activation of glial proliferation in response to damage (Eng et al., 1992; Norton et al., 1992). Studies have demonstrated reduced glial cell proliferation and reduced expression of GFAP by ethanol exposure in astrocyte cultures (Crews et al., 2004; Guerri & Renau-Piqueras, 1997). In addition, acute alcohol exposure or acute alcohol-induced brain damage results in gliosis (enlargement and increased proliferation of astrocytes) and increases in GFAP levels (Crews et al., 2004; Evrard et al., 2006). In contrast, chronic ethanol exposure results in decreased levels of GFAP (Duvernoy et al., 1981; Franke et al., 1997; Miguel-Hidalgo, 2005; Udomuksorn et al., 2011).

Postmortem studies in patients with alcohol dependence showed low glial densities in the Pre-Frontal Cortex (PFC). However, in these patients glutamine sythetase (GS) levels as well as GFAP levels were significantly higher (Miguel-Hidalgo et al., 2010). One hypothesis for this activation of astrocytes in alcoholism involving increased GS/GFAP expression may be due to the repeated acute exposure to alcohol or to periods of withdrawal that defines alcoholism. This augmentation of GS expression in astrocytes of alcoholics is supported by augmented GS immunoreactivity detected in the PFC of alcohol-consuming rats three days after withdrawal from alcohol (Miguel-Hidalgo, 2005). In this animal model, the GS immunoreactivity was significantly correlated with the amount of ethanol ingested in the days before withdrawal. It has been suggested that astrocytes play a critical role in controlling glutamatergic activity and take up most of the synaptically released glutamate that terminates neurotransmitter activity. Glutamate can then be delivered to neurons via the glutamate–glutamine cycle (Danbolt, 2001). Therefore, changes in the glial expression of GS/GFAP suggest an impairment of certain aspects of glutamatergic processing during alcohol exposure and withdrawal. Further research should determine whether the morphological plasticity and GS/GFAP expression are induced more readily in chronic alcoholics despite a paradoxical association of chronic alcohol intake with low glial or astrocyte density (Korbo, 1999; Miguel-Hidalgo et al., 2002; Miguel-Hidalgo et al., 2006).

3.4 Clinical studies: The role of NMDA receptor antagonists ketamine and memantine

Several studies have suggested that NMDA receptor antagonists are an effective method of treatment for alcohol disorders. Ketamine, a NMDA receptor antagonist, has been evaluated in subjects with a strong family history of ethanol dependence versus subjects with no such family history (Petrakis, 2004). This study demonstrated that during ketamine infusion individuals with a family history of ethanol dependence showed an attenuated response in terms of perceptual alterations and dysphoric mood relative to those without such a family history. This study reaffirms NMDAR dysfunction as an important contributing factor of alcohol dependence. Another study by Phelps et al. investigated whether a family history of alcohol dependence influences ketamine's initial antidepressant effect. The study reported that subjects with a family history of alcohol dependence showed significantly greater improvement in MADRS (Montgomery-Asberg Depression Rating Scale) scores compared with subjects who had no family history of alcohol dependence. The study concluded that a family history of alcohol dependence appears to predict a rapid initial anti-depressant response to NMDA receptor antagonists (Phelps, 2009). The precise reasons underlying the better response of the family history of alcohol dependence (FHP) group to ketamine remains unknown but reaffirms NMDARs association with LTD. Another study compared the ethanol-related effects of ketamine and thiophental on both NMDA and $GABA_A$ receptor activity. This study reported that the ethanol-like effects of ketamine were greater than that of thiopental (Dickerson, 2008). The results obtained are important because ketamine (a NMDAR antagonist) produced alcohol alterations in perception that were not produced by thiopental (a $GABA_A$ receptor agonist). This also reaffirms the role of the NMDAR in alcohol dependence.

Memantine, another NMDAR antagonist, also has been evaluated in clinical trials for the treatment of alcoholism. The first study was conducted by Bisagra et al. by evaluating the acute effects of memantine on the subjective, physiological, and performance effects of alcohol in moderate (10–30 drinks per week) alcohol drinkers. This study reported that pre-treatment with memantine attenuated the craving for alcohol before alcohol administration but not after alcohol was given. It demonstrated that memantine increased the dissociative effects of alcohol without altering its sedative, stimulant, and overall intoxicating effects. It reported that memantine had no effect on alcohol-induced impairment in performance, physiological changes, or pharmacokinetics. This study also showed that memantine increased subjective reports of dissociation, confusion, stimulation, and impaired motor coordination on the balance task (Bisaga & Evans, 2004). Due to the high comorbidity shared between alcoholism and depression Muhonen et al. also evaluated memantine as well as escitalopram, a selective serotonin reuptake inhibitor (SSRI), for the treatment of comorbid with alcohol dependence. This study reported that both treatments significantly reduced the baseline level of depression and anxiety according to Montgomery-Asberg Depression Rating Scale (MADRS) and Hamilton Rating Scale for Anxiety (HAM-A). This evidence provides safety and potential efficacy of memantine and escitalopram for major depressive disorder in patients with comorbid alcohol dependence (Muhonen, 2008).

4. Conclusion

Approximately 2 billion people world-wide consume alcoholic beverages. Alcohol use is related to a wide range of physical, mental, and social detriments. Additionally, alcohol affects almost every organ in the human body as well as the central nervous system. The protein theory is the generally accepted theory on how alcohol affects the CNS. This theory proposes that alcohol acts specifically on membrane protein receptors such as the iGluR-NMDA. The iGluR-NMDA is one of the most active molecules in the central nervous system and has been shown to be directly inhibited in a non-competitive manner by alcohol. It is a post-synaptic receptor critical in most neural activities such as learning and memory.

NMDARs are hetermeric complexes composed of three major types of subunits NR1, NR2, and NR3. Alcohol effects on the NMDAR are dependent on the NMDAR subunit composition as well as alcohol concentration. The major effects of alcohol on the NMDAR activity are thought to be conferred by alcohol's direct interaction with the NR2 subunits of the NMDA receptor. The effects of alcohol can be categorized into several stages. These stages are referred to as initiation of alcohol consumption, maintenance of alcohol consumption, craving and reinstating of alcohol seeking, and relapse to alcohol use. A combination of ionotropic receptors such as NMDAR, non-ionotropic receptors, and other receptors of the glutamatergic system are intimately involved in the acquisition of alcohol dependence. The NMDAR has a critical role in the stages of initiation of alcohol consumption and relapse to alcohol use. In response to the NMDA receptors role in alcohol addiction several NMDAR antagonists have been used in clinical trials to alleviate alcohol dependence. These antagonists include ketamine and memantine. Both have been shown to be successful in alleviating some of the symptoms of alcohol dependence. Future research should focus on the continued characterization of the NMDAR structure as well as its structural variation in different tissue compartments within the brain. Also, further studies are needed to elucidate the interactions of alcohol on specific NMDAR subunits and characterize their effects on NMDAR activity. This will be crucial in developing novel therapeutic targets against alcohol addiction.

5. References

Allgaier, C. (2002). Ethanol sensitivity of NMDA receptors. *Neurochem Int,* 41, 6 (December 2002), pp. 377–382, ISSN 0197-0186

Alvestad, R.M., Grosshans, D.R., Coultrap, S.J., Nakazawa, T., Yamamoto, T., and Rowning, M.D., (2003). Tyrosine dephosphorylation and ethanol inhibition of N-Methyl-aspartate receptor function. *J Biol Chem,* 278, 13, (March 2003), pp. 11020-11025, ISSN 0021-9258

Andersson, O., Stenqvist, A., Attersand, A. and von Euler, G. (2001). Nucleotide sequence, genomic organization, and chromosomal localization of genes encoding the human NMDA receptor subunits NR3A and NR3B. *Genomics,* 78, 3, (December 2001), pp. 178–184, ISSN 0888-7543

Bachteler, D., Economidou, D., Danysz, W., Ciccocioppo, R., Spanagel, R. (2005). The effects of acamprosate and neramexane on cue-induced reinstatement of ethanol-seeking behavior in rat. *Neuropsychopharmacology,* 30, 6 (June 2005), pp. 1104–1110, ISSN 0893-133X

Bäckström, P., Bachteler, D., Koch, S., Hyytiä, P., Spanagel, R. (2004). mGluR5 antagonist MPEP reduces ethanol-seeking and relapse behavior. *Neuropsychopharmacology,* 29, 5 (May 2004), pp. 921–928, ISSN 0893-133X

Baker, K., Harding, A., Halliday, G., Kril, J., and Harper C. (1999). Neuronal loss in functional zones of the cerebellum of chronic alcoholics with and without Wernicke's encephalopathy. *Neuroscience,* 91, 2, 429-438, ISSN 0306-4522

Belelli, D., Lambert, J.J. (2005). Neurosteroids: endogenous regulators of the GABA(A) receptor. *Nat Rev Neurosci,* 6, 7, (July 2005), pp. 565-75 ISSN 1471-0048

Bell RL, Rodd ZA, Schultz JA, Peper CL, Lumeng L, Murphy JM, McBride WJ. Effects of short deprivation and re-exposure intervals on the ethanol drinking behavior of selectively bred high alcohol-consuming rats. *Alcohol,* 42, 5, (August 2008), pp. 407-416, ISSN 0741-8329

Bezzi, P., and Volterra, A. (2001). A neuron-glia signalling network in the active brain. *Curr Opin Neurobiol,* 11, 3, (Jun 2001), pp. 387-394, ISSN 0959-4388

Biala, G., and Kotlinska, J. (1999). Blockade of the acquisition of ethanolinduced conditioned place preference by N-methyl-D-aspartate receptor antagonists. *Alcohol,* 34, 2 (March-april 1999), pp 175–182, ISSN 0735-0414

Bisaga, A., and Evans, S.M. (2004). Acute effects of memantine in combination with alcohol in moderate drinkers. *Psychopharmacology (Berl),* 172, 1, (February 2004), pp. 16-24, ISSN 0033-3158

Bison, S., and Crews, F. (2003). Alcohol withdrawal increases neuropeptide Y immunoreactivity in rat brain. *Alcohol Clin Exp Res,* 27, 7, (July 2003), pp. 1173-1183, ISSN 1530-0277

Blitzer, R.D., Gil, O., and Landau, E.M. (1990). Long-term potentiation in rat hippocampus is inhibited by low concentrations of ethanol. *Brain Res,* 24, 537, (December 1990), pp. 203-208, ISSN: 0006-8993

Boyce-Rustay, and J., Holmes, A. (2006). Ethanol-related behaviors in mice lacking the NMDA receptor NR2A subunit. *Psychopharmacology* (Berl), 187, 4 (September 2006), pp. 455–466, ISSN 0033-3158

Braithwaite, S.P., Paul, S., Nairn, A.C., and Lombroso, P.J. (2006). Synaptic plasticity: one STEP at a time. *Trends Neurosci*, 29, 8 (August 2006), pp. 452-458, ISSN 0166-2236

Butler, T.R., Smith, K.J., Self, R.L., Braden, B.B., Prendergast, M.A. (2008). Sex differences in the neurotoxic effects of adenosine A1 receptor antagonism during ethanol withdrawal: reversal with an A1 receptor agonist or an NMDA receptor antagonist. *Alcohol Clin Exp Res*, 32, 7 (July 2008), pp. 1260-1270, ISSN 1530-0277

Carpenter-Hyland, E.P., Woodward, J.J., and Chandler, L.J. (2004). Chronic ethanol induces synaptic but not extrasynaptic targeting of NMDA receptors. *J Neurosci*, 8, 24, (September 2004), pp. 7859-7868, ISSN 0270-6474.

Chandler, L.J., Dean, N., and Greg, S. (1999). Chronic Ethanol Upregulates NMDA and AMPA, but Not Kainate Receptor Subunit Proteins in Rat Primary Cortical Cultures. *Alcohol Clin Exp Res*, 23, 2, (February 1999), pp. 363-370, ISSN 1530-0277

Chandler, L.J., Carpenter-Hyland, E., Hendricson, A.W., Maldve, R.E., Morrisett, R.A., Zhou, F.C., Sari, Y., Bell, R., and Szumlinski, K.K.(2006). Structural and functional modifications in glutamateric synapses following prolonged ethanol exposure. *Alcohol Clin Exp Res*, 30, 2, (February 2006), pp. 368-376, ISSN 1530-0277

Chandler, L.J., Newsom, H., Sumners, C., and Crews, F. (1993). Chronic ethanol exposure potentiates NMDA excitotoxicity in cerebral cortical neurons. *J Neurochem*, 60, 4, (April 1993), pp. 1578-1581, ISSN 0022-3042

Chatterton, J.E., Awobuluyi, M., Premkumar, L.S., Takahashi, H., Talantova, M., Shin, Y., Cui, J., Tu, S., Sevarino, K.A., Nakanishi, N., et al. (2002). Excitatory glycine receptors containing the NR3 family of NMDA receptor subunits. *Nature*, 415 (February 2002), pp. 793–798, ISSN 0028-0836

Chen, B.-S., and Roche, K. W. (2007). Regulation of NMDA receptors by phosphorylation. *Neuropharmacology*, 53 (September 2007), pp. 362-368, ISSN 0028-3908

Chen, P.E., and Wyllie, D.J.A. (2006). Pharmacological insights obtained from structure-function studies of ionotropic glutamate receptors. *Br. J. Pharmacol*, 547 (April 2006), pp. 839–853, ISSN 0007-1188

Ciabarra, A., Sullivan, J., Gahn, L., Pecht, G., Heinemann, S., Sevarino, K. (1995). Cloning and characterization of chi-1: A developmentally regulated member of a novel class of the ionotropic glutamate receptor family. *J Neurosci*, 15, 10 (October 1995), pp. 6498–6508, ISSN 0270-6474.

Clapp, P., Gibson, E.S., Dell'acqua, M.L., and Hoffman, P.L. (2010). Phosphorylation regulates removal of synaptic N-methyl-D-aspartate receptors after withdrawal from chronic ethanol exposure. *J Pharmacol Exp Ther*, 332, 3, (Mar 2010), pp. 720-729, ISSN 0022-3565

Cochilla, A.J., and Alford, S. (1999). NMDA receptor-mediated control of presynaptic calcium and neurotransmitter release. *J Neurosci*, (January 1999), 19, 1, pp. 193-205, ISSN 0270-6474

Collins, M.A., Neafsey, E.J., Wang, K., Achille, N.J., Mitchell, R.M., Sivaswamy, S. (2010). Moderate ethanol preconditioning of rat brain cultures engenders neuroprotection against dementia-inducing neuroinflammatory proteins: possible signaling mechanisms. *Mol Neurobiol*, 41, (June 2010), pp. 420-425, ISSN: 0893-7648

Collins S., Sigtermans M.J., Dahan A., Zuurmond W.W., Perez R.S. (2010). NMDA receptor antagonists for the treatment of neuropathic pain. *Pain Med,* 11, 11, (November 2010), pp. 1726-1742, ISSN 1526-4637

Collins, M.A., and Neafsey, E.J. (2011). Neuroinflammatory Pathways in Binge Alcohol-Induced Neuronal Degeneration: Oxidative Stress Cascade Involving Aquaporin, Brain Edema, and Phospholipase A2 Activation. *Neurotox Res,* (September 2011), [Epub ahead of print], ISSN 1476-3524

Collins, M.A., Zou, J.Y., Neafsey, E.J. (1998). Brain damage due to episodic alcohol exposure in vivo and in vitro: furosemide neuroprotection implicates edema-based mechanism. *FASEB J.*, 12 (February 1998), pp. 221-230, ISSN: 1530-6860

Corso, T.D., Mostafa, H.M., Collins, M.A., and Neafsey, E.J. (1998). Brain neuronal degeneration caused by episodic alcohol intoxication in rats: effects of nimodipine, 6,7-dinitro-quinoxaline-2,3-dione, and MK-801. *Alcohol Clin Exp Res,* 22, 1, (February 1998), pp. 217-224, ISSN 1530-0277

Cowen, M.S., Djouma, E., Lawrence, A.J. (2005). The metabotropic glutamate 5 receptor antagonist 3-[(2-methyl-1,3-thiazol-4-yl)ethynyl]-pyridine reduces ethanol self-administration in multiple strains of alcohol-preferring rats and regulates olfactory glutamatergic systems. *J Pharmacol Exp Ther*, 315, 2 (November 2005), pp. 590–600, ISSN 0022-3565

Cowen, M.S., Schroff, K.C., Gass, P., Sprengel, R., Spanagel, R. (2003). Neurobehavioral effects of alcohol in AMPA receptor subunit (GluR1) deficient mice. *Neuropharmacology*, 45, 3, (September 2003), pp. 325–333, ISSN 0028-3908

Crews F.T., Steck JC, Chandler LJ, Yu CJ, Day A. (1998). Ethanol, stroke, brain damage, and excitotoxicity. *Pharmacol Biochem Behav,* 59, 4, (April 1998), pp. 981-991, ISSN 0091-3057

Crews, F.T., Collins, M.A., Dlugos, C., Littleton, J., Wilkins, L., Neafsey, E.J., Pentney, R., Snell, L.D., Tabakoff, B., Zou, J., and Noronha, A. (2004). Alcohol-induced neurodegeneration: when, where and why? *Alcohol Clin Exp Res,* 28, 2, (February 2004), pp. 350-364, ISSN 1530-0277

Crews, F.T., and Nixon, K. (2009). Mechanisms of neurodegeneration and regeneration in alcoholism. *Alcohol and Alcoholism,* 44, 2,(March 2009), pp. 115-127, ISSN 0735-0414

Cull-Candy S, Brickley S, Farrant M. (2001). NMDA receptor subunits: diversity, development and disease. *Curr Opin Neurobiol*, 11, 3, (Jun 2001), pp. 327-335, ISSN 0959-4388

Cull-Candy, S.G., and Leszkiewicz, D.N. (2004). Role of distinct NMDA receptor subtypes at central synapses. *Sci STKE,* 255, (October 2004) pp. re16, ISSN 1525-8882

Cushing, A., Price-Jones, M.J., Graves, R., Harris, A.J., Hughes, K.T., Bleakman, D., and Lodge, D. (1999). Measurement of calcium flux through ionotropic glutamate receptors using Cytostar-T scintillating microplates. *J Neurosci Methods,* 1, 90, (August 1999), pp. 33-36, ISSN 0165-0270

Danbolt, N.C. (2001). Glutamate uptake. *Prog Neurobiol,* 65, 1, (September 2001), pp. 1-105, ISSN 0301-0082

De Witte P. (2004). Imbalance between neuroexcitatory and neuroinhibitory amino acids causes craving for ethanol. *Addict Behav,* 29, 7, (September 2004), pp. 1325-1339, ISSN 0306-4603

Davidson, M.D., Wilce ,P., Shanley, B.C. (1993). Increased sensitivity of the hippocampus in ethanol-dependent rats to toxic effect of N-methyl-D-aspartic acid in vivo. *Brain Research,* 606, 1, (March 1993), pp. 5-9, ISSN 0006-8993

Deng, X. S., Deitrich R. A. (2007). Ethanol metabolism and effects: nitric oxide and its interaction. *Curr Clin Pharmacol,* 2, 2, (May 2007), pp. 145-53, ISSN 1574-8847

Dickerson, D., Pittman, B., Ralevski, E., Perrino, A., Limoncelli, D., Edgecombe, J., Acampora, G., Krystal, J.H., and Petrakis, I. (2010). Ethanol-likeeffects of thiopental and ketamine in healthyhumans. *J Psychopharmacol,* 24, 2, (February 2010), pp.203-211, ISSN 0269-8811

Dingledine, R., Borges, K., Bowie, D., and Traynelis, S.F. (1999). The glutamate receptor ion channels. *Pharmacol Rev,* 51 (March 1999), pp. 7–61, ISSN 0031-6997

Dittman, J. S., Kreitzer, A. C., and Regehr, W. G. (2000). Interplay between facilitation, depression, and residual calcium at three presynaptic terminals. *J Neurosci,* 20, 4, (February 2000), pp. 1374-85, ISSN 0270-6474

Dobrunz, L. E., and Stevens, C. F. (1997). Heterogeneity of release probability, facilitation, and depletion at central synapses. *Neuron,* 18, 6 (June 1997), pp. 995–1008, ISSN 0896-6273

Dodd, P.R. Beckmann, A.M. Davidson, M.S. Wilce, P.A. (2000). Glutamate-mediated transmission, alcohol, and alcoholism. *Neurochem Int,* 37, (2000), pp. 509-533, ISSN 0197-0186

Durand, G.M., Bennett, M.V.L., Zukin, R.S. (1993). Splice variants of the N-methyl-d-aspartate receptor NR1 identify domains involved in regulation by polyamines and protein kinase C. *Proc Natl Acad Sci USA* 90 (July 2003), pp. 6731–6735, ISSN 0027-8424

Eng, L.F., Yu, A.C., and Lee, Y.L. (1992). Astrocytic response to injury. *Prog Brain Res,* 94, pp. 353-365, ISSN 0006-8993

Evrard, S.G., Duhalde-Vega, M., Tagliaferro, P., Mirochnic, S., Caltana, L.R., and Brusco, A. (2006). A low chronic ethanol exposure induces morphological changes in the adolescent rat brain that are not fully recovered even after a long abstinence: an immunohistochemical study. *Exp Neurol,* 200, 2, (August 2006), pp. 438-459, ISSN 0014-4886

Ewald R.C., Cline H.T. (2009). NMDA Receptors and Brain Development. In: Biology of the NMDA Receptor. *Frontiers in Neuroscience,* Boca Raton (FL): CRC Press, ISBN 13: 978142004414

Farber N.B., Heinkel C., Dribben W.H., Nemmers B., Jiang X. (2004). In the adult CNS, ethanol prevents rather than produces NMDA antagonist-induced neurotoxicity. *Brain Res,* 1028, 1, (November 2004),pp. 66-74, ISSN 0006-8993

Ferko, A. (1994). Interaction between L-glutamate and ethanol on the central depressant properties of ethanol in mice. *Pharmacol Biochem Behav,* 47, 2 (February 1994), pp. 351–354, ISSN 0091-3057

Ferrani-Kile, K., Randall, P., Leslie, S. (2003). Acute ethanol affects phosphorylation state of the NMDA receptor complex: implication of tyrosine phosphatases and protein kinaseA. Brain research. *Molecular brain research,* 115, 1 (July 2003), pp. 78-86, ISSN 0169-328X

Ferreira, V.M., Frausto, S., Browning, M.D., Savage, D.D., Morato, G.S., and Valenzuela, C.F. (2001). Ionotropic glutamate receptor subunit expression in the rat hippocampus: lack of an effect of a long-term ethanol exposure paradigm. *Alcohol Clin Exp Res,* 25, 10, (October 2001), pp. 1536-1541, ISSN 0145-6008

Ferrer-Montiel, A. V. & Montal, M. (1996). Pentameric subunit stoichiometry of a neuronal glutamate receptor. *Proc. Natl. Acad. Sci. USA,* 93, 7 (April 1996), pp. 2741–2744, ISSN 0027-8424

Fitzpatrick, C.J., and Lombroso, P.J. (2011). The Role of Striatal-Enriched Protein Tyrosine Phosphatase (STEP) in Cognition. *Front Neuroanat*, 5, 47, (July 2011), Epub, ISSN 1662-5129

Floyd, D.W., Jung, K.Y., and McCool, B.A. (2003). Chronic Ethanol Ingestion Facilitates N-Methyl-D-aspartate Receptor Function and Expression in Rat Lateral/Basolateral Amygdala Neurons. *J Pharmacol Exp Ther*, 307, pp. 1020-1029, ISSN 0022-3565

Follesa, P., Ticku, M.K. (1996). Chronic ethanol-mediated up-regulation of the N-methyl-D-aspartate receptor polypeptide subunits in mouse cortical neurons in culture. *Journal of Biological Chemistry*, 271, 23, (June 1996), pp. 13297-13299.

Forcina, M., Ciabarra, A., Seravino, K. (1995). Cloning of chi-2: a putative member of the ionotropic glutamate receptor superfamily. *Soc Neurosci Abstr*, 21 (June 1995), pp. 438-3, ISSN 0190-5295

Franke, H., Kittner, H., Berger, P., Wirkner, K., and Schramek, J. (1997). The reaction of astrocytes and neurons in the hippocampus of adult rats during chronic ethanol treatment and correlations to behavioral impairments. *Alcohol*, 14, 5, (September 1997), pp. 445-454, ISSN 0741-8329

Fulton, T., Crews, F.T., and Nixon, K. (2009). Mechanisms of Neurodegeneration and Regeneration in Alcoholism. *Alcohol and Alcoholism, 44, 2,* (March-april 2009), pp. 115-127, ISSN 0735-0414

Gass, J.T., Olive, M.F. (2008). Glutamatergic substrates of drug addiction and alcoholism. *Biochem Pharmacol*, 75, 1 (January 2008), pp. 218–265, ISSN 0006-2952

Ge, Z.J., Zhang, L.C., Zeng, Y.M., Da, T.J., Wang, J.K., Cui, G.X., Tan, Y.F., Zhao, Y.P., and Liu, G.J. (2007). Involvement of NMDA receptors in thiopental-induced loss of righting reflex, antinociception and anticonvulsion effects in mice. *Pharmacology,* 80, 2-3, (May 2007), pp. 127-133, ISSN 1432-2072

Goldstein, D.B. (1986). Effect of alcohol on cellular membranes. *Ann Emer Med* 15, 9 (September 1986), pp. 1013-1018, ISSN 0196-0644

Grant, K. (1999). Strategies for understanding the pharmacological effects of ethanol with drug discrimination procedures. *Pharmacol Biochem Behav*, 64, 2 (October 1999), pp. 261–267, ISSN 0091-3057

Grant, K.A., Valverius, P., Hudspith, M., Tabakoff, B. (1990). Ethanol withdrawal seizures and the NMDA receptor complex. *European Journal of Pharmacology*, 176, 3, (November 1990), pp. 289-296, ISSN 0014-2999

Guerri, C., and Renau-Piqueras, J. (1997). Alcohol, astroglia, and brain development. *Mol Neurobiol*, 15, 1, (August 1997), pp. 65-81, ISSN 0893-7648

Gulya, K., Grant, K.A., Valverius, P., Hoffmann, P.L., Tabakoff, B. (1991). Brain regional specificity and time-course of changes in the NMDA receptor-ionophore complex during ethanol withdrawal. *Brain Research*, 547, 1, (April 1991), pp. 129-134, ISSN 0006-8993

Hallett, P.J., Dunah A.W., Ravenscroft, P., Zhou, S., Bezard, E., Crossman, A.R., Brotchie, J.M., Standaert, D.G. (2005). Alterations of striatal NMDA receptor subunits associated with the development of dyskinesia in the MPTP-lesioned primate model of Parkinson's disease. *Neuropharmacology,* 48,4, (March 2005), pp.503-516, ISSN 0028-3908

Hamelink, C., Hampson, A., Wink, D.A., Eiden, L.E., and Eskay, R.L. (2005). Comparison of cannabidiol, antioxidants, and diuretics in reversing binge ethanol-induced neurotoxicity. *J Pharmacol Exp Ther*, 314, 2, (Aug 2005), pp. 780-788, ISSN 0022-3565

Harper, C., Dixon, G., Sheedy, D., and Garrick, T. (2003). Neuropathological alterations in alcoholic brains. Studies arising from the New South Wales Tissue Resource Centre. *Prog Neuropsychopharmacol Biol Psychiatry*, 27, 6, (September 2003), pp. 951-961, ISSN 0006-3223

Hatton, C.J, and Paoletti, P. (2005). Modulation of triheteromeric NMDA receptors by N-terminal domain ligands. *Neuron*, 46 (April 2005), pp. 261–274, ISSN 0896-6273

Hendricson, A.W., Maldve, R.E., Salinas, A.G., Theile, J.W., Zhang, T.A., Diaz, L.M., and Morrisett, R.A. (2007). Aberrant synaptic activation of N-methyl-D-aspartate receptors underlies ethanol withdrawal hyperexcitability. *J Pharmacol Exp Ther*, 321, 1, (April 2007), pp. 60-72, ISSN 0022-3565

Hendricson, A.W., Miao, C.L., Lippmann, M.J., and Morrisett, R.A. (2002). Ifenprodil and ethanol enhance NMDA receptor-dependent long-term depression. *J Pharmacol Exp Ther*, 301, 3, (June 2002), pp. 938-944, ISSN 0022-3565

Henniger, M.S., Wotjak, C.T., and Hölter, S.M. (2003). Long-term voluntary ethanol drinking increases expression of NMDA receptor 2B subunits in rat frontal cortex. *European Journal of Pharmacology*, 470, 1-2, (May 2003), pp. 470-433, ISSN 0014-2999

Heyne A., Wolffgramm J. (1998). The development of addiction to d-amphetamine in an animal model: same principles as for alcohol and opiate. *Psychopharmacology (Berl)*, 140, 4, (December 1998), pp. 510-8, ISSN 1432-2072

Heyne A., May T., Goll P., Wolffgramm J. (2000). Persisting consequences of drug intake: towards a memory of addiction. *J Neural Transm*, 107, 6, (2000), pp. 613-38, ISSN 1435-1463

Heyser, C.J., Schulteis, G., Durbin, P., Koob, G.F. (1998). Chronic acamprosate treatment eliminates the alcohol deprivation effect while having limited effects on baseline responding for ethanol in rats. *Neuropsychopharmacology*, 18, 2 (February 1998), pp. 125–133, ISSN 0893-133X

Hicklin, T.R., Wu, P.H., Radcliffe, R.A., Freund, R.K., Goebel-Goody, S.M., Correa, P.R., Proctor, W.R., Lombroso, P.J., and Browning, M.D. (2011). Alcohol inhibition of the NMDA receptor function, long-term potentiation, and fear learning requires STEP. *Proc Natl Acad Sci (USA)*, 108, 16, (April 2011), pp. 6650-6655, ISSN 0027-8424

Hirai, H., Kirsch, J., Laube, B., Betz, H., and Kuhse, J. (1996). The glycine binding site of the N-methyl-D-aspartate receptor subunit NR1: identification of novel determinants of co-agonist potentiation in the extracellular M3-M4 loop region. *Proc Natl Acad Sci U S A*, 93, 12, (June 1996), pp. 6031-6036, ISSN 0027-8424

Hölter, S.M., Danysz, W., Spanagel, R. (2000). Novel uncompetitive N-methyl-D-aspartate (NMDA)-receptor antagonist MRZ 2/579 suppresses ethanol intake in long-term ethanol-experienced rats and generalizes to ethanol cue in drug discrimination procedure. *J Pharmacol Exp Ther*, 292, 2 (February 2000), pp. 545–552, ISSN 0022-3565

Husi, H,. Ward, M.A., Choudhary, J.S., Blackstock, W.P., Grant, S.G. (2000). Proteomic analysis of NMDA receptor-adhesion protein signaling complexes. *Nature Neuroscience*, 3 (July 2000), pp. 661 - 669, ISSN 1097-6256

Hyman, S.E., and Malenka, R.C. (2001). Addiction and the brain: the neurobiology of compulsion and its persistence. *Nat Rev Neurosci*, 2, 10, (Oct 2001), pp. 695-703, ISSN 1471-003X

Javitt, D.C., Zukin S.R. (1991). Recent advances in the phencyclidine model of schizophrenia. *Am J Psychiatry*, 148, 10, (October 1991), pp. 1301-1308, ISSN 1535-7228

Kalluri, H.S., Mehta, A.K., and Ticku, M.K. (1998). Up-regulation of NMDA receptor subunits in rat brain following chronic ethanol treatment. *Molecular Brain Research*, 58, 1-2, (July 1998), pp. 221-224, ISSN 0169-328X

Lack, A.K., Diaz, M.R., Chappell, A., DuBois, D.W. and McCool, B.A. (2007). Chronic ethanol and withdrawal differentially modulate pre- and postsynaptic function at glutamatergic synapses in rat basolateral amygdala. *J Neurophysiol*, 98, 6 (December 2007), pp. 3185-3196, ISSN 0022-3077

Lareo, L.R. and Corredor, C. (2006). Molecular correlate of consciousness. In: *Consciousness and Learning Research*, S. K. Turrini (Ed) Nova Publishers, New York. pp. 97–117, ISSN 0196-6006

Lau, C.G. and Zukin, R.S. (2007). NMDA receptor trafficking in synaptic plasticity and neuropsychiatric disorders. *Nat. Rev. Neurosci*, 8 (June 2007), pp. 413-426, ISSN 1471-003X

Laube, B., Kuhse, J. & Betz, H. (1998). Evidence for a tetrameric structure of recombinant NMDA receptor. *J. Neurosci*, 18, 8, (Apr 1998), pp. 2954–2961, ISSN 0270-6474

Lebel, D., Sidhu, N., Barkai, E. and Quinlan, E.M. (2006). Learning in the absence of experience-dependent regulation of NMDAR composition. *Learn. Mem*, 13, 5, (October 2006), pp. 566–570, ISSN 1072-0502

Levine, MS, Cepeda C, André VM. (2010). Location, location, location: contrasting roles of synaptic and extrasynaptic NMDA receptors in Huntington's disease. *Neuron* 28, 65, (January 2010), pp. 145-147, ISSN: 0896-6273

Liljequist, S. (1991). NMDA receptor antagonists inhibit ethanol-produced locomotor stimulation in NMRI mice. Alcohol, 8, 4, (July 1991), pp. 309-312, ISSN 0741-8329

Lovinger, D.M., White, G., Weight, F.F. (1989). Ethanol inhibits NMDA-activated ion current in hippocampal neurons. *Science*, 243 (March 1989), pp. 1721–1724, ISSN 0036-8075

Lovinger, D.M. (1995). Developmental decrease in ethanol inhibition of N-methyl-Daspartate receptors in rat neocortical neurons: Relation to the actions of ifenprodil. *J Pharmacol Exp Ther*, 274, 1, (July 1995), pp. 164-172, ISSN 0022-3565

Lovinger, D.M. (1997). Alcohols and neurotransmitter gated ion channels: past, present, and future. *Naunyn Schmiedebergs Arch Pharmacol*, 356, 3, (September 1997), pp. 267-82, ISSN 1432-1912

Lovinger, D.M. (1999). 5-HT3 receptors and the neural actions of alcohols: an increasingly exciting topic. *Neurochem Int*, 35, 2 (August 1999), pp. 125–130, ISSN 0197-0186

Low, C., Wee, K. (2010). New insights into the not-so-new NR3 subunits of N-methyl-D-aspartate receptor: localization, structure, and function. *Mol Pharmacol*, 78, 1 (July 2010), pp. 1-11, ISSN 0026-895X

Lynch, D.R., and Guttmann, R.P. (2002). Excitotoxicity: perspectives based on NMDA receptor subtypes. *J Pharmacol Exp Ther*, 300 (March 2002), pp. 717–723, ISSN 0022-3565.

MacDonald, J.F., Jackson, M.F., and Beazely, M.A. (2006). Hippocampal long-term synaptic plasticity and signal amplification of NMDA receptors. *Crit Rev Neurobiol*, 18, 1-2, pp. 71-84, ISSN 0892-0915

Mahadev, K., Vemuri, M. (1999). Effect of pre- and postnatal ethanol exposure on protein tyrosine kinase activity and its endogenous substrates in rat cerebral cortex. *Alcohol*, 17, 3 (April 1999), pp. 223-9, ISSN 0741-8329

Malenka, R.C., and Bear, M.F. (2004). LTP and LTD: an embarrassment of riches. *Neuron*, 44, 1, (September 2004), pp. 5-21. ISSN 0896-6273

Matsuda, K., Fletcher, M,. Kamiya, Y., and Yuzaki, M. (2003). Specific assembly with the NMDA receptor 3B subunit controls surface expression and calcium permeability of NMDA receptors. *J Neurosci*, 23, 31 (November 2003), pp. 10064–10073, ISSN 0270-6474

Matsumoto, I. Burke, L. Inoue, Y. Wilce, P.A. (2001). Two models of ethanol withdrawal kindling. *Nihon Arukoru Yakubutsu Igakkai Zasshi*, 36 (2001), pp. 53–64, ISSN 1341-8963

Mayer, M.L. (2005b). Glutamate receptor ion channels. *Curr Opin Neurobiol*, 15 (October 2005b), pp. 282–288, ISSN 0959-4388

Medina, A.E., Liao, D.S., Mower, A.F., and Ramoa, A.S. (2001). Do NMDA receptor kinetics regulate the end of critical periods of plasticity? *Neuron*, 32, 4, (November 2001), pp. 553-555 ISSN 0896-6273

Méndez, G., Reyes, E., Poutou, R., Quevedo, B., Lareo, L. (2008). Purification of IgY against the NR3 subunit of the rat brain NMDA receptor. *Rev.MVZ Córdoba*, 13, 1 (February 2008), pp. 1146-1156, ISSN 0122-0268

Miguel-Hidalgo, J.J. (2005). Lower packing density of glial fibrillary acidic protein-immunoreactive astrocytes in the prelimbic cortex of alcohol-naive and alcohol-drinking alcohol-preferring rats as compared with alcohol-nonpreferring and Wistar rats. *Alcohol Clin Exp Res*, 29, 5, (May 2005), pp. 766-772, ISSN 1530-0277

Miguel-Hidalgo, J.J., Alvarez, X.A., Cacabelos, R., and Quack, G. (2002). Neuroprotection by memantine against neurodegeneration induced by beta-amyloid(1-40). *Brain Res*, 958, 1, (Dec 2002), pp. 210-221, ISSN 0006-8993

Miguel-Hidalgo, J.J., and Rajkowska G. (2003). Comparison of prefrontal cell pathology between depression and alcohol dependence. *J Psychiatr Res*, 37, 5, (September 2003), pp. 411-420, ISSN 0022-3956

Miguel-Hidalgo, J.J., Overholser, J.C., Meltzer, H.Y., Stockmeier, C.A., and Rajkowska, G. (2006). Reduced glial and neuronal packing density in the orbitofrontal cortex in alcohol dependence and its relationship with suicide and duration of alcohol dependence. *Alcohol Clin Exp Res*, 30, 11, (November 2006), pp. 1845-1855, ISSN 1530-0277

Miguel-Hidalgo, J.J., Waltzer, R., Whittom, A.A., Austin, M.C., Rajkowska, G., and Stockmeier, C.A. (2010). Glial and glutamatergic markers in depression, alcoholism, and their comorbidity. *J Affect Disord*, 127, 1-3, (December 2010), pp. 230-240, ISSN 0165-0327

Mihic S.J., Harris R.A. (1997). GABA and the GABAA receptor. *Alcohol Health Res World* 21, 2 (1997), pp. 127-31, ISSN 0090-838X

Mihic, S. (1999). Acute effects of ethanol on GABAA and glycine receptor function. *Neurochem Int*, 35, 2 (August 1999), pp. 115–123, ISSN 0197-0186

Mirshahi T., and Woodward J.J. (1995) Ethanol sensitivity of heteromeric NMDA receptors: Effects of subunit assembly, glycine and NMDAR1 Mg2+-insensitive mutants. *Neuropharmacology* 34, 3 (March 1995), pp. 347-355, ISSN 0028-3908

Misra, C.h., Brickley, S., Farrant, M., and Cull-Candy, S. (2000). Identification of subunits contributing to synaptic and extrasynaptic NMDA receptors in Golgi cells of the rat cerebellum. *The Journal of Physiology*, 524 (April 2000), pp. 147-162, ISSN 0022-3751

Miyakawa, T., Yagi, T., Kitazawa, H., Yasuda, M., Kawai, N., Tsuboi, K., and Niki, H. (1997) Fyn kinase as a determinant of ethanol sensitivity: Relation to NMDA-receptor function. *Science*, 278 (October 1997), pp. 698-701, ISSN 0036-8075

Momiyama, A., Feldmeyer, D., Cull-Candy, S.G. (1996). Identification of a native low-conductance NMDA channel with reduced sensitivity to Mg2+ in rat central neurones. *J Physiol (Lond),* 494 (July 1996), pp. 479–492, ISSN 0022-3751

Monyer, H., Sprengel, R., Schoepfer, R., Herb, A., Higuchi, M., Lomeli, H., Burnashev, N., Sakmann, B., Seeburg, P.H. (1992). Heteromeric NMDA receptors: Molecular and functional distinctions of subtypes. *Science (Wash DC),* 256 (May 1992), pp. 1217–1221, ISSN 0036-8075

Moreno, F., Reyes, E., Lareo, L. (2010). Computational study of the evolutionary relationships of the ionotropic receptors NMDA, AMPA and kainate in four species of primates. *Universitas Scientiarum.* 15, 3 (October 2010), pp. 183-193, ISSN 0122-7483

Morrisett, R.A., and Swartzwelder, H.S. (1993). Attenuation of hippocampal long-term potentiation by ethanol: a patch-clamp analysis of glutamatergic and GABAergic mechanisms. *J Neurosci,* 13, 5, (May 1993), pp. 2264-2272. ISSN 0270-6474

Muhonen, L.H., Lönnqvist, J., Juva, K., and Alho, H. (2008). Double-blind, randomized comparison of memantine and escitalopram for the treatment of major depressive disorder comorbid with alcohol dependence. *J Clin Psychiatry,* 69, 3, (Mar 2008), pp. 392-399, ISSN 0160-6689

Murail, S., Wallner, B., Trudell, J.R., Bertaccini, E., Lindahl, E. (2011). Microsecond Simulations Indicate that Ethanol Binds between Subunits and Could Stabilize an Open-State Model of a Glycine Receptor. *Biophys J,* 100 (April 2011), pp. 1642-1650, ISSN 0006-3495

Nagy J, László L. (2002). Increased sensitivity to NMDA is involved in alcohol-withdrawal induced cytotoxicity observed in primary cultures of cortical neurones chronically pre-treated with ethanol. *Neurochem Int,* 40,7, (June 2002), pp. 585-591, ISSN 0364-3190

Nagy J, Kolok S, Dezso P, Boros A, Szombathelyi Z. (2003). Differential alterations in the expression of NMDA receptor subunits following chronic ethanol treatment in primary cultures of rat cortical and hippocampal neurones. *Neurochem Int,* 42, 1, (January 2003), pp. 35-43, ISSN 0364-3190

Narahashi, T., Aistrup, G.L., Marszalec, W., Nagata, K. (1999). Neuronal nicotinic acetylcholine receptors: a new target site of ethanol. *Neurochem Int,* 35, 2 (August 1999), pp. 131–141, ISSN 0197-0186

Nelson, T.E., Ur, C.L., and Gruol, D.L. (2005). Chronic intermittent ethanol exposure enhances NMDA-receptor-mediated synaptic responses and NMDA receptor expression in hippocampal CA1 region. *Brain Research,* 1048, 1-2, (Jun 2005), pp. 69-79, ISSN 00068993

Newlin, D.B., and Renton, R.M. (2010). High risk groups often have higher levels of alcohol response than low risk: the other side of the coin. *Alcohol Clin Exp Res,* 34, 2, (February 2010), pp. 199-202, ISSN 0145-6008

Nishi, M., Hinds, H., Lu, H.P., Kawata, M., and Hayashi, Y. (2001). Motoneuron-specific expression of NR3B, a novel NMDA-type glutamate receptor subunit that works in a dominant-negative manner. *J Neurosci,* 21, (December 2001), pp. 23:RC185, ISSN 0270-6474

Norton, W.T., Aquino, D.A., Hozumi, I., Chiu, F.C., and Brosnan, C.F. (1992). Quantitative aspects of reactive gliosis: a review. *Neurochem Res,* 17, 9, (September 1992), pp. 877-885, ISSN 1573-6903

Nusser, Z. (2000). AMPA and NMDA receptors: similarities and differences in their synaptic distribution. *Curr. Opin. Neurobiol.* 10, 3, (June 200), pp. 337–341, ISSN 0959-4388

Obara, M., Szeliga, M., and Albrecht, J. (2007). Regulation of pH in the mammalian central nervous system under normal and pathological conditions: facts and hypotheses. *Neurochem Int,* 52, 6, (May 2008), pp. 905-19, ISSN 0197-0186

Paoletti, P., Ascher, P., and Neyton, J. (1997). High-affinity zinc inhibition of NMDA NR1-NR2A receptors. *J Neurosci,* 17, 15, (August 1997), pp. 5711-5725, ISSN 0270-6474

Paoletti, P., and Neyton, J. (2007). NMDA receptor subunits: function and pharmacology. *Curr Opin Pharmacol,* 7 (February 2007), pp. 39–47, ISSN 1471-4892

Paoletti P. (2011). Molecular basis of NMDA receptor functional diversity. *Eur J Neurosci,* 33, 8, (April 2011), pp. 1351-1365, ISSN 1359-5962

Paul, S., Olausson, P., Venkitaramani, D.V., Ruchkina, I., Moran, T.D., Tronson, N., Mills, E., Hakim, S., Salter, M.W., Taylor, J.R., and Lombroso, P.J. (2007). The striatal-enriched Protein tyrosine phosphatase gates long-term potentiation and fear memory in the lateral amygdala. *Biol Psychiatry,* 61, 9 (May 2007), pp. 1049-1061, ISSN 0006-3223

Pelkey, K.A., Askalan, R., Paul, S., Kalia, L.V., Nguyen, T.H., Pitcher, G.M., Salter, M.W., and Lombroso P.J. (2002). Tyrosine phosphatase STEP is a tonic brake on induction of long-term potentiation. *Neuron,* 34, 1 (March 2002), pp. 127-138, ISSN 0896-6273

Peoples R.W., Weight FF. (1992). Ethanol inhibition of N-methyl-D-aspartate-activated ion current in rat hippocampal neurons is not competitive with glycine. *Brain Res,* 7,571, (February 1992), pp. 342-344, ISSN 0006-8993

Perez-Otano, I., Schulteis, C. T., Contractor, A., Lipton, S. A., Trimmer, J. S., Sucher, N. J. and Heinemann, S.F. (2001). Assembly with the NR1 subunit is required for surface expression of NR3A-containing NMDA receptors. *J. Neurosci,* 21, 4, (February 2001), pp. 1228–1237, ISSN 0270-6474

Perin-Dureau, F., Rachline, J., Neyton, J., Paoletti, P. (2002). Mapping the binding site of the neuroprotectant ifenprodil on NMDA receptors. *J Neurosci,* 22, 14 (July 2002), pp. 5955-65, ISSN 0270-6474

Petrakis, I.L., Limoncelli, D., Gueorguieva, R., Jatlow, P., Boutros, N.N., Trevisan, L., et al. (2004). Altered NMDA glutamate receptor antagonist response in individuals with a family vulnerability to alcoholism. *Am J Psychiatry,* 161, 10 (October 2004) 1776–1782, ISSN 0002-953X

Phelps, L.E., Brutsche, N., Moral, J.R., Luckenbaugh, D.A., Manji, H.K., and Zarate, C.A. Jr. (2009). Family history of alcohol dependence and initial antidepressant response to an N-methyl-D-aspartate antagonist. *Biol Psychiatry,* 65, 2, (January 2009), pp. 181-184, ISSN 0006-3223

Popp, R.L., Lickteig, R., Browning, M.D., and Lovinger, D.M. (1998). Ethanol sensitivity and subunit composition of NMDA receptors in cultured striatal neurons. *Neuropharmacology,* 37, 1, pp. 45-56, ISSN 0028-3908

Prybylowski, K., Wenthold, R. (2004). N-Methyl-D-aspartate receptors: subunit assembly and trafficking to the synapse. *J Biol Chem,* 279, 11 (March 2004), pp. 9673-6, ISSN 0021-9258

Qin, L., He, J., Hanes, R.N., Pluzarev, O., Hong, J.S., and Crews, F.T. (2008). Increased systemic and brain cytokine production and neuroinflammation by endotoxin following ethanol treatment. J *Neuroinflammation,* 18, (March 2008), pp. 5-10, ISSN 1742-2094

Reyes-Montaño, E.A, Lareo, L.R., Chow, D-C., Pérez-Gómez, G. (2006). Immunolocalization and Biochemical Characterization of N-methyl-D-aspartate Receptor Subunit NR1 from Rat Brain. *The Protein Journal,* 25, 2 (February 2006), pp. 95-108, ISSN 1572-3887

Ripley, T.L., Little, H.J. (1995). Effects on ethanol withdrawal hyperexcitability of chronic treatment with a competitive N-methyl-D-aspartate receptor antagonist. J *Pharmacol Exper Therap,* 272, 1, (January 1995), pp. 112-118, ISSN. 0022-3565

Roberto, M., Bajo, M., Crawford, E., Madamba, S.G., and Siggins, G.R. (2006). Chronic Ethanol Exposure and Protracted Abstinence Alter NMDA Receptors in Central Amygdala. *Neuropsychopharmacology,* 31,5, (May 2006), pp. 988-996, ISSN 0893-133X

Roberto, M., Schweitzer, P., Madamba, S.G., Stouffer, D.G., Parsons, L.H., Siggins, G.R. (2004) Acute and chronic ethanol alter glutamatergic transmission in rat central amygdala: An in vitro and in vivo analysis. *J Neurosci,* 24, 7 (February 2004), pp. 1594-1603, ISSN 0270-6474

Rodd ZA, Bell RL, Kuc KA, Murphy JM, Lumeng L, McBride WJ. Effects of concurrent access to multiple ethanol concentrations and repeated deprivations on alcohol intake of high alcohol-drinking (HAD) rats. *Addict Biol,* (2008), Submitted, ISSN 1369-1600

Ron, D. (2004). Signaling Cascades Regulating NMDA Receptor Sensitivity to Ethanol. *Neuroscientist,* 10 (August 2004), pp. 325–336, ISSN 0306-4522

Saft C, Epplen JT, Wieczorek S, Landwehrmeyer GB, Roos RA, de Yebenes JG, Dose M, Tabrizi SJ, et al. (2011). NMDA receptor gene variations as modifiers in Huntington disease: a replication study. *PLoS Curr,* 4, 3, (October 2011), RRN1247, ISSN 2157-3999

Salter, M.W., and Kalia, L.V. (2004). Src kinases: a hub for NMDA receptor regulation. *Nat. Rev. Neurosci.,* 5 (April 2004), pp. 317–328, ISSN 1471-003X

Sanchis-Segura, C., Spanagel, R. (2006). Behavioural assessment of drug reinforcement and addictive features in rodents: an overview. *Addict Biol,* 11, 1 (March 2006), pp. 2–38, ISSN 1355-6215

Sander T., Ball D., Murray R., Patel J., Samochowiec J., Winterer G., Rommelspacher H., Schmidt L.G., Loh E.W. (1999). Association analysis of sequence variants of GABA(A) alpha6, beta2, and gamma2 gene cluster and alcohol dependence. *Alcohol Clin Exp Res* 23 (March 1999), pp. 427-31, ISSN 1720-8319

Schroeder, J.P., Overstreet, D.H., Hodge, C.W. (2005). The mGluR5 antagonist MPEP decreases operant ethanol self-administration during maintenance and after repeated alcohol deprivations in alcohol-preferring (P) rats. *Psychopharmacology (Berl),* 179, 1 (April 2005), pp. 262–270, ISSN 0033-3158

Schuckit, M.A., and Smith, T.L. (2001). The clinical course of alcohol dependence associated with a low level of response to alcohol. *Addiction,* 96, 6 (June 2001), pp. 903-910, ISSN 0965-2140

Sevarino, K., Ciabarra, A., Forcina, M. (1996). χ-1 and χ-2, members of a novel class of the glutamate receptor superfamily. *Soc Neurosci Abstr*, 22 (October 1995), pp. 59219, ISSN 0190-5295

Smith, K.J., Butler, T.R., Self, R.L., Braden, B.B., Prendergast, M.A. (2008). Potentiation of N-methyl-D-aspartate receptor-mediated neuronal injury during methamphetamine withdrawal in vitro requires co-activation of IP3 receptors. *Brain Res*, 1187, 2, (January 2008), pp. 67-73, ISSN: 0006-8993

Smothers, C.T., Clayton, R., Blevins, T., and Woodward, J.J. (2001). Ethanol sensitivity of recombinant human N-methyl-D-aspartate receptors. *Neurochem Int*, 38, 4, (April 2001), pp. 333-340, ISSN 0197-0186

Snell, L.D., Nunley, K.R., Lickteig, R.L., Browning, M.D., Tabakoff, B., and Hoffman, P.L. (1996). Regional and subunit specific changes in NMDA receptor mRNA and immunoreactivity in mouse brain following chronic ethanol ingestion. *Mol Brain Res*, 40, 1, (August 1996), pp. 71-78, ISSN 0169-328X

Snyder, E.M., Nong, Y., Almeida, C.G., Paul, S., Moran, T., Choi, E.Y., Nairn, A.C., Salter, M.W., Lombroso, P.J., Gouras, G.K., and Greengard, P. (2005). Regulation of NMDA receptor trafficking by amyloid-beta. *Nat Neurosci*, 8 (March 2005), pp. 1051-1058, ISSN 0896-6273

Spanagel, R. (2009). Alcoholism: A Systems Approach From Molecular Physiology to Addictive Behavior. *Physiol Rev*, 89 (April 2009), pp. 649–705, ISSN 0031-9333

Spanagel, R., Hölter, S., Allingham, K., Landgraf, R., Zieglgänsberger, W. (1996). Acamprosate and alcohol: I. Effects on alcohol intake following alcohol deprivation in the rat. *Eur J Pharmacol*, 305, 1-3, (June 1996), pp. 39–44, ISSN 0014-2999

Spanagel, R., Sigmund, S., Cowen, M., Schroff, K.C., Schumann, G., Fiserova, M. et al. (2002). The neuronal nitric oxide synthase (nNOS) gene is critically involved in neurobehavioral effects of alcohol. *J Neurosci*, 22, 19, (October 2002), pp. 8676–8683, ISSN 0270-6474

Sucher, N., Brose, N., Deitcher, D., Awobuluyi, M., Gasic, G., Bading, H., Cepko, C., Greenberg, M., Jahn, R., Heinemann, S. (1993). Expression of endogenous NMDAR1 transcripts without receptor protein suggests post-transcriptional control in PC12 cells. *J Biol Chem*, 268 (October 1993), pp. 22299–22304, ISSN 0021-9258

Suvarna, N., Borgland, S.L., Wang, J., Phamluong, K., Auberson, Y.P., Bonci, A., and Ron, D. (2005). Ethanol alters trafficking and functional N-methyl-D-aspartate receptor NR2 subunit ratio via H-Ras. *J Biol Chem*, 280, 36, (September 2005), pp. 31450-31459, ISSN 0021-9258

Suzdak P.D., Schwartz R.D., Skolnick P., Paul S.N. (1986). Ethanol stimulates gamma-aminobutyric acid receptor-mediated chloride transport in rat brain synaptoneurosomes. *Proc Natl Acad Sci U S A*, 83 (1986), pp. 4071-5 ISSN 0027-8424

Taffe, M.A., Kotzebue, R.W., Crean, R.D., Crawford, E.F., Edwards, S., and Mandyam, C.D. (2010). Long-lasting reduction in hippocampal neurogenesis by alcohol consumption in adolescent nonhuman primates. *Proc Natl Acad Sci U S A*, 107, 24, (June 2010), pp. 11104-11109, ISSN 0027-8424

Takadera, T., Ohyashiki. T. (2008). Benzyl alcohol inhibits N-methyl-D-aspartate receptor-mediated neurotoxicity and calcium accumulation in cultured rat cortical neurons. *J Biomed Sci*, 15 (August 2008), pp. 767-770, ISSN 1937-6871

Tang, T., Badger, J., Roche, P., Roche, K. (2010). Novel Approach to Probe Subunit-specific Contributions to N-Methyl-D-aspartate (NMDA) Receptor Trafficking Reveals a Dominant Role for NR2B in Receptor Recycling. *J Biol Chem*, 285, 27 (July 2010), pp. 20975-81, ISSN 0021-9258

Trujillo KA, Akil H. (1995). Excitatory amino acids and drugs of abuse: a role for N-methyl-D-aspartate receptors in drug tolerance, sensitization and physical dependence. *Drug Alcohol Depend*, 38, 2, (May 1995), pp. 139-154, ISSN 0376-8716

Tsai G., Gastfriend D.R., Coyle J.T. (1995). The glutamatergic basis of human alcoholism. *Am J Psychiatry*, 152 (March 1995), pp. 332-40, ISSN 1535-7228

Tsai, G., Coyle, J.T. (1998) The role of glutamatergic neurotransmission in the pathophysiology of alcoholism. *Annu Rev Med*, 49, (February 1998), pp. 173-184, ISSN 0066-4219

Udomuksorn, W., Mukem, S., Kumarnsit, E., Vongvatcharanon, S., and Vongvatcharanon, U. (2011). Effects of alcohol administration during adulthood on parvalbumin and glial fibrillary acidic protein immunoreactivity in the rat cerebral cortex. *Acta Histochem*, 113, 3, (May 2011), pp. 283-289, ISSN 0044-5991

Ulbrich, M., Isacoff, E. (2008). Rules of engagement for NMDA receptor subunits. *Proc Natl Acad Sci U S A*, 105, 37 (September 2008), pp. 14163-8, ISSN 0027-8424

Ułas J, Weihmuller FB, Brunner LC, Joyce JN, Marshall JF, Cotman CW. (1994). Selective increase of NMDA-sensitive glutamate binding in the striatum of Parkinson's disease, Alzheimer's disease, and mixed Parkinson's disease/Alzheimer's disease patients: an autoradiographic study. J Neurosci. 14, 11, (November 1994), pp. 6317-6324, ISSN-0270-6474

Vargas, N., Reyes, E., Lareo, L. (2010). In silico approach to the evolution of ionotropic glutamate receptor gene family in four primate species. *Universitas Scientiarum*, 15, 3 (October 2010), pp. 194-205, ISSN 0122-7483

Vastagh C, Gardoni F, Bagetta V, Stanic J, Zianni E, Giampa' C, Picconi B, Calabresi P,. (2012). NMDA receptor composition modulates dendritic spine morphology in striatal medium spiny neurons. *J Biol Chem*, (April 2012), [Epub ahead of print], ISSN 0021-9258

Vengeliene, V., Bachteler, D., Danysz, W., Spanagel, R. (2005). The role of the NMDA receptor in alcohol relapse: a pharmacological mapping study using the alcohol deprivation effect. *Neuropharmacology*, 48 (May 2005), pp. 822-829, ISSN 0028-3908

Vengeliene, V., Bilbao, A., Molander, A., and Spanagel, R. (2008). Neuropharmacology of alcohol addiction. Br *J Pharmacol*. 154, 2 (May 2008), pp. 299–315, ISSN 0007-1188

Vicini, S., Wang, J.F., Li, J.H., Zhu, W.J., Wang, Y.H., Luo, J.H., Wolfe, B.B., and Grayson, D.R. (1998). Functional and pharmacological differences between recombinant N-methyl-D-aspartate receptors. *J Neurophysiol*, 79 (February 1998), pp. 555–566, ISSN 0022-3077

Volterra, A., and Meldolesi, J. (2005). Astrocytes, from brain glue to communication elements: the revolution continues. *Nat Rev Neurosci*, 6, 8, (August 2005), pp. 626-640, ISSN 1471-003X

Wallner, M., Hanchar, H.J., Olsen, R.W. (2003). Ethanol enhances alpha 4 beta 3 delta and alpha 6 beta 3 delta gamma-aminobutyric acid type A receptors at low concentrations known to affect humans. *Proc Natl Acad Sci USA*, 100, 25 (December 2003), pp. 15218–15223, ISSN 0027-8424

Wang, J., Carnicella, S., Phamluong, K., Jeanblanc, J., Ronesi, J.A., Chaudhri, N., Janak, P.H., Lovinger, D.M., and Ron, D. (2007). Ethanol induces long-term facilitation of NR2B NMDA receptor activity in the dorsal striatum: implications for alcohol drinking behavior. *J Neurosci*, 27, 13, (March 2007), pp. 3593-3602, ISSN 0270-6474

Weitlauf, C., Egli, R.E., Grueter, B.A., and Winder, D.G. (2004). High-frequency stimulation induces ethanol-sensitive long-term potentiation at glutamatergic synapses in the dorsolateral bed nucleus of the stria terminalis. *J Neurosci*, 24, 25, (June 2004), pp. 5741-5747, ISSN 0270-6474

Weitlauf C., Woodward J.J. (2008). Ethanol selectively attenuates NMDAR-mediated synaptic transmission in the prefrontal cortex. Alcohol Clin Exp Res. (April 2008), 32, 4, pp. 690-698, ISSN 0145-6008

Wirkner, K., Eberts, C., Poelchen, W., Allgaier, C., and Illes, P. (2000). Mechanism of inhibition by ethanol of NMDA and AMPA receptor channel functions in cultured rat cortical neurons. *Naunyn Schmiedebergs Arch Pharmacol*, 362, 6, (December 2000), pp. 568-576, ISSN 0028-1298

Wolffgramm J., Galli G., Thimm F., Heyne A. (2000). Animal models of addiction: models for therapeutic strategies? *J Neural Transm*, 107, 6, (2000), pp. 649-68, ISSN 1435-1463

World Health Organization. (2004). Departamental of Mental Health and Substance abuse. WHO Global Status Report on Alcohol 2004. Geneva. 2004

Wu, P., Coultrap, S., Browning, M., Proctor, W. (2011) Functional Adaptation of the NMDA receptor to acute ethanol inhibition is modulated by striatal-enriched protein tyrosine phosphatase and p38 mitogen activated protein kinase. *Molecular Pharmacology*, 80, 3 (September 2011), pp. 529-37, ISSN 0026-825X

Wu, P.H., Coultrap, S., Browning, M.D., and Proctor, W.R. (2010). Correlated changes in NMDA receptor phosphorylation, functional activity, and sedation by chronic ethanol consumption. *J Neurochem*, 115, 5, (December 2010), pp 1112-1122, ISSN 1471-4159

Wyllie, D. (2008). 2B or 2B and 2D? - That is the question. *J. Physiol*, 586, 3 (February 2008), pp. 693, ISSN 0022-3751

Wyllie, D.J.A., Béhé, P., and Colquhoun, D. (1998). Single-channel activations and concentration jumps: comparison of recombinant NR1a/NR2A and NR1a/NR2D NMDA receptors. *J Physiol*, 510 (July 1998), pp. 1–18, ISSN 0022-3751

Xu, J., Kurup, P., Zhang, Y., Goebel-Goody, S.M., Wu, P.H., Hawasli, A.H., Baum, M.L., Bibb, J.A., and Lombroso, P.J. (2009). Extrasynaptic NMDA receptors couple preferentially to excitotoxicity via calpain-mediated cleavage of STEP. *J Neurosci*, 29, 29, (July 2009), pp. 9330-9343, ISSN 0270-6474

Yaka, R., Phamluong, K., and Ron, D. (2003). Scaffolding of Fyn kinase to the NMDA receptor determines brain region sensitivity to ethanol. *J Neurosci*, 23, 9, (May 2003), pp. 3623-3632, ISSN 0270-6474

Zhou, M., and Baudry, M. (2006), Developmental Changes in NMDA Neurotoxicity Reflect Developmental Changes in Subunit Composition of NMDA Receptors. *J. Neurosci*, 26, 11, (March 2006), pp. 2956-2963, ISSN 0270-6474

7

Role of Multifunctional FADD (Fas-Associated Death Domain) Adaptor in Drug Addiction

Alfredo Ramos-Miguel, María Álvaro-Bartolomé, M. Julia García-Fuster and Jesús A. García-Sevilla
University of the Balearic Islands
Spain

1. Introduction

Human drug addictions are chronic medical disorders characterized by tolerance and dependence to the abused substance, incentive sensitization, loss of control over drug use that becomes compulsive, relapse (Belin & Everitt, 2010), and in some cases high mortality. A large body of research has established that the majority of drugs leading to addiction stimulate dopamine release through the meso-cortico-limbic circuit in laboratory animals and humans (e.g. see Badiani et al., 2011). Brain neuroadaptations along the reward system are a focus of current research, especially those induced in the prefrontal cortex of human addicts (Goldstein & Volkow, 2011). These persistent neuroplastic events appear to be major causes for compulsive drug-seeking behavior despite the negative effects (e.g., neurotoxicity) induced by drugs of abuse in humans (Nutt et al., 2007).

It is generally accepted that some addictive drugs can induce cell death in the human brain, following observations that neurons and astrocytes die when exposed to drugs of abuse (Cunha-Oliveira et al., 2008; Büttner, 2011). Neurotoxicity and neuroplasticity acting together in the addicted brain might explain the dampened cognition and the reinforced behaviors driving to drug consumption. The best-studied cell-killing machinery is the so-called programmed cell death or apoptosis (Galluzzi et al., 2011). *In vivo* studies have reported controversial data for drugs of abuse regulating the apoptotic machinery in the brain (Tegeder & Geisslinger, 2004). Moreover, other findings have revealed important roles of pro-apoptotic proteins in the molecular mechanisms mediating synaptic and structural plasticity in the brain (Gilman & Mattson, 2002). Indeed, proteins belonging to the extrinsic apoptotic pathway have gained special interest in the study of neuroplastic machinery for their functional duality, promoting either apoptosis or cell survival and differentiation (Park et al., 2005; Tourneur and Chiocchia, 2010). Thus, Fas-associated death domain (FADD) protein is the most proximal adaptor molecule that mediates the signaling of death receptors belonging to the tumor necrosis factor receptor superfamily (TNFRSF), such as Fas or TNFRSF6 receptor (Tourneur and Chiocchia, 2010). Although the main role of FADD adaptor is to engage cell death through the extrinsic apoptotic pathway (Galluzzi et al., 2011), it also mediates non-apoptotic actions in cell systems *in vitro* (Park et al., 2005) and has a critical role in embryogenesis (Imtiyaz et al., 2009). In the CNS, Fas receptor dysregulation is associated with a number of disease states, including neurodegenerative disorders (Sharma et al., 2000). Fas stimulation can also promote neurite outgrowth and neuronal branching, which suggests the induction of neuroplastic responses in neurons (Lambert et al., 2003; Reich et al., 2008). Notably, FADD can translocate to the nucleus, a process favoured by its phosphorylation, and regulate nuclear factors, possibly altering the genetic profile of the cell, and promoting differentiation, neuroplasticity, and/or other anti/non-apoptotic actions.

All these features made of FADD an intriguing molecule for the study of brain neurotoxicity and/or neuroplasticity induced by drugs of abuse. This chapter reviews current evidence on the new roles of brain FADD in the complex neurobiology of drug addiction. After a brief overview on Fas/FADD complex and specific features of FADD protein, the involvement of multifunctional FADD and associated signalling in the acute and chronic effects of opiates, cocaine and cannabinoids are summarized from biochemical and behavioral studies performed in rat, mouse and human brains.

2. Relevant features of FADD protein

2.1 Fas/FADD complex: Pro-apoptotic function

In the standard model of Fas-mediated cell death (binding of FasL resulting in receptor trimerization; Algeciras-Schimnich et al., 2002), Fas and FADD are bound through homotypic death domain (DD) interactions (Fas/FADD complex) (Fig. 1A). Then FADD can recruit death effector domain (DED)-containing initiator pro-caspase 8 (and other molecules such as FLIP and PEA-15) to form a death inducing signalling complex (DISC), which finally promotes the activation of death-effector caspases (mainly caspase-3) with the final cleavage of downstream vital cellular substrates. Recently, two models of Fas/FADD-DISC (Scott et al., 2009; Wang et al., 2010) and a likely 5 Fas:5 FADD stoichiometry (Fig. 1A; Wang et al., 2010) have been proposed based on the crystal structures of the proteins. Therefore, FADD

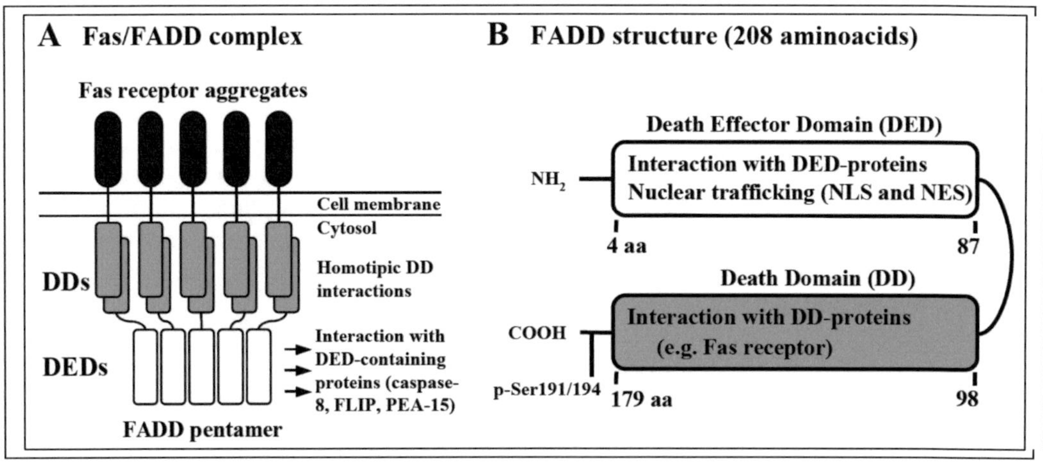

Fig. 1. (A) Fas/FADD-DISC complex. (B) FADD protein structure and domains (DD and DED). NLS: nuclear localization signals; NES: nuclear export signals. FLIP: FADD-like interleukin-1β-converting enzyme-inhibitory protein; PEA-15: phosphoprotein enriched in astrocytes of 15 kDa.

can form functional homo-oligomers of high molecular mass (oligomeric signalling complexes) which have been shown to increase the efficiency of Fas apoptotic signalling in normal and cancer cells (Sandu et al., 2006). Cell death in the CNS shares the same basic mechanisms operating in peripheral cells. Thus, brain apoptosis can be initiated through the extrinsic (Fas receptor) and intrinsic (mitochondrial) pathways, which converge to the activation of executioner caspases (Sastry and Rao, 2000).

2.2 FADD phosphorylation: Nuclear localization and functional implications

The structure of FADD displays, outside its C-terminal DD region (Fig. 1B), a single serine phosphorylation site (p-Ser191 in mouse, p-Ser194 in human; p-Ser194 or p-Ser195 in rat; Zhang et al., 2004; García-Fuster et al., 2008a). This phosphorylation of FADD, mainly mediated by casein kinase 1α (CK1α), is essential for the non-apoptotic actions of this multifunctional protein, such as the regulation of cell growth and differentiation (Alappat et al., 2005).

Although FADD was initially thought to be a cytoplasmic protein, it contains nuclear localization and export signals (NLS/NES; Fig. 1B) that allow its nuclear translocation (Gómez-Angelats and Cidlowski, 2003). Some studies have even reported that FADD is predominantly stored in the nucleus of resting cells, being redistributed to the cytoplasm upon Fas receptor activation (Föger et al., 2009). In any case, p-FADD is the main protein species translocated to the nucleus (Screaton et al., 2003). Nuclear p-FADD is involved in the anti-apoptotic actions of the molecule through the modulation of critical factors (Screaton et al., 2003; Alappat et al., 2005).

2.3 FADD adaptor in the brain: Immunodetection of protein forms and regional distribution

In rat, mouse and human brain tissue, various commercially available antibodies tested against FADD (up to seven) readily immunolabeled a ≈51-kDa band corresponding to its dimeric form (Fig. 2A, left panel). To a lesser extent, these antibodies also reacted against the monomeric (≈20-23 kDa) and other FADD species of higher magnitude (≈92-116 kDa) (García-Fuster et al., 2008a). In contrast, different antibodies against p-FADD recognized 92-116-kDa bands corresponding to oligomeric p-FADD species (Fig. 2A, right panel). Noteworthy, these higher FADD structures fit well with the recently proposed pentameric model of DISC association (see Fig. 1A; Wang et al., 2010). In addition, some of these antibodies immunodetected the monomeric p-FADD species (García-Fuster et al., 2008a; Ramos-Miguel et al., 2009) (Fig. 2A, right panel). The ability of these phospho-directed antibodies to label p-FADD species was challenged with the alkaline phosphatase assay, which demonstrated the specificity of these antibodies to bind to the p-sites of the protein (Fig. 2A, right panel). Therefore, in brain tissue, it is likely that non-p-FADD is more stable as a dimer, and its phosphorylation switches FADD self-associative properties. Thus, these FADD (dimers) and p-FADD (monomers and oligomers) forms were initially selected to assess the role of multifunctional FADD protein in the molecular mechanisms of drug addiction. To note that some p-FADD species (e.g. ≈45 kDa form; Fig. 2A. right) most probably represent degradation products of higher mass p-oligomers. These and other technical issues are largely discussed in previous reports (García-Fuster et al., 2008a).

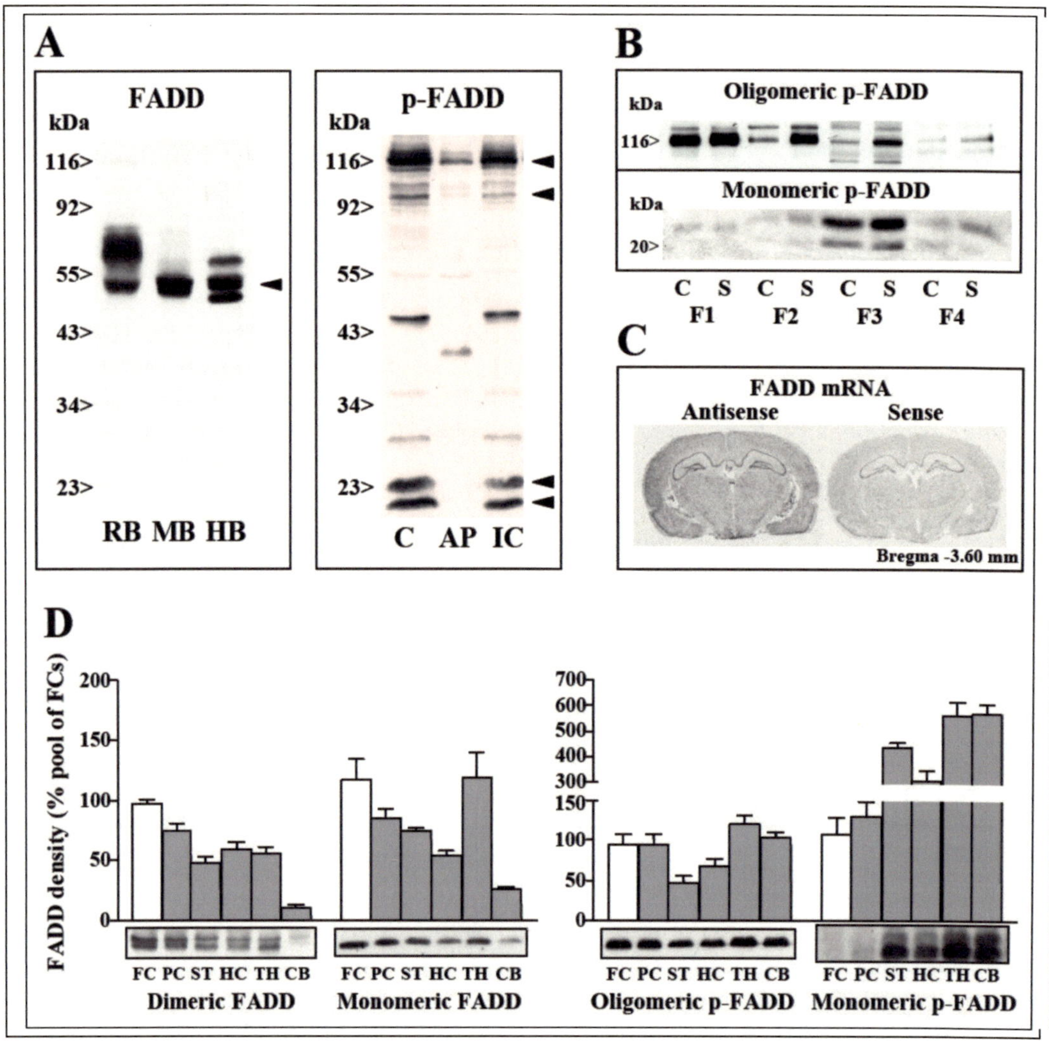

Fig. 2. (A/B) Immunodetection of FADD protein forms (arrow heads: monomeric, dimeric and oligomeric nonphosphorylated and phosphorylated species) in brain total homogenate (RB: rat cortex; MB: mouse cortex; HB: human cortex; C: rat striatum, control sample; AP: alkaline phosphatase; IC: inhibited control, alkaline phosphatase plus sodium pyrophosphate) and subcellular compartments (rat cortex; F1: cytosol; F2: membranes; F3: nucleus; F4: cytoskeleton), in which the acute effect of sufentanil (S: 0.015 mg/kg, s.c., 30 min) on p-FADD is shown (C: control saline). Protein sizes (kDa) as visualized in Western blots. (Modified from García-Fuster et al., 2007a, 2008a). (C) Detection of FADD mRNA in rat brain (anatomical level: Bregma -3.60 mm) by in situ hybridization. Note that FADD mRNA (antisense probe) showed very low expression in the brain, except for hippocampal regions and cortex (see García-Fuster et al., 2009). To verify specificity of binding a sense control probe was hybridized in test tissue. (Modified from García-Fuster et al., 2006). (D) Regional distribution of FADD protein forms in the rat brain (FC: frontal cortex, region of reference; PC: parietal cortex; ST: corpus striatum; HC: hippocampus; TH: thalamus; CB: cerebellum).

FADD is expressed in neurons and glial cells (Hartmann et al., 2002; Bi et al., 2008; Tewari et al., 2008). FADD mRNA expression is homogeneous along the brain tissue, as visualized by *in situ* hybridization (Fig. 2C), with slight increased labeling in cortical areas and hippocampus. However, the distribution of FADD protein (monomeric and dimeric species) in rat brain regions is uneven, with a greater content in the cerebral cortex than in cerebellum (Fig. 2D, left). In contrast, p-FADD (monomeric and oligomeric p-species) is highly expressed in cerebellum (Fig. 2D, right). Thus, the ratio of p-FADD to FADD (monomeric species) was much greater in the cerebellum (CB: 22.4) than in cortical areas (FC: 0.91; PC: 1.58) (Fig. 2D). Subcortical regions also display high p-FADD/FADD ratios (ST: 5.87; HC: 5.61; TH: 4.98) (Fig. 2D). The physiological relevance of the marked variation of p-FADD/FADD ratio across brain regions remains to be determined. To note that FADD and p-FADD are well expressed in brain regions (e.g., the frontal cortex and corpus striatum) more closely associated with the behavioral effects of drug of abuse (Fig. 2D). In the human brain, a dynamic relationship between monomeric and oligomeric p-FADD forms has been observed (Ramos-Miguel et al., 2009). Notably, some opiate and cannabinoid drugs, but not cocaine, have been shown to induce the interconversion between FADD and p-FADD (increasing the ratio p-FADD/FADD), which may favor the induction of non-apoptotic (neuroplastic) actions (see below and Fig. 6).

At the subcelullar level, FADD and p-FADD (rat, mouse and human brains) are expressed in cytosol and nucleus, and to a lesser extent in membranes (García-Fuster et al., 2007a, 2008a; Ramos-Miguel et al., 2009; Álvaro-Bartolomé et al., 2010) (Fig. 2B and 11D). To note that the monomeric form of p-FADD is particularly well expressed in the nucleus (Fig. 2B) (Ramos-Miguel et al., 2009). Nuclear p-FADD has been reported to play important roles in the molecular mechanisms of opiate addiction in humans (Ramos-Miguel et al., 2009), possibly by regulating nuclear factors such as methyl-CpG binding domain protein 4 (Screaton et al., 2003) and nuclear factor kappaB (Schinske et al., 2011).

2.4 FADD adaptor: Apoptotic and non-apoptotic signalling pathways

Besides the role of FADD in the cascades of apoptotic signaling in drug addiction (García-Fuster et al., 2007a, 2008b; Ramos-Miguel et al., 2009; Álvaro-Bartolomé et al., 2011), several pathways have been postulated to link FADD with some forms of behavioral plasticity induced by drugs of abuse, especially heroin/morphine (Ramos-Miguel et al., 2009, 2010, 2011) and cocaine (García-Fuster et al., 2009, 2011; Álvaro-Bartolomé et al., 2011) (Fig. 3).

These signalling pathways involve, *inter alia*, the extracellular signal-regulated kinase (ERK), the kinase Akt1 or protein kinase B (PKB), and phosphoprotein enriched in astrocytes of 15 kDa (PEA-15), which interactions with FADD are discussed below (see section 3.3) in the context of the acute/chronic effects of opiates, cocaine and cannabinoids (Fig. 3).

3. Role of FADD adaptor in opiate addiction

Opiate addiction is associated with various forms of neurotoxicity, which can result in serious brain dysfunction in most subjects (Yücel et al., 2007; Bütnner, 2011). Moreover, heroin addicts often develop severe immunodeficiencies that could be the result of apoptotic cell death in the immune system (Kreek, 1990; Govitrapong et al., 1998). In fact, morphine was reported to increase, through a naloxone-sensitive mechanism, the expression of Fas receptor mRNA in mouse splenocytes and in human blood lymphocytes (Yin et al., 1999). However, the possibility of opiate-induced cell death in the mature brain, including the brains of human addicts, still is a debated issue (Boronat et al., 2001; Tegeder and Geisslinger, 2004; Liao et al., 2005; Cunha-Oliveira et al., 2008; García-Fuster et al., 2008b; Tramullas et al., 2008; Zhang et al., 2008).

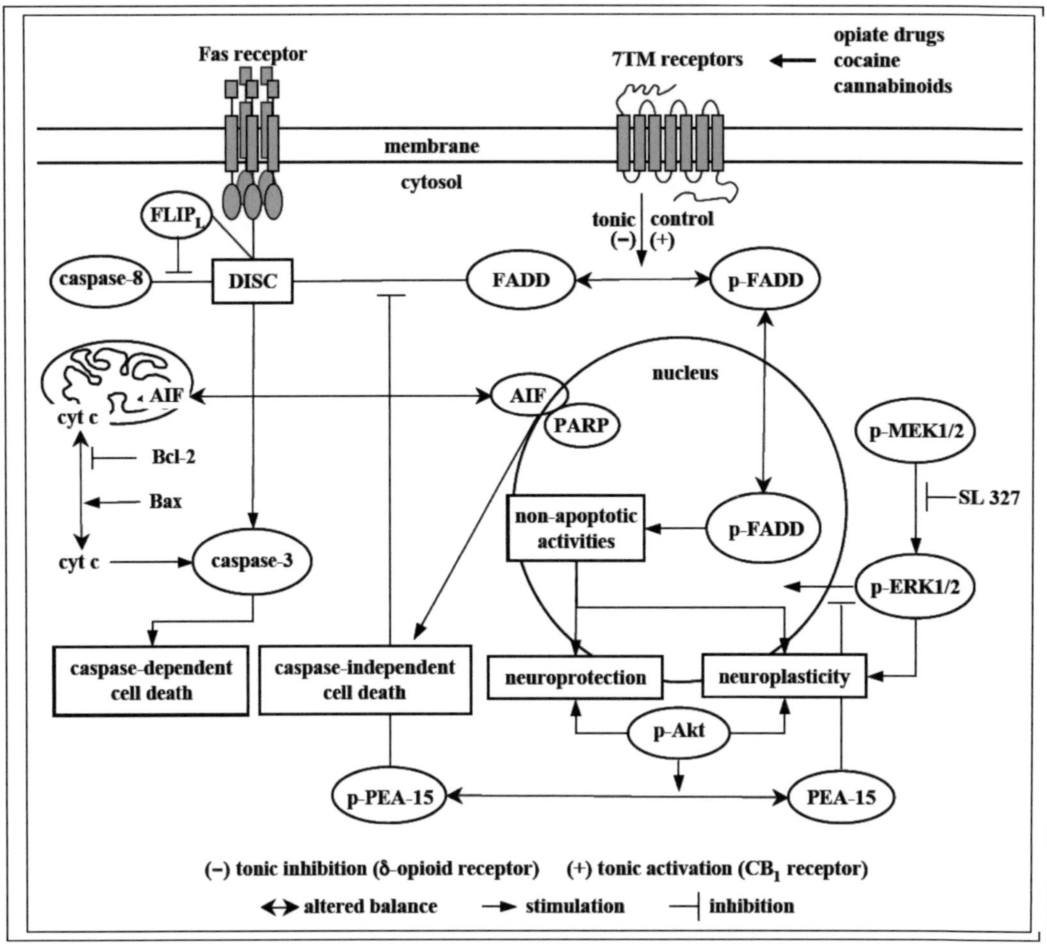

Fig. 3. Schematic diagram illustrating the complex interactions between the multifunctional protein FADD (pro-apoptotic, anti-apoptotic and/or neuroplastic actions) and pro-survival MAP kinases (MEK-ERK) and Akt1/PEA-15 signalling in opiate, cocaine and cannabinoid addiction. See the main text for specific details and comments.

3.1 Regulation of basal Fas/FADD complex by opioid receptors: Anti-apoptotic δ-opioid receptor tone

A relevant interaction between the opioid system and Fas/FADD complex in the brain was disclosed using gene-targeted mice lacking μ-, δ-, or κ-opioid receptors (García-Fuster et al., 2007b). Thus, wild-type (WT) and knock-out (KO) mice were compared to investigate the existence of endogenous opioid tones regulating the basal contents of Fas receptor and FADD adaptor in the brain.

The results indicated that μ- and κ-receptors do not exert a significant tonic control on Fas/FADD complex expression levels in the mouse brain (i.e., no major target changes in μ- and κ-KO mice). In δ-KO mice, however, Fas aggregates (Fas forms triggering receptor signalling) and FADD adaptor were markedly increased in the cortex (Fig. 4) and corpus striatum. Moreover, the basal content of monomeric p-FADD (the FADD species implicated in non-apoptotic signals) was also up-regulated in the cortices of δ-KO mice, which is in line with the observed increase of FADD in these animals (Fig. 4). In this context, it is worth mentioning that inhibitory δ-opioid receptors possess a high level of constitutive (ligand-independent) activity (Costa and Herz, 1989; Neilan et al., 1999), which could control the basal level of some associated signalling molecules such as the Fas/FADD complex.

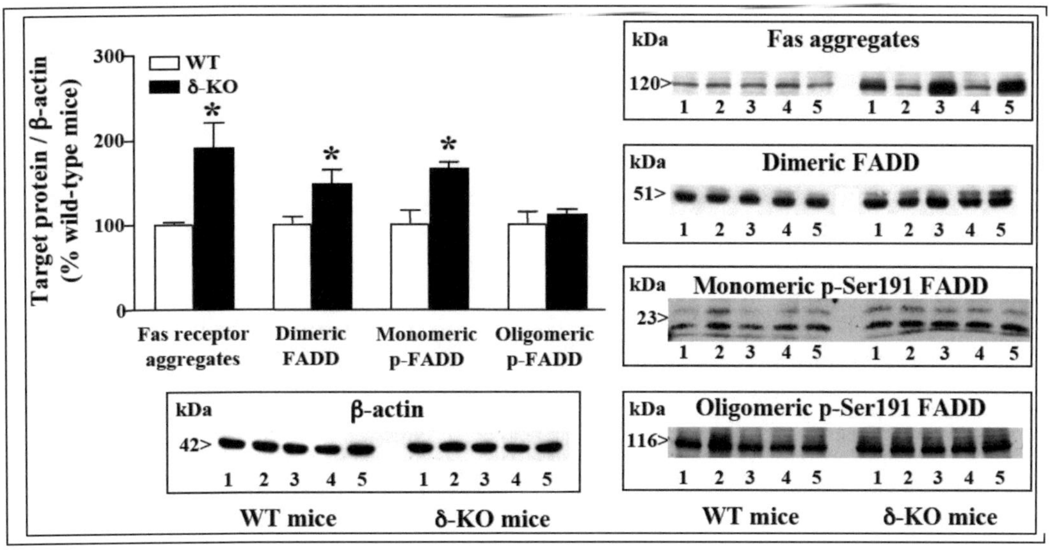

Fig. 4. Fas receptor aggregates, FADD adaptor, and p-FADD (monomeric and oligomeric forms) in the cerebral cortex of WT mice and δ-opioid receptor KO mice. *At least $p<0.05$ *versus* WT. (Modified from García-Fuster et al., 2007b).

Taken together, the findings in δ-KO mice strongly suggest that the functioning of pro-apoptotic Fas/FADD complex *in vivo* is partly under an inhibitory tonic control of brain δ-opioid receptors (i.e., removal of a negative endogenous opioid tone results in Fas/FADD up-regulation; see Fig. 3) (García-Fuster et al., 2007b). The anti-apoptotic δ-opioid receptor tone on Fas/FADD complex could play an important role in the neuroprotection afforded by δ-opioid receptor agonists (Narita et al., 2006).

3.2 Acute, chronic and withdrawal effects of opiate drugs on FADD and associated signalling in the brain

Acute and chronic treatments of rats with various opiate drugs (heroin, morphine, SNC-80, U-50488-H, pentazocine), as well as the induction of opiate withdrawal states, were initially shown to result in increases or decreases of various Fas receptor forms in the brain (Boronat et al., 2001q; García-Fuster et al., 2003, 2004). Thus, heroin/morphine addiction in rats was associated with up-regulation of both native and aggregated forms, thereby suggesting the induction of pro-apoptotic actions in the brain (García-Fuster et al., 2003, 2004). In contrast, similar treatments with morphine and selective μ-(fentanyl, sufentanil), δ-(SNC-80) and κ-(U-50488-H) opioid receptor agonists were associated with receptor-specific reductions of FADD, except for the chronic treatments that show tachyphylaxis to the acute drug effects in the brain (Fig. 5) (García-Fuster et al., 2007a).

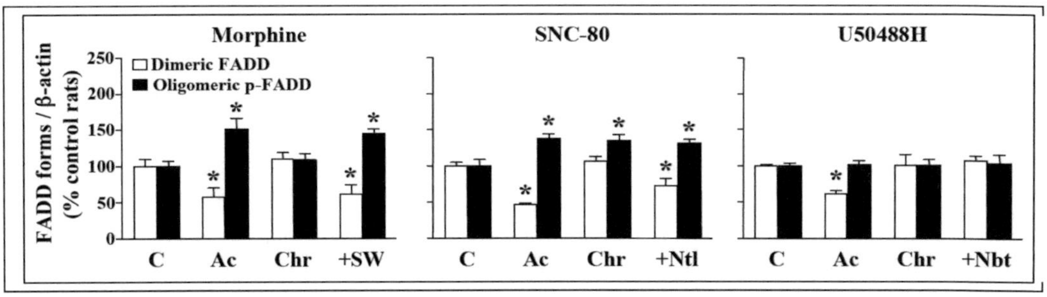

Fig. 5. Acute (Ac), chronic (Chr) and spontaneous (+SW) or antagonist precipitated (naltrindole, Ntl; nor-binaltorphimine, Nbt) withdrawal effects of μ-(morphine), δ-(SNC-80) and κ-(U50488H) opioid receptor agonists on FADD and p-FADD in rat brain cortex. *At least $p<0.05$ *versus* control (C). (Modified from García-Fuster et al., 2007a, 2008a).

As a matter of fact, the modulation of FADD by opiate drugs is opposite to that of Fas receptor, which suggests that possible apoptotic signals engaged by Fas activation would be offset by a lesser signal transduction through FADD adaptor. Indeed, μ/δ-opiate agonists increased the content of p-FADD in the brain (Fig. 5; see also Fig. 2B for the acute effect of sufentanil on p-FADD in subcellular compartments), which suggests the induction of non-apoptotic (neuroplastic) effects by these drugs (see Fig. 3) (García-Fuster et al., 2007a, 2008a). On the other hand, SNC-80-induced down-regulation of FADD in rat brain (cortex and striatum) was blunted after the inhibition of the MEK-ERK pathway *in vivo*, which demonstrates the direct involvement of this anti-apoptotic signalling in FADD regulation (García-Fuster et al., 2007a). On the other hand, the molecular mechanism by which seven transmembrane (7TM) receptors interact with FADD (i.e., G protein dependent or independent process; see Fig. 3) remains to be fully determined (see García-Fuster et al., 2008a).

Remarkably, morphine, sufentanil and SNC-80 (acute, chronic and/or withdrawal effects) up-regulated the content of p-FADD with a concomitant decrease of total FADD in rat brain cortex (Fig. 6A), indicating that these drugs promote an increase in the ratio of p-FADD to FADD (a proposed index of non-apoptotic activity). The inverse relationship between p-FADD and FADD is likely to be due to changes in the phosphorylation status, possibly mediated by CK1α, of the adaptor molecule induced by opiate drugs (García-Fuster et al., 2008a; Ramos-Miguel et al., 2009). These findings support the concept of an interconversion between non-phosphorylated FADD and phosphorylated FADD after exposure to opiate drugs, which appears to be a relevant molecular mechanism in morphine-induced neuroplasticity (see below). A similar inverse correlation between p-FADD and FADD has been observed for the acute effects of the CB_1 receptor agonist WIN55212-2 (Fig. 6B), but not for the psychostimulant cocaine (Fig. 6C).

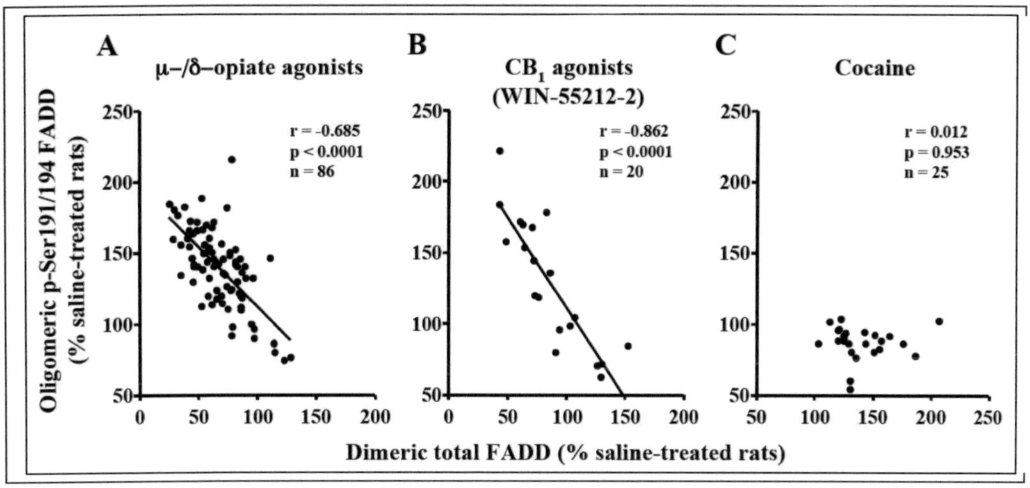

Fig. 6. Inverse correlation between the contents of p-FADD and FADD in rat or mouse brain cortex (each point corresponds to an animal). (A) Opiate agonists: effects of acute (30 and 100 mg/kg) and chronic (10-100 mg/kg; 6 days) morphine, and spontaneous morphine withdrawal (1-3 days); effects of acute sufentanil (15-30 mg/kg); effects of acute SNC-80 (10-30 mg/kg). (B) CB_1 receptor agonist: effects of acute WIN55212-2 (0.5-8 mg/kg). (C) Effects of acute cocaine (3-30 mg/kg). (Modified from García-Fuster et al., 2008a, 2009; Álvaro-Bartolomé et al., 2010).

3.3 FADD phosphorylation correlates with morphine-evoked behaviors

Recent findings have revealed a direct role of p-FADD in the molecular mechanisms leading to the expression of unconditioned morphine-induced psychomotor sensitization (Ramos-Miguel et al., 2010) and to the expression of spontaneous morphine abstinence syndrome (Ramos-Miguel et al., 2011) in rats.

To develop sensitization to morphine (Ramos-Miguel et al., 2010), rats were subjected to a standard treatment protocol (Fig. 7A, left) in which they received saline (controls) or morphine (10 mg/kg/day) for 5 days in absence of environmental cues. After 3 (day 8 of the treatment; Fig. 7A) or 14 days of spontaneous saline/morphine withdrawal (SW3 and SW14, respectively), all rats received a morphine challenge (10 mg/kg) to assess the expression of locomotor sensitization, which was observed at SW3 (Fig. 7A) but not at SW14 (Ramos-Miguel et al., 2010). In parallel to morphine-induced behavioral sensitization, striatal FADD was modulated at SW3, but not at SW14. Thus, p-FADD was up-regulated (Fig. 7A, right) whereas FADD content was decreased (not shown) at SW3. Therefore, the ratio p-FADD/FADD (a postulated marker of neuroplasticity) was increased (2.6-fold) in rat striatum. Similarly, ERK activity was also enhanced in the same striatal samples (Fig. 7A, right). Notably, inhibition of MEK-ERK signalling attenuated the expression of morphine-induced psychomotor sensitization and fully prevented the up-regulation of p-FADD at SW3 (Fig. 7A). The Akt1/PEA-15 pathway, which may link ERK and FADD functions (see Fig. 3), was also activated at SW3, being dependent on the integrity of MEK-ERK signalling (Fig. 7A, right). Taken together, these findings reveal a major role of p-FADD, interacting with MEK/ERK and Akt1/PEA-15, in mediating the short-lasting expression of unconditioned psychomotor sensitization induced by morphine in rats.

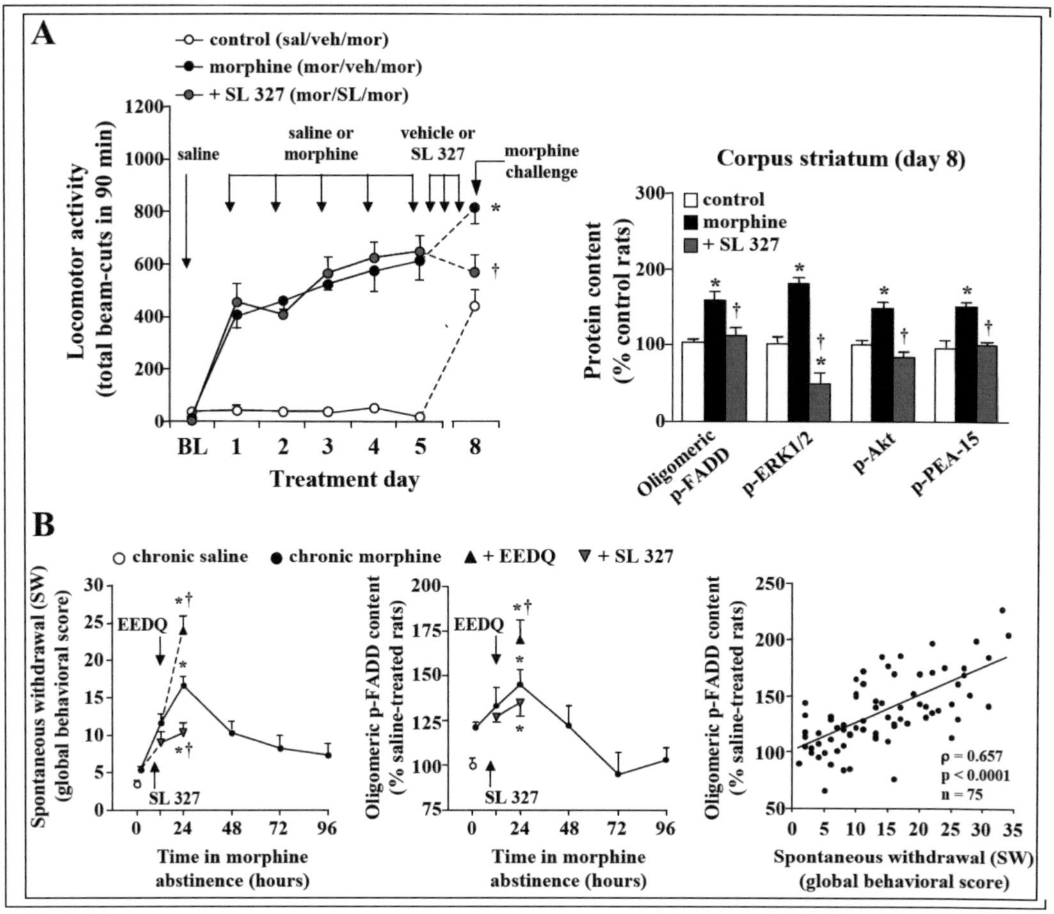

Fig. 7. (A) FADD phosphorylation and expression of unconditioned morphine-induced psychomotor sensitization. Note that day 8 of the treatment corresponds to SW3 (see text). (B) FADD phosphorylation and intensity of spontaneous morphine abstinence syndrome. BL, baseline; SL327, an inhibitor of MEK in vivo; EEDQ, an alkylating of α_2-adrenoceptors. *At least $p<0.05$ *versus* controls, †at least $p<0.05$ *versus* morphine-treated rats. (Modified from Ramos-Miguel et al., 2010, 2011).

To explore the role of FADD in the mechanisms of morphine-induced physical dependence, the regulation of cortical p-FADD was investigated during the development of spontaneous opiate withdrawal (SW) in morphine-dependent rats (10-100 mg/kg for 6 days) (Ramos-Miguel et al., 2011). Notably, cortical p-FADD mirrored the time course of morphine SW (12-96 h; peak at 24 h) (Fig. 7B, left), which resulted in a striking correlation between p-FADD and the intensity of morphine abstinence (Fig. 7B, right). On the other hand, the involvement of α_2-adrenoceptors in opiate addiction is well-known, and the stimulation of these inhibitory receptors induces anti-withdrawal effects in morphine-dependent animals and in human addicts. Interestingly, the inactivation of brain α_2-adrenoceptors (EEDQ at SW12) (Fig. 7B, left) further enhanced morphine abstinence intensity and cortical p-FADD content at SW24 (Fig. 7B, right and middle panels). The disruption of ERK signalling (SL 327 at SW4 and SW8) did not alter morphine abstinence at SW12, but did attenuate the behavioral syndrome at SW24 (Fig. 7B, left). ERK inhibition, however, did not prevent the up-regulation of p-FADD at SW12 and SW24 (Fig. 7B, middle panel). Taken together, these findings reveal that cortical p-FADD, mainly through an interaction with α_2-adrenoceptors, plays a functional role in the behavioral expression of morphine abstinence in rats.

Together, these studies indicate that relevant behavioral adaptations induced by repeated morphine exposure in rats correlate with an increased p-FADD/FADD ratio in the cerebral cortex, which strongly suggests that multifunctional FADD is involved in the complex molecular mechanisms of opiate-induced neuroplasticity.

3.4 Regulation of apoptotic pathways and associated signalling in brains of opiate addicts: p-FADD and neuroplasticity

Recent studies have investigated the role of Fas receptor, FADD adaptor and its phosphorylation, other pro- and anti-apoptotic proteins, and FADD-associated signalling pathways, in postmortem brains of long-term opiate addicts (García-Fuster et al., 2008b; Ramos-Miguel et al., 2009). The prefrontal cortex (Brodmann's area 9, middle frontal gyrus; PFC/BA9) was the region selected for examination because it is directly related with the mesocorticolimbic dopaminergic system and the rewarding and addictive properties of opiates and other drugs of abuse.

First, the hypothesis was tested that human opiate addiction is associated with an increased cell death in the brain (García-Fuster et al., 2008b). In a well-characterized cohort (n=48) of heroin or methadone abusers (including the assessment of opiates and metabolites in blood, urine, and hair samples), the content of Fas receptor in PFC/BA9 did not differ from that in age-, gender-, and postmortem delay-matched controls (Fig. 8A). In contrast, FADD adaptor was down-regulated in the same brain samples of short- and long-term opiate addicts (Fig. 8A). Furthermore, initiator caspase-8 was not altered, but $FLIP_L$ content, a dominant inhibitor of caspase-8, was increased in long-term opiate addicts.

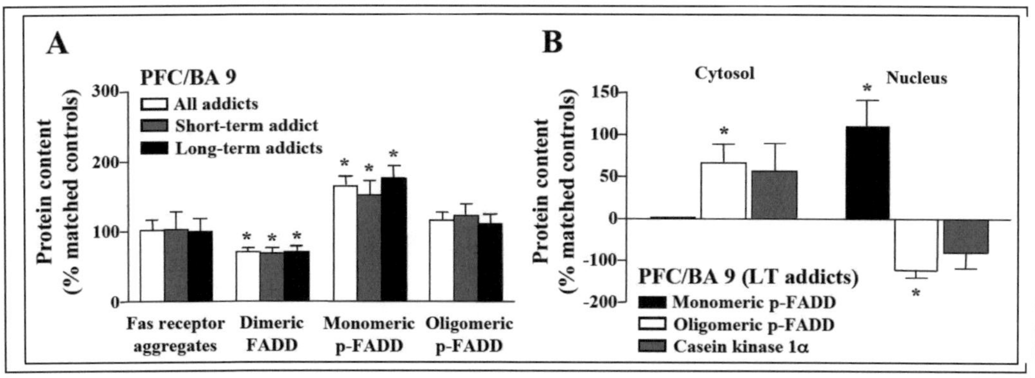

Fig. 8. (A) Contents of Fas receptor aggregates, FADD adaptor, and p-FADD in the prefrontal cortex/Brodmann's area 9 (PFC/BA 9; total homogenate samples) of short- and long-term opiate abusers. (B) Subcellular content (increases or decreases in cytosol and nucleus) of p-FADD and CK1α in the PFC/BA9 of long-term (LT) opiate addicts. *At least $p<0.05$ *versus* matched controls. (Modified from García-Fuster et al., 2008b; Ramos-Miguel et al., 2009).

In the intrinsic mitochondrial pathway, pro-apoptotic Bax and AIF (apoptosis-inducing factor) were unchanged, cytochrome c (a potent caspase-3 activator) was reduced, and anti-apoptotic Bcl-2 augmented in long-term opiate addicts. Importantly, the content of executioner caspase-3/active fragments and the pattern of cleavage of nuclear PARP-1 (poly-(ADP-ribose)-polymerase-1), a hallmark of apoptosis, were very similar in opiate addicts and control subjects.

Taken together, these findings indicate that the molecular machineries of canonical apoptotic pathways are not abnormally activated enough in the PFC/BA9 of opiate abusers to suggest higher rates of cell death in this brain region. Instead, the long-term adaptations of FADD and cytochrome c (down-regulation) and those of $FLIP_L$ and Bcl-2 (up-regulation) could be related to the induction of non-apoptotic actions including phenomena of neuroplasticity in brains of opiate addicts.

Therefore, the role of p-FADD and FADD-associated signalling pathways involved in neuroplasticity was investigated (Ramos-Miguel et al., 2009) in the same cohort and brain region of opiate abusers (García-Fuster et al., 2008b). In these subjects, the content of monomeric, but not oligomeric, p-FADD was markedly increased in the PFC/BA9 of short- and long-term opiate abusers (Fig. 8A, total homogenate samples). At the subcellular level (PFC/BA9), long-term opiate addiction was associated with up-regulation of monomeric p-FADD and down-regulation of oligomeric p-FADD in the nucleus (Fig. 8B). In the cytosol, in contrast, oligomeric p-FADD was increased (Fig. 8B). Along this line, CK1α, the enzyme that mediates p-FADD, was found co-localized with FADD in cytosol and nucleus (Fig. 8B). These findings appear to indicate that FADD is phosphorylated (and oligomerized) in the cytosol of cortical cells (PFC/BA9), and translocates to the nucleus, where it is disaggregated to monomers to develop its nuclear functions (see Fig. 3).

In long-term opiate addicts, on the other hand, marked down-regulation of ERK1/2, JNK1/2 (c-Jun N-terminal Kinase), PEA-15 and Akt1 signalling were observed in the PFC/BA9 (total homogenate and subcellular compartments) (Ferrer-Alcón et al., 2004; Ramos-Miguel et al., 2009). Remarkably, down-regulation of ERK1/2 and Akt1 in the PFC of chronic opiate addicts could also play a major role in the induction of tolerance to opiate reward (Ramos-Miguel et al., 2009). A complex cross-talk between FADD/p-FADD and Akt1/PEA-15 and ERK1/2 signalling would take place in the brain to finally result in the induction of neuroplasticity without an abnormal rate of cell death in the PFC/BA9 of chronic opiate addicts (see Fig. 3).

Taken together, the results of these studies (García-Fuster et al., 2008b; Ramos-Miguel et al., 2009) clearly indicate that opiate addiction in humans is associated with an altered balance between p-FADD (content increased) and FADD (content decreased) in brain, which may favor the neuroplastic actions of FADD adaptor (ratio p-FADD/FADD: a 3.3-fold increase over matched controls). In fact, relevant roles of p-FADD in modulating morphine-induced behavioral plasticity have been demonstrated in the rat brain (see subheading 3.3.).

4. Role of FADD adaptor in cocaine addiction

Cocaine and/or its oxidative metabolites (e.g. norcocaine) can induce various forms of neurotoxicity (Büttner, 2011), including apoptotic effects in both cultured cells (Xiao et al.,

2000; Cunha-Oliveira et al., 2008) and the developing brain (Novikova et al., 2005). However, the aberrant activation of several cell death mechanisms by cocaine, including those mediated by the Fas/FADD complex, in the adult rat brain remains inconclusive (Dietrich et al, 2005; García-Fuster et al., 2009). Nevertheless, self-exposure to cocaine in humans was recently shown to enhance the degradation of a DNA-repairing enzyme in the PFC/BA9 of long-term addicts, which is compatible with the induction of aberrant cell death by the psychostimulant (Álvaro-Bartolomé et al., 2011).

4.1 Acute, chronic and withdrawal effects of cocaine on FADD and associated signalling in the brain

Acute treatments of rats with cocaine (7.5-30 mg/kg) modulated FADD protein forms in brain cortex, increasing the content of FADD and moderately decreasing that of p-FADD with the lower doses (Fig. 9A) (García-Fuster et al., 2009; Álvaro-Bartolomé et al., 2011). In contrast to opiate and cannabinoid drugs, cortical FADD and p-FADD do not correlate after acute cocaine (Fig. 6C), suggesting that psychostimulants favours the expression of pro-apoptotic FADD form (increased). Acute cocaine increased FADD in all subcellular compartments where it was expressed, with the greater effects in the cytosol and nucleus (García-Fuster et al., 2009). Dopamine D_2 receptors were involved in FADD activation by cocaine as pretreatment with raclopride, a D_2-type receptor antagonist, fully prevented the acute cocaine-induced increase of FADD in rat brain cortex (Fig. 9B). Pretreatment with a D_1-type receptor antagonist (SCH-23390) did not block the acute effect of cocaine on FADD (Fig. 9B). In fact, SCH-23390 by itself increased cortical FADD (Fig. 9B), an effect possibly mediated by its agonistic properties at 5-HT1c/2c receptors (García-Fuster et al., 2009).

A non-contingent experimenter-administered regimen of chronic cocaine in rats (15 or 40 mg/kg, for 6-7 days), known to induce behavioral sensitization, induced tachyphylaxis to the acute modulatory effect of the psychostimulant on cortical FADD (Fig. 9C). Cocaine withdrawal (1-7 days) was associated with a transient reduction in cortical FADD, which was significant 3 days after discontinuation of the chronic treatment (Fig. 9C) (García-Fuster et al., 2009; Álvaro-Bartolomé et al., 2011). It is worth noting that there was a positive correlation between FADD protein and the levels of FADD mRNA in rat brain cortex ($r=0.43$; $n=29$; $p<0.05$, see García-Fuster et al., 2009).

Acute cocaine (20 mg/kg) stimulated p-Thr34 DARPP-32 (dopamine- and cAMP-regulated phosphoprotein of 32 kDa) in rat brain cortex, consistent with the engagement of dopamine signalling. Chronic cocaine (40 mg/kg for 6 days) and cocaine withdrawal (3 days), however, were not associated with activation of cortical p-DARPP-32 (tachyphylaxis after the repeated treatment). Interestingly, chronic cocaine and abstinence, but not acute cocaine, increased the content of t-DARPP (a truncated 30 kDa isoform of DARPP-32 with striking anti-apoptotic actions; El-Rifai et al., 2002) in rat brain cortex. Moreover, acute cocaine, but not the chronic/abstinence treatments, stimulated Akt1 in rat brain cortex. Neither treatment with cocaine (acute, chronic, and abstinence) altered the basal stimulation of anti-apoptotic PEA-15 and pro-apoptotic JNK1/2 signaling (Álvaro-Bartolomé et al., 2011).

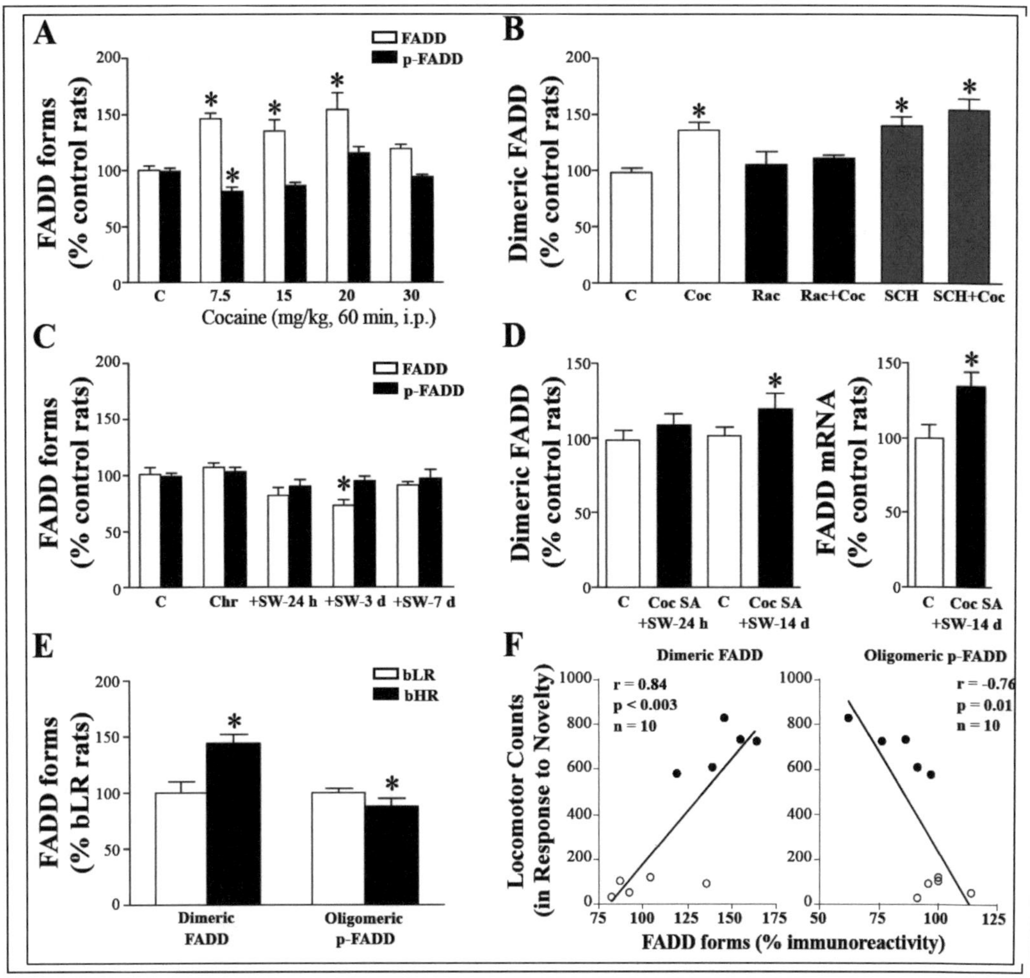

Fig. 9. (A) Acute dose-response effects of cocaine (7.5-30 mg/kg) on FADD and p-FADD in rat brain cortex. (B) FADD is modulated by acute cocaine (Coc, 7.5 mg/kg) through the activation of dopamine D_2 receptors in rat cortex. Rac: raclopride (0.5 mg/kg), SCH: SCH-23390 (0.5 mg/kg). (C) Non-contingent chronic cocaine (Chr, 15 mg/kg for 7 days) and spontaneous withdrawal (+SW) time course effects on cortical FADD and p-FADD. (D) Effects of spontaneous withdrawal (+SW) following contingent cocaine self-administration (Coc SA) on hippocampal FADD protein and mRNA. (E) Basal cortical differences in FADD and p-FADD in bred low-responder (bLR) and high-responder (bHR) rats. (F) Individual differences in locomotor response to novelty correlated (Pearson's r) with basal contents of FADD and p-FADD in rat cortex; non-parametric analysis (Spearman's ρ) also resulted in significant correlations for FADD ($\rho=0.85$; $p<0.003$; n=10) and p-FADD ($\rho=-0.70$; $p<0.05$; n=10) (open circle: bLR rats; closed circles: bHR rats). *At least $p<0.05$ *versus* control (C) or bLR rats. (Modified from García-Fuster et al., 2009, 2011; Álvaro-Bartolomé et al., 2011).

It is unlikely that cocaine-induced up-regulation of pro-apoptotic FADD in rat brain (Fig. 9A) could result in the induction of aberrant cell death. In fact, neither acute and chronic cocaine treatments nor cocaine spontaneous withdrawal altered the content of Fas receptor forms or mitochondrial cytochrome c (a potent caspase-3 activator) and AIF (a mitochondrial mediator of caspase-independent apoptosis) in rat cortex (Álvaro-Bartolomé et al., 2011). Moreover, none of these cocaine treatments altered the pattern of cleavage of nuclear PARP-1 in rat brain cortex (García-Fuster et al., 2009; Álvaro-Bartolomé et al., 2011).

A recent study has examined how a contingent extended daily access to cocaine self-administration impacts the hippocampus at the cellular and molecular levels, and how these alterations can change over the course of cocaine withdrawal (García-Fuster et al., 2011). This animal model has good validity in that it results in the escalation of drug intake (as controlled by the animal, see Ahmed and Koob, 1998) and in cognitive deficits (Briand et al., 2008) similar to those seen in human addicts. Moreover, hippocampal plasticity likely plays an important role in addiction-related behaviors. For example, suppression of hippocampal neurogenesis enhanced resistance to extinction of drug-seeking behavior (Noonan et al., 2010). The results of this study indicated that 5-hour of extended daily access to cocaine for 14 days elicits a profound increase in drug intake from the first self-administration session to the last (García-Fuster et al., 2011), providing a model to study the hippocampal adaptations associated with cocaine withdrawal after abuse of the psychostimulant. This cocaine paradigm led to alterations of hippocampal cell fate regulation (in various hippocampal subregions) during the course of withdrawal (1, 14 and 28 days) with significant changes observed at 14 days (García-Fuster et al., 2011). Notably, FADD adaptor (protein and mRNA; Fig. 9D) was increased in the hippocampus of rats with impaired cell proliferation rates (Ki-67+ mitotic progenitor cells and NeuroD+ neural progenitor cells). The increase in hippocampal FADD (14 days of cocaine withdrawal) did not parallel changes in apoptotic cell death, as measured by cleavage of nuclear PARP-1 (García-Fuster et al., 2011). These data suggest that FADD adaptor is an important hippocampal cell fate regulator during cocaine withdrawal in rats.

4.2 Relevance of FADD in novelty-seeking behaviour and cocaine abuse

Selectively breeding for divergence in locomotor reactivity to a novel environment (bred high-responder (bHR) and low-responder (bLR) lines of Sprague-Dawley rats) has been shown to display reliable differences across multiple behavioural and neurochemical dimensions (Stead et al., 2006). For example, bHR compared to bLR rats have shown an increased behavioural sensitization to cocaine (García-Fuster et al., 2010) and a greater initial propensity to self-administer cocaine (Davis et al., 2008). Interestingly, bHR and bLR rats showed significant basal differences in cortical FADD (higher content in bHR) and p-FADD (lower content in bHR) (Fig. 9E) (García-Fuster et al., 2009). However, bHR/bLR rats showed similar levels of basal nuclear PARP-1 cleavage, indicating similar rates of basal induction of cell death in the cortex (García-Fuster et al., 2009). Moreover, locomotion in a novel environment (bLR *versus* bHR) correlated with the basal content of cortical FADD (positive relation) and p-FADD (inverse relation) (Fig. 9F, n=10). Similarly to the acute, chronic and withdrawal cocaine effects observed in commercially purchased Sprague-Dawley rats (see Fig. 9A/C), the basal differences observed between bHR and bLR rats were maintained post-cocaine (i.e., increased FADD after acute cocaine with a reversal following 3 days of withdrawal) for both phenotypes (García-Fuster et al., 2009). These results suggest that FADD signalling could represent a molecular correlate for the bHR and/or bLR phenotype and therefore the initial propensity to initiate cocaine use (Belin et al., 2008).

4.3 Regulation of apoptotic pathways and associated signalling in brains of cocaine addicts: Increased degradation of nuclear PARP-1

In a recent study (Álvaro-Bartolomé et al., 2011), the hypothesis was tested that cocaine addiction in humans results in abnormal activation of canonical (extrinsic and intrinsic) apoptotic pathways leading to increased cell death in the brain (Fig. 10).

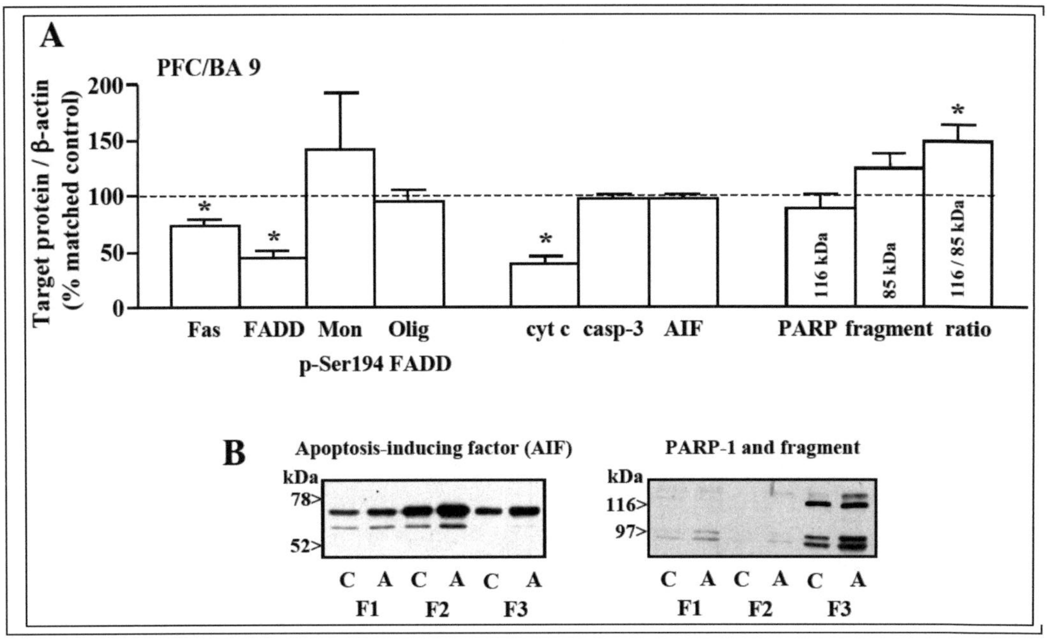

Fig. 10. (A) Contents of apoptotic proteins of the intrinsic (Fas receptor, FADD adaptor and p-FADD) and intrinsic (cytochrome c, caspase-3 and AIF) pathways, as well as the cleavage of nuclear PARP-1 in the prefrontal cortex/Brodmann's area 9 (PFC/BA9; total homogenate samples) of cocaine abusers. (B) Subcellular content of AIF and PARP-1 (F1: cytosol; F2: membranes; F3: nucleus) in the PFC/BA9 of a representative chronic cocaine addict. *At least $p<0.05$ *versus* matched controls. (Modified from Álvaro-Bartolomé et al., 2011).

In a small (n=10) and well-characterized cohort of "pure" cocaine abusers (including the assessment of cocaine and metabolites in blood, urine, and hair samples), Fas aggregates and FADD adaptor were down-regulated in the PFC/BA9 (Fig. 10A), which was associated with a modest increase in p-FADD/FADD ratio. Moreover, mitochondrial cytochrome c was also reduced, but not caspase-3 or AIF (Fig. 10A) (AIF, however, was increased in the nuclear fraction, Fig. 10B). Importantly, the proteolytic cleavage of nuclear PARP-1 (ratio of 85 kDa fragment to 116 kDa PARP-1) was augmented in the same brain samples of cocaine addicts (Fig. 10A), including an increase in the cortical nuclear fraction (Fig. 10B). In chronic cocaine abusers (PFC/BA9), several signalling molecules associated with cocaine/dopamine and/or apoptotic pathways (Akt1, PEA-15, JNK1/2) were found unaltered, with the exception of DARPP-32 and anti-apoptotic t-DARPP whose contents were decreased.

These findings indicate that cocaine addiction in humans is not associated with abnormal upregulation of major components of the extrinsic and intrinsic apoptotic machineries in the

PFC/BA9. On the contrary, the downregulation of Fas–FADD receptor complex and cytochrome c could reflect the induction of contraregulatory adaptations or non-apoptotic (neuroplastic) actions induced by the repeated abuse of the psychostimulant. In any case, the enhanced degradation of nuclear PARP-1 (Fig. 10B), a hallmark of apoptosis, clearly indicates the possibility of aberrant cell death in brains of chronic cocaine addicts. The molecular mechanism appears to involve the induction of oxidative stress by cocaine metabolites (norcocaine and derivatives) and the activation of the mitochondrial death effector AIF after its translocation to the nucleus (Fig. 10B) (Álvaro-Bartolomé et al., 2011), where it interact with PARP-1 and induces chromatin condensation and large-scale DNA fragmentation (Strosznajder et al., 2010). This particular (caspase-independent) cell death subroutine, involving the nuclear interaction of AIF and PARP-1, has been named *parthanatos* and has a role in multiple pathophysiological conditions (Galluzzi et al., 2011), which could include the induction of neurotoxic effects in the brain of human cocaine addicts (see Fig. 3).

5. Role of FADD adaptor in the neurobiology of the cannabinoid system

Among the many effects induced by natural and synthetic cannabinoids (Pertwee, 1997), their beneficial or deleterious actions on neuronal survival remain a controversial topic (Guzmán et al., 2002; Álvaro-Bartolomé et al., 2010). Although cannabinoids can induce pro-apoptotic activity in several cellular models (Maccarrone and Finazzi-Agró, 2003), recent evidence also demonstrates that these compounds, acting through cannabinoid CB_1 (Aguado et al., 2007) or CB_2 receptors (Viscomi et al., 2009) can also protect neurons from death. It is conceivable therefore that the neuroprotection induced by some cannabinoids *in vivo* could be the result of a favorable balance between the relative activation of anti- and pro-apoptotic signalling pathways in the brain.

5.1 Regulation of basal Fas/FADD complex by cannabinoid receptors: Pro-apoptotic CB_1 receptor tone

CB_1 receptors are highly expressed in the CNS (Howlett et al., 2002) and display a high level of constitutive activity (Gifford and Ashby, 1996). This contrasts with brain CB_2 receptors, which pharmacological activation has been questioned in conscious rats (Chin et al., 2008) and, therefore, the presence of any receptor constitutive activity is uncertain. Similarly to δ-opioid receptors (see Fig. 4; García-Fuster et al., 2007b), the remarkable constitutive activity of CB_1 receptors was also postulated to be involved in the tonic control of pro-apoptotic Fas/FADD complex. This possibility was investigated using gene-targeted mice lacking CB_1 or CB_2 receptors (Álvaro-Bartolomé et al., 2010).

In brain regions of CB_1-KO mice (cerebral cortex, corpus striatum and cerebellum), the content of Fas receptor and/or FADD was reduced (Fig. 11A), suggesting that endocannabinoids acting on CB_1 receptors stimulate the expression of pro-apoptotic Fas/FADD complex. In these mice, non-apoptotic p-FADD and p-FADD/FADD ratio are increased (Fig. 11A), indicating that CB_1 receptors tonically inhibit the phosphorylation of brain FADD, which could also favour the induction of pro-apoptotic actions. In brain regions of CB_2-KO mice, in contrast, the changes of Fas receptor, FADD and p-FADD (somehow opposite to those observed in CB_1-KO mice) did not indicate that CB_2 receptors are involved in the tonic regulation of Fas/FADD complex. The alterations of Fas/FADD in brains of CB_1 and CB_2 receptors KO mice did not appear to result in an increased cell death because the pattern of cleavage of nuclear PARP-1 was very similar to that measured in WT mice (Álvaro-Bartolomé et al., 2010).

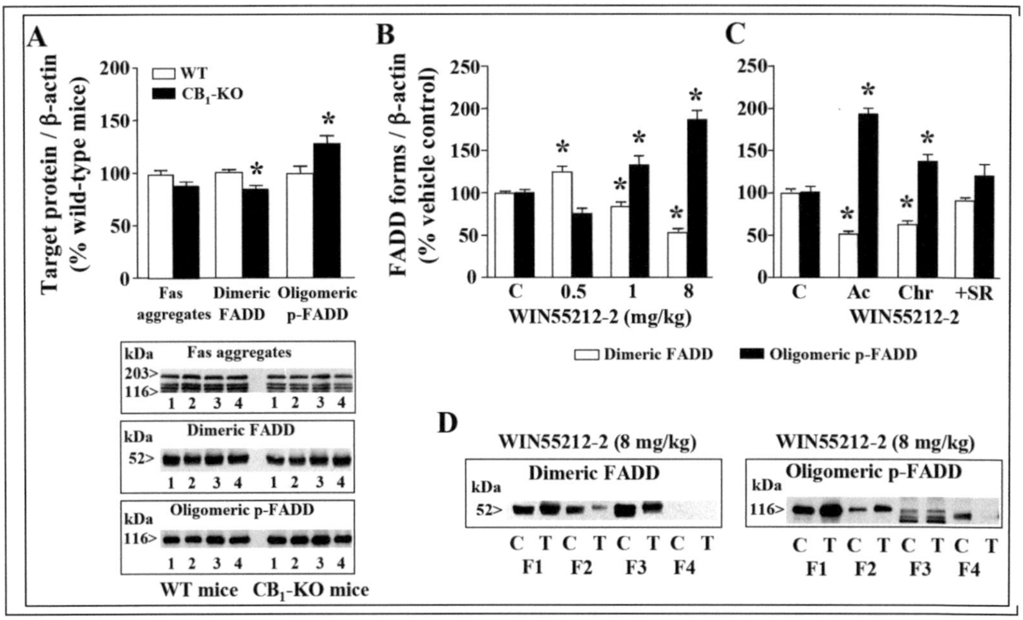

Fig. 11. (A) Fas receptor aggregates, FADD adaptor, and p-FADD in the cerebral cortex of WT mice and cannabinoid CB_1 receptor KO mice. (B) Acute (dose-response) effects of the CB_1 receptor agonist WIN55212-2 on the content of FADD and p-FADD in mouse brain cortex. (C) Acute (Ac, 8 mg/kg), chronic (Chr, 1-8 mg/kg, increasing doses for 5 days) and withdrawal effects (SR, 10 mg/kg; precipitated with the antagonist SR141716A or rimonabant) of WIN55212-2 on FADD and p-FADD content in mouse brain cortex. (D) Effects of WIN55212-2 (8 mg/kg) on the content of FADD and p-FADD at the subcellular level (F1: cytosol; F2: membranes; F3: nucleus; F4: cytoskeleton). *At least $p<0.05$ *versus* WT or control (C). (Modified from Álvaro-Bartolomé et al., 2010).

Therefore, CB_1 receptors appear to exert a tonic activation of Fas/FADD complex in brain (Fig. 11A) that is opposite to that induced by δ-opioid receptors (inhibitory tonic control; Fig. 4). Given the interactions between cannabinoids and opiates (Bushlin et al., 2010), and particularly between CB_1 receptors and δ-opioid receptors (Urigüen et al., 2005), the opposite tonic control of these inhibitory receptors on pro-apoptotic Fas/FADD complex could be of relevance in drug mechanisms leading to neuronal cell death or neuroprotection.

5.2 Acute, chronic and withdrawal effects of cannabinoid drugs on FADD and associated signalling in the brain

Acute treatment of mice with the CB_1 receptor agonist WIN55212-2 (0.5, 1 and 8 mg/kg) did not alter the content of Fas receptor forms in the cerebral cortex. However, a low dose of WIN55212-2 (0.5 mg/kg) increased FADD, whereas higher doses of the agonist (1 and 8 mg/kg) decreased FADD content in mouse brain cortex (Fig. 11B). WIN55212-2 also induced bell-shaped dose effects on p-FADD, but in the opposite direction (Fig. 11B). Pretreatment of mice with the antagonist rimonabant prevented the opposite effects of WIN55212-2 on FADD and p-FADD, indicating a CB_1 receptor-related mechanism. At the subcellular level, WIN55212-2 increased p-FADD in the cytosol and membranes, and to a lesser extent in the nucleus (Fig. 11D right). In contrast, WIN55212-2 decreased FADD in membranes and nucleus, and increased its content in cytosol (Fig. 11D left). WIN55212-2 also increased CK1α in cytosol, which was coincident with the marked enhancement of p-FADD in this compartment (Fig. 11D right). In marked contrast to the activation CB_1 receptors, high doses of the CB_2 receptor agonist JWH133 were not associated with significant changes of Fas receptor forms, FADD or p-FADD in mouse brain cortex (Álvaro-Bartolomé et al., 2010).

These data indicate that the activation of CB_1 receptors decreases (lower dose) or increases (higher doses) the ratio of cortical p-FADD/FADD (an index of non-apoptotic activity). Interestingly, and as observed for opiate drugs, acute WIN55212-2 treatment induced opposite changes on p-FADD and FADD (Fig. 6B), and this interconversion of FADD forms associated with the activation of CB_1 receptors could be important in the actions of cannabinoids in the brain. For example and consistent with the findings observed in the cerebral cortex of CB_1 receptor KO mice (Fig. 11A: decreased FADD and increased p-FADD), a low dose of WIN55212-2 (0.5 mg/kg) increased FADD and decreased p-FADD in mouse brain cortex (Fig. 11B). This opposite regulation of FADD forms is also consistent with the existence of a pro-apoptotic CB_1 receptor tone. However, the selective CB_1 receptor antagonist/inverse agonist rimonabant (10 mg/kg) did not alter FADD or p-FADD in brains of mice, suggesting that the receptor tonic control on this system is moderate (Álvaro-Bartolomé et al., 2010).

It is noteworthy that chronic WIN55212-2 administration (1-8 mg/kg for 5 days) also resulted in down-regulation of FADD and up-regulation of p-FADD in mouse brain cortex (Fig. 11C), which indicates a sustained attenuation of apoptotic signalling in spite of the induction of some tolerance (tachyphylaxis) upon the repeated stimulation of CB_1 receptors. Rimonabant-precipitated WIN55212-2 withdrawal did not cause a rebound of FADD or p-FADD over control values (Fig. 11C). Along this line, the acute and chronic treatments of mice with WIN55212-2, as well as rimonabant-precipitated withdrawal, did not alter the contents of mitochondrial cytochrome c, AIF, or the cleavage of nuclear PARP-1 in the cerebral cortex. These negative findings further discount the induction of cell death after the activation of CB_1 receptors in the mouse brain.

On the other hand, acute, but not chronic, treatment with WIN55212-2 markedly stimulated the activation of anti-apoptotic ERK1/2 and Akt1/PEA-15, as well as pro-apoptotic JNK1/2 and p38 MAPK in the mouse cerebral cortex. This suggests that the acute neuroprotection *in vivo* induced by some cannabinoids could be the result of a favorable balance between the relative activation of anti- and pro-apoptotic signalling pathways. In contrast to FADD and p-FADD, the lack of a sustained stimulation of anti- and pro-apoptotic cascades upon chronic WIN55212-2 treatment probably reflects the rapid induction of CB_1 receptor desensitization in the regulation of these systems (Álvaro-Bartolomé et al., 2010).

The current findings indicate that the chronic stimulation of CB_1 receptors is associated with a marked downregulation of brain FADD, a major pro-apoptotic molecule of the extrinsic cell death pathway. This may represent a relevant molecular mechanism to explain, in part, the neuroprotective effects induced by natural and synthetic cannabinoids (Guzmán et al., 2002). In addition, the chronic stimulation of CB_1 receptors is also associated with up-regulation of p-FADD, the protein form that mediates non-apoptotic actions including brain plasticity (see Fig. 3). The link between CB_1 receptors and the multifunctional FADD adaptor provides new insights into the complex neurobiology of the cannabinoid system.

6. General conclusions

The modulation of FADD adaptor by drugs of abuse is a new and relevant molecular process in the complex neurobiology of addictions. The regulation of FADD and associated signalling by opiate drugs (heroin/methadone) and the psychostimulant cocaine can lead to neurotoxicity and/or neuroplasticity in brains of human addicts. The ratio of p-Ser194 FADD (anti-apoptotic form) to FADD (pro-apoptotic form) appears to represent a novel marker of cortical plasticity.

In the prefrontal cortex of long-term opiate addicts, the observed down-regulation of FADD (i.e. attenuation of Fas signals), the up-regulation of $FLIP_L$ and Bcl-2 (greater anti-apoptotic effects), the increased Bcl-2/Bax ratio (positive balance for cell survival), the reduction of cytochrome c (lesser activation of other pro-apoptotic factors), the lack of abnormal caspase-3 activation, and the normal pattern of nuclear PARP-1 cleavage (Fig. 3) clearly indicate the absence of aberrant cell death. In contrast, p-FADD and p-FADD/FADD ratio are increased in brains of opiate addicts, which suggests the induction of neuroplastic actions. In fact, other studies in laboratory rats have shown that the behavioural response to morphine-induced psychomotor sensitization, as well as the severity of opiate abstinence syndrome (two well-known neuroplastic responses) correlated with increased p-FADD and reduced FADD in the brain, which further supports the role of p-FADD/FADD ratio as a marker of neuronal plasticity.

In the prefrontal cortex of long-term cocaine addicts, Fas/FADD receptor complex and mitochrondrial cytochrome c are down-regulated, suggesting contraregulatory adaptations or non-apoptotic actions (Fig. 3). Importantly, however, the degradation of nuclear PARP-1 is increased in the absence of caspase-3 activation. This type of caspase-independent cell death (named *parthanatos*) involves the induction of oxidative stress by cocaine metabolites (norcocaine and derivatives) and the nuclear translocation of the mitochondrial death effector AIF (Fig. 3). Therefore, cocaine addiction in humans appears to be associated with aberrant cell death in the brain. However, p-FADD/FADD ratio is also increased which also suggest the induction of neuroplastic changes in brains of cocaine addicts. In fact, other studies in laboratory rats have shown that p-FADD and FADD in the cortex represent a molecular correlate of the initial brain plasticity that might predispose to some facets of addictive-like behaviours such as locomotor response to novelty.

7. Acknowledgments

The studies performed in the Laboratory of Neuropharmacology, IUNICS, UIB, were funded by MICINN/MINECO/FEDER (SAF2004-03685, SAF2008-011311, SAF2011-29918),

Plan Nacional Sobre Drogas (2007I061) and RETICS/RTA (RD06/0001/0003) ISCIII-MICINN/MINECO/FEDER, Spain. MJGF is a 'Ramón y Cajal' Researcher (MICINN/MINECO-UIB). JAGS is a member of the Institut d'Estudis Catalans (Barcelona, Catalonia, Spain).

8. References

Aguado, T.; Romero, E.; Monory, K.; Palazuelos, J.; Sendtner, M.; Marsicano, G.; Lutz, B.; Guzmán, M. & Galve-Roperh, I. (2007) The CB1 cannabinoid receptor mediates excitotoxicity-induced neural progenitor proliferation and neurogenesis. *Journal of Biological Chemistry*, Vol.282, No.33, pp. 23892-23898.

Ahmed, S.H. & Koob, G.F. (1998) Transition from moderate to excessive drug intake: change in hedonic set point. *Science*, Vol.282, No.5387, pp. 298-300.

Alappat, E.C.; Feig, C.; Boyerinas, B.; Volkland, J.; Samuels, M.; Murmann, A.E.; Thorburn, A.; Kidd, V.J.; Slaughter, C.A.; Osborn, S.L.; Winoto, A.; Tang, W.J. & Peter, M.E. (2005) Phosphorylation of FADD at serine 194 by CKIα regulates its nonapoptotic activities. *Molecular Cell*, Vol.19, No.3, pp. 321-332.

Algeciras-Schimnich, A.; Shen, L.; Barnhart, B.C.; Murmann, A.E.; Burkhardt, J.K. & Peter, M.E. (2002) Molecular ordering of the initial signaling events of CD95. *Molecular and Cellular Biology*, Vol.22, No.1, pp. 207-220.

Álvaro-Bartolomé, M.; Esteban, S.; García-Gutiérrez, M.S.; Manzanares, J.; Valverde, O. & García-Sevilla, J.A. (2010) Regulation of Fas receptor/Fas-associated protein with death domain apoptotic complex and associated signaling systems by cannabinoid receptors in the mouse brain. *British Journal of Pharmacology*, Vol.160, No.3, pp. 643-656.

Álvaro-Bartolomé, M.; La Harpe, R.; Callado, L.F.; Meana, J.J. & García-Sevilla, J.A. (2011). Molecular adaptations of apoptotic pathways and signaling partners in the cerebral cortex of human cocaine addicts and cocaine-treated rats. *Neuroscience*, Vol.196, No.1, pp.1-15.

Badiani, A.; Belin, D.; Epstein, D.; Calu, D. & Shaham, Y. (2011) Opiate versus psychostimulant addiction: the differences do matter. *Nature Reviews Neuroscience*, Vol.12, No.11, pp. 685-700.

Belin, D.; Mar, A.C.; Dalley, J.W.; Robbins, T.W. & Everitt, B.J. (2008) High impulsivity predicts the switch to compulsive cocaine taking. *Science*, Vol.320, No.5881, pp. 1352-1355.

Belin, D. & Everitt, N.J. (2010) Drug Addiction: The neural and psychological basis of a compulsive incentive habit. In Handbook of Basal Ganglia Structure and Function (Eds. H. Steiner & K. Tseng). New York, Academic Press. Chapter 33, pp. 571-592.

Bi, F.F.; Xiao, B.; Hu, Y.Q.; Tian, F.F.; Wu, Z.G.; Ding, L. & Zhou X.F. (2008) Expression and localization of Fas-associated proteins following focal cerebral ischemia in rats. *Brain Research*, Vol.1191, pp. 30-38.

Boronat, M.A.; García-Fuster, M.J. & García-Sevilla, J.A. (2001) Chronic morphine induces up-regulation of the pro-apoptotic Fas receptor and down-regulation of the anti-apoptotic Bcl-2 oncoprotein in rat brain. *British Journal of Pharmacology*, Vol.134, No.6, pp. 1263-1270.

Briand, L.A.; Flagel, S.B.; García-Fuster, M.J.; Watson, S. J.; Akil, H.; Sarter, M.; Robinson, T.E. (2008) Persistent alterations in cognitive function and prefrontal dopamine D2 receptors following extended, but not limited, access to self-administered cocaine. *Neuropsychopharmacology*, Vol.33, No.12, pp. 2969-2980.

Bushlin, I.; Rozenfeld, R.; Devi, L.A. (2010) Cannabinoid-opioid interactions during neuropathic pain and analgesia. *Current Opinion in Pharmacology*, Vol.10, No.8, pp. 80-86.

Büttner, A. (2011) Review: The neuropathology of drug abuse. *Neuropathology and Applied Neurobiology*, Vol.37, No.2, pp. 118-134.

Chin, C.L.; Tovcimak, A.E.; Hradil, V.P.; Seifert, T.R.; Hollingsworth, P.R.; Chandran, P. et al. (2008) Differential effects of cannabinoid receptor agonists on regional brain activity using pharmacological MRI. *British Journal of Pharmacology*, Vol.153, No.2, pp. 367-379.

Costa, T. & Herz, A. (1989) Antagonists with negative intrinsic activity at delta opioid receptors coupled to GTP-binding proteins. *Proceedings of the National Academy of Sciences of the United States of America*, Vol.86, No.19, pp. 7321-7325.

Cunha-Oliveira, T.; Rego A.C. & Oliveira, C.R. (2008) Cellular and molecular mechanisms involved in the neurotoxicity of opioid and psychostimulant drugs. *Brain Research Reviews*, Vol.58, No.1, pp.192-208.

Davis, B.A.; Clinton, S.M.; Akil, H.; Becker, J.B. (2008) The effects of novelty-seeking phenotypes and sex differences on acquisition of cocaine self-administration in selectively bred high-responder and low-responder rats. *Pharmacology, Biochemistry and Behavior*, Vol.90, No.3, pp. 331-338.

Dietrich, J.B.; Mangeol, A.; Revel, M.O.; Burgun, C.; Aunis, D. & Zwiller, J. (2005) Acute or repeated cocaine administration generates reactive oxygen species and induces antioxidant enzyme activity in dopaminergic rat brain structures. *Neuropharmacology*, Vol.48, No.7, pp. 965-974.

El-Rifai, W.; Smith, M.F. Jr.; Li, G.; Beckler, A.; Carl, V.S.; Montgomery, E.; Knuutila, S.; Moskaluk, C.A.; Frierson, H.F. Jr.; Powell, S.M. (2002) Gastric cancers overexpress DARPP-32 and a novel isoform, t-DARPP. *Cancer Research*, Vol.62, No.14, pp. 4061-4064.

Ferrer-Alcón, M.; García-Fuster, M.J.; La Harpe, R. & García-Sevilla, J.A. (2004) Long-term regulation of signalling components of adenylyl cyclase and mitogen-activated protein kinase in the pre-frontal cortex of human opiate addicts. *Journal of Neurochemistry*, Vol.90, No.1, pp. 220-230.

Föger, N.; Bulfone-Paus S.; Chan, A.C. & Lee, K.H. (2009) Subcellular compartmentalization of FADD as a new level of regulation in death receptor signaling. *The FEBS Journal*, Vol.276, No.15, pp. 4256-4265.

Galluzzi, L.; Vitali, I.; Abrams, J.M.; Alnemri, E.S.; Baehrecke, E.H.; Blagosklonny, M.V.; et al. (2011) Molecular definitions of cell death subroutines: recommendations of the Nomenclature Committee on Cell Death 2012. *Cell Death & Differentiation*, in press. doi: 10.1038/cdd.2011.96.

García-Fuster, M.J.; Ferrer-Alcón, M.; Miralles, A. & García-Sevilla, J.A. (2003) Modulation of Fas receptor proteins and dynamin during opiate addiction and induction of opiate withdrawal in rat brain. *Naunyn-Schmiedeberg's Archives of Pharmacology*, Vol.368, No.5, pp. 421-431.

García-Fuster, M.J.; Ferrer-Alcón, M.; Miralles, A. & García-Sevilla, J.A. (2004) Deglycosylation of Fas receptor and chronic morphine treatment up-regulate high molecular mass Fas aggregates in the rat brain. *European Journal of Pharmacology*, Vol.496, No.1-3, pp. 63-69.

García-Fuster, M.J.; Watson, S.J. & Akil, H. (2006). Effect of cocaine on Fas-Associated protein with Death Domain (FADD) in the rat brain. *Society for Neuroscience Annual Meeting*. Poster 294.19. Atlanta, USA.

García-Fuster, M.J.; Miralles, A. & García-Sevilla, J.A. (2007a) Effects of opiate drugs on Fas-associated protein with death domain (FADD) and effector caspases in the rat brain: Regulation by the ERK1/2 MAP kinase pathway. *Neuropsychopharmacology*, Vol.32, No.2, pp. 399-411.

García-Fuster, M.J.; Ferrer-Alcón, M.; Martín, M.; Kieffer, B.L.; Maldonado, R. & García-Sevilla, J.A. (2007b) Effects of constitutive deletion of opioid receptors on the basal densities of Fas and Fas-associated protein with death domain (FADD) in the mouse brain: A δ-opioid tone inhibits FADD. *European Neuropsychopharmacology*, Vol.17, No.5, pp. 366-374.

García-Fuster, M.J.; Ramos-Miguel, A.; Miralles, A. & García-Sevilla, J.A. (2008a) Opioid receptor agonists enhance the phosphorylation state of Fas-associated death domain (FADD) protein in the rat brain: Functional interactions with casein kinase Iα, $G\alpha_i$ proteins, and ERK1/2 signaling. *Neuropharmacology*, Vol.55, No.5, pp. 886-99.

García-Fuster, M.J.; Ramos-Miguel, A.; Rivero, G.; La Harpe, R.; Meana, J.J. & García-Sevilla, J.A. (2008b) Regulation of the extrinsic and intrinsic apoptotic pathways in the prefrontal cortex of short- and long-term human opiate abusers. *Neuroscience*, Vol.157, No.1, pp. 105-119.

García-Fuster, M.J.; Clinton, S.M.; Watson, S.J. & Akil, H. (2009) Effect of cocaine on Fas-associated protein with death domain in the rat brain: Individual differences in a model of differential vulnerability to drug abuse. *Neuropsychopharmacology*, Vol.34, No.5, pp. 1123-1134.

García-Fuster, M.J.; Perez, J.A.; Clinton, S.M.; Watson, S.J. & Akil, H. (2010) Impact of cocaine on adult hippocampal neurogenesis in an animal model of differential propensity to drug abuse. *European Journal of Neuroscience*, Vol.31, No.1, pp. 79-89.

García-Fuster, M.J.; Flagel, S.B.; Mahmood, S.T.; Mayo, L.M.; Thompson, R.C.; Watson, S.J. & Akil, H. (2011). Decreased proliferation of adult hippocampal stem cells during cocaine withdrawal: Possible role of the cell fate regulator FADD. *Neuropsychopharmacology*, Vol.36, No.11, pp. 2303-2317.

Gifford, A.N. & Ashby, C.R. Jr. (1996) Electrically evoked acetylcholine release from hippocampal slices is inhibited by the cannabinoid receptor agonist, WIN 55212-2, and is potentiated by the cannabinoid antagonist, SR 141716A. *Journal of Pharmacology and Experimental Therapeutics*, Vol.277, No.3, pp. 431-436.

Gilman, C.P. & Mattson, M.P. (2002) Do apoptotic mechanisms regulate synaptic plasticity and growth-cone motility? *Neuromolecular Medicine*, Vol.2, No.2, pp. 197-214.

Goldstein, R.Z. & Volkow, N.D. (2011) Dysfunction of the prefrontal cortex in addiction: neuroimaging findings and clinical implications. *Nature Reviews Neuroscience*, Vol.12, No.11, pp. 652-669.

Gómez-Angelats, M. & Cidlowski, J.A. (2003) Molecular evidence for the nuclear localization of FADD. *Cell Death & Differentiation*, Vol.10, No.7, pp. 91-97.

Govitrapong, P.; Suttitum, T.; Kotchabhakdi, N. & Uneklabh, T. (1998) Alterations of immune functions in heroin addicts and heroin withdrawal subjects. *Journal of Pharmacology and Experimental Therapeutics*, Vol.286, No.2, pp. 883-889.

Guzmán, M.; Sánchez, C. & Galve-Roperh, I. (2002) Cannabinoids and cell fate. *Pharmacology and Therapeutics*, Vol.95, No.2, pp. 175-184.

Hartmann, A.; Mouatt-Prigent, A.; Faucheux, B.A.; Agid, Y. & Hirsch, E.C. (2002) FADD: A link between TNF family receptors and caspases in Parkinson's disease. *Neurology*, Vol.58, No.2, pp. 308-310.

Howlett, A.C.; Barth, F.; Bonner, T.I.; Cabral, G.; Casellas, P; Devane, W.A.; Felder, C.C.; Herkenham, M.; Mackie, K.; Martin, B.R.; Mechoulam, R. & Pertwee, R.G. (2002) International Union of Pharmacology. XXVII. Classification of cannabinoid receptors. *Pharmacological Reviews*, Vol.54, No.2, pp. 161-202.

Imtiyaz, H.Z.; Zhou, X.; Zhang, H.; Chen, D.; Hu, T. & Zhang, J. (2009) The death domain of FADD is essential for embryogenesis, lymphocyte development, and proliferation. *Journal of Biological Chemistry*, Vol.284, No.15, pp. 9917-9926.

Kreek, M.J. (1990) Immune function in heroin addicts and former heroin addicts in treatment: pre- and post-AIDS epidemic. *NIDA Research Monographs*, Vol. 96, pp.192-219.

Lambert, C.; Landau, A.M. & Desbarats, J. (2003) Fas-beyond death: a regenerative role for Fas in the nervous system. *Apoptosis*, Vol.8, No.6, pp. 551-562.

Liao, D.; Lin, H.; Law, P.Y. & Loh, H.H. (2005) Mu-opioid receptors modulate the stability of dendritic spines. *Proceedings of the National Academy of Sciences of the United States of America*, Vol.102, No.5, pp. 1725-1730.

Maccarrone, M. & Finazzi-Agrò, A. (2003) The endocannabinoid system, anandamide and the regulation of mammalian cell apoptosis. *Cell Death & Differentiation*, Vol.10, No.9, pp. 946-955.

Narita, M.; Kuzumaki, N.; Miyatake, M.; Sato, F.; Wachi, H.; Seyama, Y. & Suzuki, T. (2006) Role of δ-opioid receptor function in neurogenesis and neuroprotection. *Journal of Neurochemistry*, Vol.97, No.5, pp. 1494-1505.

Neilan, C.L.; Akil, H.; Woods, J.H. & Traynor, J.R. (1999) Constitutive activity of the δ-opioid receptor expressed in C6 glioma cells: identification of non-peptide δ-inverse agonists. *British Journal of Pharmacology*, Vol.128, No.3, pp. 556-562.

Noonan, M.A.; Bulin, S.E.; Fuller, D.C. & Eisch, A.J. (2010) Reduction of adult hippocampal neurogenesis confers vulnerability in an animal model of cocaine addiction. *Journal of Neuroscience*, Vol.30, No.1, pp. 304-315.

Novikova, S.I.; He, F.; Bai, J.; Badan, I.; Lidow, I.A. & Lidow, M.S. (2005) Cocaine-induced changes in the expression of apoptosis-related genes in the fetal mouse cerebral wall. *Neurotoxicology & Teratology*, Vol.27, No.1, pp. 3-14.

Nutt, D.; King, L.A.; Saulsbury, W.; Blakemore, G. (2007) Development of a rational scale to assess the harm of drugs of potential misuse. *Lancet*, Vol. 369, No.9566, pp. 1047-1053.

Park, S.M.; Schickel, R. & Peter, M.E. (2005) Nonapoptotic functions of FADD-binding death receptors and their signaling molecules. *Current Opinion in Cell Biology*, Vol.17, No.6, pp. 610-616.

Pertwee, R.G. (1997) Pharmacology of cannabinoid CB_1 and CB_2 receptors. *Pharmacology & Therapeutics*, Vol.74, No.2, pp. 129-180.

Ramos-Miguel A.; García-Fuster, M.J.; Callado, L.F.; La Harpe, R.; Meana, J.J. & García-Sevilla, J.A. (2009) Phosphorylation of FADD (Fas-associated death domain protein) at serine 194 is increased in the prefrontal cortex of opiate abusers: Relation to mitogen activated protein kinase, phosphoprotein enriched in astrocytes of 15 kDa, and Akt signaling pathways involved in neuroplasticity. *Neuroscience*, Vol.161, No.1, pp. 23-38.

Ramos-Miguel, A.; Esteban, S. & García-Sevilla, J.A. (2010) The time course of unconditioned morphine-induced psychomotor sensitization mirrors the phosphorylation of FADD and MEK/ERK in rat striatum: Role of PEA-15 as a FADD-ERK binding partner in striatal plasticity. *European Neuropsychopharmacology*, Vol.20, No.1, pp. 49-64.

Ramos-Miguel, A.; Miralles, A. & García-Sevilla, J.A. (2011) Correlation of rat cortical Fas-associated death domain (FADD) protein phosphorylation with the severity of spontaneous morphine abstinence syndrome: Role of α_2-adrenoceptors and extracellular signal-regulated kinases. *Journal of Psychopharmacology*, Vol.25, No.12, pp. 1691-1702.

Reich, A.; Spering, C. & Schulz, J.B. (2008) Death receptor Fas (CD95) signaling in the central nervous system: tuning neuroplasticity? *Trends in Neuroscience*, Vol.31, No.9, pp. 478-486.

Sandu, C.; Morisawa, G.; Wegorzewska, I.; Huang, T.; Arechiga, A.F.; Hill, J.M.; Kim, T.; Walsh, C.M. & Werner, M.H. (2006) FADD self-association is required for stable interaction with an activated death receptor. *Cell Death & Differentiation*, Vol.13, No.12, pp. 2052-2061.

Sastry, P.S. & Rao, K.S. (2000) Apoptosis and the nervous system. *Journal of Neurochemistry*, Vol.74, No.1, pp. 1-20.

Scott, F.L.; Stec, B.; Pop, C.; Dobaczewska, M.K.; Lee, J.J.; Monosov, E.; Robinson, H.; Salvesen, G.S.; Schwarzenbacher, R. & Riedl, S.J. (2009) The Fas-FADD death domain complex structure unravels signalling by receptor clustering. *Nature*, Vol.457, No.7232, pp. 1019-1022.

Screaton, R.A.; Kiessling, S.; Sansom, O.J.; Millar, C.B.; Maddison, K.; Bird, A.; Clarke, A.R. & Frisch, S.M. (2003) Fas-associated death domain protein interacts with methyl-CpG binding domain protein 4: a potential link between genome surveillance and apoptosis. *Proceedings of the National Academy of Sciences of the United States of America*, Vol.100, No.9, pp. 5211-5216.

Sharma, K.; Wang, R.X.; Zhang, L.Y.; Yin, D.L.; Luo, X.Y.; Solomon, J.C.; Jiang, R.F.; Markos, K.; Davidson, W.; Scott, D.W. & Shi, Y.F. (2000) Death the Fas way: regulation and pathophysiology of CD95 and its ligand. *Pharmacology & Therapeutics*, Vol.88, No.3, pp. 333-347.

Stead, J.D.; Clinton, S.; Neal, C.; Schneider, J.; Jama, A.; Miller, S.; Vazquez, D.M.; Watson, S.J. & Akil, H. (2006) Selective breeding for divergence in novelty-seeking traits: heritability and enrichment in spontaneous anxiety-related behaviors. *Behavior Genetics*, Vol.36, No.5, pp. 697-712.

Strosznajder, R.P.; Czubowicz, K.; Jesko, H. & Strosznajder, J.B. (2010) Poly(ADP-ribose) metabolism in brain and its role in ischemia pathology. *Molecular Neurobiology*, Vol.41, No.2-3, pp. 187-196.

Tegeder, I. & Geisslinger, G. (2004) Opioids as modulators of cell death and survival--unraveling mechanisms and revealing new indications. *Pharmacological Reviews*, Vol.56, No.3, pp. 351-369.

Tewari, R.; Sharma, V.; Koul, N. & Sen, E. (2008) Involvement of miltefosine-mediated ERK activation in glioma cell apoptosis through Fas regulation. *Journal of Neurochemistry*, Vol.107, No.3, pp. 616-627.

Tourneur, L. & Chiocchia, G. (2010) FADD: a regulator of life and death. *Trends in Immunology*, Vol.31, No.7, pp. 260-269.

Tramullas, M.; Martínez-Cué, C. & Hurlé, M.A. (2008) Chronic administration of heroin to mice produces up-regulation of brain apoptosis-related proteins and impairs spatial learning and memory. *Neuropharmacology*, Vol.54, No.4, pp. 640-652.

Urigüen, L.; Berrendero, F.; Ledent, C.; Maldonado, R. & Manzanares, J. (2005) Kappa- and delta-opioid receptor functional activities are increased in the caudate putamen of cannabinoid CB1 receptor knockout mice. *European Journal of Neuroscience*, Vol.22, No.8, pp.2106-1210.

Viscomi, M.T.; Oddi, S.; Latini, L.; Pasquariello, N.; Florenzano, F.; Bernardi, G.; Molinari, M. & Maccarrone, M. (2009) Selective CB_2 receptor agonism protects central neurons from remote axotomy-induced apoptosis through the PI3K/Akt pathway. *Journal of Neuroscience*, Vol.29, No.14, pp. 4564-4570.

Wang, L.; Yang, J.K.; Kabaleeswaran, V.; Rice, A.J.; Cruz, A.C.; Park, A.Y.; Yin, Q.; Damko, E.; Jang, S.B.; Raunser, S.; Robinson, C.V.; Siegel, R.M.; Walz, T. & Wu, H. (2010) The Fas-FADD death domain complex structure reveals the basis of DISC assembly and disease mutations. *Nature Structural & Molecular Biology*, Vol.17, No.11, pp. 1324-1329.

Xiao, Y.; He, J.H.; Gilbert, R.D. & Zhang, L. (2000). Cocaine induces apoptosis in fetal myocardial cells through a mitochondria-dependent pathway. *Journal of Pharmacology and Experimental Therapeutics*, Vol.292, No.1, pp. 8-14.

Yin, D.; Mufson, R.A.; Wang, R. & Shi Y. (1999). Fas-mediated cell death promoted by opioids. *Nature*, Vol.397, No.6716, p. 218.

Yücel, M.; Lubman, D.I.; Harrison, B.J.; Fornito, A.; Allen, N.B.; Wellard, R.M.; Roffel, K.; Clarke, K.; Wood, S.J.; Forman, S.D. & Pantelis, C. (2007) A combined spectroscopic and functional MRI investigation of the dorsal anterior cingulate region in opiate addiction. *Molecular Psychiatry*, Vol.12, No.7, pp. 691-702.

Zhang, J.; Zhang, D. & Hua, Z. (2004) FADD and its phosphorylation. *IUBMB Life*, Vol.56, No.7, pp. 395-401.

Zhang, Y.; Chen, Q. & Yu, L.C. (2008) Morphine: a protective or destructive role in neurons? *Neuroscientist*, Vol.14, No.6, pp. 561-570.

8

Polydrug Use in Adolescence

Marta Rodríguez-Arias and María Asunción Aguilar
University of Valencia
Spain

1. Introduction

1.1 Drug and polydrug use among adolescents

The 2010 Monitoring the Future survey conducted by the US government raises concerns about an increase in drug use among teenagers, particularly those of a younger age. A similar trend has been reflected by European surveys, such as the 2010 Annual report on the state of the drugs problem in Europe, EMCDDA. According to this study, commissioned by the European Council, the use of multiple substances – polydrug use – is widespread and represents a major challenge. A recent survey by the Spanish government (EDADES 2009/2010) revealed that approximately 50% of drug users consumed two or more substances simultaneously. The objective of users is to increase or reverse the effects of the different drugs taken, but greater health risks and problems and a poor treatment response are also inherent in polydrug consumption. Almost all patterns of polydrug use include alcohol, and the use of amphetamines or ecstasy among frequent or heavy alcohol consumers is much higher than the average. A study by the Spanish government (Encuesta Estatal sobre uso de drogas en estudiantes de enseñanzas secundarias, ESTUDES, 2008) revealed that Spanish students between 14-18 years old who used drugs generally consumed more than one drug at the same time. 96.2% of students who had taken ecstasy in the previous year had simultaneously consumed alcohol and 86.1% had simultaneously consumed cannabis. An association between consumption of stimulants and hallucinogen drugs was also reported. For example, among students who had used ecstasy in the previous year, 71.4% had also consumed cocaine, while 38.5% of those who had used cocaine in the same period had also consumed ecstasy.

2. The adolescent brain

Adolescence is the period of gradual physiological, cognitive, behavioural and psychosocial transition from childhood to adulthood (Pickles et al., 1998) during which individuals experience physical changes, new interests, greater independence and heightened responsibility. Since adolescence is a process, it is difficult to characterize its ontogenetic time course, and no single event signals its onset or termination. In humans, adolescence is often considered to begin with the onset of the biological changes associated with puberty (the period during which an individual becomes sexually mature), although the timing of puberty within the adolescent period varies notably among humans. Adolescence ends when the individual assumes adult social roles, with a change in the sleep pattern having been proposed as a physiological marker of its termination (Abbott, 2005). The adolescent age span in humans is commonly considered to be from 12 to 18 years, although the entire second decade is sometimes considered adolescence, with up to 25 years being considered late adolescence (Baumrind, 1987).

Adolescent subjects exhibit certain characteristic behaviours (some of which are common among adolescents across species), including hyperphagia, shorter periods of sleep, increases in peer-directed social interactions and affiliation with peers, an increase in the number of conflicts with parents, egocentrism, a lack of 'common sense' in decision-making, rigidity in reasoning, impulsivity, including a preference for actions that offer immediate rewards (cognitive impulsivity), reduced self-control, enhanced novelty-seeking and risk-taking behaviours (Spear, 2011a; Sturman & Moghaddam, 2011). All of these behaviours can lead to a higher incidence of risky behaviours such as misconduct at school, drink driving, unsafe sex, use of illegal drugs, and antisocial behaviours (Doremus-Fitzwater et al., 2010; Eaton et al., 2010; Spear, 2011b). Although cognitive control improves throughout adolescence (Luna et al., 2010), youths show differences in cognitive strategies in relation to adults. According to the "fuzzy trace theory" adolescents process the risk and benefits of choices more explicitly than adults, which, paradoxically, leads to greater risk-taking (Rivers et al., 2008). The characteristic irresponsibility of adolescents may be due to differences in the way in which they experience risk and reward, especially under conditions of heightened emotional arousal (Sturman & Moghaddam, 2011). Thus, the risk-taking behaviour of adolescents is probably related to the fact that their decision-making capacity is more vulnerable to disruption by stress. Adolescence is generally considered to be a stressful stage of life, and individuals are more likely to perceive events as stressful at this age, with adolescents exhibiting higher rates of depressed mood, sleep problems, emotional instability, anxiety and self-consciousness (Buchanan et al., 1992). Moreover, some aspects of neurobehavioural and hormonal responses to stressors also vary when adolescents are compared to younger or older individuals (Allen & Matthews, 1997). Similarly, behavioural experiments in laboratory animals have revealed that adolescents are more disrupted by stressors than younger or older counterparts and that they differ behaviourally and physiologically in their response to stressors when compared to animals of other ages (Buwalda et al., 2011; Stone & Quartermain, 1998; Vázquez, 1998). For example, the rise in plasma corticosterone levels induced by restraint stress is prolonged in adolescent rats in comparison with adult animals. Moreover, while adult male rats, which are repeatedly exposed to daily restraint stress, show a clear habituation in their neuroendocrine response, adolescent male rats actually exhibit a facilitation of this response (Romeo, 2010).

The characteristic behaviour of adolescence can be explained in neurobiological terms (Brenhouse & Andersen, 2011; Casey et al., 2011; Sturman & Moghaddam, 2011). Indeed, the features of an adolescent brain predispose individuals to behaving in the way referred to above. Maturational alterations of the brain contribute to these age-specific behavioural characteristics, including the increase in risk-taking and propensity to use drugs of abuse (Doremus-Fitzwater et al., 2010). Recent research has demonstrated the importance of gonadal hormones for neurobehavioural maturation during adolescence in laboratory animals and an association between gonadal hormones and adolescent behaviour/mood in humans (see Vigil et al., 2011, for review). Adolescence represents a stage of development of the nervous system (as does embryonic development) in which steroid hormones trigger various organizational phenomena related to structural brain circuit remodelling:

myelination, apoptosis, neural pruning, and dendritic spine remodelling, thus determining the adult behavioural response to steroids or sensory stimuli (Vigil et al., 2011).

The adolescent brain undergoes dramatic changes in gross morphology. During this phase there is a massive loss of gray matter and synapses in neocortical brain regions (Gogtay et al., 2004), and the most characteristic ontogenetic change, which occurs across a variety of species, is an alteration of the prefrontal cortex. Throughout human adolescence there is a marked increase in hemispheric asymmetry and in the degree to which the two cerebral hemispheres can process information independently (Merola & Liederman, 1985). In the primate cortex, the density of receptors of different neurotransmitter systems (dopamine, serotonine, acetylcholine, and GABA) decreases as adolescence progresses (Lidow et al., 1991; Brenhouse & Andersen, 2011). Most of the synapses that undergo pruning during adolescence are excitatory, which results in a decline in N-methyl-D-aspartate (NMDA) receptors and the extension of glutaminergic excitatory stimulation to the cortex (Insel et al., 1990). There is a body of evidence to show that the balance of excitatory and inhibitory neurotransmission varies between adolescents and adults, suggesting that the increased inhibition associated with development of the prefrontal cortex promotes greater neural coordination (Sturman & Moghaddam, 2011).

Maturational changes are also evident during adolescence in limbic regions such as the hippocampus (Insel et al., 1990; Wolfer and Lipp, 1995), and gray matter reductions also take place in the striatum and other subcortical structures (Sowell et al., 2002). Conversely, white matter increases in cortical and subcortical fiber tracts (Paus et al., 2001) and in circuits connecting the amygdala and striatum with the prefrontal cortex (Asato et al 2010). A decrease is observed in glutamate receptors in the hippocampus (Insel et al., 1990) and DA receptors in the striatum (Seeman et al., 1987; Teicher et al, 1995). Cannabinoid binding peaks in the limbic forebrain of rats during adolescence before declining to adult levels (Rodriguez de Fonseca et al., 1993). Experimental evidence supports a shift during adolescence from a relative balance between subcortical and cortical DA systems toward a greater predominance of cortical DA. In contrast to this enhanced DA tone in the prefrontal cortex during adolescence, DA activity in the accumbens and other subcortical DA terminal regions seems to be less noticeable in adolescents than in adults (Andersen & Gazzara, 1993). Basal levels of synaptic DA are lower during this phase of development, although adolescents show a greater and faster increase in drug-induced DA release (Badanich et al. 2006; Laviola et al. 2001). Consistent with this, adolescents are generally subject to a less positive impact from stimuli with moderate to low incentive value, and thus seek additional appetitive reinforcers (Spear, 2000).

Neuroimaging studies have shown variations in human adolescent functional activity in different forebrain regions, including the amygdala, orbitofrontal cortex and striatum (Bjork et al., 2010). For example, the amygdala and accumbens of adolescents exhibit more activity than those of adults (Ernst et al., 2002). Similarly, in comparison to adults, adolescents show a lower response to reward in the lateral orbitofrontal cortex and a higher activity in the nucleus accumbens (Galvan et al., 2006). Neural coordination within and between brain regions as well as processing efficiency are reduced in adolescents due to a less-effective information transfer between regions, incomplete myelination, and imbalances in neuronal inhibition/excitation within critical brain regions (Sturman & Moghaddan, 2011). Human and animal studies have revealed a differential development of subcortical limbic systems related to top-down control systems during adolescent brain development, with subcortical limbic systems developing earlier than control systems. It has been proposed that the mechanisms underlying adolescent changes in behaviour (impulsiveness, risky choices, drug taking, etc.) could underlie an imbalance between an increased sensitivity to motivational cues and immature cognitive control (Casey et al., 2011). In summary, immature neuronal processing in the prefrontal cortex and other cortical and subcortical regions, and their interaction, lead to a behaviour that is biased toward risk and emotional reactivity during the adolescent period (Sturman & Moghaddan, 2011).

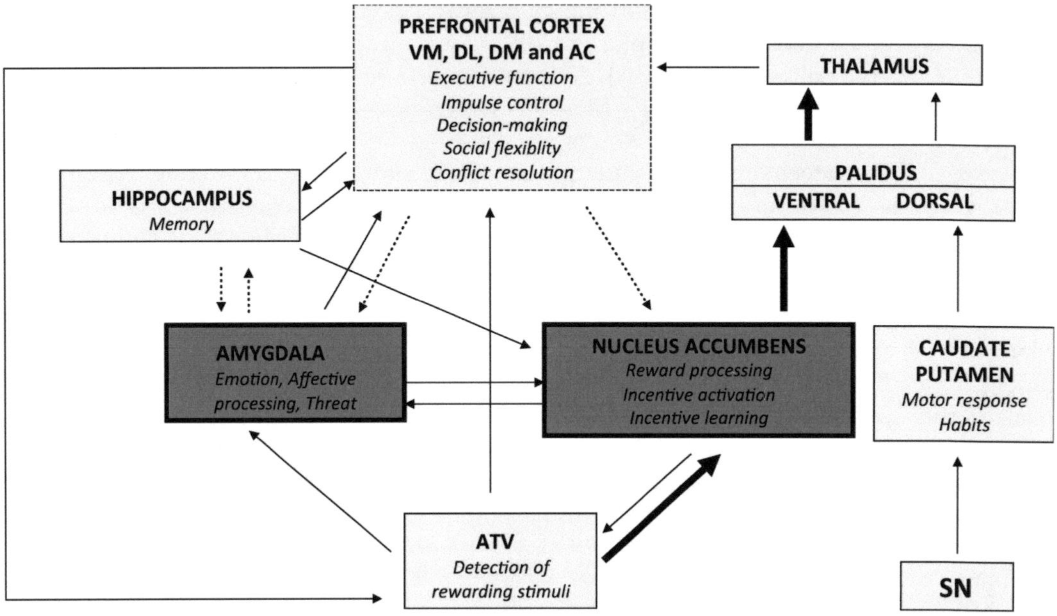

Fig. 1. Neural circuit involved in motivated behaviour. Thick lines represent hyperactive brain areas or connections and faint and dashed lines represent brain areas that are more hypoactive in adolescent subjects than in adults.

The adolescent brain operates in a promotivational state due to the combination of three factors:

a. limited inhibitory capacity and poor regulatory control (due to the lack of cortical maturation)
b. DA hyperactivity in the nucleus accumbens when processing appetitive stimuli
c. Amygdala hyperactivity, which explains affective intensity and liability, and a weaker harm-avoidance system (Ernst et al., 2009).

The relatively early development of bottom-up limbic regions (nucleus accumbens and amygdala), along with an immaturity of top-down regulatory systems (PFC), biases behavior toward risk-taking, risk-seeking, impulsive choice, sensation-seeking and novelty preference.

3. Effects of drugs on adolescents

In addition to increases in sensation- and novelty-seeking, drug use is more common during adolescence (2010 Annual report on the state of the drugs problem in Europe, EMCDDA;

Doremus-Fitzwater et al., 2010; Spear, 2011b). Youngsters differ from adults in their response to a variety of drugs (Schramm-Sapyta et al., 2009). These ontogenetic variations in drug responsiveness may be related with age differences in pharmacokinetics, particularly with respect to the functioning of the neural substrates upon which these drugs act, and also with social enhancement. As discussed previously, the neural systems involved in the effects exerted by drugs (mesolimbic DA system) differ considerably between adolescents and adults. These ontogenetic differences in drug responsiveness may have significant consequences for adolescents, who exhibit a reduced sensitivity to various drugs of abuse. This insensitivity can promote greater use per occasion in relation to more mature individuals (Schramm-Sapyta et al., 2009). After peer substance use, the next most powerful predictor of adolescent alcohol and drug use is perceived stress (Wagner et al., 1999). In animal models, stress has been shown to increase the rewarding effects of drugs of abuse (Piazza & LeMoal, 1998; Ribeiro Do Couto et al., 2006). On the other hand, experimental data suggest that drugs of abuse induce stronger effects in adolescents than in adults, although the literature is not conclusive regarding these differences (for review see Schramm-Sapyta et al., 2009). The developmental stage of adolescence can promote early experimentation with drugs, as addictive substances are generally more rewarding and less aversive (Schramm-Sapyta et al., 2009).

Moreover, adolescent substance use disrupts the normal development of an adolescent brain. Exposure to drugs of abuse can induce neurobehavioural, neurochemical and neuroendocrinal effects in the adolescent rat brain, thereby affecting the growth process and systems involved in plasticity and cognition (Jain & Balhara, 2010). Since adolescents undergo structural and functional dynamic changes in brain areas implicated in the reinforcing properties of drugs of abuse (prefrontal cortex and ventral striatum) and habit formation (dorsal striatum), drug-taking during this period could increase susceptibility to drug dependence, although there is a lack of studies that demonstrate causality.

4. Animal models of drug addiction

The use of animal models to study drug addiction has the advantage of experimental control of variables (age of initial exposure, drug, dose, duration, timing of exposure, etc.) and has provided much valuable information. The main drawback to animal studies is that no model completely reproduces all the stages in the development of drug addiction. Results obtained with multiple behavioural and neurobiological models are necessary to achieve a deeper understanding of this disorder (Ahmed, 2010; Belin et al. 2010; Sanchis-Segura & Spanagel, 2006; Schramm-Sapyta et al., 2009; Shippenberg & Koob, 2002; Weiss, 2010).

There are several animal models with a high predictive value, though most studies are performed with one of two paradigms: self-administration or conditioned place preference (CPP) (Aguilar et al., 2009). The most direct procedure for evaluating the reinforcing properties of a substance is self-administration (the animal works to obtain the substance: for example by pressing a lever), which assesses the intrinsic rewarding properties of a substance; and both oral and intravenous routes have been used to assess the relevance of age in voluntary intake. Animals that acquire drug-taking behaviour more quickly or indulge in it more frequently can be considered to resemble human drug addicts. However, drug taking, even when acquired quickly, is not equivalent to drug dependence (Ahmed, 2010). Another shortcoming of the self-administration paradigm is the complexity of the technique and the lack of a standardized procedure for evaluating substances with different potencies, reinforcement properties and pharmacokinetics. The choice of training substance, species and procedural parameters can radically affect the results obtained (Moser et al., 2011). Variations of the self-administration model have been developed to study the main features of addiction. For example, the progressive ratio method designed by Hodos (1961), in which the sweetness and volume of a milk is varied in order to measure reward strength, has been used to assess motivation to seek a drug (Depoortere et al., 1993). On the other hand, extinction and reinstatement paradigms are employed to model relapse. Following acquisition of self-administration, animals undergo a process by which the response is extinguished and reinstatement is induced by drug priming, stress or drug-associated cues (Shaham et al., 2003; Epstein et al., 2006). Time-out and punished responding model compulsive use (Deroche-Gamonet et al., 2004; Vanderschuren and Everitt, 2004) and long-access training schedules model high-level use (Knackstedt & Kalivas, 2007). Additionally, models of habitual drug-seeking have also been developed (Everitt et al., 2008).

The CPP paradigm (in which rodents repeatedly exposed to a distinct environment in the presence of a positively reinforcing substance show preference for that environment) evaluates the conditioned rewarding properties of a substance, and is also frequently used due to its procedural simplicity and rapidity. This model is dose-sensitive, and drugs of abuse are typically rewarding at low to moderate doses and aversive at high doses. CPP is sensitive to a wide range of substances. In general, CPP is useful for measuring the level and persistence of drug-induced reward (Tzschentke, 1998), but not for modelling pathological drug-seeking or taking. For this reason, variations of this procedure (adding an extinction and reinstatement of the extinguished conditioned preference) have been developed to model addiction-like behaviours (Aguilar et al., 2009).

Other animal models are employed to study motor behaviour, conditioned aversion, withdrawal, sensitization and compulsive drug-seeking (Belin et al., 2009; Schramm-Sapyta et al., 2009; Weiss, 2010). Most drugs of abuse stimulate locomotor behaviour through activation of the dopaminergic circuits that contribute to their reinforcing effects. At lower doses locomotor activity is generally increased, whereas at higher doses, locomotion falls and stereotypical behaviour can emerge. Conditioned place and taste aversion are designed to assess the aversive effects of drugs of abuse (which are assumed to discourage intake). Animals are trained to associate a place or a palatable flavour with the aversive sensations induced by a drug injected by the experimenter (generally lithium), which causes the place or flavour to be subsequently avoided. These tests measure the use-limiting effects of drugs of abuse but do not model pathological drug-seeking or taking (Schramm-Sapyta et al., 2009), since experimenter-delivered injections greatly differ from volitional intake even for the aversive effects of the drug (Galici et al., 2000).

Withdrawal is a constellation of affective and physiological changes that occurs after cessation of intake of some drugs of abuse and is used to evaluate dependence. Symptoms generally reflect the reversal of initial drug effects, although they vary with the drug, duration and extent of exposure. This, together with the kind of observations made and the choice of end points, can obstruct the interpretation of withdrawal effects (Moser et al., 2011). In the case of ethanol or opioids, withdrawal effects (including autonomic and behavioural activation) can be easily quantified in animal models. Withdrawal from psychostimulants and most other drugs of abuse results in a generalized "negative motivational state" which can be assessed using an intracranial self-stimulation procedure (Bauzo & Bruijnzeel, 2012) or an anxiety-like state which can be assessed using many models, including the social interaction test and elevated plus maze (Hall et al. 2010). Repeated exposure to any of the aforementioned drugs can lead to a phenomenon called sensitization, in which the ambulatory, stereotypic or rewarding effect of a repeated low dose is augmented. Sensitization reflects lasting neuroplastic changes in response to repeated exposure, and is hypothesized to be a behavioural correlate of increased drug craving and development of dependence (Robinson and Berridge, 2008), though its relevance to drug dependence is debatable. However, since data from sensitization studies have led to the development of pharmacotherapies that have been tested in animal models of relapse and in human addicts, some authors support sensitisation as a useful model for determining the neural basis of addiction (Steketee & Kalivas, 2011). Compulsive drug-seeking is analysed by the more complex methods of self-administration (progressive ratio, extinction, reinstatement, punishment, long-access, etc.), which tend to be more informative regarding vulnerability to addiction. However, it is difficult to employ these new techniques in developmental studies that aim to examine the behaviour of adolescent vs adult rodents, partly due to the prolonged duration of the experimental procedures.

5. Animal models of adolescent polydrug consumption

Recent advances in imaging have made it easier to study the human brain, but many questions about the effect of drugs in the adolescent brain require experimental manipulation in experimental animals in order to be answered. Given the across-species similarities in neurobehavioural features of adolescence, non-human animals undergoing this developmental transition can be used as models of human adolescence (Spear, 2000). There is growing evidence that adolescent humans and rodents experience many similar structural and functional changes in the brain as they progress towards adulthood. Behavioural changes characteristics of adolescence (increased social behaviour, novelty- and sensation-seeking, risk-taking, emotional instability and impulsivity) are also observed in rodents (Jain & Balhara, 2010). However, the use of adolescent rodent models does have some limitations. There are numerous areas of adolescent functioning in humans that cannot be addressed using animal models (peer pressure and self esteem, impact of parenting styles, obsession about weight, etc.). Moreover, the increases in adrenal hormones/neuroactive steroids during adrenarche in humans are generally not evident in other mammalian species. Furthermore, forebrain systems of rodents are less prominent than in humans, their social organization is simpler, and the time course of adolescence is briefer. The time frame of adolescence in non-human animals such as the rat is even more difficult to characterize than in humans. Among researchers who study adolescence in rats, opinions differ somewhat (Spear, 2000). The problem is further magnified by the limited amount of research to have focused on adolescence in laboratory animals. Animals of both genders exhibit neurobehavioural characteristics typical of adolescence during the period between postnatal days 28 and 42. According to hormonal, physical and social criteria, this development phase corresponds with age 12-18 in humans (Spear 2000). Moreover, different physiological changes (growth spurt, loss of excitatory input to prefrontal cortex, vaginal opening in females and increases in maturing spermatids in males) occur during this period. Indeed, some ontogenetic changes that signal the early onset of adolescence in female rats can emerge as early as 20 days of age, with later development taking place up until 55-60 days of age in males. Taking into account the abovementioned limitations, adolescent rodent models can be considered to possess good face and construct validity, since there are strong similarities between human adolescents and various animal models of adolescence in terms of developmental history, behavioural traits and neural and hormonal characteristics (Spear, 2011a). As more information is generated, stronger evidence of these forms of validity, and of predictive validity, will no doubt be obtained.

Moreover, there are several methodological difficulties that are encountered when using experimental animals to model the complex pattern of drug abuse observed in humans. A polydrug animal model of drug abuse allows a situation that is closer to reality than the simple effect produced by one drug. However, a number of variables need to be taken into account when using such a model. Comparison of the studies published in the literature is difficult, since practically each one of them represents a different model of polydrug administration. This is to be expected given the high number of variables involved in this kind of study (Schensul et al., 2005). The first variable to bear in mind is the combination of drugs employed. In most studies only two drugs are employed; in many cases cocaine or alcohol. Another important aspect is the temporal pattern of drug administration employed. Until now, most studies have focused on acute administration (Braida & Sala, 2002; Daza-Losada et al., 2009a; Diller et al., 2007; Manzanedo et al., 2010; Robledo et al., 2007), though there is a growing number of studies employing repeated administration and studying long-term effects (Achat-Mendes et al., 2003; Daza-Losada et al., 2008a, 2008b, 2009; Estelles et al., 2006; Jones et al., 2010; Ribeiro Do Couto et al., 2011a, 2011b; Rodriguez-Arias et al., 2011). This is another point of discrepancy; some studies have measured effects after very short periods post-administration (only 2 or 3 days), while others have assessed effects weeks or even months after the last administration. Finally, the effect under evaluation can vary considerably between purely physiological studies and those focusing exclusively on behavioural changes. All these discrepancies point to the fact that polydrug models simplify the complex reality of human consumption, in which each the pattern of drug use of each individual is unique.

Most of the studies that have assessed polydrug use have employed adult animals and acute administration. Thus, it is necessary to design models of adolescent polydrug consumption that reflect the human reality, despite the intrinsic difficulties they may pose. Our research group has been working for several years in this field during which we have studied different drug combinations and different patterns of drug administration.

The aim of the present chapter is to offer a detailed review of the experiments performed in this area. With this purpose in mind we will discuss not only the key results obtained in our experiments but also those of other studies of adolescent polydrug use. In an attempt to provide a clear overview of the evidence obtained to date, studies have been classified according to the pattern of drug administration employed. In this way, studies employing acute administration of drugs and studying immediate effects have been grouped together. Studies evaluating the binge pattern of drug administration, commonly employed by users of psychostimulants, constitute a second group. This section also represents a recently employed model developed with the aim of replicating the binge drinking that is so common among adolescents and young people of many cultures. Finally, we will discuss several studies in which a specific drug has triggered the reinstatement of drug-seeking behaviour of a different pharmacological kind of drug, known as the cross-reinstatement phenomenon and also the phenomenon of sensitization.

6. Principal results

6.1 Acute polydrug studies

6.1.1 MDMA plus cocaine

Preclinical studies have until now focused mainly on the long-term consequences of drug pre-treatment in terms of subsequent changes in spontaneous behaviour or in the response to other drugs of abuse. For instance, a substantial number of studies have focused on the long-term consequences of MDMA pre-treatment on subsequent cocaine administration (Achat-Mendes et al., 2003; Åberg et al., 2007; Daza-Losada et al., 2008, 2009b). However, hardly any have examined the interactive profile of concomitant exposure to MDMA and cocaine. Diller and coworkers (2007) studied the effects of concurrent administration of MDMA and cocaine on CPP in adult rats, finding that both drugs induced CPP when administered alone. Co-administration, on the other hand, produced an antagonism, except when higher doses were employed. These results highlight how the neurochemical and behavioural effects of MDMA and cocaine consumed separately are dramatically altered when taken together. Based on the inverse relation between serotonin and DA activity (in general, decreases in serotonin neurotransmission produce an increase of DA function) (Di Giovanni et al., 2010), these authors speculated that cocaine had undermined MDMA-mediated serotonin release more than MDMA-mediated DA release, thereby increasing the overall reward.

In a more recent study, we focused on the interaction of acute MDMA and cocaine administration in adolescent mice (Daza-Losada et al., 2009a), studying the acute interaction of both drugs on motor activity, anxiety, memory and brain monoamines. One of the most important results of this study was that acutely administered cocaine plus MDMA induced an anxiolytic response in the elevated plus maze that was not present when the drugs were administered separately. Mice treated with cocaine and MDMA spent significantly more time in the open arms of the plus maze than controls or animals treated with just one of the drugs. This result was not due to an unspecific increase of motor activity, as no increase in the number of total or closed entries was observed in animals treated with both drugs. Although numerous studies have indicated that MDMA causes anxiety problems in drug users (for review see Baylen et al., 2006), our results revealed that MDMA alone does not exert a strong effect on levels of anxiety in adolescent mice. The few studies performed in the plus maze with mice have shown that acute MDMA administration induces anxiogenic or anxiolytic effects that vary depending on the dose employed (Navarro et al. 2002). Although all the available evidence supports an anxiogenic effect of acute cocaine administration in adult mice (Erhardt et al., 2006), cocaine did not affect the behaviours studied in the plus maze in our study. One possible explanation could be the different experimental conditions of the studies compared or a different dose-response curve to cocaine in adolescent versus adult mice. These results endorse the hypothesis that adolescent animals are more "protected" from adverse psychostimulant-related properties than older subjects (Laviola et al., 1999), and highlight the importance of employing adolescent animals in studies.

Another important observation of our study was that an increase in DA turnover in the striatum was observed only when both drugs were administered together, due to a substantial increase in DOPAC concentration that was not accompanied by alterations of

DA levels. Neither serotonin nor its metabolites were altered in the striatum, but there was an increase in the concentration of serotonin in the cortex (total cortex, including the frontal cortex), which led to a decrease in its turnover. Although MDMA and cocaine act on the same neurotransmitter systems, the mechanisms involved differ, as do the effects produced. MDMA provokes an acute release of both serotonin and dopamine from nerve terminals (review in Colado et al., 2004) and is more potent in inhibiting serotonin and norepinephrine than dopamine transporters, while cocaine blocks these three monoamine transporters at similar concentrations (Han et al., 2006). One report suggested that serotonin plays a more prominent role in the psychotropic effects of MDMA than in those of cocaine (Itzhak et al., 2006). As in our study, both drugs were administered together, cocaine appeared to block MDMA entry into the nerve terminals, thereby inhibiting MDMA-mediated monoamine release, which mainly affects serotonin. On the other hand, the reuptake-blocking effects of these compounds may have been an added factor that made DA more available to the synapse, which could have been responsible for the increase in dopaminergic turnover observed. This DA/serotoninergic balance, which occurred only in the groups treated with both drugs, could be, in part, responsible for the anxiolytic effect observed when cocaine and MDMA were administered together. Our results endorse the hypothesis of Diller and coworkers (2007), since we have observed an increase in DA turnover and lower levels of serotonin turnover in the striatum and cortex. These findings point to an increase in DA availability in conjunction with the release of serotonin in small amounts or at a slow rate, leading to a decrease in its turnover. These studies demonstrate that the combined use of MDMA and cocaine produces a specific neurochemical and behavioural profile different to that observed when each drug is administered alone.

6.1.2 MDMA plus cannabinoids

Several studies have highlighted that the prolonged combined use of MDMA and cannabis is associated with a variety of psychological problems, including elevated impulsiveness, anxiety and psychotic behaviour (Daumann et al., 2004). The cannabinoid system interacts with a variety of neurotransmitters, including DA and serotonin (Nakazi et al., 2000), and represents a common neurobiological substrate for the addictive properties of different drugs of abuse (Maldonado et al., 2006). In line with this, many of the physiological responses provoked by MDMA are modulated by the endocannabinoid system (Piomelli et al., 2005).

Few studies have clarified the effects of exposure to cannabinoids on liability to MDMA abuse, and most of them suggest that cannabinoid agonists potentiate the rewarding effects of MDMA (Braida & Sala, 2002). However, studies performed recently have demonstrated that cannabinoid agonists modify sensitivity to the behavioural effects of MDMA in different ways (increase/decrease) depending on the dose employed. We have observed that a low dose of the specific CB1 agonist WIN 55212-2 increases the rewarding effects of an ineffective dose of MDMA administered during acquisition of the CPP. However, higher doses of the cannabinoid agonist weaken the preference induced by effective doses of MDMA (Manzanedo et al., 2010). Our results are in accordance with those of Robledo and co-workers (2007), who reported that a sub-threshold dose of THC produced CPP in mice when combined with a non-rewarding dose of MDMA but decreased the CPP induced by an effective dose of MDMA.

Cannabinoids participate in the regulation of DA synthesis, release and turnover (Gardner et al., 1998). The overlapping expression of cannabinoid and dopamine receptors in some brain areas such as the nucleus accumbens (Hermann et al., 2002) may represent a neuroanatomical substrate for such an interaction. At doses that neither WIN 55212-2 nor MDMA alter brain monamines, animals treated with both drugs exhibited decreases of striatal DA and serotonin in the cortex (Manzanedo et al., 2010). Despite the anti-inflammatory and anti-oxidative properties of cannabinoids (Pazos et al., 2008; Aggarwal et al., 2009), animal studies have revealed that chronic administration of THC causes hippocampal damage (Fisk et al., 2006) and that exposure to low concentrations of cannabinoids over a prolonged period is likely to have a neurotoxic effect (Rubovitch et al., 2002; Sarne & Keren, 2004). This evidence points to the capacity of cannabinoids to increase the neurotoxic potential of MDMA. We must keep in mind that, due to the crucial role that the DA system plays in the reinforcing effects of drugs of abuse, the neurotoxic effect of MDMA on mice could modulate the response of lesioned brains to these drugs. For instance, mice pre-exposed to neurotoxic doses of MDMA exhibit a higher consumption of, and a preference for, EtOH than saline-treated animals (Izco et al. 2007).

6.2 Binge pattern

6.2.1 MDMA plus cocaine

Epidemiological data reveal that the majority of MDMA users cease taking the drug spontaneously in their twenties (von Sydow et al., 2002), which highlights the relevance of using adolescent subjects in animal models. In addition to presenting a distinctive behavioural profile (Spear, 2000; Adriani & Laviola, 2003), young rats and mice are highly sensitive to the administration of psychostimulant agents (Laviola et al., 1999; Spear, 2000).

Both MDMA and cocaine have been proved to induce long-term response after their consumption. MDMA users present weeks after discontinuation of intake, a reduced hormonal response to drug challenge and a combination of depressive pattern, dysphoria, high levels of aggressiveness and elevated scores of novelty-seeking behaviour (Gerra et al., 1998). These long-term effects have also been described in mice and rats exposed to MDMA during adolescence, among which changes in social behaviour (Morley-Fletcher et al., 2002), motor activity (Balogh et al., 2004) and anxiety levels (Faria et al., 2006; Clemens et al., 2007) have been detected. On the other hand, cocaine administration also induces long-term effects in adolescent mice, which are expressed through increased flee and avoidance behaviour and fewer social contacts (Estelles et al., 2006). However, the long-lasting effect of the combination of two drugs taken during adolescence has received little attention. Furthermore, it should be taken into consideration that human MDMA and cocaine consumers commonly adhere to a binge pattern, which has been associated with a higher occurrence of stimulant-induced psychosis and addiction (Gawin, 1991; Segal & Kuczenski, 1997; Belin et al., 2011). To explore these effects, we performed a series of studies using a model that mimics a binge pattern of MDMA and cocaine consumption. This model consists of two daily injections (at 8 am and 8 pm) of an identical dose of MDMA alone or plus cocaine, for 3 days (6 administrations), between postnatal day 28 and 30. Mice were evaluated three weeks after the last treatment, on postnatal day 51. MDMA administration decreased the concentration of striatal DA when administered at high doses (20 mg/kg) in agreement with previous reports (for review see Colado et al., 2004), but cocaine inhibited this decrease in DA concentration three weeks later (Daza-Losada et al., 2008a). In accordance with these results, pretreatment with the dopamine uptake inhibitor GBR 12909 prevented long-term loss in the striatal concentration of DA (O'Shea et al., 2001). This lack of neurotoxicity could have been due to the effect exerted on body temperature by the two drugs together, as cocaine is known to counteract the increase produced by neurotoxic doses of MDMA. Most evidence suggests that merely preventing MDMA-induced hyperthermia is enough to produce significant neuroprotection (Colado et al., 2001). Although a rise in temperature is an important element in MDMA-induced neurotoxicity, this phenomenon appears to involve more than MDMA metabolites, including dopamine deamination and/or autooxidation (Sprague & Nichols, 2005). As we administered both drugs together, it is also feasible that cocaine interfered with the dopamine uptake system by inhibiting the entry of MDMA into the nerve terminal. By affecting one or several of these processes, cocaine is capable of blocking dopamine neurodegeneration in the mouse brain.

Since many MDMA users employ opiates in order to relieve the psychostimulant effects of ecstasy, it is of relevance to evaluate whether such individuals are subject to an increase in the well-known rewarding properties of morphine. We have observed that, following MDMA binges during adolescence, sensitivity to reinstatement of an extinguished preference is increased, as a morphine-induced preference was reinstated with lower priming doses in MDMA-treated mice than in non-treated animals (Daza-Losada et al., 2008b). In the literature regarding learning, reinstatement refers to the recovery of a learned response when a subject is non-contingently exposed to either a conditioned or an unconditioned stimulus after extinction. This recovery of a learned response, which represents a return to drug seeking, occurs when rats or mice are exposed to drugs, drug cues or stressors following extinction. In the CPP version of the reinstatement model, an extinguished CPP is robustly reinstated by non-contingent administration of a priming dose of the drug (Aguilar et al., 2009). Contrasting results were obtained when adolescent mice were treated with cocaine alone or plus MDMA. These animals need higher priming doses of morphine than non-treated mice in order to reinstate the preference. The ability of repeated treatment with psychomotor stimulants to enhance the response to subsequent challenge by an opiate seems to be affected by the route and timing of administration of each drug. Prenatal treatment with cocaine decreases the rewarding actions of morphine in adult offspring (Estelles et al., 2006), while, in adult rats, doses of morphine that fail to produce CPP have been shown to induce a marked preference in those which have previously received cocaine (Shippenberg et al., 1998). However, when acute challenge with heroin takes place 3 weeks after daily systemic injections of cocaine, locomotor cross-sensitization does not occur (DeVries et al., 1998). When cocaine is administered during gestational development, the development of brain reward systems can be altered, resulting in a long-term attenuation of the rewarding properties of morphine. Nevertheless, the possibility that such animals are unable to form the necessary association between a particular environment and morphine cannot be ruled out (Heyser et al., 1990; Inman-Wood et al., 2000). Additionally, prenatal exposure to cocaine can reduce the duration of pregnancy, gestational weight gain and food intake in the dams, factors that can contribute to an abnormal response to morphine. Finally, an association between prenatal cocaine exposure and the effect of altered maternal behaviour on later cognitive functions cannot be ruled out.

Thus, MDMA-treated mice are more vulnerable to relapse after receiving a priming administration of morphine, but this tendency is completely blocked in animals exposed to cocaine, in which an opposite effect is exhibited. Cocaine induces modifications in DA receptor function and transduction events mainly in the mesocorticolimbic dopamine pathway, where it induces an up-regulation of the cAMP-signalling pathway (Nestler, 2004) and augments the activity of the transcription factor cAMP response element-binding protein (CREB) (Walters et al., 2003). Increased CREB expression in the nucleus accumbens undermines the rewarding effects of both cocaine (Carlezon et al., 1998) and morphine (Barrot et al., 2002). In addition, repeated exposure to cocaine upregulates DYN/KOPr systems (Shippenberg et al., 2007).. This increase may initially serve as a homeostatic response that opposes the alteration in neurotransmission that occurs after exposure to this drug use. However, following the discontinuation of drug use, the unopposed actions of this system are likely to result in dysregulation of basal DA and glutamate transmission, thereby contributing to aberrant activity within the prefrontal-cortico-striatal loop (Shippenberg et al., 2007). These could represent some of the mechanisms responsible for the way in which cocaine affects the response of the dopaminergic system by altering the intensity of the response to priming.

MDMA and cocaine are often first consumed at an early age, and the response to MDMA of users in their twenties can be affected by previous exposure to these or other drugs. Similarly to the observations reported with morphine, Achat-Mendes and co-workers (2003) found that a priming injection of cocaine after extinction reinstated a significantly higher CPP in mice previously exposed during adolescence to a comparable regimen of MDMA. Comparable results have been described in adolescent (Aberg et al., 2007) and adult rats (Horan et al., 2000). These results are also in accordance with the finding that the acquisition of cocaine self-administration is facilitated in rats pre-exposed to MDMA (Fletcher et al., 2001). Concurring with these results, we have demonstrated that exposure to MDMA or cocaine binges during adolescence induces long-lasting changes that increase the reinforcing effects of MDMA (Daza-Losada et al., 2009b). We observed that only mice previously exposed to MDMA developed CPP after being conditioned with a sub-threshold dose of MDMA. On the other hand, although all the groups developed CPP after conditioning with 10 mg/kg of MDMA, the extinguished preference was reinstated only in animals exposed to MDMA or cocaine during adolescence, in which it also took longer for the preference to be extinguished. Extinction provides a measurement of the motivational properties of drugs, which are evident in the persistence of drug-seeking behaviour in the absence of the drug (Aguilar et al., 2009). This is a powerful means of assessing the incentive motivational properties of drug-paired stimuli or non-contingent drug administration in the reinstating response (Pulvirenti, 2003). However, when the two drugs were administered together, cocaine blocked the increases that MDMA induced in sensitivity to the MDMA-induced CPP and in vulnerability to reinstatement of the preference. Once again, as the two drugs were administered simultaneously, the competition for the same molecular target could have affected their action, leading to a weaker effect.

Most authors believe that increases in drug-induced CPP or self-administration observed in animals exposed to MDMA are due to the actions that MDMA exerts on the serotoninergic system (Horan et al. 2000; Fletcher et al. 2001). However, in many cases, it has been reported that the MDMA regimen employed did not induce dopaminergic or serotoninergic neurotoxicity, which was indeed the case in the studies mentioned above. None of the drugs, whether administered alone or together, induced significant changes in the concentration of these monoamines in the striatum, cortex or hippocampus 3 weeks later, at which time CPP was initiated (Daza-Losada et al. 2008b). Moreover, the chosen CPP schedule did not affect the concentration of monoamines (Daza-Losada et al. 2007).

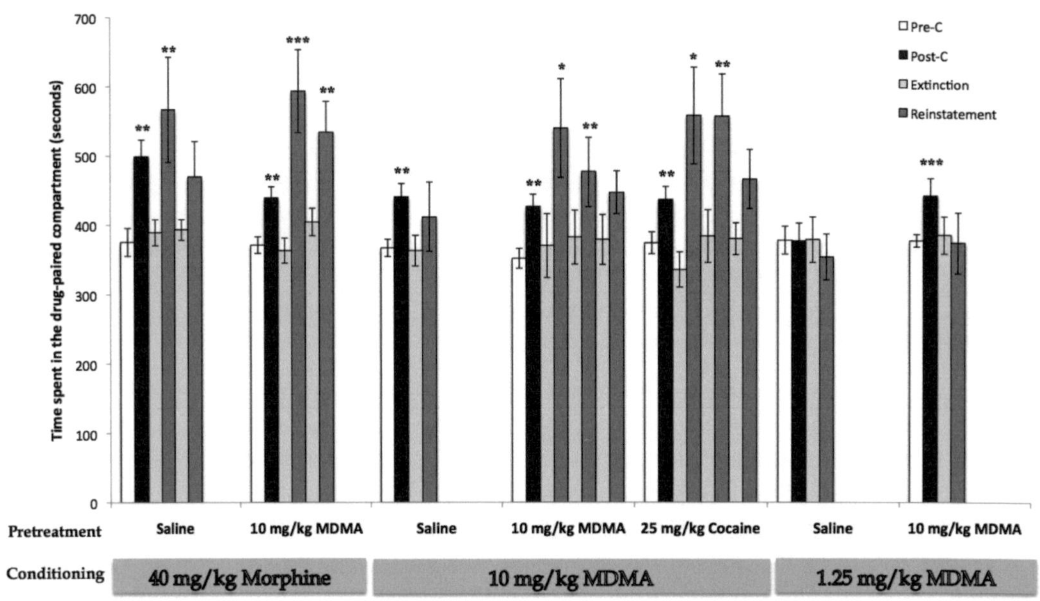

Fig. 2. Effects of MDMA or cocaine administration during adolescence on the acquisition and reinstatement of morphine or MDMA-induced CPP in adult mice. Bars represent mean (±SEM) time spent in the drug-paired compartment before conditioning session (□), after conditioning session (■), in the last extinction session (light grey), and in the reinstatement test (dark grey). During adolescence, mice were treated with six injections of physiological saline, 10 mg/kg of MDMA, or 25 mg/kg of cocaine. Three weeks later mice were conditioned with 40 mg/kg of morphine, or 10 mg/kg or 1.25 mg/kg of MDMA. After conditioning and extinction procedures, all animals received a priming injection of 50% of the drug dose administered during conditioning. In the subsequent reinstatement test, the priming doses employed were 25 and 12.5% that used during conditioning. MDMA exposure during adolescence increased the vulnerability to reinstatement of the extinguished preference induced by morphine and MDMA. This effect was also induced by administration of cocaine during adolescence. Pre-treatment with MDMA also increased its rewarding effects. * $p< 0,05$, ** $p<0.01$, *** $p<0.001$ significant difference in time spent in Post-C or Reinstatement tests vs. Pre-C session. Modified from Daza-Losada et al 2008b, 2009b).

6.2.2 MDMA and ethanol binges

Another drug often taken by adolescents in combination with ecstasy is alcohol (Riley et al., 2001; Barrett et al., 2006). Physiological and behavioural studies in humans and rodents have demonstrated an interaction between these two drugs (Mohamed et al., 2009). In humans, ethanol enhances and prolongs the euphoria and feelings of well-being induced by MDMA

(Hernández-López et al., 2002), but moderates some of its physiological effects, such as fluid retention and hyperthermia (Dumont et al., 2010). In addition, animal models have demonstrated that the hyperpyretic effect of MDMA is modulated by Ethanol according to the moment of ethanol administration and ambient temperature (Cassel et al., 2004, 2005 and 2007).

Research has only recently begun to use animal models to evaluate ethanol–MDMA interactions. Ethanol was shown to increase MDMA concentrations not only in blood but also, and to a greater extent, in the striatum and cortex than in the hippocampus (Hamida et al. 2009). On the other hand, levels of alcohol dehydrogenase 2, which metabolizes ethanol to acetaldehyde, were found to be 35% lower in MDMA-treated rats than in controls (Upreti et al. 2009). EthOH significantly potentiates the MDMA-induced outflow of serotonin and DA in rat striatal slices (Riegert et al., 2008). EthOH also affects the neurotoxicity induced by MDMA, although discrepant results have been reported. In rats, EtOH treatment before MDMA administration enhances long-term neurotoxicity, while in mice, EtOH protects DA neurons from the toxic effects of MDMA when evaluated 72 h after the first injection (Johnson et al., 2004). At the behavioural level, EtOH administration potentiates MDMA-induced hyperlocomotion in rats (Cassel, et al. 2004; Riegert, et al. 2008), and repeated co-administration of the two drugs results in a pronounced sensitization of hyperactivity (Hamida et al., 2007, 2008). Recently, Jones and co-workers (2010) have reported CPP in rats that received MDMA plus ethOH but not in those administered just with one of these drugs. These results suggest that acute co-administration of EtOH plus MDMA potentiates the reinforcing effects of each drug alone. Moreover, administration of EtOH would appear to increase the risk of compulsive use of MDMA.

A small number of studies have evaluated chronic exposure to both ethOH and MDMA, and none have explored this interaction in adolescent animals. Employing a model of binge drinking in which animals are treated during adolescence with intermittent doses of ethOH (a total of 16 doses administered intraperitoneally; two per day for two days, followed by a two-day interval without drugs), we aimed to imitate the pattern of weekend binge drinking that is currently so common among adolescents.

Mice were injected twice per day on postnatal day 29, 30, 33, 34, 37, 38, 41, and 42 and with MDMA twice daily on postnatal day 33, 34, 41, and 42. The behavioural and neurochemical test took place three weeks after the last drug administration. Pascual and co-workers (2007) demonstrated that this pattern of ethOH administration during adolescence enhances neural cell death in several brain regions (neocortex, hippocampus, and cerebellum) and induces long-lasting neurobehavioural impairments in conditional discrimination learning as well as motor learning and discrimination between novel and familiar objects. We too have observed that exposure to ethOH during adolescence increases the anxiogenic response induced by MDMA in the elevated plus maze, with adult treated-mice spending less time in the open arms of the maze than non treated littermates. In addition, although ethOH undermines the hyperthermic response induced by MDMA, animals exposed to ethOH plus MDMA exhibit lower concentrations of DA in the striatum than those treated with MDMA only (Rodriguez-Arias et al., 2011). In the study in question, though ethanol efficiently decreased the hyperthermic response induced by MDMA, it did not protect mice treated with 20 mg/kg of MDMA and actually increased the toxic effect in those treated with 10 mg/kg of MDMA, in which a hypothermic response was observed. This effect could be the result of binge pattern ethOH administration enhancing MDMA-induced long-term neurotoxicity through a mechanism that is unrelated to changes in acute hyperthermia and which is thought to involve hydroxyl radical formation (Izco et al., 2007). All the groups that presented reduced levels of striatal DA exhibited increased levels of anxiety. We have previously observed that adolescent mice treated with a schedule of MDMA that provoked a similar decrease in DA concentration without alterations in DOPAC levels behave normally in the elevated plus maze (Daza-Losada et al. 2008b). However, in our study, the decrease in DA was accompanied by a considerable decrease in DOPAC levels, which may have been responsible for the behavioural differences observed. Dopamine plays an important role in anxiety by modulating a cortical brake that the medial prefrontal cortex exerts on the anxiogenic output of the amygdala. It also has a considerable influence on the trafficking of impulses between the basolateral and central nuclei of the amygdala. Intra-amygdaloid infusion of D1 agonists and antagonists elicits anxiogenic and anxiolytic effects, respectively, suggesting an anxiogenic role for D1 receptors in the amygdala. Analyses of the effects of D2 agonists and antagonists suggest that, depending on the model of anxiety in question, either anxiogenic or anxiolytic effects are elicited (de la Mora et al., 2010).

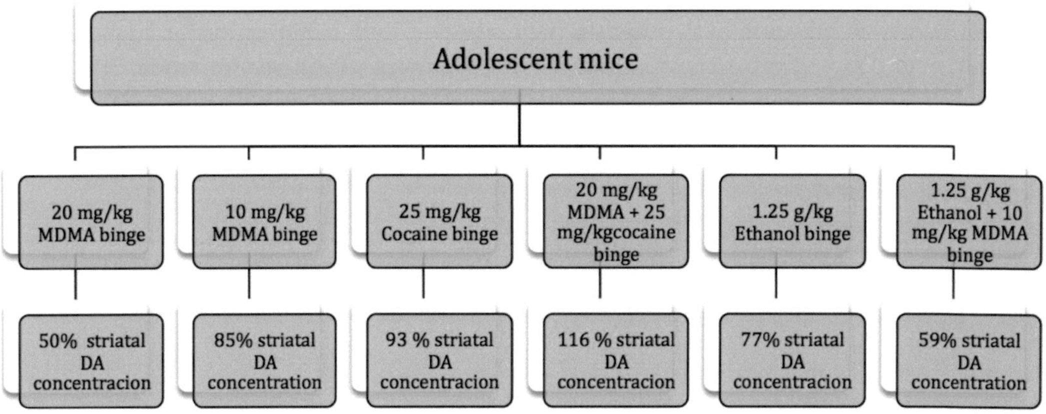

Fig. 3. Effects of MDMA, cocaine or ethanol binge administration during adolescence on the striatal DA concentration three weeks after the last drug administration. Co-administration of cocaine counteracted the neurotoxic effect of binge administration of 20 mg/kg of MDMA. However, intermittent ethanol administration increased the dopaminergic decrease induced by a non-neurotoxic dose (10 mg/kg) of MDMA. *** $p<0.001$ differences with respect to the saline group. Modified from Daza-Losada et al 2008a, and Rodriguez-Arias et al., 2011.

In addition to inducing long-term consequences for the rewarding effects of drugs, any manipulation or intervention during adolescence can produce other changes, such as the reactivity of the HPA axis to different stressful situations. In a series of recent reports (Ribeiro do Couto et al., 2011a, 2011b), we observed that exposure during adolescence to intermittent injections of ethOH or MDMA modify the response of mice to MDMA administration in adulthood, in addition to previous reports that pointed out long-term behavioural (an increase in anxiety) and neurochemical (a rise in MDMA-induced neurotoxicity) effects (Rodriguez-Arias et al., 2011). Pre-exposure to ethOH, MDMA or both increased the rewarding effects of an ineffective dose of MDMA (1.25 mg/kg). Although these pre-treatments did not affect acquisition of the CPP induced by higher doses, the preference was more persistent in mice pre-exposed to MDMA, ethOH or to both drugs. In addition, reinstatement of the extinguished preference was achieved with lower priming doses of MDMA in the groups pre-exposed to ethOH or MDMA (Ribeiro do Couto et al., 2011a). These effects appear to be due to the changes in the rewarding effects of MDMA rather than unspecific effects such as changes in basal motor activity or stress levels. After conditioning adults mice with an effective (but non neurotoxic) dose of MDMA (10 mg/kg), we once again observed that MDMA or ethanol exposure during adolescence increased the time required to extinguish the preference induced by MDMA and that these effects were related with an increase in either brain monoamine or corticosterone levels in response to MDMA (Ribeiro do Couto et al., 2011b). Mice treated with ethanol after the priming injection presented a significant increase in striatal DA. It is possible that this stronger neurochemical response to the priming dose of MDMA increased the efficacy of conditioning, reflected in a greater resistance to extinction. Similarly, the administration of 10 mg/kg of MDMA led to higher corticosterone values in mice exposed to MDMA during adolescence, while the response to low-mild stressors or to 5 mg/kg of MDMA did not differ, which could produce a stronger learning during conditioning.

In these series of studies, the combination of intermittent administration of ethOH+MDMA did not produce synergistic effects at either behavioural or neurochemical levels. In fact, the combination of the two drugs would seem to counteract the behavioural and hormonal effects of MDMA observed when each is administered alone. These results are in line with the previously discussed observation that adolescent exposure to MDMA exerts more powerful and longer-lasting effects on an MDMA-induced CPP than exposure to cocaine+MDMA (Daza-Losada et al., 2009). In this case, it is possible that ethanol interferes with the metabolism of MDMA and with its penetration of, and/or elimination, from the brain, and that this is responsible for the lack of effects observed after co-administration. Evidence that ethanol increases brain and blood concentrations of MDMA (Johnson et al., 2004) implies an enhanced MDMA-based neurotoxicity and an increased liability to abuse (Hamida et al., 2009). Since no neurotoxic effects were observed after any of the drug pre-treatments measured in the first reinstatement test, our results could be explained by the fact that ethanol increases the concentration of MDMA in the brain. Indeed, we found that the rewarding effects of MDMA produced an inverted U-curve in function of dose, with high doses proving to be devoid of motivational effects (Daza-Losada et al., 2007).

6.3 Cross-reinstatement and sensitization studies

This last section is dedicated to other kinds of drug interaction, cross-reinstatement and sensitization phenomena. Cross-reinstatement can be defined as the reinstatement of extinguished drug-seeking by drugs other than the previously self-administered or conditioning drug. This phenomenon has been widely demonstrated in self-administration and CPP studies. Cross-reinstatement with drugs from different classes to that of the self-administered drug has been demonstrated using the self-administration model. Cannabinoid agonists, DA agonists and re-uptake inhibitors and morphine, among others, produce reinstatement of cocaine-seeking after self-administration of cocaine has ended (reviewed by Shalev et al., 2002). Similarly, amphetamine and cocaine produce reinstatement of heroin self-administration (De Vries et al., 1998). Some studies have also demonstrated cross-reinstatement using the CPP paradigm. An extinguished cocaine-induced CPP can be reinstated by a priming injection of related psychostimulants (Itzhak & Martin, 2002), and of other drugs of abuse of different pharmacological classes (Romieu et al., 2004). In the same way, we observed that a cocaine or amphetamine priming following extinction reinstated morphine-induced CPP (Ribeiro Do Couto et al., 2005). In a series of recent studies, we have also observed cross-reinstatement between cannabinoids and MDMA in adolescent animals. Extinguished MDMA-induced CPP was reinstated after a priming injection of the CB1 cannabinoid agonist WIN 55212-2, but this phenomenon only occurred in animals exposed to the cannabinoid agonist during adolescence (Rodríguez-Arias et al., 2010). However, in mice conditioned with WIN 55212-2, a priming injection of MDMA was capable of reinstating the extinguished preference without pre-exposure (Manzanedo et al., 2010). Most authors agree that the mesocorticolimbic DA system is involved in cross-reinstatement. For instance, Wang et al. (2000) suggested that opiates and psychostimulants can all activate the mesolimbic DA system to release DA, which is a mechanism underlying the relapse to drug-seeking behaviour induced by morphine, cocaine or amphetamine. It is possible that one drug cross-primes the other via this common pathway, which is involved in incentive motivation and appetitive goal-directed behaviour (Wang et al., 2000). Such evidence of cross-reinstatement between drugs of different pharmacological classes has also been found in adolescents and suggests that, in drug-abstinent individuals, exposure to an addictive drug can produce intense craving for the previously abused drug and thus lead to relapse to drug-taking and dependence.

The repeated, intermittent administration of a variety of potentially addictive drugs produces persistent increases in their incentive motivational properties (Manzanedo et al., 2004, 2005; Shippenberg & Heidbreder, 1995). Age-related differences in psychostimulant sensitization profiles have been described (Laviola et al., 1995, 1999), with adolescent rats proving to be less vulnerable to MDMA-induced sensitization, only developing this response to MDMA when administered with a high dose and within a narrow margin of time (Aberg et al., 2007). In a recent study, we have evaluated for the first time the effect of adolescent exposure to cannabinoids on the reinforcing effects of MDMA (Rodriguez-Arias et al., 2010). On postnatal day 27, animals received the first of five daily injections of the cannabinoid agonist WIN55212-2, and three days later the place conditioning procedure for MDMA was initiated. In mice pre-exposed to cannabinoids, sub-threshold doses of MDMA induced CPP and reinstatement of an extinguished preference. In the same way, delta-9-tetrahydrocannabinol administration increased hedonic reactions to sucrose and the rise of dialysate DA in the shell of the NAc (de Luca et al., in press). These results endorse the gateway hypothesis, which is sustained by numerous epidemiological studies and suggests that prior exposure to cannabinoids encourages use of other illicit drugs such as psychostimulants (Lynskey et al., 2003). Few studies have tested this hypothesis in animal models, and those that have done so do not provide firm support for it. However, the adolescent brain is particularly sensitive to external and internal variables such as drug exposure, since this phase of development is characterized by active neural changes in, for example, synapse formation and elimination, in brain areas essential for behavioural and cognitive functions (Charmandari et al., 2003; Rice & Barone, 2000). Consequently, exposure to cannabis during the adolescent period may increase vulnerability to subsequent drug abuse disorders.

Authors	Treatment employed	Specie	Age	Behaviour studied/ model employed	Drugs of abuse	Results
Diller et al 2007	acute treatment	rats	adult	MDMA- or cocaine-induced CPP	MDMA and cocaine	Both drugs induced CPP when administered alone. Co-administration produced an antagonism, except at high doses
Daza-Losada et al., 2009a	acute treatment	mice	adolescent	Anxiety (EPM) and striatal monoamine levels	MDMA and cocaine	Anxiolytic response in the elevated plus maze and increased DA turnover in the striatum only when the two drugs were administered together
Braida & Sala, 2002	acute treatment	rats	adult	Self-administration of MDMA (ICV)	MDMA and cannabinoid agonist	Cannabinoid agonists potentiated the rewarding effects of MDMA
Manzanedo et al., 2010	acute treatment	mice	adolescent	MDMA- induced CPP	MDMA and cannabinoid agonist	Low dose of the CB1 agonist increased the rewarding effects of an ineffective dose of MDMA, but higher doses of the cannabinoid agonist weakened the preference induced by effective doses of MDMA
Robledo et al (2007)	acute treatment	mice	adult	THC-induced CPP	Δ9-THC and MDMA	A sub-threshold dose of THC produced CPP in mice when combined with a non-rewarding dose of MDMA, but decreased the CPP induced by an effective dose of MDMA
Daza-Losada et al., 2008a	MDMA and cocaine binge during adolescence	mice	adolescent	Striatal monoamine levels	MDMA and cocaine	MDMA-induced long-lasting decreases in the concentration of striatal DA at high doses, but cocaine inhibited this effect
Daza-Losada et al., 2008b	MDMA binge during adolescence	mice	adolescent	Morphine-induced CPP	MDMA and morphine	Sensitivity to reinstatement of an extinguished preference was increased in morphine-induced CPP
Estelles et al., 2006	Prenatal cocaine administration	mice	adult	Morphine-induced CPP	Cocaine and morphine	Prenatal treatment with cocaine decreased the rewarding actions of morphine in adult offspring
Achat-Mendes et al., 2003	MDMA binge during adolescence	mice	adolescent	Cocaine-induced CPP	Cocaine and MDMA	A priming injection of cocaine after extinction reinstated a significantly higher CPP in mice previously exposed to MDMA during adolescence
Daza-Losada et al., 2009b	MDMA and cocaine binge during adolescence	mice	adolescent	MDMA- induced CPP	Cocaine and MDMA	Only mice previously exposed to MDMA developed CPP after conditioning with a sub-threshold dose of MDMA. The extinguished preference was reinstated only in animals exposed to MDMA or cocaine during adolescence
Jones et al (2010)	acute treatment	rats	adult	MDMA- and EtOH-induced CPP	MDMA and EtOH	CPP was detected in rats that had received MDMA plus ethanol but not in those that had been administered just one of the drugs
Rodriguez-Arias et al., 2011	MDMA and EtOH binge during adolescence	mice	adolescent	Anxiety (EPM) and striatal monoamine levels	MDMA and EtOH	An increase was observed in the anxiogenic response induced by MDMA in adult mice treated with MDMA plus EtOH. EtOH increased the neurotoxic effect of MDMA
Ribeiro do Couto et al., 2011a, 2011b	MDMA and EtOH binge during adolescence	mice	adolescent	MDMA-induced CPP	MDMA and EtOH	Pre-exposure to EtOH, MDMA or both drugs increased the rewarding effects of an ineffective dose of MDMA. Reinstatement of the extinguished preference was achieved with lower priming doses of MDMA in the groups pre-exposed to ethanol or MDMA

Table 1. Synthesis of the most relevant interactions observed in the different models explained within the text.

7. Conclusion

In conclusion, the risks associated with multi-drug exposure during adolescence are still unclear. The high frequency of the combined used of several drugs in human adolescent users demands an in-depth evaluation of their interaction. It is obvious that the developing brain is highly vulnerable to the damaging effects of drugs; effects that can be irreversible. Studies performed to date demonstrate that the combined use of drugs produces a specific neurochemical and behavioural profile which differs to that observed when each drug is administered alone. These kinds of studies are more complicated to perform than those employing only one drug and involve many more variables that need to be controlled. Nevertheless, despite their complexity and the limitations inherent in their design, each of these studies constitutes a piece of a giant jigsaw puzzle which, as it is gradually put together, provides an increasingly clearer image of the reality of drug use.

8. Acknowledgement

This work was supported by the following grants: Ministerio de Economia y Competitividad.

Dirección General de Investigación (PSI2011-24762), Instituto de Salud "Carlos III" (FIS), RETICS, Red de Trastornos Adictivos (RD06/001/0016) and Generalitat Valenciana, Conselleria de Educación (PROMETEO/2009/072), Spain.

9. References

2010 Monitoring the Future (MTF) NIDA. National Institutes of Health. US Department of Health & Human Services.
http://drugabuse.gov/drugpages/MTF.html

2010 Annual report on the state of the drugs problem in Europe. EMCDDA, Lisbon, November 2009.
http://www.emcdda.europa.eu/attachements.cfm/att_93236_EN_EMCDDA_AR2009_EN.pdf

Abbott, A. (2005). Physiology: an end to adolescence. Nature, Vol.433, No.7021, (January, 2005), p. 27, ISSN 0028-0836

Åberg, M.; Wade, D.; Wall, E. & Izenwasser, S. (2007). Effect of MDMA (ecstasy) on activity and cocaine conditioned place preference in adult and adolescent rats. Neurotoxicology and Teratology, Vol.29, No.1, (January-February, 2007), pp. 37–46, ISSN 0892-0362

Achat-Mendes, C.; Anderson, K.L. & Itzhak, Y. (2003). Methylphenidate and MDMA adolescent exposure in mice: long-lasting consequences on cocaine-induced reward and psychomotor stimulation in adulthood. Neuropharmacology, Vol.45, No.1, (July, 2003), pp. 106–115, ISSN 0028-3908

Adriani, W. & Laviola, G. (2003). Elevated levels of impulsivity and reduced place conditioning with d-amphetamine: two behavioral features of adolescence in mice. Behavioral Neuroscience, Vol.117, No.4, (August, 2003), pp.695–703, ISSN 0735-7044

Aggarwal, S.K.; Carter, G.T.; Sullivan, M.D.; ZumBrunnen, C.; Morrill, R. & Mayer, J.D. (2009). Medicinal use of cannabis in the United States: historical perspectives, current trends, and future directions. Journal of Opioid Management, Vol.5, No.3, (May-June, 2009), pp. 153-168. ISSN 1551-7489

Aguilar, M.A.; Rodríguez-Arias, M. & Miñarro, J. (2009). Neurobiological mechanisms of the reinstatement of drug-conditioned place preference. Brain Research Reviews, Vol.59, No.2, (March, 2009), pp. 253-277, ISSN 0165-017

Ahmed, S.H. (2010). Validation crisis in animal models of drug addiction: Beyond non-disordered drug use toward drug addiction. Neuroscience and Biobehavioral Reviews, Vol. 35, No.2, (November, 2010), pp. 172–184, ISSN 0149-7634

Allen, M.T. & Matthews, K.A. (1997). Hemodynamic responses to laboratory stressors in children and adolescents: the influences of age, race, and gender. Psychophysiology, Vol.34, No.3, (May, 1997), pp. 329-339, ISSN 0048-5772

Andersen, S.L. & Gazzara, R.A. (1993). The ontogeny of apomorphine-induced alterations of neostriatal dopamine release: effects on spontaneous release. Journal of Neurochemistry, Vol.61, No.6, (December, 1993), pp. 2247-2255, ISSN 0022-3042

Asato, M.R.; Terwilliger, R.; Woo, J. & Luna, B. (2010). White matter development in adolescence: a DTI study. Cerebral Cortex, Vol.20, No.9, (September, 2010), pp. 2122–2131, ISSN 1047-3211

Badanich, K.A.; Adler, K.J. & Kirstein, C.L. (2006). Adolescents differ from adults in cocaine conditioned place preference and cocaine-induced dopamine in the nucleus accumbens septi. European Journal of Pharmacology, Vol.550, No.1-3, (November, 2006), pp. 95–106, ISSN 0014-2999

Balogh, B.; Molnar, E.; Jakus, R.; Quate, L.; Olverman, H.J.; Kelly, P.A.; Kantor, S. & Bagdy, G. (2004). Effects of a single dose of 3,4-methylenedioxymethamphetamine on circadian patterns, motor activity and sleep in drug-naive rats and rats previously exposed to MDMA. Psychopharmacology, Vol. 173, No.3-4, (May, 2004), pp. 296–309, ISSN 0033-3158

Barrett, S.P.; Darredeau, C. & Pihl, R.O. (2006). Patterns of simultaneous polysubstance use in drug using university students. Human Psychopharmacology, Vol.21, No.4, (June, 2006), pp. 255–63. ISSN 0885-6222

Barrot, M.; Olivier, J.D.; Perrotti, L.I.; DiLeone, R.J.; Berton, O.; Eisch, A.J.; Impey, S.; Storm, D.R.; Neve, R.L.; Yin, J.C.; Zachariou, V. & Nestler, E.J. (2002). CREB activity in the nucleus accumbens shell controls gating of behavioral responses to emotional stimuli. Proceeding of the National Academy of Sciences USA, Vol.99, No.17, (August, 2002), pp. 11435–11440, ISSN 0027-8424

Baumrind, D. (1987). A developmental perspective on adolescent risk taking in contemporary America. In: Adolescent social behavior and health, Irwin Jr. CE, editor, pp. 93–125, Jossey-Bass, ISBN-10: 1555429394, San Francisco, CA.

Bauzo, R.M. & Bruijnzeel, A.W. (2012). Animal models of nicotine withdrawal: intracranial self-stimulation and somatic signs of withdrawal. Methods in Molecular Biology, Vol.829, No. 3, (2012), pp.257-268, ISSN 1064-3745

Baylen, C.A. & Rosenberg, H. (2006). A review of the acute subjective effects of MDMA/ ecstasy, Addiction, Vol.101, No.7, (July, 2006) 933–947, ISSN 0965-2140

Belin, D., Besson, M., Bari, A., & Dalley, J. (2009). Multi-disciplinary investigations of impulsivity in animal models of attention-deficit hyperactivity disorder and drug addiction vulnerability. In S. Granon (Ed.), Endophenotypes of Psychiatric and Neurodegenerative Disorders in Rodent Models. New York: Oxford University Press. ISBN: 8178954028

Belin, D., Economidou, D., Pelloux, Y., & Everitt, B. J. (2010). Habit Formation and Compulsion. In M. C. Olmstead (Ed.), Animal models of drug addiction. Humana Press. ISBN-13 9781607619338

Belin, D.; Berson, N.; Balad, E.; Piazza, P.V.; Deroche-Gamonet, V. (2011) High-novelty-preference rats are predisposed to compulsive cocaine self-administration. Neuropsychopharmacology, Vol. 36, No. 3 (February, 2011), pp. 569-579 , ISSN 0893-133X

Bjork, J.M.; Smith, A.R.; Chen, G. & Hommer, D.W. (2010). Adolescents, Adults and Rewards: Comparing Motivational Neurocircuitry Recruitment Using fMRI. PLoS ONE Vol.5, No.7, (July, 2010), pp. e11440, ISSN 1932-6203

Braida, D. & Sala, M. (2002). Role of the endocannabinoid system in MDMA intracerebral self-administration in rats. British Journal of Pharmacology, Vol.136, No.8, (August, 2002), pp. 1089-1092, ISSN 0007-1188

Brenhouse, H.C. & Andersen S.L. (2011). Developmental trajectories during adolescence in males and females: A cross-species understanding of underlying brain changes Neuroscience and Biobehavioral Reviews, Vol.35, No.8, (August, 2011), pp. 1687–1703, ISSN 0149-7634

Buchanan, C.M.; Eccles, J.S. & Becker, J.B. (1992). Are adolescents the victims of raging hormones: evidence for activational effects of hormones on moods and behavior at adolescence. Psychological Bulletin, Vol.111, No.1, (January, 1992), pp. 62–107, ISSN 0033-2909

Buwalda, B.; Geerdink, M.; Vidal, J. & Koolhaas, J.M. (2011). Social behavior and social stress in adolescence: A focus on animal models. Neuroscience and Biobehavioral Reviews, Vol.35, No.8, (August, 2011), pp. 1713–1721, ISSN 0149-7634

Carlezon, W.A. Jr.; Thome, J.; Olson, V.G.; Lane-Ladd, S.B.; Brodkin, E.S.; Hiroi, N.; Duman, R.S.; Neve, R.L. & Nestler, E.J. (1998). Regulation of cocaine reward by CREB. Science, Vol.282, No.5397, (December, 1998), pp. 2272–2275, ISSN 0036-8075

Casey, B.; Jones, R.M. & Somerville, L.H. (2011). Braking and Accelerating of the Adolescent Brain. Journal of Research on Adolescence, Vol.21, No.1, (March, 2011), pp. 21-33, ISSN 1532-7795

Cassel, J.C.; Ben Hamida, S. & Jones, B.C. (2007). Attenuation of MDMA-induced hyperthermia by ethanol in rats depends on ambient temperature. European Journal of Pharmacology, Vol.571, No.2-3, (October, 2007), pp. 152–155. ISSN 0014-2999

Cassel, J.C.; Jeltsch, H.; Koenig, J. & Jones, B.C. (2004). Locomotor and pyretic effects of MDMA ethanol associations in rats. Alcohol, Vol.34, No.2-3, (October-November, 2004), pp. 285–289. ISSN 0741-8329

Cassel, J.C.; Riegert, C.; Rutz, S.; Koenig, J.; Rothmaier, K.; Cosquer, B.; Lazarus, C.; Birthelmer, A.; Jeltsch, H.; Jones, B.C. & Jackisch, R. (2005). Ethanol, 3, 4-methylenedioxymethamphetamine (ecstasy) and their combination: long-term behavioral, neurochemical and neuropharmacological effects in the rat. Neuropsychopharmacology, Vol.30, No.10, (October, 2005), pp. 1870–1882, ISSN 0893-133X

Charmandari, E.; Kino, T.; Souvatzoglou, E. & Chrousos, G.P. (2003). Pediatric stress: hormonal mediators and human development. Hormones Research, Vol.59, No.4, (2003), pp. 161–179. ISSN 0301-0163

Clemens, K.J.; Cornish, J.L.; Hunt, G.E. & McGregor, I.S. (2007). Repeated weekly exposure to MDMA, methamphetamine or their combination: long-term behavioural and neurochemical effects in rats. Drug & Alcohol Dependence, Vol.86, No.2-3, (January, 2007), pp. 183–190, ISSN 0376-8716

Colado, M.I.; O'Shea, E. & Green, A.R. (2004). Acute and long-term effects of MDMA on cerebral dopamine biochemistry and functions. Psychopharmacology, Vol.173, No.3-4, (May, 2004), pp. 249-263, ISSN 0033-3158

Colado, M.I.; Camarero, J.; Mechan, A.O.; Sanchez, V.; Esteban, B.; Elliott, J.M. & Green, A.R. (2001). A study of the mechanisms involved in the neurotoxic action of 3,4-methylenedioxymethamphetamine (MDMA, 'ecstasy') on dopamine neurones in mouse brain. British Journal of Pharmacology, Vol.134, No.8, (December, 2001), pp. 1711–1723, ISSN 1476-5381

Colado, M.I.; O'Shea, E. & Green, A.R. (2004). Acute and long-term effects of MDMA on cerebral dopamine biochemistry and function, Psychopharmacology, Vol.173, No.3-4, (May, 2004), pp. 249–263, ISSN 0033-3158

Cunningham, M.G.; Bhattacharyya, S. & Benes, F.M. (2002). Amygdalo-cortical sprouting continues into early adulthood: implications for the development of normal and abnormal function during adolescence. Journal of Comparative Neurology, Vol.453, No2., (November, 2002), pp. 116–130, ISSN 0021-9967

Daumann, J.; Hensen, G.; Thimm, B.; Rezk, M.; Till, B. & Gouzoulis-Mayfrank, E. (2004). Self-reported psychopathological symptoms in recreational ecstasy (MDMA) users are mainly associated with regular cannabis use: further evidence from a combined cross-sectional/longitudinal investigation. Psychopharmacology, Vol.173, No.3-4, (May, 2004), pp. 398-404. ISSN 0033-3158

Daza-Losada, M.; Ribeiro Do Couto, B.; Manzanedo, C.; Aguilar, M.A.; Rodríguez-Arias, M. & Miñarro, J. (2007). Rewarding effects and reinstatement of MDMA-induced CPP in adolescent mice. Neuropsychopharmacology, Vol.32, No.8, (August, 2007), pp. 1750–1759. ISSN 0893-133X

Daza-Losada, M.; Rodríguez-Arias, M.; Maldonado, C.; Aguilar, M.A. & Miñarro, J. (2008a). Behavioural and neurotoxic long-lasting effects of MDMA plus cocaine in adolescent mice. European Journal of Pharmacology, Vol.590, No.1-3, (August, 2008), pp. 204-211. ISSN 0014-2999

Daza-Losada, M.; Rodríguez-Arias, M.; Aguilar, M.A. & Miñarro, J. (2008b). Effect of adolescent exposure to MDMA and cocaine on acquisition and reinstatement of morphine-induce CPP. Progress in Neuro-Psychopharmacology & Biological Psychiatry, Vol.32, No.3, (April, 2008), pp. 701–709, ISSN 0278-5846

Daza-Losada, M.; Rodríguez-Arias, M.; Maldonado, C.; Aguilar, M.A.; Guerri, C. & Miñarro, J. (2009a). Acute behavioural and neurotoxic effects of MDMA plus cocaine in adolescent mice. Neurotoxicology & Teratology, Vol.31, No.1, (January-February, 2009), pp. 49-59, ISSN 0892-0362

Daza-Losada, M.; Rodríguez-Arias, M.; Aguilar, M.A. & Miñarro, J. (2009b). Acquisition and reinstatement of MDMA-induced conditioned place preference in mice pre-treated with MDMA or cocaine during adolescence. Addiction Biology, Vol.14, No.4, (September, 2009), pp. 447-456. ISSN 1369-1600

de la Mora, M.P.; Gallegos-Cari, A.; Arizmendi-García, Y.; Marcellino, D.; Fuxe, K. (2010) Role of dopamine receptor mechanisms in the amygdaloid modulation of fear and anxiety: Structural and functional analysis. Proggress in Neurobiology Vol.90, No.2, (February, 2010), pp. 198-216. ISSN 0301-0082

De Luca, M.A.; Solinas, M.; Bimpisidis, Z.; Goldberg, S.R.; Di Chiara, G. (2012) Cannabinoid facilitation of behavioral and biochemical hedonic taste responses. Neuropharmacology, in press.

Deroche-Gamonet, V., Belin, D. & Piazza, P,V. (2004). Evidence for addiction-like behavior in the rat. Science, Vol. 305, No.5686, (August, 2004), pp. 1014-1017, ISSN 0036-8075

De Vries, T.J.; Schoffelmeer, A.N.; Binnekade, R.; Mulder, A.H. & Vanderschuren, L.J. (1998). Drug-induced reinstatement of heroin- and cocaine-seeking behaviour following long-term extinction is associated with expression of behavioural sensitization. European Journal of Neuroscience, Vol.10, No.11, (November, 1998), pp. 3565–71, ISSN 1460-9568

Di Giovanni, G., Esposito, E., Di Matteo, V. (2010) Role of serotonin in central dopamine dysfunction. CNS Neurosci Ther. Vol.16, No. 3, pp. 179-194, DOI: 10.1111/j.1755-5949.2010.00135.x

Diller, A.J.; Rocha, A.; Cardon, A.L.; Valles, R.; Wellman, P.J. & Nation, J.R. (2007). The effects of concurrent administration of +/−3,4-methylenedioxymethamphetamine and cocaine on conditioned place preference in the adult male rat. Pharmacology, Biochemistry & Behavior, Vol.88, No.2, (December, 2007), pp. 165–170, ISSN 0091-3057

Doremus-Fitzwater, T.L.; Elena I. Varlinskaya, E.I. & Spear, L.P. (2010). Motivational systems in adolescence: Possible implications for age differences in substance abuse and other risk-taking behaviors. Brain & Cognition, Vol.72, No.1 (February, 2010), pp. 114, ISSN 0278- 2626

Dumont, G.; Kramers, C.; Sweep, F.; Willemsen, J.; Touw, D.; Schoemaker, R.; van Gerven, J.; Buitelaar, J. & Verkes, R. (2010). Ethanol co-administration moderates 3,4-methylenedioxymethamphetamine effects on human physiology. Journal of Psychopharmacology, Vol.24, No.2, (February, 2010), pp. 165-174, ISSN 0269-8811

Eaton, D.K.; Kann, L.; Kinchen, S.; Shanklin, S.; Ross, J.; Hawkins, J.; Harris, W.A.; Lowry, R.; McManus, T.; Chyen, D.; Lim, C.; Whittle, L.; Brener, N.D. & Wechsler, H. (2010). Youth risk behavior surveillance - United States, 2009. Morbidity and Mortality Weekly Report (MMWR) Surveillance Summaries, Vol.59 No.5, (Jun, 2010), pp. 1-142, ISSN 1546-0738

Encuesta domiciliaria sobre alcohol y drogas en España (EDADES) 2009/2010. Delegación del gobierno para el plan nacional sobre drogas. Ministerio de sanidad, política social e igualdad.
http://www.pnsd.msc.es/Categoria2/observa/estudios/home.htm

Encuesta Estatal sobre Uso de Drogas en Estudiantes de Enseñanzas Secundarias (ESTUDES) (2008). Ministerio de Sanidad y Política Social, Delegación del Gobierno para el Plan Nacional sobre Drogas
http://www.pnsd.msc.es/Categoria2/observa/estudios/home.htm

Epstein, D.H.; Preston, K.L.; Stewart, J. & Shaham, Y. (2006). Toward a model of drug relapse: an assessment of the validity of the reinstatement procedure. Psychopharmacology, Vol.189, No.1, (November, 2006), pp. 1-16, ISSN 0033-3158

Erhardt, E.; Zibetti, L.C.; Godinho, J.M.; Bacchieri, B. & Barros, H.M. (2006). Behavioral changes induced by cocaine in mice are modified by a hyperlipidic diet or recombinant leptin. Brazilian Journal of Medical & Biological Research, Vol.39, No.12, (December, 2006), pp. 1625–1635, ISSN 0100-879X

Ernst, M.; Bolla, K.; Mouratidis, M.; Contoreggi, C.; Matochik, J.A.; Kurian, V.; Cadet, J.L.; Kimes, A.S. & London, E.D. (2002). Decision-making in a risk-taking task: a PET study. Neuropsychopharmacology, Vol.26, No.5, (May, 2002), pp. 682-691, ISSN 0893-133X

Ernst, M., Romeo R.D. & Andersen S.L. (2009). Neurobiology of the development of motivated behaviors in adolescence: A window into a neural systems model. Pharmacology, Biochemistry and Behavior, Vol.93, No.3, (September, 2009), pp. 199–211, ISSN 0091-3057

Estelles, J.; Rodriguez-Arias, M.; Maldonado, C.; Manzanedo, C.; Aguilar, M.A. & Minarro, J. (2006). Prenatal cocaine alters later responses to morphine in adult male mice.

Progress in Neuropsychopharmacology & Biological Psychiatry, Vol.30, No.6, (August, 2006), pp. 1073–1082, ISSN 0278-5846

Everitt, B.J.; Belin, D.; Economidou, D.; Pelloux, Y.; Dalley, J.W. & Robbins, T.W. (2008). Neural mechanisms underlying the vulnerability to develop compulsive drug-seeking habits and addiction. Philosophical Transactions of the Royal Society of London B Biological Sciences, Vol.363, No.1507, (October, 2008), pp.3125-35. ISSN 0080-4622

Faria, R.; Magalhaes, A.; Monteiro, P.R.; Gomes-Da-Silva, J.; Amelia Tavares, M. & Summavielle, T. (2006). MDMA in adolescent male rats: decreased serotonin in the amygdala and behavioral effects in the elevated plus-maze test. Annals of the New York Academy of Science, Vol.1074, (August, 2006), pp. 643–649, ISSN 0077-8923

Fisk, J.E.; Montgomery, C.; Wareing, M. & Murphy, P.N. (2006). The effects of concurrent cannabis use among ecstasy users: neuroprotective or neurotoxic? Human Psychopharmacology, Vol.21, No.6, (August, 2006), pp. 355-366, ISSN 0885-6222

Fletcher, P.J.; Robinson, S.R. & Slippoy, D.L. (2001). Pre-exposure to (+/-) 3,4-methylenedioxy-methamphetamine (MDMA) facilitates acquisition of intravenous cocaine self-administration in rats. Neuropsychopharmacology, Vol.25, No.2, (August, 2001), pp. 195–203, ISSN 0893-133X

Galici, R., Pechnick, R.N., Poland, R.E. & France, C.P. (2000). Comparison of noncontingent versus contingent cocaine administration on plasma corticosterone levels in rats. European Journal of Neuroscience, Vol.387, No.1, (January, 2000), pp. 59–62, ISSN 0953-816X

Galvan, A.; Hare, T.A.; Parra, C.E.; Penn, J.; Voss, H.; Glover, G. & Casey,B.J. (2006). Earlier development of the accumbens relative to orbitofrontal cortex might underlie risk-taking behavior in adolescents. Journal of Neuroscience, Vol.26, No.25, (June, 2006), pp. 6885–6892, ISSN 0270-6474

Gardner, E.L. & Vorel, S.R. (1998). Cannabinoid transmission and reward-related events. Neurobiology of Disease, Vol.5, No.6, (December, 1998), pp 502-533, ISSN 0969-9961

Gawin, F.H. (1991). Cocaine addiction: psychology and neurophysiology. Science, Vol.251, No.5001, (March, 1991), pp. 1580–1586, ISSN 0036-8075

Gerra, G.; Zaimovic, A.; Giucastro, G.; Maestri, D.; Monica, C.; Sartori, R.; Caccavari, R. & Delsignore, R. (1998). Serotonergic function after (+/−)3,4-methylene-dioxymethamphetamine ('Ecstasy') in humans. International Clinical Psychopharmacology, Vol.13, No.1, (January, 1998), pp. 1–9, ISSN 0271-0749

Gogtay, N.; Giedd, J.N.; Lusk, L.; Hayashi, K.M.; Greenstein, D.; Vaituzis, A.C.; Nugent 3rd, T.F.; Herman, D.H.; Clasen, L.S.; Toga, A.W.; Rapoport, J.L. & Thompson, P.M. (2004). Dynamic mapping of human cortical development during childhood through early adulthood. Proceedings of the National Academy of Sciences of the United States of America, Vol. 101, No.21, (May, 2004), pp.8174–8179, ISSN 0027-8424

Hall, B.J.; Pearson, L.S. & Buccafusco, J.J. (2010). Effect of the use-dependent, nicotinic receptor antagonist BTMPS in the forced swim test and elevated plus maze after cocaine discontinuation in rats. Neuroscience Letters, Vol.474 No.2, (April, 2010) pp. 84-87, ISSN 0304-3940

Hamida, S.B.; Plute, E.; Bach, S.; Lazarus, C.; Tracqui, A.; Kelche, C.; de Vasconcelos, A.P.; Jones, B.C. & Cassel, J.C. (2007). Ethanol-MDMA interactions in rats: the importance of interval between repeated treatments in biobehavioral tolerance and sensitization to the combination. Psychopharmacology, Vol.192, No.4, (July, 2007), pp. 555–569, ISSN 0033-3158

Hamida, S.B.; Plute, E.; Cosquer, B.; Kelche, C.; Jones, B.C. & Cassel, J.C. (2008). Interactions between ethanol and cocaine, amphetamine, or MDMA in the rat: thermoregulatory and locomotor effects. Psychopharmacology, Vol.197, No.1, (March, 2008), pp. 67–82, ISSN 0033-3158

Hamida, S.B.; Tracqui, A.; de Vasconcelos, A.P.; Szwarc, E.; Lazarus, C.; Kelche, C.; Jones, B.C. & Cassel, J.C. (2009). Ethanol increases the distribution of MDMA to the rat brain: possible implications in the ethanol-induced potentiation of the psychostimulant effects of MDMA. International Journal of Neuropsychopharmacology, Vol.12, No.6, (July, 2009), pp. 749–759, ISSN 1461-1457

Han, D.D. & Gu, H.H. (2006). Comparison of the monoamine transporters from human and mouse in their sensitivities to psychostimulant drugs. BMC Pharmacology, Vol.3, No.6, p. 6, ISSN 1471-2210

Hermann, H.; Marsicano, G. & Lutz, B. (2002). Coexpression of the cannabinoid receptor type 1 with dopamine and serotonin receptors in distinct neuronal subpopulations of the adult mouse forebrain. Neuroscience, Vol.109, No.3, (February, 2002), pp. 451-480, ISSN 0306-4522

Hernández-López, C.; Farré, M.; Roset, P.N.; Menoyo, E.; Pizarro, N.; Ortuño, J.; Torrens, M.; Camí, J. & de La Torre, R. 3, 4-Methylenedioxymethamphetamine (ecstasy) and alcohol interactions in humans: psychomotor performance, subjective effects, and pharmacokinetics. Journal of Pharmacology & Experimental Therapeutics, Vol.300, No.1, (January, 2002), pp. 236–44, ISSN 0022-3565

Heyser, C.J.; Chen, W.J.; Miller, J.; Spear, N.E. & Spear, L.P. (1990). Prenatal cocaine exposure induces deficits in Pavlovian conditioning and sensory preconditioning among infant rat pups. Behavioral Neuroscience, Vol.104, No.6, (December, 1990), pp. 955–963, ISSN 0735-7044

Hodos, W. (1961). Progressive ratio as a measure of reward strength. Science, Vol.134, No.3483, (September, 1961), pp. 943-944, ISSN 0036-8075

Horan, B.; Gardner, E.L. & Ashby, C.R. (2000). Enhancement of conditioned place preference response to cocaine in rats following subchronic administration of 3,4-methylenedioxymethamphetamine (MDMA). Synapse, Vol.35, No.2, (February, 2000), pp. 160–162, ISSN 0887-4476

Inman-Wood, S.L.; Williams, M.T.; Morford, L.L. & Vorhees, C.V. (2000). Effects of prenatal cocaine on Morris and Barnes maze tests of spatial learning and memory in the offspring of C57BL/6J mice. Neurotoxicology & Teratology, Vol.22, No.4, (July-August, 2000), pp. 547–557, ISSN 0892-0362

Insel, T.R.; Miller, L.P. & Gelhard, R.E. (1990). The ontogeny of excitatory amino acid receptors in rat forebrain: I. N-methyl-d-aspartate and quisqualate receptors. Neuroscience, Vol.35, No.1, pp. 31–43, ISNN 0306-4522

Itzhak, Y. & Martin, J.L. (2002). Effect of the neuronal nitric oxide synthase inhibitor 7-nitroindazole on methylphenidate-induced hyperlocomotion in mice. Behavioural Pharmacology, Vol.13, No.1, (February, 2002), pp. 81-86, ISSN 0091-3057

Itzhak, Y. & Ali, S.F. (2006). Role of nitrergic system in behavioral and neurotoxic effects of amphetamine analogs. Pharmacology & Therapeutics, Vol.109, No.1-2, (January, 2006), pp. 246–262, ISSN 0163-7258

Izco, M.; Marchant, I.; Escobedo, I.; Peraile, I.; Delgado, M.; Higuera-Matas, A.; Olias, O.; Ambrosio, E.; O'Shea, E. & Colado, M.I. (2007). Mice with decreased cerebral dopamine function following a neurotoxic dose ofMDMA (3, 4-methylenedioxymethamphetamine, "Ecstasy") exhibit increased ethanol consumption and preference. Journal of Pharmacology & Experimental Therapeutics, Vol. 322, No.3, (September, 2007), pp. 1003–1012, ISSN 0022-3565

Jain, R. & Balhara, Y.P. (2010). Impact of alcohol and substance abuse on adolescent brain: a preclinical perspective. Indian Journal of Physiology & Pharmacology, Vol.54, No.3, pp. 213-234, ISSN 0019-5499

Johnson, E.A.; O'Callaghan, J.P. & Miller, D.B. (2004). Brain concentrations of d-MDMA are increased after stress. Psychopharmacology, Vol.173, No.3-4, (May, 2004), pp. 278–286, ISSN 0033-3158

Jones, B.C.; Ben-Hamida, S.; de Vasconcelos, A.P.; Kelche, C.; Lazarus, C.; Jackisch, R. & Cassel, J.C. (2010). Effects of ethanol and ecstasy on conditioned place preference in the rat. Journal of Psychopharmacology, Vol.24, No.2, (February, 2010), pp. 275–279, ISSN 0269-8811

Knackstedt, L.A. & Kalivas, P.W. (2007). Extended access to cocaine self-administration enhances drug-primed reinstatement but not behavioral sensitization. Journal of Pharmacology and Experimental Therapeutics, Vol.322, No.3, (September, 2007), pp. 1103-1109. ISSN 0022-3565

Laviola, G., Adriani, W.; Terranova, M.L. & Gerra, G. (1999). Psychobiological risk factors for vulnerability to psychostimulants in human adolescents and animal models. Neuroscience & Biobehavioral Reviews, Vol.23, No.7, (November, 1999), pp. 993–1010, ISSN 0149-7634

Laviola, G.; Wood, R.D.; Kuhn, C. & Francis, R.L.P. (1995). Cocaine sensitization in periadolescent and adult rats. Journal of Pharmacology & Experimental Therapeutics, Vol.275, No.1, (October, 1995), pp. 345–357, ISSN 0022-3565

Laviola, G.; Pascucci, T. & Pieretti, S. (2001). Striatal dopamine sensitization to d-amphetamine in periadolescent but not in adult rats. Pharmacology, Biochemistry & Behavior, Vol.68, No.1, (January, 2001), pp. 115–124, ISSN 0091-3057

Lidow, M.S.; Goldman-Rakic, P.S. & Rakic, P. (1991). Synchronized overproduction of neurotransmitter receptors in diverse regions of the primate cerebral cortex. Proceedings of the National Academy of Sciences of USA, Vol.88, No.22, (November, 1991), pp. 10218–10221, ISSN 0027-8424

Luna, B.; Padmanabhan, A. & O'Hearn K. (2010) What has fMRI told us about the Development of Cognitive Control through Adolescence? Brain & Cognition, Vol. 72, No.1, (February, 2010), pp.101, ISSN 0278-2626

Lynskey, M.T.; Heath, A.C.; Bucholz, K.K.; Slutske, W.S.; Madden, P.A.; Nelson, E.C.; Statham, D.J. & Martin, N.G. (2003). Escalation of drug use in early-onset cannabis users vs co-twin controls. Journal of the American Medical Association, Vol.289, No.4, (January, 2003), pp. 427-433, ISSN 0098-7484

Maldonado, R.; Valverde, O. & Berrendero, F. (2006). Involvement of the endocannabinoid system in drug addiction. Trends in Neurosciences, Vol.29, No.4, (April, 2006), pp. 225-232, ISSN 0166-2236

Manzanedo, C.; Aguilar, M.A.; Rodríguez-Arias, M.; Navarro, M. & Miñarro, J. (2004). Cannabinoid agonist-induced sensitisation to morphine place preference in mice. NeuroReport, Vol.15, No.8, (June, 2004), pp. 1373-1377, ISSN 0959-4965

Manzanedo, C.; Aguilar, M.A.; Rodriguez-Arias, M. & Minarro, J. (2005). Sensitization to the rewarding effects of morphine depends on dopamine. NeuroReport, Vol.16, No.2, (February, 2005), pp. 201–205, ISSN 0959-4965

Manzanedo, C.; Rodríguez-Arias, M.; Daza-Losada, M.; Maldonado, C.; Aguilar, M.A. & Miñarro, J. (2010). Effect of the CB1 cannabinoid agonist WIN 55212-2 on the acquisition and reinstatement of MDMA-induced conditioned place preference in mice. Behavioral & Brain Functions, Vol.6, (March, 2010), p. 19. ISSN 1744-9081

Merola, J.L. & Liederman, J. (1985). Developmental changes in hemispheric independence. Child Development, Vol.56, No.5, (October, 1985), pp. 1184–1194, ISSN 0009-3920

Mohamed, W.M.; Hamida, S.B.; de Vasconcelos, A.P.; Cassel, J.C. & Jones, B.C. (2009). Interactions between 3, 4-methylenedioxymethamphetamine and ethanol in humans and rodents. Neuropsychobiology, Vol.60, No.3-4, pp. 188–194, ISSN 0302-282X

Morley-Fletcher, S.; Bianchi, M.; Gerra, G. & Laviola, G. (2002). Acute and carryover effects in mice of MDMA ("ecstasy") administration during periadolescence. European Journal of Pharmacology, Vol.448, No.1, (July, 2002), pp. 31–38, ISSN 0014-2999

Moser, P.; Wolinsky, T.; Duxon, M. & Porsolt, R.D. (2011). How Good Are Current Approaches to Nonclinical Evaluation of Abuse and Dependence? Journal of Pharmacology & Experimental Therapeutics, Vol.336, No.3, (March, 2011), pp. 588–595, ISSN 0022-3565

Nakazi, M.; Bauer, U.; Nickel, T.; Kathmann, M. & Schlicker, E. (2000). Inhibition of serotonin release in the mouse brain via presynaptic cannabinoid CB1 receptors. Naunyn-Schmiedeberg´s Archives of Pharmacoogy, Vol.361, No.1, (January, 2000), pp. 19-24, ISSN 0028-1298

Navarro, J.F. & Maldonado, E. (2002). Acute and subchronic effects of MDMA ("ecstasy") on anxiety in male mice tested in the elevated plus-maze, Progress in Neuropsychopharmacology & Biological Psychiatry, Vol.26, No.6, (October, 2002), pp. 1151–1154, ISSN 0278-5846

Nestler, E.J. (2004). Historical review: Molecular and cellular mechanisms of opiate and cocaine addiction. Trends in Pharmacological Sciences, Vol.25, No.4, (April, 2004), pp. 210–218, ISSN 0165-6147

O'Shea, E.; Esteban, B.; Camarero, J.; Green, A.R. & Colado, M.I. (2001). Effect of GBR 12909 and fluoxetine on the acute and long term changes induced by MDMA ('ecstasy') on the 5-HT and dopamine concentrations in mouse brain. Neuropharmacology, Vol.40, No.1, pp. 65–74, ISSN 0028-3908

Pascual, M.; Blanco, A.M.; Cauli, O.; Miñarro, J. & Guerri, C. (2007). Intermittent ethanol exposure induces inflammatory brain damage and causes long-term behavioural alterations in adolescent rats. European Journal of Neuroscience, Vol.25, No.2, (January, 2007), pp. 541–550, ISSN 0953-816X

Paus, T.; Collins, D.L.; Evans, A.C.; Leonard, G.; Pike,B. & Zijdenbos,A. (2001). Maturation of white matter in the human brain: a review of magnetic resonance studies. Brain Research Bulletin, Vol.54, No.3, (February, 2001), pp. 255–266, ISSN 0361-9230

Pazos, M.R.; Sagredo, O. & Fernández-Ruiz, J. (2008). The endocannabinoid system in Huntington's disease. Current Pharmaceutical Design, Vol.14, No.23, pp. 2317-2325, ISSN 1381-6128

Piazza, P.V. & LeMoal, M. (1998). The role of stress in drug self-administration. Trends in Pharmacological Sciences, Vol.19, No.2, (February, 1998), pp. 67–74, ISSN 0165-6147

Pickles, A.; Pickering, K.; Simonoff, E.; Silberg, J.; Meyer, J. & Maes, H. (1998). Genetic clocks and soft events: A twin model for pubertal development and other recalled sequences of developmental milestones, transitions, or ages at onset. Behavior Genetics, Vol.28, No.4, (July, 1998), pp. 243–253, ISSN 0001-8244

Piomelli, D. (2005). The endocannabinoid system: A drug discovery perspective. Current Opinion on Investigational Drugs, Vol.6, No.7, (July, 2005), pp. 672-679, ISSN 1472-4472

Pulvirenti, L., (2003). Glutamate neurotransmission in the course of cocaine addiction. In: Glutamate and Addiction, Herman, B.H. (Ed.), Humana Press, New Jersey, pp. 171–181 ISBN-10: 0896038793

Ribeiro Do Couto, B.; Aguilar, M.A.; Rodríguez-Arias, M. & Miñarro, J. (2005). Cross-reinstatement by cocaine and amphetamine of morphine-induced place preference in mice. Behavioral Pharmacology, Vol.16, No.4, (July, 2005), pp. 253-259, ISSN 0955-8810

Ribeiro Do Couto, B.; Aguilar, M.A.; Manzanedo, C.; Rodríguez-Arias, M.; Armario, A. & Miñarro, J. (1996). Social stress is as effective as physical stress in reinstating morphine-induced place preference in mice. Psychopharmacology, Vol.185, No.4, (May, 2006), pp. 459-470, ISSN 0033-3158

Ribeiro Do Couto, B.; Rodríguez-Arias, M.; Fuentes, S.; Gagliano, H.; Armario, A.; Miñarro, J. & Aguilar, MA. (2011). Adolescent pre-exposure to ethanol or MDMA prolongs the conditioned rewarding effects of MDMA. Physiology & Behavior, Vol.103, No.5, (July, 2011), pp.585-593, ISSN 0031-9384

Ribeiro Do Couto, B.; Daza-Losada, M.; Rodríguez-Arias, M.; Nadal, R.; Guerri, C.; Summavielle, T.; Miñarro, J. & Aguilar, M.A. (2011). Adolescent pre-exposure to ethanol and MDMA increases conditioned rewarding effects of MDMA and drug-induced reinstatement. Addiction Biology, in press, ISSN 1369-1600

Rice, D. & Barone, S. Jr. (2000). Critical periods of vulnerability for the developing nervous system: evidence from humans and animal models. Environment Health Perspectives, Vol.108, No.3, (June, 2000), pp. 511–533, ISSN 0091-6765

Riegert, C.; Wedekind, F.; Hamida, S.B.; Rutz, S.; Rothmaier, A.K.; Jones, B.C.; Cassel, J.C. & Jackisch, R. (2008). Effects of ethanol and 3, 4-methylenedioxymethamphetamine (MDMA) alone or in combination on spontaneous and evoked overflow of dopamine, serotonin and acetylcholine in striatal slices of the rat brain. International Journal of Neuropsychopharmacology, Vol.11, No.6, (September, 2008) pp. 743–763, ISSN 1461-1457

Riley, S.C.; James, C.; Gregory, D.; Dingle, H. & Cadger, M. (2001). Patterns of recreational drug use at dance events in Edinburgh, Scotland. Addiction, Vol.96, No.7, (July, 2001), pp. 1035–1047, ISSN 0965-2140

Rivers, S.E.; Reyna, V.F. & Mills, B. (2008). Risk taking under the influence: a fuzzy-trace theory of emotion in adolescence. Developmental Review, Vol.28, No.1, (March, 2008), pp. 107–144, ISSN 0273-2297

Robinson, T.E. & Berridge, K.C. (2008). Review. The incentive sensitization theory of addiction: some current issues. Philosophical Transactions of the Royal Society B: Biological Sciences, Vol.363, No.1507, (October, 2008), pp. 3137–3146, ISSN 0080-4622

Robledo, P.; Trigo, J.M.; Panayi, F.; de la Torre, R. & Maldonado, R. (2007). Behavioural and neurochemical effects of combined MDMA and THC administration in mice. Psychopharmacology, Vol.195, No.2, (December, 2007), pp. 255-264, ISSN 0033-3158

Rodríguez-Arias, M.; Manzanedo, C.; Roger-Sánchez, C.; Do Couto, B.R.; Aguilar, M.A. & Miñarro, J. (2010). Effect of adolescent exposure to WIN 55212-2 on the acquisition and reinstatement of MDMA-induced conditioned place preference. Progress in Neuropsychopharmacology & Biological Psychiatry, Vol.34, No.1, (February, 2010), pp. 166-171, ISSN 0278-5846

Rodríguez-Arias, M.; Maldonado, C.; Vidal-Infer, A.; Guerri, C.; Aguilar, M.A. & Miñarro, J. (2011). Intermittent ethanol exposure increases long-lasting behavioral and neurochemical effects of MDMA in adolescent mice. Psychopharmacology, May 10. DOI: 10.1007/s00213-011-2329-x, ISSN 0033-3158

Rodrıguez de Fonseca, F.; Ramos, J.A.; Bonnin, A. & Fernandez-Ruiz, J.J. (1993). Presence of cannabinoid binding sites in the brain from early postnatal ages. NeuroReport, Vol.4, No., (mes, 1993), pp. 135–138, ISSN 0959-4965

Romieu, P.; Meunier, J.; Garcia, D.; Zozime, N.; Martın-Fardon, R.; Bowen, W.D. & Maurice, T. (2004). The sigma1 (□1) receptor activation is a key step for the reactivation of cocaine conditioned place preference by drug priming. Psychopharmacology, Vol.175, No.2, (September, 2004), pp. 154–162, ISSN 0033-3158

Rubovitch, V.; Gafni, M. & Sarne, Y. (2002). The cannabinoid agonist DALN positively modulates L-type voltage-dependent calcium channels in N18TG2 neuroblastoma cells. Molecular Brain Research, Vol.101, No.1-2, (May, 2002), pp. 93-102, ISSN 0169-328X

Sanchis-Segura, C. & Spanagel, R. (2006). Behavioural assessment of drug reinforcement and addictive features in rodents: an overview. Addiction Biology, Vol.11, No.1, (March, 2006), pp. 2-38, ISSN 1369-1600

Sarne, Y. & Keren, O. (2004). Are cannabinoid drugs neurotoxic or neuroprotective? Medical Hypotheses, Vol.63, No.2, pp. 187-192, ISSN 0306-9877

Schensul, J.J.; Convey, M. & Burkholder, G. (2005) Challenges in measuring concurrency, agency and intentionality in polydrug research. Addictive Behaviours, Vol.30, No.3, (March, 2005), pp. 571-574, ISSN 0306-4603

Schramm-Sapyta, N.L.; Walker, Q.D.; Caster, J.M.; Levin, E.D. & Kuhn, C.M. (2009). Are adolescents more vulnerable to drug addiction than adults? Evidence from animal models. Psychopharmacology, Vol.206, No.1, (September, 2009), pp. 1-21, ISSN 0033-3158

Seeman, P.; Bzowej, N.H.; Guan, H-C; Bergeron, C.; Becker, L.E.; Reynolds, G.P.; Bird, E.D.; Riederer, P.; Jellinger, K.; Watanabe, S. & Tourtellotte, W.W. (1987). Human brain dopamine receptors in children and aging adults. Synapse, Vol.1, No.5, pp. 399–404, ISSN 0887-4476

Segal, D.S. & Kuczenski, R. (1997). An escalating dose "binge" model of amphetamine psychosis: behavioral and neurochemical characteristics. Journal of Neuroscience, Vol.17, No.7, (April, 1997), pp. 2551–2566, ISSN -0270-6474

Shalev, U.; Grimm, J.W. & Shaham, Y (2002). Neurobiology of relapse to heroin and cocaine seeking: a review. Vol. Pharmacological Reviews, Vol.54, No.1, (March, 2002), pp. 1–42, ISSN 0031-6997

Shippenberg, T.S. & Heidbreder, C. (1995). Sensitization to the conditioned rewarding effects of cocaine: pharmacological and temporal characteristics. Journal of Pharmacology & Experimental Therapeutics, Vol.273, No.2, (May, 1995), pp. 808–815, ISSN 0022-3565

Shippenberg, T.S. & Koob (2002) Recent Advances in Animal Models of Drug Addiction, In: *Neuropsychopharmacology: The Fifth Generation of Progress*, Kenneth L. Davis, Dennis Charney, Joseph T. Coyle, and Charles Nemeroff (Eds), pp.1381-1397, American College of Neuropsychopharmacology, ISBN-10: 0781728371, Nashville, TN.

Shippenberg, T.S.; LeFevour, A. & Thompson, A.C. (1998). Sensitization to the conditioned rewarding effects of morphine and cocaine: differential effects of the kappa opioid receptor agonist U69593. European Journal of Pharmacology, Vol.345, No.1, (March, 1998), pp. 27–34, ISSN 0014-2999

Shippenberg, T.S.; Zapata, A.; Chefer, V.I. (2007) Dynorphin and the pathophysiology of drug addiction. Pharmacology and Therapeutics, Vol. 116, No. 2 (November, 2007) pp. 306-321, ISSN 0163-7258

Sowell, E.R.; Trauner, D.A.; Gamst, A. & Jernigan, T.L. (2002). Development of cortical and subcortical brain structures in childhood and adolescence: a structural MRI study. Developmental Medicine & Child Neurology, Vol.44, No.1, (January, 2002), pp. 4–16, ISSN 0012-1622

Spear, L.P. (2000). The adolescent brain and age-related behavioral manifestations. Neuroscience & Biobehavioral Reviews, Vol.24, No.4, (June, 2000), pp. 417-463, ISSN 0149-7634

Spear, L.P. (2011a). Rewards, aversions and affect in adolescence: Emerging convergences across laboratory animal and human data. In: Developmental Cognitive Neuroscience, Ron Dahl and Louk Vanderschuren (Eds), Vol. 1, No.4, pp.390-403. ISSN: 1878-9293.

Spear, L.P. (2011b). Adolescent neurobehavioral characteristics, alcohol sensitivities, and intake: Setting the stage for alcohol use disorders?. In: Child Development Perspectives, Vol.5, No.4, pp.231-238. ISSN 1750-8606.

Sprague, J.E. & Nichols, D.E. (2005). Neurotoxicity of MDMA (ecstasy): beyond metabolism. Trends in Pharmacological Sciences, Vol. 26, No.2, (February, 2005), pp. 59–60, ISSN 0165-6147

Steketee, J.D. & Kalivas, P.W. (2011). Drug Wanting: Behavioral Sensitization and Relapse to Drug-Seeking Behavior. Pharmacological Reviews, Vol.63, No.2, (June, 2011) pp. 348–365, ISSN 0031-6997

Stone, E.A. & Quartermain, D. (1998). Greater behavioral effects of stress in immature as compared to mature male mice. Physiology & Behavior, Vol.63, No.1, (December, 1998), pp. 143–145, ISSN 0031-9384

Sturman, D.A. & Moghaddam, B. (2011). The neurobiology of adolescence: Changes in brain architecture, functional dynamics, and behavioral tendencies. Neuroscience & Biobehavioral Reviews, Vol.35, No.8, (August, 2011), pp. 1704-1712, ISSN 0149-7634

Teicher, M.H.; Andersen, S.L. & Hostetter, J.C. Jr. (1995). Evidence for dopamine receptor pruning between adolescence and adulthood in striatum but not nucleus accumbens. Developmental Brain Research, Vol.89, No.2, (November, 1995), pp. 167–172, ISSN 0165-3806

Tzschentke, T.M. (1998). Measuring reward with the conditioned place preference paradigm: a comprehensive review of drug effects, recent progress and new issues. Progress in Neurobiology, Vol.56, No.6, (December, 1998), pp. 613–672, ISSN 0301-0082

Upreti, V.V.; Eddington, N.D.; Moon, K.H.; Song, B.J. & Lee, I.J. (2009). Drug interaction between ethanol and 3,4-methylenedioxymethamphetamine ("ecstasy"). Toxicology Letters, Vol.188, No.2, (July, 2009), pp. 167–172, ISSN 0378-4274

Vázquez, D.M. (1998). Stress and the developing limbic–hypothalamic- pituitary–adrenal axis. Psychoneuroendocrinology, Vol.23, No.7, (October, 1998), pp. 663–700, ISSN 0306-4530

Vigil, P.; Orellana, R.F.; Cortes, M.E.; Molina, C.T.; Switzer, B.E. & Klaus, H. (2011). Endocrine Modulation of the Adolescent Brain: A Review. Journal of Pediatric and Adolescent Gynecology, (April 20), doi:10.1016/j.jpag.2011.01.061 ISSN 1083-3188

von Sydow, K.; Lieb, R.; Pfister, H.; Hofler, M. & Wittchen, H.U. (2002). Use, abuse and dependence of ecstasy and related drugs in adolescents and young adults—a transient phenomenon? Results from a longitudinal community study. Drug & Alcohol Dependence, Vol.66, No.2, (April, 2002), pp. 147–159, ISSN 0376-8716

Wagner, E.F., Myers, M.G. & McIninch. J.L. (1999). Stress-coping and temptation-coping as predictors of adolescent substance use. Addictive Behaviors, Vol.24, No.6, (November-December, 1999), pp. 769-779, ISSN 0306-4603

Walters, C.L.; Kuo, Y.C. & Blendy, J.A. (2003). Differential distribution of CREB in the mesolimbic dopamine reward pathway. Journal of Neurochemistry, Vol.87, No.5, (December, 2003), pp. 1237–1244, ISSN 0022-3042

Wang, B.; Luo, F.; Zhang, W.T. & Han, J.S. (2000). Stress or drug priming induces reinstatement of extinguished conditioned place preference. NeuroReport, Vol.11, No.12, (August, 2000), pp. 2781–2784, ISSN 0959-4965

Weiss, F. (2010). Advances in Animal Models of Relapse for Addiction Research. In: Advances in the Neuroscience of Addiction. Kuhn CM, Koob GF, (Eds). CRC Press, Frontiers in Neuroscience. ISBN-10: 0849373913 Boca Raton (FL)

Wolfer, D.P. & Lipp, H-P. (1995). Evidence for physiological growth of hippocampal mossy fiber collaterals in the guinea pig during puberty and adulthood. Hippocampus, Vol.5, No.4, pp. 329–340, ISSN 1098-1063

9

Food Addiction, Obesity and Neuroimaging

Karen M. von Deneen[1] and Yijun Liu[2]
[1]*Xidian University,*
[2]*University of Florida,*
[1]*China*
[2]*USA*

1. Introduction

This chapter will be dedicated to addressing various aspects of food addiction (where food is portrayed as being an addictive substance). It will encompass our group's and colleagues' newest neuroimaging research results and methods with respect to the findings of other researchers in the field. The chapter will attempt to elucidate the mechanisms of food addiction (FA) leading to obesity. It will begin with a brief introduction on the major points relating to obesity and FA. The first section will address the neurobiology and neurophysiology of addiction as well as the causes of obesity and its global impacts, concluding with therapeutic measures and future research.

2. Food addiction and obesity: Health problems

Obesity-related deaths rank second in the world (Mokdad et al., 2004). Obesity is linked with stroke, heart disease, diabetes mellitus, osteoarthritis, and certain cancers (Raman, 2002). Developing countries have also been affected by this global epidemic (Zemmet, 2000). The number of adults over the age of 20 with a BMI over 30 has increased rapidly over the past 20 years (Pi-Sunyer, 2002). Although the etiology of obesity has been predominantly correlated with eating behavior, other factors such as individual preferences, mental disorders, genetic makeup, or addictive tendencies have been suggested to play contributing roles (von Deneen and Liu, 2011). Among some known etiological factors, the intrauterine environment plays a role in placing children at risk for becoming obese and having diabetes and high cholesterol levels (Blumenthal & Gold, 2010). McMillen et al. (2009) suggested that specific periods during pregnancy predisposed individuals to obesity, therefore maternal nutrition and perinatal lifestyle played a major role in fetal programming. Over-nutrition during pregnancy led to larger offspring or gestational diabetes associated with obesity, while breastfeeding could counter the effects of obesity (Martorell et al., 2001).

New insights into the obesity issue involved developing an FA model that states food is eaten for pleasure and hedonistic intake of food can be linked with drug addiction and eating disorders.

This section will assess childhood obesity etiology, metabolic syndrome, dietary and behavioral causes with a specific impetus on the Han Chinese population (von Deneen et al.,

2011). Obesity particularly in China has led to worldwide attention and is becoming a pandemic disease resulting from a shift in energy balance caused by altered genes, a sedentary lifestyle, and neurohormonal imbalances as a result of Western influence. Obesity is spreading to low income and middle-income countries, such as China, as a result of novel dietary habits, promoting chronic diseases and premature mortality (Cecchini et al., 2010). Work-related activities declined, whereas leisure time is dominated by television/computer programs and other physically inactive pursuits (Popkin, 2001). The vicious obesity cycle begins with excess adipose leading to chronic low grade inflammation that results in insulin resistance (IR) along with hypertension, atherosclerosis, dyslipidemia and type 2 diabetes mellitus (T2DM), which are consistent findings of metabolic syndrome (MetS) (Achike et al., 2011). Studies have shown that obesity can be linked to lower ghrelin concentrations in obese individuals (Groschl et al., 2005). As a result, ghrelin levels have been found to be negatively correlated with body fat and waist circumference (WC) (Fagerberg, Hulten & Hulthe, 2003).

Metabolic syndrome (MetS) is defined as "a combination of clinical disorders that increase the risk for diabetes and cardiovascular disease, including atherosclerosis, stroke and hypertension" (Achike et al., 2011). The components of MetS include abdominal fat, atherogenic dyslipidemia, hypertension, pro-inflammatory state, pro-thrombic state and IR with or without glucose intolerance (Grundy et al., 2004). Obesity, dyslipidemia and hyperglycemia are all risk factors for colorectal cancer (Giovannucci, 2002). Increased plasma free fatty acids (FFA) in obese Chinese people acted as an important link between obesity and IR, and plasma FFA levels were negatively correlated with insulin sensitivity (Li et al., 2005). The Chinese were five times more likely to have a family history of T2DM than non-Chinese subjects (Xu et al., 2010). Finally, in middle-aged and elderly Chinese living in northeast China, there was a higher incidence of MetS and cardiovascular disease, especially atherosclerosis (Liu et al., 2010), which is increasing as influenced by a Westernized lifestyle (Mi et al., 2008).

2.1 Social and cultural influence on obesity

Parents and extended family members play a crucial role in shaping their children's eating and exercise habits (Rhee, 2008). This is a global phenomenon, but the best example to describe the state the world is in with regards to obesity is China. Even though the Western world (first world countries) has had the greatest problems with obesity and FA, China is following in its footsteps. Approximately 22% of Chinese parents regarded their children as being underweight even if their children weren't. Meanwhile, 23% of overweight children were perceived by their parents as being normal (Shi et al., 2007). Parental assessment of the weights of their children was associated with the physical appearance of the parents themselves (Huang, Becerra & Oda, 2007). Overweight daughters were more likely to be criticized by their mothers (Maynard et al., 2003). Chinese parents tended to misperceive their sons' weights more than their daughters'. Mothers had a better ability to discriminate their children's size. This gender difference could be related to social values and status (Campbell et al., 2006), hence exacerbating the obesity problem. For example, girls with slim and graceful bodies were deemed acceptable by Chinese society, while overweight boys were regarded as "strong and healthy" (Maynard et al., 2003). Parents' and other family members' 'pressure to eat' strategy was correlated with children's caloric consumption (Drucker et al., 1999). Another important factor leading to childhood obesity is that a high portion of Hong-Kong school children spend too many hours watching television (TV) and playing computer or video games (Kong & Chow, 2010). Overweight or obese adolescents had a tendency to view TV programs and become less physically active. In China, access to Westernized TV programming and food advertising has increased (Hong, 1998). Advertisements for food products, such as soft drinks and salty snacks, constituted more than 80% of commercials in China (Ji & McNeal, 2001). According to mothers surveyed in urban areas in China, many children have their own spending money, and they often use this money to buy snacks and beverages (Zhang & Harwood, 2004). Chinese parents stated that their children influenced most of their purchases, especially of snacks (McNeal & Yeh, 1997). This can be witnessed in most Chinese cities with large supermarkets today. Food products and restaurant chains seen in TV programs and commercials provide food cues to children, thus enhancing the need to snack while watching TV (Coon et al., 2001). TV is present in almost every Chinese household, and TV advertising in China increasingly promotes high-calorie foods (Parvanta et al., 2010). Low-income families spend more hours watching TV than their counterparts (Livingstone, 2002). However, snacks seen on TV tended to be purchased more by those with higher incomes (Wang et al., 2008b). All in all, this evidence portrays that non-physical entertainment does play a major role in weight management in young people all over the world.

China can be portrayed as a "double burden of malnutrition" where under-nutrition coexists with obesity (Popkin et al., 1995). The food selection and consumption in China has resulted in a diet that is more energy-dense and laden with saturated animal fat and processed sugars, and is low in complex carbohydrates, fiber, fresh fruits and vegetables (Zhai et al., 2009). Underprivileged individuals tend to stock up on non-nutritious, high-calorie foods as low-budget staples, whereas nutrient-rich foods and high-quality diets are consumed by more affluent customers (Jones et al., 2007). In China, sugar-sweetened beverages (SSB) are a major food source with a high glycemic index (Murakami et al., 2006), thus are easily exploitable as a form of addictive substance. Another study found associations between frequent SSB intake and obesity predominantly in Chinese women, while lack of exercise, smoking, and high meat consumption increased the risk for greater weight gain in both genders (Ko et al., 2010). One study found that overweight children and adolescents consumed more energy, protein, and fat and ate fewer carbohydrates than did the controls (Guldan, 2010). They consumed less grain, fewer vegetables, more fruits, meats and cooking oil, eggs, fish, milk, and legumes. Those who ate at least 25g of cooking oil, 200g of meat, and 100g of dairy products had a higher chance of being overweight (Li et al., 2007).

From a recent cross-sectional survey done in Jiangsu Province, researchers found that a higher socio-economic status and urban residency were associated with energy-dense foods such as animal and dairy products, soft drinks, Western food, and increased snacking/breakfast skipping behaviors (Shi et al., 2005). Rural and lower income students normally consumed rice porridge, a traditional, thin breakfast gruel. However, they also preferred hamburgers, ice cream, milk, fruits, chocolate, and SSB (Shi et al., 2005). The traditional Chinese high-glycemic diet consists of a variety of high-glycemic staple rice products such as boiled rice, rice congee, and glutinous rice which pose adverse cardiovascular and MetS risks (Ding & Malik, 2008). When the Chinese population was lean and active, this diet did not pose as much risk. However, China today has an obesity epidemic and a dietary transition shifting toward more processed foods such as SSB (Ding & Malik, 2008).

The reason is that these foods are "appetizing, convenient and ready to eat, portable, affordable in single portions," and widely marketed for the younger generation, allowing them to be addicted to these foods. These addictive substances include soft drinks, biscuits, snacks, and fast-food sandwiches (Guldan, 2010). Higher incomes in China allow families to purchase SSB, snacks, and fast food. Supermarkets are packed with highly-processed, energy-dense, nutrient-poor, and lower-priced foods. Preferences include polished grains/white rice products, because Chinese consumers are unaware of the benefits from whole grains (Guldan, 2010). Another major dietary component is glutamate, which is a major taste ingredient of dietary protein described as 'Umami' (Kurihara & Kashiwayangani, 2000). Increasing concern with the rise of obesity in Westernized nations with the addition of monosodium glutamate (MSG) to commercially prepared foods is evident (Shi et al., 2010). There was a positive association between MSG consumption and the socio-economic status in rural China (Shi et al., 2010). Along those lines, Kazaks, Uyghurs and Mongolians are the major minorities in Xinjiang. The Kazaks have been reported to have hypertension (Jumabay et al., 2001), while obesity is common in the Uyghurs and Mongolians (Wang et al., 2006). Significant differences in mean blood pressure between Han, Kazaks, Uyghurs and Tibetan ethnic groups were deemed to be caused by different diet-related habits. It is well-known that alcohol, high-sodium foods and meat are traditionally popular among these groups, which are associated with surviving the cold weather in Xinjiang. Traditionally among Kazaks, Uyghurs and Mongolians in Xinjiang, alcohol consumption is paired with eating large amounts of animal fat or salty dishes, which could lead to an increase in fibrinogen levels. Males in particular traditionally drink spirits to deal with the cold. Additionally, salted milk tea is consumed in large amounts; vegetables are also rare in this region, hence they are not commonly consumed (Xi & Mi, 2009).

Eating disorders ranged from 1.3% to 5.21% among young Chinese females (Fu et al., 2005). However, these data do not represent the entire population. Currently, there is little knowledge about weight control concerns and behaviors in China. Body mass index (BMI), dieting, and eating disorder symptoms are not clearly defined (Fan et al., 2010). Another important study of adolescents in China found a strong association between smoking and the belief that smoking was important in weight control (Ge et al., 1994).

Overall, there are numerous problems arising from this epidemic such as psychosocial, emotional, neurological, cardiovascular, endocrine, musculoskeletal, gastrointestinal and pulmonary issues (Ebbeling, Pawlak & Ludwig, 2002). The costs of healthcare "associated with being overweight or obese projected exceed 850 billion dollars annually by 2030 in United States alone (Wang et al., 2008a)." As a result, this leads to a significant financial burden.

3. Biology and neurobiology of food intake

Food consumption is regulated via peripheral signals and central neuronal circuits (Wang et al., 2009) including the hypothalamus (HYP), amygdala (AMY), hippocampus (HIPP), insula, orbitofrontal cortex (OFC), and striatal brain regions (Dagher, 2009). These pathways regulate mechanisms of food reward, environmental stimuli perception, and integration of homeostasis of energy and gastrointestinal tract contents with food availability (Dagher, 2009). Most importantly, midbrain dopamine (DA) reward circuits motivate food ingestion and hedonistic sensations resulting from eating (Dagher, 2009) as well as brain opioid peptides (Barbano et al., 2005), which in turn work in tandem with other circuits responsible for enforcing feeding behaviors and weight regulation (Wang et al., 2009), as seen in Figure 1.

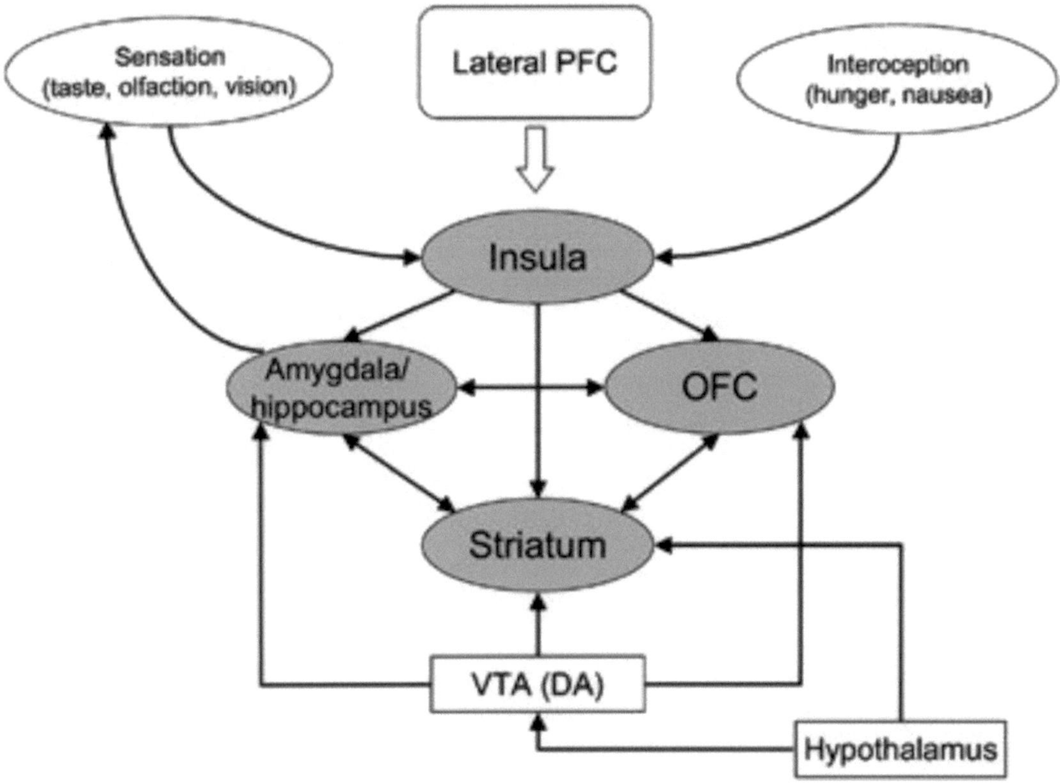

Fig. 1. A generalized brain network for regulation of hunger as depicted from Dagher (2009). PFC, prefrontal cortex; OFC, orbitofrontal cortex; VTA, ventral tegmental area; DA, dopamine.

The HYP and its circuits include orexin (ORX) and melanin concentrating hormone producing neurons in the lateral HYP as well as neuropeptide Y (NPY)/agouti related protein and alpha-melanocyte stimulating hormone producing neurons in the arcuate nucleus (ARC) known as the principal homeostatic brain regions responsible for regulating body weight (Wang et al., 2009). At the cellular level, important factors involved in communicating with the ARC in hunger regulation include ORX, melanin, NPY, and alpha-melanocyte-stimulating hormone (Wang et al., 2009). Ghrelin, leptin, insulin, and peptide YY all regulate hunger, satiety, and metabolism by stimulating neurons in the HYP (Wang et al., 2009). Ghrelin interacts with HYP depending on food intake, while leptin relays information to the HYP as well with regards to adipose storage (Wang et al., 2009). Insulin and peptide YY regulate metabolic changes (Wang et al., 2009). A useful summary of the neuropeptides that have the most dramatic influence on weight and eating regulation is listed in Table 1 and is also described in more detail by Wang et al. (2009).

Stimulate feeding	Inhibit feeding
Decrease energy expenditure	Increase energy expenditure
Anandamide	Calcitonin, Amylin, Bombesin, Somatostatin, Cytokines
β-endorphin	Cholecystokinin
Dynorphin	CRF
GABA	Dopamine
Galanin	Insulin
Ghrelin	Leptin
GHRH	Neurotensin
Neuropeptide Y	Serotonin
Norepinephrine	TRH, MSH, Glucagon, Enterostatin

Table 1. Neuropeptides That Regulate Food Intake (Sahu & Kalra, 1993)

4. Food addiction: Failure in self-regulation

Overeating and obesity are related to other substance addictions, not only in terms of overlapping neural substrates, but also in terms of genetic and environmental influences on eating behaviors and the implications that these influences have on treatment (Joranby, Pineda & Gold, 2005). The interaction between central satiety signals and reward responses to food stimuli with regards to failure in self-regulation will be discussed.

There are two primary circuits depicting reward behavior. The first one is the connected regions of the prefrontal cortex and the AMY. The second one is the limbic system involving the AMY, HYP, septal nuclei, ventral striatum, and dopaminergic innervations (Augustine, 1996). In most addictions, long-term is associated with drastic physiological alterations in the reward circuitry (Goldstein & Volkow, 2002) such as down-regulation of motivation, higher cognition and self-monitoring. Most importantly, emotions are correlated with the strength of the addiction (Shapira et al., 2003). One study found that hunger signals in the right OFC caused cravings and memories of food in fasting patients (Morris & Dolan, 2001). In more detail, those that fasted recognized previously viewed food faster. This is interesting because it implies dissociable roles of the OFC and left AMY in recognition of previously viewed food, while the nucleus accumbens (NA_c) responds to internal reward (Morris & Dolan, 2001).

4.1 Homeostatic substrates of over-eating

Hyperphagia is primarily due to continuous stimulation of NPY receptors (Kalra & Kalra, 1996). An imbalance of NPY signaling at a local level in the hypothalamus (ARC and paraventricular nucleus (PVN)) results in unregulated eating (Kalra & Kalra, 2004a). The neurotransmitter γ-aminobutyric acid (GABA) has also been known to enhance feeding behavior via its receptors, causing decreased melanocortin signaling to the PVN, which in turn results in hyperphagia (Cowley et al., 2001). Furthermore, it is possible that mutations or disturbances of α-melanocyte stimulating hormone (α-MSH) and other peptides involved in satiety can lead to hyperphagia and obesity (Kalra et al., 1999). Finally, in the case of abnormal hypothalamic function that accounts for a variety of eating disorders, it may lead to hyperglycemia, which in turn causes other endocrine problems (Liu & Gold, 2003). This may be explained by one dietary example where fructose was consumed. Fructose promotes insulin production but blocks its release (Sato et al., 1996). Insulin is known to inhibit feeding by increasing leptin which in turn leads to weight gain (Saad et al., 1998).

Hence, this would be a good model to explain why individuals with FA are obese and are more vulnerable to develop addiction-like behavior towards high carbohydrate foods containing high fructose corn syrup.

From a neurohormonal perspective, glutamate is believed to be the neurotransmitter responsible for transmitting information between the areas depicted above, although the exact mechanism is still not understood (Swanson & Petrovich, 1998). It may be plausible that potential feeding mechanisms involve direct glutamatergic connections from the basolateral amygdala (BLA) to the lateral hypothalamic area (LHA), although the exact LHA neurons involved in this process remain unidentified. Nevertheless, it may be safe to assume that BLA outputs could influence LHA subsystems required for feeding initiation. For example, groups of LHA neurons express two recently discovered neuropeptides, melanin-concentrating hormone (MCH) and ORX, which are regulated by the hunger–satiety state and are linked to initiation of feeding (Elmquist, Elias & Saper, 1999). There is still more information with regards to the interaction between ORX and FA that is outside the realm of this chapter, so refer to Kalra & Kalra (2004b). However, hunger caused by food cues is an adaptive mechanism for survival, but at the same time, learned cues can serve as a harmful force to promote overindulgence in food despite satiety. These particular learned cues can overcome specific satiety signals in order to promote continued eating (De Castro, 1997).

4.2 Metabolic substrates

The gene-environment interaction, as part of the metabolic substrates contributing to obesity, is defined as "the response or the adaptation to an environmental agent, a behavior, or a change in behavior is conditional on the genotype of the individual" (Bouchard, 2009). For example, in Fujian province, the rate of obesity has increased due to poor nutrition before and during pregnancy, economic development, urbanization and improved living standards (McAuley et al., 2001). The genetic loci associated with obesity are: *NEGR1, SEC16B-RASAL2, TMEM18, SFRS10-ETV5-DGKG, GNPDA2, NCR3-AIF1-BAT2, LGR4-LIN7CBDNF, MTCH2, BCDIN3DFAIM2, SH2B1-ATP2A1, KCTD15*, and *FTO* (fat mass and obesity associated) (Scuteri et al., 2007). The *FTO* gene is present in all tissues and encodes a non-heme (FeII)-dioxygenase that adapts to hypoxia, lipolysis, or DNA methylation (Gerken et al., 2007). This key protein may serve as a link between the central nervous system and energy homeostasis. *FTO* variants (rs8050136 and rs9939609) were associated with obesity and body mass index (BMI) in Hong Kong, Taiwan, and Singapore populations (Frayling et al., 2007). Further research needs to be done on obesity susceptibility genes for clinical applications. One study found a relationship between *FTO* SNP rs8050136 and BMI. It showed that the combined genetic risk of single-nucleotide polymorphisms (SNPs) may be useful in predicting obesity (Cheung et al., 2010). The A allele was indeed linked to obesity in Chinese adults (Li et al., 2010). Future studies need to be done if there is a link between FA and these obesity genes as well as with other addictions. For further discussion on this topic, please refer to these specific studies (Chen et al., 2009; Ruiz et al., 2010).

Prader-Willi syndrome (PWS) is the primary model for failure in self-regulation and the most important metabolic substrate with regards to hedonic food addiction (von Deneen, Gold & Liu, 2009). Our group has worked in both of these areas and believes that there are many shared neurohormonal pathways as well as distinct differences that may clue researchers in on why certain individuals overeat and become obese. Neuroimaging studies have shown that highly palatable food has characteristics similar to that of drugs of abuse. Many of the brain changes reported for hedonic eating and obesity are also seen in various forms of addictions (von Deneen et al., 2011). Most importantly, overeating and obesity may have an acquired drive such as for alcohol or drugs, and motivation and incentive craving, wanting, and liking occur after early and repeated exposures to stimuli. The acquired drive for great food and relative weakness of the satiety signal would cause an imbalance in drive and hunger centers of the HYP and their regulation. Prader-Willi may be a genetic model of the disease we are seeing on a daily basis. New hypotheses can yield new screening tests for new treatments.

4.3 Increased drive

Volkow & Fowler (2000) believe that reward circuits (NAc, AMY) have been central to drug addiction mechanisms, where the addictive state also involves disruption of circuits involved with compulsive behaviors and with increased drive. Intermittent activation of reward circuitry involving DA leads to dysfunction of the OFC via the striato-thalamo-orbitofrontal circuit. The OFC is hypermetabolic in proportion to the intensity of the craving seen after last cocaine use or during drug-induced craving (Volkow & Fowler, 2000). Since the OFC is directly involved with drive and compulsive repetitive behaviors, abnormal activation in addicted individuals could explain compulsive drug use despite adverse reactions. This indicates that pleasure by itself cannot maintain compulsive substance abuse and drugs that could interfere with the activation of the striato-thalamo-orbitofrontal circuit could be beneficial in the treatment of drug addiction (Volkow & Fowler, 2000).

Carbohydrates, as one of the most commonly abused food substances in FA, have been found to have an interesting psychological effect. For instance, women who craved and sought high-carbohydrate foods did so to alleviate negative feelings and emotions, showing that this food group depicts compulsive behavior (Corsica & Pelchat, 2010). More so, being chronically or acutely stressed led to consumption of high-fat or sugary foods, predisposing these individuals to bingeing and a failure in dieting (Dagher & Robbins, 2009; Dagher, 2009). An interesting concept is the "refined food hypothesis" in which processed foods such as sugars, fat, salt, flour, and caffeine are the source of addiction (Ifland et al., 2009) as well as salty foods which mimic opiate agonists (Cocores & Gold, 2009). Finally, interesting findings have shown that motivation circuits relating to drinking alcohol and eating fat lead to the release of hypothalamic orexigenic peptides, such as ghrelin, which increase the consumption of these foods and raise triglyceride levels (Barson et al., 2009). In a study utilizing rats, the level of triglycerides predicted increased caloric consumption and orexigenic peptide expression following a high-fat meal (Karatayev et al., 2009).

Drugs and food exert their reinforcing effects in part by increasing DA in limbic regions, which may explain how drug abuse/addiction relates to obesity (Volkow et al., 2008). Eating craved food and drug addiction result in reward circuitry activation involving DA pathways. However, these actions activate these pathways in different ways. FA affects reward circuitry through endogenous opioids and cannabinoids, while drugs share the same circuitry through direct effects on DA neurons or via indirect effects through neurotransmitters (Volkow & Wise, 2005). Overstimulation of DA leads to more compulsive behavior and loss of control of food and drug intake due to increased availability of DAD2 receptors in the striatum (Volkow & Li, 2004). However, FA can be considered more complex than drug abuse due to involvement of peripheral, endocrine and central pathways outside of the reward circuitry (Levine, Kotz & Gosnell, 2003).

The fundamental idea of the reward system hypothesis is that there must be an explicit emotional state connected with the addiction, such as seen in PWS. The stronger the emotional link, the stronger the addiction. There exist a couple of primary circuits for the reward system. The first one involves a reciprocal connection between the prefrontal areas of the brain and the AMY. The second is the limbic system that links the AMY with the HYP and septal nuclei. The Papez limbic system also joins the HYP with the hippocampus and thalamus (Joranby, Pineda & Gold, 2005). Therefore, the reward system hypothesis states that appetizing food and addictive behaviors compete for reward regions such as the NA_C . The act of overeating and obesity can lead to decreasing food reward and addiction (Kleiner et al., 2004). On the other hand, obesity is a "reward deficiency syndrome" (Blum et al., 1996). Most importantly, increased activation in the somatic parietal areas in food addicted individuals suggests that enhanced activity in these regions involves sensory processing of food, making food even more rewarding (Wang et al., 2001), which is not typical in PWS cases. The reward hypothesis was best explained through sugar-dependent rat studies (Avena, Long & Hoebel, 2005; Rada, Avena & Hoebel, 2005; Avena, Rada & Hoebel, 2008). These rats had a disrupted Acetylcholine (ACh) response to hunger, ingested greater amounts of sugar, and produced more DA than control rats (Avena, Long & Hoebel, 2005). This may explain why PWS and obese individuals may be addicted to certain palatable foods that cause a delayed, prolonged increase in ACh levels. In drug addiction, the ventral striatum and midbrain were associated with immediate rewards and the hippocampus responded to reward consequences. The globus pallidus, thalamus, and subgenual cingulate were associated with immediate rewards, while the caudate, insula, and ventral prefrontal cortex (vPFC) responded to reward consequences (Elliott, Friston & Dolan, 2000). The mesolimbic reward system is a common pathway that food and drugs follow in order to reinforce craving behavior (Tartar, Ammerman & Ott, 1998). This pathway is also affected by PWS causing aberrant reward circuitry (James et al., 2007). We are still unable to differentiate the reward system mechanisms in PWS and other addictions.

There are specific circuits and networks in the brain that regulate cravings, appetite, and cue-induced ingestion of addictive foods. The NA_C and DA are specifically responsible for food reward and motivated eating (Cardinal et al., 2002). There are a variety of pathways that depict appetite and food craving regulation (Kalra & Kalra, 2004b). The ability of food-related cues and a food-associated environment to induce eating in healthy humans can shed light on why PWS individuals overeat and become obese. In animal models, brain regions consisting of the BLA, medial prefrontal cortex (mPFC), and LHA act as a network to regulate eating by learned, motivational cues (Elmquist, Elias & Saper, 1999). The AMY has been shown to be crucial in cue-enhanced eating (Arana et al., 2003). The OFC is also involved in food-related cues (Arana et al., 2003). The mPFC regulates eating due to environmental cue pressure (O'Doherty, 2004). Activations of the AMY and medial OFC occur when food-deprived individuals are shown food items, and greater activations are seen when food items are viewed (Arana et al., 2003). Our group has seen similar activations in PWS (James et al., 2007). The ventral mPFC has a significant role in appetite influenced by motivational cues, as reported by our group in PWS patients who had increased blood oxygen level-dependent (BOLD) responses in the ventral mPFC while viewing pictures of food (James et al., 2007). This would explain the excessive hunger due to increased reward values when viewing food, as well as the importance of the frontal cortex in its role in food responses. This data is also supported by findings of our group (James et al., 2002). Similarly, regions of the PFC may also participate in brain networks involved in cue-induced drug cravings. Other regions overlapping the ventral mPFC are also activated by chocolate- and nicotine-associated contextual cues in rats (Schroeder, Binzak & Kelley, 2001). The ventral mPFC was correlated with decreased consumption of high caloric, sweet and fatty foods, as in the case of PWS. A dysfunctional ventral mPFC could mechanistically depict feeding behavior in PWS or obese humans relevant to overeating, appetite, cues and cravings (O'Doherty et al., 2000). This may be a key point as to why food addicted obese individuals continue to overeat despite satiety. In PWS patients, obsession and preoccupation with food, lack of satiation, and incessant food seeking are typical behaviors as compared to normal obese humans (Ogura et al., 2008). PWS adults show preference for sweet or high carbohydrate foods over any other type of food. This is sometimes the case in normal obese individuals (Ogura et al., 2008). PWS patients will often eat the most desirable foods first, such as sweet, high caloric foods, and the least preferred foods last. Oftentimes, this is a ritualistic procedure in which the PWS-afflicted individual will gather the food and line it up in order of preference and ingest it sequentially (Singh et al., 2008). PWS cases are most susceptible to visual cues, thus passing by a bakery or restaurant, or even seeing sweet or highly palatable foods on television, will cause an enormous increase in craving and appetite despite satiety as compared to normal obese people. PWS patients will often have tantrums and aberrant behavior after seeing or smelling delicious, inviting food (Singh et al., 2008), which is highly uncommon in non-PWS individuals. In PWS, food cues (visual) have a very high emotional attachment and significance leading to bingeing episodes (Simmons, Martin & Barsalou, 2005). PWS is a biological model for hyperphagia and the reward system utilized to explain human obesity using functional magnetic resonance imaging (fMRI). Neuroimaging would be the most logical tool in precisely locating the brain regions responsible for controlling appetite and for being the reward centers specifically for FA (Tataranni & DelParigi, 2003). Using food-related pictures or other visual means to elicit brain responses has been a standard method of determining valid mechanisms that delineate the path to obesity (Jansen, 1998). Hence, the fMRI-supported hypothesis that PWS is a naturally occurring human model for FA or loss of control of eating or absence of satiety would be crucial for further studies. In the end, what remains is how logical and effective past, present, and future research can aid and treat abnormal eating behavior and brain responses to internal and external food cues in individuals afflicted with obesity.

4.4 Increased incentive

Compulsive drug-seeking and drug-taking behaviors are not always motivated by pleasure or by the desire to relieve withdrawal. The question remains, why do addicts compulsively seek drugs? Several groups have attempted to address this question by proposing the concept of "incentive-sensitization" (Robinson & Berridge, 1993; Berridge & Robinson, 1995). The essential concepts of the incentive-sensitization theory are: (1) potentially addictive drugs produce long-term adaptations in neural systems, hence altering the brain; (2) the brain systems that are altered are involved in the process of incentive motivation and reward; (3) the critical neuroadaptations for addiction hypersensitize these brain reward systems to drugs and drug-associated stimuli; and (4) the brain systems that become sensitized do not mediate the pleasurable effects of addictive substances, but instead they mediate a subcomponent of the reward system known as incentive salience or "wanting" (Robinson & Berridge, 1993; Berridge & Robinson, 1995; Berridge & Robinson, 1998).

A study has shown that low D2 receptor availability places people at risk for FA and obesity (Allison et al., 1999). In morbidly obese individuals, prefrontal regions were responsible for the correlation between D2 receptor availability and glucose metabolism (Volkow et al., 2008). Food cues increased striatal DA production which in turn caused increased hunger and craving for that particular food; this indicated regulation by the NAc (Volkow et al., 2002). The four major circuits involved in drug and food addictions are reward/saliency, motivation/drive, learning/conditioning and inhibitory control/emotional regulation/executive function (Volkow et al., 2008). Disruption of these circuits leads to decreased motivation for good behavior and potentiates bad behavior that ends with negative results (weight gain in FA and drug overdose in substance abuse). This results in linking new memories of expected pleasurable responses when consuming the addictive substance or viewing similar stimuli (Volkow et al., 2008).

4.5 Food addiction as an addiction

Food addiction results from craving certain food or food-substances so as "to obtain a state of heightened pleasure, energy or excitement (Tartar, Ammerman & Ott, 1998)." It is important to understand the general pathophysiology of obesity in that metabolic alterations are not necessarily a cause of this disease, as seen in other eating disorders. Investigations into non-drug related addictions such as gambling, sex and food have provided insightful findings in understanding the neural mechanisms behind the addiction process (Comings et al., 2001; Bancroft & Vukadinovic, 2004; Petry, 2006; Warren & Gold, 2007; Avena et al., 2008; Cocores & Gold, 2009; Blumenthal & Gold, 2010; Liu et al., 2010; Potenza et al., 2012) .

FA is a chronic relapsing disorder associated with food cravings or food-related substances that lead to euphoria (Gold & Stembach, 1984) or amend negative emotions (Ifland et al., 2009). As a result, the new DSM-V (http: //www.dsm5.org) will revise the category 'Eating Disorders' to 'Eating and Feeding Disorders.' Most food addicts crave carbohydrates or specific foods (Spring et al., 2008). FA is predominantly influenced by compulsive behavior instigated by emotional and environmental factors such as stress, pressure from family to be thinner, religious traditions, etc. (Gold, 1999). Most importantly, FA is related to drug addiction in that DA levels regulate this type of psychological dependence by activating DA pathways responsible for addictive behavior (Warren & Gold, 2007; Wang et al., 2009; Blumenthal & Gold, 2010). In one study, Wang et al. (2009) stated that drug addiction hijacks neurobiological pathways that regulate reward, motivation, decision-making, learning, and memory. Withdrawal results in anti-reward effects due to a loss of brain reward system function and stress when the addictive substance is not available (Dackis & O'Brien, 2005; Koob, 2009).

High-fat and high-sugar foods are being exploited by developed and developing countries (Davis & Carter, 2009) resulting in increased numbers of food addicts. These foods are linked to increasing neurochemicals such as DA (Liu et al., 2010), as demonstrated in animal studies (Rada & Hoebel, 2005), which can be applied to fMRI studies that have shown delayed satiety in obese people, meaning they consume more food despite being full than do normal individuals (Liu et al., 2000). Sugar craving caused a decrease in serotonin levels as well (Wurtman & Wurtman, 1995). As a result, FA is associated with the formation of pathological brain pathways that are reinforced by abnormal eating patterns and behaviors.

Current research in FA and other disorders has shown that there were similar neurobiological pathways as those found in drug addiction (Berry & Mechoulam, 2002; Gearhardt et al., 2009a; Wang et al., 2009; Blumenthal & Gold, 2010). Animal studies attributed addiction to specific foods (Avena et al., 2004; Avena et al., 2005; Avena et al., 2008), although humans have a tendency to respond to external food cues (Benarroch et al., 2007; James et al., 2007; von Deneen et al., 2009). Food and drugs cause DA to be released from dopaminergic neurons, originating from the mesencephalon and projecting to forebrain structures in the ventral striatum depending on the amount of reward obtained (Volkow et al., 2002; Volkow et al., 2008). Brain regions known to be associated with reward circuitry include the OFC, AMY, insula, striatum, anterior cingulate cortex (ACC), and dorsolateral prefrontal cortex (DLPFC) (McBride et al., 2006; Franklin et al., 2007). FA can be diagnosed using the Yale Food Addiction Scale (YFAS) based on the Diagnostic Statistical Manual (DSM)-IV-TR substance dependence criteria. This would then allow direct comparison between FA and drug abuse (Gearhardt et al., 2009b). There are numerous current reviews that would be helpful references in explaining the neurobiology and neurophysiology of addiction (please see Detar, 2011; Avena et al., 2102; Urban & Martinez, 2012).

4.6 Neuroimaging of addiction: Main findings

Most imaging projects studied DA involvement in the process of drug addiction because the ability of drugs of abuse to increase limbic DA is considered crucial for their reinforcing effects (Koob et al., 1994; Di Chiara, 1999). However, increased DA does not account for the process of addiction, since drugs of abuse increase DA in non-addicted as well as addicted subjects (Goldstein & Volkow, 2002). In the case of cocaine addiction, drug-induced DA increases and the intensity of self-reports of the drug's reinforcing properties is smaller in addicted subjects (Volkow et al., 1997). This means DA involvement in drug addiction is likely to be mediated by changes in neurocircuitry modulated by DA, including the frontal cortex. Current structural/volumetric MRI studies depicted morphological changes in the frontal lobe in various forms of drug addiction (Goldstein & Volkow, 2002). In one study, frontal lobe volume losses were shown in cocaine-dependent subjects (Liu et al., 1998; Franklin et al., 2002), alcoholic subjects (Jernigan et al., 1991; Pfefferbaum et al., 1997), and heroin-dependent subjects (Liu et al., 1998). The latter study indicated there were negative correlations between normalized prefrontal volumes and prolonged cocaine or heroin use, meaning there was a cumulative effect of substance abuse on frontal volumes. DA activation, as seen during amphetamine administration, also prevented inhibition of the AMY by the medial prefrontal cortex (Rosenkranz & Grace, 2001). A similar process may be occurring in human drug addiction, in which prefrontal top-down processes are diminished (see Miller & Cohen, 2001). Therefore, if the frontal cortex and its functions become down-regulated in human drug addiction, the motivational, higher cognitive, and self-monitoring processes become affected (Goldstein & Volkow, 2002).

5. Neuroimaging of food addiction: Main findings

This section will briefly examine the neural correlates of addictive-like eating behavior using fMRI as compared to those with substance dependence (Gearhardt et al., 2011c). Other studies of interest relating to FA deal with the addiction potential of hyperpalatable foods (Gearhardt et al., 2011a), the public health and policy implications of FA (Gearhardt et al., 2011b), the diagnostic criteria for FA (Gearhardt et al., 2009a), and the psychological correlates of obesity (Friedman & Brownell, 1995).

Researchers may benefit from functional neuroimaging results depicting shared neural and hormonal pathways to determine similarities between substance abuse and hedonistic overeating, such as in FA and drug abuse individuals who continue to have cravings despite a dysfunctional satiety signal (Zhang et al., 2011). Functional neuroimaging studies have further revealed that good or great smelling, looking, tasting, and reinforcing food has characteristics similar to that of drugs of abuse (James et al., 2002; James et al., 2007). Many of the brain changes in fMRI studies showed that both food and drugs activated the AMY, insula, OFC, and striatum (Jonas & Gold, 1986; Matsuda et al., 1999). Food and drug cravings also showed signal activation in the HIPP, insula, and caudate (Matsuda et al., 1999).

In Brownell's group study (Gearhardt et al., 2011c), the relationship between high food addiction scores and blood oxygen level–dependent (BOLD) functional magnetic resonance imaging activation in response to receiving palatable food was evaluated. FA scores were positively correlated with activation in the ACC, medial OFC, and AMY when anticipating eating highly palatable food such as a chocolate milkshake. There was greater activation in the DLPFC and caudate when anticipating highly palatable food and decreased activation in the lateral OFC when eating palatable foods (Gearhardt et al., 2011c). These regions are associated with positive rewards from food cues (Rolls, 2000) and satiety (Small et al., 2001). Similar patterns of neural activation were seen in substance dependence (Gearhardt et al., 2011c) in response to visual cues. Another interesting finding showed that the urge to cease consumption of a palatable food or drug is suppressed in the lateral OFC (Berridge & Kringelbach, 2008; Schoenbaum & Shaham, 2008). There has been some thought that food addicts eat compulsively but have compensatory behaviors to reduce weight (Fuhrer et al., 2008). Recent functional neuroimaging studies have found abnormal brain activations in obese people. We found that before food intake, obese men had significantly increased baseline activity in the left putamen, left posterior insula, left medial temporal cortex and bilateral parietal cortex relative to lean men using a regional homogeneity (ReHo) analysis method. In this method, we measured temporal homogeneity of the regional BOLD signals. Decreased activity was also found in the medial orbitofrontal lobe, left DPFC, right inferior temporal lobe and right cerebellum in the obese subjects. After food intake, the obese men had remarkably elevated brain activity in the left putamen and bilateral parietal lobe, and reduced activity in the left superior frontal lobe and bilateral middle temporal lobe. These results indicated that, either before or after food intake, obese men might have a stronger desire to eat. This study provided strong evidence supporting the hypothesis that there is hypo-functioning reward circuitry in obese individuals, in which the prefrontal cortex may fail to inhibit the striatum and insula, and consequently lead to overeating and obesity.

This study (Zhang et al., unpublished results) found a difference in BOLD activation between obese individuals versus controls especially in the left hemisphere as shown in Figure 2. It has been shown that a higher BMI was correlated with decreased gray matter in the left OFC and right cerebellum (Walther et al., 2010), indicating that obese individuals have limited inhibitions than controls (Baylis & Moore, 1994). In this study (Zhang et al., unpublished results), obese men had decreased neural activity in the left DLPFC prior to liquid ingestion, meaning they could not inhibit their hunger and found eating to be more desirable. The obese men also had higher activation in the left insula indicating that the insula could have affected satiety and eating (Zhang et al., unpublished results). Furthermore, greater ReHo activation in the bilateral parietal cortex in obese individuals showed that food was more palatable and enjoyable (Volkow, Fowler & Wang, 2004). Overall, it was found that the obese have hypo-functioning reward circuitry where the medial prefrontal cortex (MPFC) and left DLPFC fail to inhibit the left putamen and insula causing overeating (Zhang et al., unpublished results). fMRI was thus useful in determining the mechanisms of obesity with regards to neural activity.

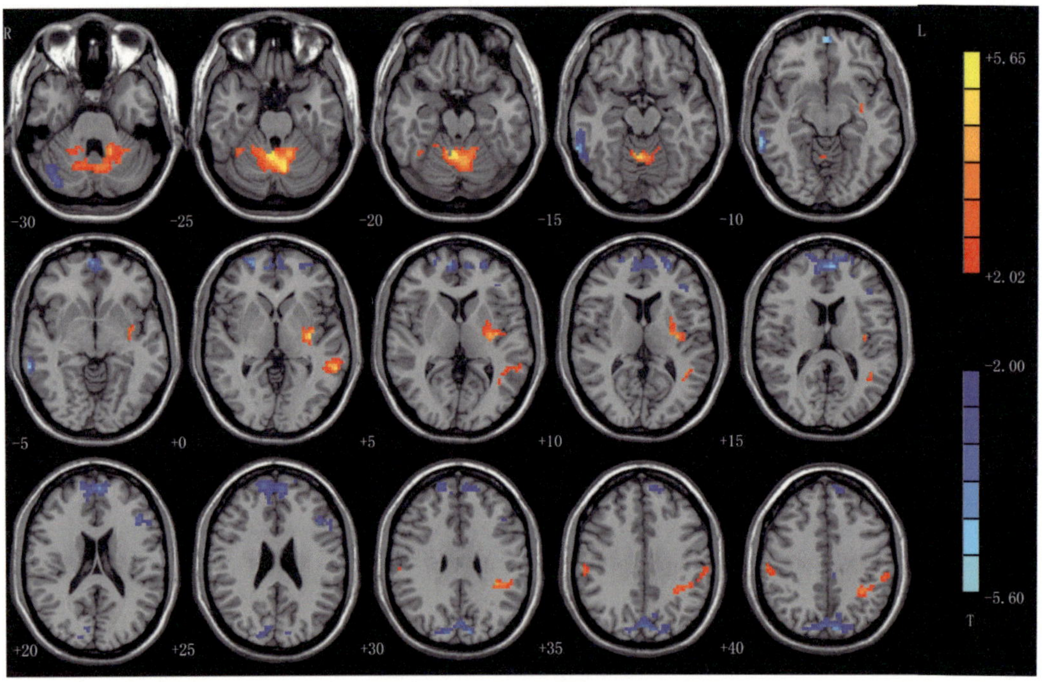

Fig. 2. A T-statistical difference map between obese subjects and controls before liquid ingestion ($p<0.05$, corrected). Warm and cold colors indicate obese subject-related ReHo increases and decreases, respectively (Zhang et al., unpublished).

6. Food addiction versus drug addiction

This section will introduce similarities and differences between food and drugs of abuse (Blumenthal & Gold, 2010). The DSM fifth edition has been prepared to address addiction with new terminologies and approaches. For example, the term substance dependence was replaced with substance-use disorder. This is defined as 'A maladaptive pattern of substance-use leading to clinically significant impairment or distress, as manifested by two (or more) of the listed criteria occurring within a 12-month period (http://www.dsm5.org/ProposedRevisions/Pages/Substance-RelatedDisorders.aspx).' Substance-abuse disorder progresses from bingeing to withdrawal, and finally leading to craving the substance (Koob & Volkow, 2010). This cyclic behavior can be sustained and entertained by stress. Substance-use disorder stems from taking over neurobiological pathways regulating reward, motivation, decision-making, learning and memory in order to become responsive to the drug of choice (Everitt & Robbins, 2005; Wise, 2006; Belin et al., 2009; Hyman et al., 2009; Wang et al., 2009). Various neural networks, such as in the dorsolateral striatum, AMY, OFC and midbrain, regulate drug-seeking behavior which depends on feelings associated with using and craving that particular drug (Zapata et al., 2003; Belin & Everitt, 2008; Everitt et al., 2008; Koob, 2009). For a thorough review of this process and the neural structures involved, please see Robbins & Everitt (1999). Furthermore, DA seems to be the essential regulator of dependence, particularly in stimulants, while alcohol, opioids, and nicotine act upon opioid receptors (Koob & Volkow, 2010). This can be seen in individuals with Parkinson's disease who become addicted to dopamine-containing medications (Dagher & Robbins, 2009).

A general figure (Figure 3) of the neurobiology of addiction is provided below.

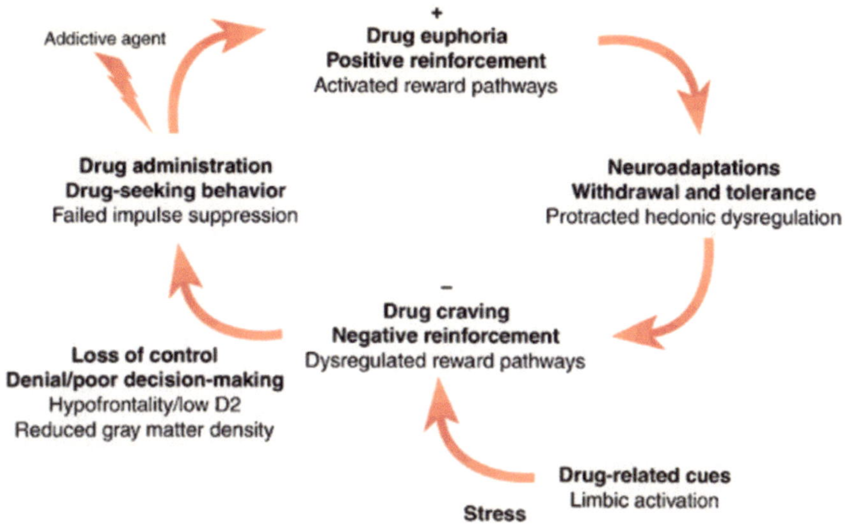

Fig. 3. Neurobiology of addiction that can be applied to food addiction as depicted by Dackis & O'Brien (2005).

The figure clearly depicts how the cycle of drug addiction is positively reinforced by euphoria from drug intake and negatively reinforced during withdrawal, craving for the drug and hedonic dysregulation. This cycle becomes more uncontrollable as the brain becomes more addicted. Drug-related cues and stress increase this craving leading to a loss of control stemming from dysfunction of the prefrontal cortex. Neuronal mechanisms for these components of addiction have been delineated in animal models and human neuroimaging studies (Dackis & O'Brien, 2005).

Accumulating evidence has shown that there are many shared neural and hormonal pathways as well as distinct differences that may help researchers find why certain individuals overeat and become addicted. The FA criteria that provide this evidence are listed in Table 2 below.

Tolerance	Starting out with a single cookie, gradually increasing to several or a whole box
Withdrawal symptoms	Habitually eating to relieve depression, anxiety, and other emotional states; unpleasant physical sensations when cutting back on carbohydrates
Taking in larger amounts or for a longer duration	Intending to eat a single serving but instead eating a whole package; binges extending several hours
Attempts to cut back	Frequent attempts to eat 'correctly'(e.g. avoid overeating or eating certain foods)
Excessive time spent pursuing, using, or recovering from use	Frequent thinking about food, planning intake, preparing, and/or resting or sleeping after excessive intake
Reduction/discontinuation of important activities because of use	Eating instead of spending time with friends; feeling too sick after overeating to do anything
Continued use despite consequences	Overeating in spite of overweight, physical illness, and/or distress about overeating

Table 2. Food addiction characteristics compared with substance abuse criteria based on Ifland et al. (2009).

Most importantly, overeating and obesity may have an acquired drive such as drug addiction with respect to motivation and incentive craving, wanting, and liking which occur after early and repeated exposures to stimuli. The acquired drive for great food and relative weakness of the satiety signal would cause an imbalance between the drive and hunger/reward centers in the brain described earlier and their regulation when conditioned via visual cues (Liu et al., 2010). As mentioned before, FA can be defined as a chronic relapsing problem caused by various fundamental factors that encourage craving for food or food-related substances so as "to obtain a state of heightened pleasure, energy, or excitement (Tartar, Ammerman & Ott, 1998)." An example of this would be carbohydrate cravers that have learned to consume high carbohydrate foods to improve their mood caused by a drop in serotonin levels (Spring et al., 2008). Most FA and eating disorders are the result of loss of control, impulsive and/or compulsive behavior stemming from emotional and environmental conditions and a psychological dependence on food. Abnormal eating behaviors along with other addictions affect the levels of DA in the mesolimbic dopaminergic system (Mogenson, 1982; Blum et al., 1996; Goldstein & Volkow, 2002; Everitt & Robbins, 2005). FA is defined by a system as follows: bingeing consists of "unusually large bouts of intake" (Colantuoni et al., 2001); withdrawal is "indicated by signs of anxiety and behavioral depression" (Colantuoni et al., 2002); craving is "measured during sugar abstinence as enhanced by responding to sugar" (Avena, Long & Hoebel, 2005); and cross-sensitization results "from sugar to drugs of abuse" (Avena et al., 2004). Furthermore, bingeing is also defined as "escalation of intake with a high proportion of intake at one time, usually after a period of voluntary abstinence or forced deprivation" (Avena, Rada & Hoebel, 2008). FA consists of sensitization and tolerance phases, which initiate addiction (Koob & Le Moal, 2005). Withdrawal resulting from the addictive food or foods has been known to be caused by alterations in the opioid system (Colantuoni et al., 2002). This phase consists of two parts, in which DA decreases and ACh is released from the NAc.

When sugar was analyzed with regards to withdrawal symptoms, it was stated that it was capable of producing DA, ACh, and opioids similar to most narcotic substances (Avena, Rada & Hoebel, 2008). Withdrawal is marked by anxiety (File et al., 2004) and depression (Avena, Rada & Hoebel, 2008). For more information on using sugar as an addictive substance please refer to the following references (Colantuoni et al., 2001; Colantuoni et al., 2002; Avena et al., 2004; Avena et al., 2005; Avena, Rada & Hoebel, 2008). Food craving can happen after a prolonged period of abstinence since "craving" is better defined by "increased efforts to obtain a substance of abuse or its associated cues as a result of dependence and abstinence" (Avena, Rada & Hoebel, 2008). Cross-sensitization is the last phase of FA and is predominantly defined as "an increased locomotor response to a different drug or substance" (Avena, Rada & Hoebel, 2008). All of these definitions play a major role in helping define and classify food (especially sugar) as a true addictive substance in comparison to the criteria for drug dependence as shown at least in rats (Haddock et al., 2000). People becoming addicted to food may be overweight and may possibly have leptin resistance as well that leads to overeating (Liu & Gold, 2003).

Finally, the most problematic group for an increase in addictive behavior and obesity has been young adults and adolescents in the past 30 years (Dietz, 2001). One study showed that binge eating and drug abuse were linked (Ross & Ivis, 1999). Interestingly, those that smoked had an increased body mass index (BMI) than non-smokers, and they were also at a risk for gaining weight when not using drugs (Hodgkins et al., 2004). Therefore, it is reasonable to conclude that teenagers used food to replace the reinforcement behavior of drug addiction to compensate for the reward systems of the brain. Eating disorders are a form of addiction in a way that individuals are obsessed with body image and compulsively crave certain foods such as in binge eating.

6.1 Intervention and prevention

Besides altering the endocrine makeup of individuals affected by FA via drug therapies, alternative and complementary approaches could play a major role in the intervention and possible prevention of obesity. Decreasing access to highly palatable and addicting foods is necessary (and restriction to all foods and small inanimate objects for patients with PWS) (von Deneen, Gold & Liu, 2009). Management includes 24 hour or constant supervision, planned physical activities, a strict diet (≤ 1200 cal/day) divided into structured, portioned meals at set times, and a static, predictable way of life (Benarroch et al., 2007). Encouraging afflicted groups to exercise or do other enjoyable activities will discourage them from their usual eating behaviors, as well as maintaining a highly controlled eating environment and food regimen with strict, consistent and reinforced rules. There are two common types of non-medicinal methods to decreasing body weight and/or improving the health condition of the individual. The first one is the undieting approach which discourages the use of food restriction or dieting due to its ineffectiveness and possible health risks (Foster, 2001). The second type is isolated dieting in which one consumes less of a particular type of food or food group such as seen in the Adkins diet where carbohydrates are almost completely eliminated from the diet. Experimental treatments in animals may have practical application in treatment and prevention of obesity. There is a possibility such drugs can be marketed for use in human medicine. Another suggested experimental treatment is the aid of central leptin gene therapy (Kalra & Kalra, 2002), where an injection of recombinant adeno-associated virus vector encoding leptin into the HYP of prepubertal and adult rats resulted in weight gain and suppressed diet-induced obesity. The explanation was that it promoted loss of fatty deposits caused by a decrease in NPY and an increase in MCH and thermogenesis. This is a novel approach that may not be suitable for humans at this point. Indeed, disrupting NPYergic signaling at multiple loci without affecting normal hypothalamic function would be ideal, but more research needs to be done in this area (Kalra & Kalra, 2004a). Another experimental method is based on the theory that ACh inhibits feeding through the M1 receptors if a muscarinic agonist, arecholine, is injected into the NA_C. This can be reversed by using an M1 antagonist pirenzapine (Rada & Hoebel, unpublished). Thus, it would be interesting to determine if arecholine would be a safe and effective method to prevent hyperphagia in individuals with FA and PWS patients. Some studies showed that taste aversion was a very useful therapy in which ACh levels were increased while decreasing DA levels (Mark et al., 1995). Others have found that baclofen, a GABA-B agonist, is useful for those that over-indulge on fatty foods (Buda-Levin, Wojnicki & Corwin, 2005). Other treatments utilized naloxone (an opioid antagonist) to block the opioid system, and rimonabant (a CB1 receptor antagonist) to block the cannabinoid system (Kenny, 2011); these systems have been shown to reinforce feeding behavior, and when used together, they act synergistically to treat obesity (Berry & Mechoulam, 2002). The still-investigational drug is Lorcaserin, a combination of benzazepine and hydrochloride, two neurological agents. Lorcaserin is a selective 5-HT2C receptor agonist, working through the serotonin system, which regulates appetite, mood, and motor behavior. Two other investigational obesity drugs target the DA reward system-Contrave, which is a combination of bupropion and naltrexone, and Qnexa, which combines phentermine and topiramate (Solinas & Goldberg, 2005).

7. Conclusion

Obesity continues to place a tremendous burden on healthcare systems. Our current and future research on the neurobiological systems that motivate appetitive behavior strongly suggests that an acquired drive for highly energy-dense, reinforcing foods is contributing to weight gain. The limitations of current treatments compel healthcare professionals to develop more effective ways based on neurobiological addiction models to curb the obesity epidemic.

Future studies should examine the relation between FA, hunger, and reward circuitry response with food intake and anticipated intake. The use of fMRI technology directly measures DA release or its receptors. It will be important to examine induced DA release and D2 receptor availability in those with FA. Other neurotransmitters are also likely to play an important role. Thus, future studies connecting FA and neural activation associated with these neurotransmitters will also be important. Understanding the mechanisms of hedonic eating is essential for developing and implementing treatment and management strategies that address the root causes of obesity. In addition, cognitive factors such as social environment, emotional state, or intentional efforts to control consumption can also influence food intake. Most of what we know about these regulatory systems is derived from animal models, but our understanding of the control of eating behavior in humans is very limited. Consistent with the biological imperative to identify and consume food, neuroimaging studies have begun to document the responsiveness of the human brain to food cues such as odors and/or taste samples of food (Wang et al., 2004; Rosenbaum et al., 2008). Future positron emission tomography (PET) and fMRI studies will provide neurobiological insights in brain alterations during addiction. fMRI is ideal for investigating activation in regions involved in a specific function, because scans can detect these simultaneously. It also provides temporal-spatial resolution and anatomical accuracy to be able to describe the interaction between major CNS components. This allows the monitoring of dynamic activities in the brain while processing visual cues (Zhang et al., 2011). Our group has future studies planned to determine brain responses when viewing photographs of food and non-food objects, where we will specifically examine brain regions important to the regulation of appetite and food intake in overweight and normal individuals. For example, one such fMRI study is to scan young healthy subjects of normal weight to measure different brain activation by visual images of highly rewarding-foods (high caloric foods such as hamburgers and chips) compared with images of non-rewarding objects during various physiological states; in particular, we are interested in effects of fast food-branding on the brain and the effects in Chinese children with and without exposure to the Golden Arches (McDonald's®) or the Kentucky Colonel (KFC®). The study tests the hypothesis of 'food addiction' that the fast food brands such as McDonald's® may have reinforcing effects in the brain and such effects may be related to children's drive to eat (Zhang et al., 2011). Using the Chinese population who has never been exposed to such food brands as controls (this CANNOT be done in the USA), this study would have a strong impact in the areas of addiction and obesity. Another research paradigm proposed is mostly based on a bottom-up approach to test the relationship between chronic subcutaneous recombinant leptin injections and weight loss (Benoit et al., 2004). fMRI techniques are powerful tools to probe leptin neurological function in modulation of human ingestive behavior and are ideal for investigating the concerted activity among the ensemble of regions involved in a specific function, because scans can detect all regions of brain activation simultaneously. Many recent studies have employed fMRI techniques to gain neuroanatomical insights into the effects of leptin in brain processing hunger, satiety and food reward in obese human subjects (Farooqi et al., 2007; Baicy et al., 2007). As a result, we propose to assess brain activation in response to acute subcutaneous leptin injection by examining the resting-state and exposure to stimuli consisting of food cues using an fMRI experiment (Zhang et al., 2011). We will also attempt to correlate the fMRI leptin brain response with weight gain based on a cafeteria diet. Positive results from this study will provide an invaluable diagnostic guideline for initiating early adulthood nutritional and behavioral intervention on an individualized basis to temper obesity development. This would constitute a realistic and meaningful cost-effective approach. An obesity-prevention strategy will help curb rising obesity treatment-related health expenditures. Positive study outcomes will also highlight a technological breakthrough for fMRI investigation of region-specific neural activity in an acutely stimulated brain reactive state rather than in a chronically adapted state following long-term drug treatment or other types of intervention. Thus, we hope to illuminate promising methods that use visual food cues to investigate mechanisms of human eating behavior, and to facilitate a more unified and reproducible approach to neuroimaging studies of FA and obesity. Results from this study can go far beyond obesity studies and could extend to the field of pharmacological research (Zhang et al., 2011). Furthermore, more research needs to be conducted world-wide especially in the Chinese population. Obesity in China is a multifactorial disease where intervention is not always clear-cut or applicable. For instance, specific gene therapy may be available in the future to prevent childhood and adulthood weight gain and endocrine disorders. Lifestyle and behavioral changes need to be addressed and applied to prevent unhealthy physiques. Alternative medicine intervention, such as acupuncture and Traditional Chinese Medicine remedies, may be most appropriate for this part of the world. Overall, obesity is preventable and now is the ideal time in implementing current scientific methods and techniques to battle this epidemic (von Deneen & Liu, 2011).

8. Acknowledgment

This research was supported by the Project for the National Key Basic Research and Development Program (973) under Grant Nos. 2011CB707702 and 2012CB518501, the National Natural Science Foundation of China under Grant Nos. 30930112, 30970774, 60901064, 30873462, 81000640, 81000641, 81071217, 81101036, 81101108 and 31150110171, the Fundamental Research Funds for the Central Universities and the Knowledge Innovation Program of the Chinese Academy of Sciences under Grant No. KGCX2-YW-129.

9. References

Achike, FI.; To, NH.; Wang, H. & Kwan, CY. (2011). Obesity, metabolic syndrome, adipocytes and vascular function: a holistic viewpoint. *Clin Exp Pharmacol Physiol*, Vol.38, No.1, pp. 1-10.

Allison, DB.; Mentore, JL.; Heo, M.; Chandler, LP.; Cappelleri, JC.; Infante, MC. & Weiden, PJ. (1999). Antipsychotic-induced weight gain: a comprehensive research synthesis. *Am. J. Psychiatry*, Vol.156, pp. 686–696.

Arana, FS.; Parkinson, JA.; Hinton, E.; Holland, AJ.; Owen, AM. & Roberts, AC. (2003). Dissociable contributions of the human amygdala and orbitofrontal cortex to incentive motivation and goal selection. *J Neurosci*, Vol.23, No.29, pp. 9632-9638.

Augustine, JR. (1996). Circuitry and functional aspects of the insular lobe in primates including humans. *Brain Research. Brain Research Reviews*, Vol.22, pp. 229–244.

Avena, NM.; Carrillo, CA.; Needham, L.; Leibowitz, SF. & Hoebel, BG. (2004). Sugar-dependent rats show enhanced intake of unsweetened ethanol. *Alcohol*, Vol.34, No.2-3, pp. 203-209.

Avena, NM.; Gold, JA.; Kroll, C. & Gold, MS. (2012). Further developments in the neurobiology of food and addiction: update on the state of the science. *Nutrition*, Vol.28, No.4, pp. 341-343.

Avena, NM.; Long, KA. & Hoebel, BG. (2005). Sugar-dependent rats show enhanced responding for sugar after abstinence: evidence of a sugar deprivation effect. *Physiol Behav*, Vol.84, No.3, pp. 359-362.

Avena, NM.; Rada, P. & Hoebel, BG. (2008). Evidence for sugar addiction: behavioral and neurochemical effects of intermittent, excessive sugar intake. *Neurosci Biobehav Rev*, Vol.32, No.1, pp. 20-39.

Baicy, K.; London, ED.; Monterosso, J.; Wong, ML.; Delibasi, T.; Sharma, A. & Licinio, J. (2007). Leptin replacement alters brain response to food cues in genetically leptin-deficient adults. *Proc Natl Acad Sci USA*, Vol.104, No.46, pp. 18276-18279.

Bancroft, J. & Vukadinovic, Z. (2004). Sexual addiction, sexual compulsivity, sexual impulsivity, or what? Toward a theoretical model. *J Sex Res*, Vol.41, No.3, pp. 225-234.

Barbano, MF.; Stinus, L.; Cador, M. & Ahmed, SH. (2005). Mesolimbic dopamine drives the diurnal variation in opiate-induced feeding. *Pharmacol Biochem Behav*, Vol.81, No.3, pp. 569-574.

Barson, JR.; Karatayev, O.; Chang, GQ.; Johnson, DF.; Bocarsly, ME.; Hoebel, BG. & Leibowitz, SF. (2009). Positive relationship between dietary fat, ethanol intake, triglycerides, and hypothalamic peptides: counteraction by lipid-lowering drugs. *Alcohol*, Vol.43, pp. 433–441.

Baylis, GC. & Moore, BO. (1994). Hippocampal lesions impair spatial response selection in the primate. *Exp Brain Res*, Vol.98, pp. 110-118.

Belin, D. & Everitt, BJ. (2008). Cocaine seeking habits depend upon dopamine-dependent serial connectivity linking the ventral with the dorsal striatum. *Neuron*, Vol.57, No.3, pp. 432-441.

Belin, D.; Jonkman, S.; Dickinson, A.; Robbins, TW. & Everitt, BJ. (2009). Parallel and interactive learning processes within the basal ganglia: relevance for the understanding of addiction. *Behav Brain Res*, Vol.199, No.1, pp. 89-102.

Benarroch, F.; Hirsch, HJ.; Genstil, L.; Landau, YE. & Gross-Tsur, V. (2007). Prader-Willi syndrome: medical prevention and behavioral challenges. *Child Adolesc Psychiatr Clin N Am*, Vol.16, No.3, pp. 695-708.

Benoit, SC.; Clegg, DJ.; Seeley, RJ. & Woods, SC. (2004). Insulin and leptin as adiposity signals. *Recent Prog Horm Res*, Vol.59, pp. 267-285.

Berridge, KC. & Kringelbach, ML. (2008). Affective neuroscience of pleasure: reward in humans and animals. *Psychopharmacology (Berl)*, Vol.199, No.3, pp. 457-480.

Berridge, KC. & Robinson, TE. (1995). The mind of an addicted brain: neural sensitization of wanting versus liking, *Current Directions in Psychological Science*, Vol.4, pp. 71–76.

Berridge, KC. & Robinson, TE. (1998). What is the role of dopamine in reward: hedonic impact, reward learning, or incentive salience? *Brain Research Reviews*, Vol.28, pp. 309–369.

Berry, EM. & Mechoulam, R. (2002). Tetrahydrocannabinol and endocannabinoids in feeding and appetite. *Pharmacol Ther*, Vol.95, No.2, pp. 185-190.

Blum, K.; Sheridan, PJ.; Wood, RC.; Braverman, ER.; Chen, TJ.; Cull, JG. & Comings, DE. (1996). The D2 dopamine receptor gene as a determinant of reward deficiency syndrome. *J R Soc Med*, Vol.89, No.7, pp. 396-400.

Blumenthal, DM. & Gold, MS. (2010). Neurobiology of food addiction. *Current Opinion in Clinical Nutrition and Metabolic Care*, Vol.13, No.4, pp. 359–365.

Bouchard C. (2009). Childhood obesity: are genetic differences involved? *Amer J Clin Nut,* Vol.89, pp. 1494S-1501S.

Buda-Levin, A.; Wojnicki, FH. & Corwin, RL. (2005). Baclofen reduces fat intake under binge- type conditions. *Physiol Behav,* Vol.86, No.1-2, pp. 176-184.

Campbell, MW.; Williams, J.; Hampton, A. & Wake, M. (2006). Maternal concern and perceptions of overweight in Australian preschool-aged children. *Med J Aust,* Vol.184, pp. 274-277.

Cardinal, RN.; Parkinson, JA.; Hall, J. & Everitt, BJ. (2002). Emotion and motivation: the role of the amygdala, ventral striatum, and prefrontal cortex. *Neurosci Biobehav Rev,* Vol.26, No.3, pp. 321-352.

Cecchini, M.; Sassi, F.; Lauer, JA.; Lee, YY.; Guajardo-Barron, V. & Chisholm, D. (2010). Tackling of unhealthy diets, physical inactivity, and obesity: health effects and cost-effectiveness. *Lancet,* Vol.376, pp. 1775-1784.

Chen, H.; Simar, D. & Morris, MJ. (2009). Hypothalamic neuroendocrine circuitry is programmed by maternal obesity: interaction with postnatal nutritional environment. *PLoS One,* Vol.4, pp. e6259.

Cheung, CY.; Tso, AW.; Cheung, BM.; Xu, A.; Ong, KL.; Fong, CH.; Wat, NM.; Janus, ED.; Sham, PC. & Lam, KS. (2010). Obesity susceptibility genetic variants identified from recent genome-wide association studies: implications in a Chinese population. *J Clin Endocrinol Metab,* Vol.95, No.3, pp. 1395-1403.

Cocores, JA. & Gold, MS. (2009). The Salted Food Addiction Hypothesis may explain overeating and the obesity epidemic. *Med Hypotheses,* Vol.73, No.6, pp. 892–899.

Colantuoni, C.; Rada, P.; McCarthy, J.; Patten, C.; Avena, NM.; Chadeayne, A. & Hoebel, BG. (2002). Evidence that intermittent, excessive sugar intake causes endogenous opioid dependence. *Obes Res,* Vol.10, No.6, pp. 478-488.

Colantuoni, C.; Schwenker, J.; McCarthy, J.; Rada, P.; Ladenheim, B.; Cadet, JL.; Schwartz, GJ.; Moran, TH. & Hoebel, BG. (2001). Excessive sugar intake alters binding to dopamine and mu-opioid receptors in the brain. *Neuroreport,* Vol.12, No.16, pp. 3549-3552.

Comings, DE.; Gade-Andavolu, R.; Gonzalez, N.; Wu, S.; Muhleman, D.; Chen, C.; Koh, P.; Farwell, K.; Blake, H.; Dietz, G.; MacMurray, JP.; Lesieur, HR.; Rugle, LJ. & Rosenthal, RJ. (2001). The additive effect of neurotransmitter genes in pathological gambling. *Clin Genet,* Vol.60, No.2, pp. 107-116.

Coon, KA.; Goldberg, J.; Rogers, BL. & Tucker, KL. (2001). Relationships between use of television during meals and children's food consumption patterns. *Pediatrics,* Vol.107, pp. E7.

Corsica, JA. & Pelchat, ML. (2010). Food addiction: true or false? *Curr Opin Gastroenterol,* Vol.26, pp. 165–169.

Cowley, MA.; Smart, JL.; Rubinstein, M.; Cerdan, MG.; Diano, S.; Horvath, TL.; Cone, RD. & Low, MJ. (2001). Leptin activates anorexigenic POMC neurons through a neural network in the arcuate nucleus. *Nature,* Vol.411, No.6836, pp. 480-484.

Dackis, C. & O'Brien, C. (2005). Neurobiology of addiction. *Nature Neuroscience,* Vol.8, pp. 1431-1436.

Dagher, A. & Robbins, TW. (2009). Personality, addiction, dopamine: insights from Parkinson's disease. *Neuron,* Vol.61, pp. 502–510.

Dagher, A. (2009). The neurobiology of appetite: hunger as addiction. *Int J Obes*, Vol.33, No.2, pp. S30–S33.

Davis, C. & Carter, JC. (2009). Compulsive overeating as an addiction disorder. A review of theory and evidence. *Appetite*, Vol.53, pp. 1–8.

Di Chiara, G. (1999). Drug addiction as dopamine-dependent associative learning disorder. *Eur J Pharmacol*, Vol.375, pp. 13–30.

De Castro, JM. (1997). How can energy balance be achieved by free-living human subjects? *Proc Nutr Soc*, Vol.56, No.1A, pp. 1-14.

Detar, DT. (2011). Understanding the disease of addiction. *Prim Care*. Vol.38, No.1, pp. 1-7.

Dietz, W. (2001). Childhood obesity. In: *Modern nutrition in health and disease* (9th Ed.) M. Shils, J. Olsen, M. Shike, et al. (Eds.), 1071–1080, Williams and Wilkins, Baltimore, MD, USA.

Ding, EL. & Malik, VS. (2008). Convergence of obesity and high glycemic diet on compounding diabetes and cardiovascular risks in modernizing China: an emerging public health dilemma. *Globalization and Health*, Vol.4, pp. 4.

Drucker, RR.; Hammer, LD.; Agras, WS. & Bryson, S. (1999). Can mothers influence their child's eating behavior. *J Dev Behav Pediatr*, Vol.20, pp. 88-92.

Ebbeling, CB.; Pawlak, DB. & Ludwig, DS. (2002). Childhood obesity: Public health crisis, common sense cure. *Lancet*, Vol.360, pp. 473–482.

Elliott, R.; Friston, KJ. & Dolan, RJ. (2000). Dissociable neural responses in human reward systems. *J Neurosci*, Vol.20, No.16, pp. 6159-6165.

Elmquist, JK.; Elias, CF. & Saper, CB. (1999). From lesions to leptin: hypothalamic control of food intake and body weight. *Neuron*, Vol.22, No.2, pp. 221-232.

Everitt, BJ.; Belin, D.; Economidou, D.; Pelloux, Y.; Dalley, JW. & Robbins, TW. (2008). Review. Neural mechanisms underlying the vulnerability to develop compulsive drug- seeking habits and addiction. *Philos Trans R Soc Lond B Biol Sci*, Vol.363, No.1507, pp.3125-3135.

Everitt, BJ. & Robbins, TW. (2005). Neural systems of reinforcement for drug addiction: from actions to habits to compulsion. *Nat Neurosci*, Vol.8, No.11, pp.1481-1489.

Fagerberg, B.; Hulten, LM. & Hulthe, J. (2003). Plasma ghrelin, body fat, insulin resistance, and smoking in clinically healthy men: the atherosclerosis and insulin resistance study. *Metabolism*, Vol.52, pp. 1460-1463.

Fan, Y.; Li, Y.; Liu, A.; Hu, X.; Ma, G. & Xu, G. (2010). Associations between body mass index, weight control concerns and behaviors, and eating disorder symptoms among non- clinical Chinese adolescents. *BMC Public Health*, Vol.10, pp. 314.

Farooqi, IS.; Bullmore, E.; Keogh, J.; Gillard, J.; O'Rahilly, S. & Fletcher, PC. (2007). Leptin regulates striatal regions and human eating behavior. *Science*, Vol.317, No.5843, pp. 1355.

File, SE.; Lippa, AS.; Beer, B. & Lippa, MT. (2004). Animal tests of anxiety. *Curr Protoc Neurosci*, Chapter 8, Unit 83.

Foster, GD.; Brownell, KD. & Fairburn, CG. (Eds). (2001). Non-dieting approaches. *Eating disorders and obesity: a comprehensive handbook*. Gulford, NY, USA.

Franklin, TR.; Acton, PD.; Maldjian, JA.; Gray, JD.; Croft, JR.; Dackis, CA.; O'Brien, CP. & Childress, AR. (2002). Decreased gray matter concentration in the insular, orbitofrontal, cingulate, and temporal cortices of cocaine patients. *Biol Psychiatry*, Vol.51, pp. 134–142.

Franklin, TR.; Wang, Z.; Wang, J.; Sciortino, N.; Harper, D.; Li, Y.; Ehrman, R.; Kampman, K.; O'Brien, CP.; Detre, JA. & Childress, AR. (2007). Limbic activation to cigarette smoking cues independent of nicotine withdrawal: a perfusion fMRI study. *Neuropsychopharmacology,* Vol.32, No.11, pp. 2301-2309.

Frayling, TM.; Timpson, NJ.; Weedon, MN.; Zeggini, E.; Freathy, RM.; Lindgren, CM.; Perry, JR.; Elliott, KS.; Lango, H.; Rayner, NW.; Shields, B.; Harries, LW.; Barrett, JC.; Ellard, S.; Groves, CJ.; Knight, B.; Patch, AM.; Ness, AR.; Ebrahim, S.; Lawlor, DA.; Ring, SM.; Ben-Shlomo, Y.; Jarvelin, MR.; Sovio, U.; Bennett, AJ.; Melzer, D.; Ferrucci, L.; Loos, RJ.; Barroso, I.; Wareham, NJ.; Karpe, F.; Owen, KR.; Cardon, LR.; Walker, M.; Hitman, GA.; Palmer, CN.; Doney, AS.; Morris, AD.; Smith, GD.; Hattersley, AT. & McCarthy, MI. (2007). A common variant in the FTO gene is associated with body mass index and predisposes to childhood and adult obesity. *Science,* Vol.316, pp. 889- 894.

Friedman, MA. & Brownell, KD. (1995). Psychological correlates of obesity: moving to the next research generation. *Psychol Bull,* Vol.117, No.1, pp. 3-20.

Fu, D.; Wang, J.; Chen, W. & Bi, Y. (2005). Disordered eating attitudes and behaviours and related mood states among female university students in Beijing. *Chin Ment Health J,* Vol.19, No.8, pp. 25-28.

Fu¨hrer, D.; Zysset, S. & Stumvoll, M. (2008). Brain activity in hunger and satiety: an exploratory visually stimulated FMRI study. *Obesity (Silver Spring),* Vol.16, No. 5, pp. 945-950.

Ge, K.; Weisell, R.; Guo, X.; Cheng, L.; Ma, H.; Zhai, F. & Popkin, BM. (1994). The body mass index of Chinese adults in the 1980s. *Eur J Clin Nutr,* Vol.48, No.3, pp. S148-154.

Gearhardt, AN.; Corbin, WR. & Brownell, KD. (2009a). Food addiction: an examination of the diagnostic criteria for dependence. *J Addict Med,* Vol.3, No.1, pp. 1-7.

Gearhardt, AN.; Corbin, WR. & Brownell, KD. (2009b). Preliminary validation of the Yale Food Addiction Scale. *Appetite,* Vol.52, No.2, pp. 430-436.

Gearhardt, AN.; Davis, C.; Kuschner, R. & Brownell, KD. (2011a). The addiction potential of hyperpalatable foods. *Curr Drug Abuse Rev,* Vol.4, No.3, pp. 140-145.

Gearhardt, AN.; Grilo, CM.; DiLeone, RJ.; Brownell, KD. & Potenza, MN. (2011b). Can food be addictive? Public health and policy implications. *Addiction,* Vol.106, No.7, pp. 1208- 1212.

Gearhardt, AN.; Yokum, S.; Orr, PT.; Stice, E.; Corbin, WR. & Brownell, KD. (2011c). Neural correlates of food addiction. *Arch Gen Psychiatry,* Vol.68, No.8, pp. 808-816.

Gerken, T.; Girard, CA.; Tung, YC.; Webby, CJ.; Saudek, V.; Hewitson, KS.; Yeo, GS.; McDonough, MA.; Cunliffe, S.; McNeill, LA.; Galvanovskis, J.; Rorsman, P.; Robins, P.; Prieur, X.; Coll, AP.; Ma, M.; Jovanovic, Z.; Farooqi, IS.; Sedgwick, B.; Barroso, I.; Lindahl, T.; Ponting, CP.; Ashcroft, FM.; O'Rahilly, S. & Schofield, CJ. (2007). The obesity-associated FTO gene encodes a 2-oxoglutarate-dependent nucleic acid demethylase. *Science,* Vol.318, No.5855, pp. 1469-1472.

Giovannucci, E. (2002). Modifiable risk factors for colon cancer. *Gastroenterol Clin North Am,* Vol.31, pp. 925-943.

Gold, MS. & Stembach, HA. (1984). Endorphins in obesity and in the regulation of appetite and weight. *Integrative Psychiatry,* Vol.2, No.6, pp. 1549-1555.

Gold, MS. (1999). Etiology and management of obesity. *Direction in Psychiatry,* Vol.19, No.20, pp. 1549-1555.

Goldstein, RZ. & Volkow, ND. (2002). Drug addiction and its underlying neurobiological basis: Neuroimaging evidence for the involvement of the frontal cortex. *American Journal of Psychiatry,* Vol.129, pp. 1642–1652.

Groschl, M.; Topf, HG.; Bohlender, J.; Zenk, J.; Klussmann, S.; Dötsch, J.; Rascher, W. & Rauh, M. (2005). Identification of ghrelin in human saliva: production by the salivary glands and potential role in proliferation of oral keratinocytes. *ClinChem,* Vol.51, pp. 997-1006.

Grundy, SM.; Brewer, B.; Cleeman, JI.; Smith, SC. & Lenfant, C. (2004). Definition of metabolic syndrome: Report of the national heart, lung, and blood institute/American heart association conference on scientific issues related to definition. *Circulation,* Vol.109, pp. 433-438.

Guldan, GS. (2010). Asian children's obesogenic diets—time to change this part of the energy balance equation? *Res Sports Med,* Vol.18, No.1, pp. 5-15.

Haddock, CK.; Dill, PL.; Poston, WSC. & Haddock, CK. (Eds.). (2000). *The effects of food on mood and behavior: implications for the addictions model of obesity and eating disorders. Food as a drug,* The Haworth Press, Inc., New York, NY.

Hodgkins, CC.; Cahill, KS.; Seraphine, AE.; Frost-Pineda, K. & Gold, MS. (2004). Adolescent drug addiction treatment and weight gain. *J Add Dis.,* Vol.23, No.3, pp. 55–66.

Hong, J. (1998). *The internationalization of television in China: an evolution of ideology, society, and media since the reform,* Praeger Publishers, Westport, CT.

Huang, JS.; Becerra, K. & Oda, T. (2007). Parental ability to discriminate the weight status of children: results of a survey. *Pediatrics,* Vol.120, pp. e112-119.

Hyman, SM.; Hong, KI.; Chaplin, TM.; Dabre, Z.; Comegys, AD.; Kimmerling, A. & Sinha, R. (2009). A stress-coping profile of opioid dependent individuals entering naltrexone treatment: a comparison with healthy controls. *Psychol Addict Behav,* Vol.23, No.4, pp. 613-619.

Ifland, JR.; Preuss, HG.; Marcus, MT.; Rourke, KM.; Taylor, WC.; Burau, K.; Jacobs, WS.; Kadish, W. & Manso, G. (2009). Refined food addiction: a classic substance use disorder. *Med Hypotheses,* Vol.72, No.5, pp. 518-526.

James, GA.; He, G.; Miller, AW.; Taeb, Y. & Liu, Y. (2002). MRI of hunger and insula activation during a fasting paradigm. *ISMRM,* Abstract.

James, GA.; Miller, JL.; Goldstone, AP.; Couch, JA.; He, G.; Driscoll, DJ. & Liu, Y. (2007). Enhanced activation of reward mediating prefrontal regions in response to food stimuli in Prader-Willi syndrome. *J Neurol Neurosurg Psychiatry,* Vol.78, No.6, pp. 615-619.

Jansen, A. (1998). A learning model of binge eating: cue reactivity and cue exposure. *Behav Res Ther,* Vol.36, No.3, pp. 257-272.

Jernigan, TL.; Butters, N.; DiTraglia, G.; Schafer, K.; Smith, T.; Irwin, M.; Grant, I.; Schuckit, M. & Cermak, LS. (1991). Reduced cerebral grey matter observed in alcoholics using magnetic resonance imaging. *Alcohol Clin Exp Res,* Vol.15, pp. 418–427.

Ji, MF. & McNeal, JU. (2001). How Chinese children's commercials differ from those of the United States: a content analysis. *J Advert,* Vol.30, pp. 79.

Jonas, JM. & Gold, MS. (1986). Cocaine abuse and eating disorders. *Lancet,* Vol.1, pp. 390-391.

Jones, N.; Furlanetto, DL.; Jackson, JA. & Kinn, S. (2007). An investigation of obese adults' views of the outcomes of dietary treatment. *J Human Nutr Diet,* Vol.20, pp. 486-494.

Joranby, L.; Pineda, K. & Gold, MS. (2005). Addiction to food and brain reward systems. *Sexual Addiction and Compulsivity*, Vol.12, No.2-3, pp. 201-217.

Jumabay, M.; Kawamura, H.; Mitsubayashi, H.; Ozawa, Y.; Izumi, Y.; Kasamaki, H.; Shimabukuro, Z.; Cheng, M.; Aisa & Wang, S. (2001). Urinary electrolytes and hypertension in elderly Kazakhs. *Clin Exp Nephrol*, Vol.5, pp. 217-221.

Kalra, PS. & Kalra, SP. (2002). Obesity and metabolic syndrome: long-term benefits of central leptin gene therapy. *Drugs Today (Barc)*, Vol.38, No.11, pp. 745-757.

Kalra, SP. & Kalra, PS. (1996). Nutritional infertility: the role of the interconnected hypothalamic neuropeptide Y-galanin-opioid network. *Front Neuroendocrinol*, Vol.17, No.4, pp. 371-401.

Kalra, SP. & Kalra, PS. (2004a). NPY and cohorts in regulating appetite, obesity and metabolic syndrome: beneficial effects of gene therapy. *Neuropeptides*, Vol.38, No.4, pp. 201-211.

Kalra, SP. & Kalra, PS. (2004b). Overlapping and interactive pathways regulating appetite and craving. *J Addict Dis*, Vol.23, No.3, pp. 5-21.

Kalra, SP.; Dube, MG.; Pu, S.; Xu, B.; Horvath, TL. & Kalra, PS. (1999). Interacting appetite-regulating pathways in the hypothalamic regulation of body weight. *Endocr Rev*, Vol.20, No.1, pp. 68-100.

Karatayev, O.; Gaysinskaya, V.; Chang, GQ. & Leibowitz, SF. (2009). Circulating triglycerides after a high-fat meal: predictor of increased caloric intake, orexigenic peptide expression, and dietary obesity. *Brain Res*, Vol.1298, pp. 111–122.

Kenny, PJ. (2011). 'Macrophage' cannabinoid receptor goes up in smoke. *Nat Neurosci*, Vol.14, No.9, pp. 1100-1102.

Kleiner, KD.; Gold, MS.; Frost-Pineda, K.; Lenz-Brunsman, B.; Perri, MG. & Jacobs, WS. (2004). Body mass index and alcohol use. *J Addict Dis*, Vol.23, No.3, pp. 105-118.

Ko, GT.; So, WY.; Chow, CC.; Wong, PT.; Tong, SD.; Hui, SS.; Kwok, R.; Chan, A.; Chan, CL.; Chan, JC. & BHBHK Research Committee. (2010). Risk associations of obesity with sugar-sweetened beverages and lifestyle factors in Chinese: the 'Better Health for Better Hong Kong' health promotion campaign. *Eur J Clin Nutrition*, Vol.64, pp. 1386-1392.

Kong, AP. & Chow, CC. (2010). Medical consequences of childhood obesity: a Hong Kong perspective. *Res Sports Med*, Vol.18, No.1, pp. 16-25.

Koob, GF.; Caine, B.; Markou, A.; Pulvirenti, L. & Weiss, F. (1994). Role for the mesocortical dopamine system in the motivating effects of cocaine. *NIDA Res Monogr*, Vol.145, pp. 1–18.

Koob, GF. & Le Moal, M. (2005). *Neurobiology of Addiction*. Academic Press, San Diego, CA.

Koob, GF. & Volkow, ND. (2010). Neurocircuitry of addiction. *Neuropsychopharmacology*, Vol.35, pp. 217–238.

Koob, GF. (2009). Dynamics of neuronal circuits in addiction: reward, antireward, and emotional memory. *Pharmacopsychiatry*, Vol.42, No.1, pp. S32–S41.

Kurihara, K. & Kashiwayanagi, M. (2000). Physiological studies on umami taste. *J Nutr*, Vol.130, No.4, pp. 931S-934S.

Levine, AS.; Kotz, CM. & Gosnell, BA. (2003). Sugars: hedonic aspects, neuroregulation, and energy balance. *Am J Clin Nutr*, Vol.78, pp. 834S–842S.

Li, HL.; Yu, YR.; Yu, HL.; Wang, C. & Zhang, XX. (2005). Relationship between peripheral insulin resistance and beta-cell function in obese subjects. *Sichuan Da Xue Xue Bao Yi Xue Ban*, Vol.36, pp. 378-381.

Li, X.; Song, F.; Jiang, H.; Zhang, M.; Lin, J.; Bao, W.; Yao, P.; Yang, X.; Hao, L. & Liu, L. (2010). A genetic variation in the fat mass-and obesity-associated gene is associated with obesity and newly diagnosed type 2 diabetes in a Chinese population. *Diabetes Metab Res Rev*, Vol.26, No.2, pp. 128-132.

Li, Y.; Zhai, F.; Yang, X.; Schouten, EG.; Hu, X.; He, Y.; Luan, D. & Ma, G. (2007). Determinants of childhood overweight and obesity in China. *British J Nutr*, Vol.97, pp. 210-215.

Liu, X.; Matochik, JA.; Cadet, JL. & London, ED. (1998). Smaller volume of pre-frontal lobe in polysubstance abusers: a magnetic resonance imaging study. *Neuropsychopharmacology*, Vol.18, pp. 243–252.

Liu, Y. & Gold, MS. (2003). Human functional magnetic resonance imaging of eating and satiety in eating disorders and obesity. *Psych Annals*, Vol.33, No.2, pp. 127-132.

Liu, Y.; Gao, JH.; Liu, HL. & Fox, PT. (2000). The temporal response of the brain after eating revealed by functional MRI. *Nature*, Vol.405, pp. 1058–1062.

Liu, Y.; von Deneen, KM.; Kobeissy, F. & Gold, MS. (2010). Food Addiction and obesity: Evidence from bench to bedside. *J of Psychoactive Drugs*, Vol.42, No.2, pp. 133-145.

Livingstone, S. (2002). *Young People and New Media*. Sage Publications, Thousand Oaks, CA.

Mark, GP.; Weinberg, JB.; Rada, PV. & Hoebel, BG. (1995). Extracellular acetylcholine is increased in the nucleus accumbens following the presentation of an aversively conditioned taste stimulus. *Brain Res*, Vol.688, No.1-2, pp. 184-188.

Martorell, R.; Stein, AD. & Schroeder, DG. (2001). Early nutrition and later adiposity. *J Nutr*, Vol.131, pp. 874S-880S.

Matsuda, M.; Liu, Y.; Mahankali, S.; Wang, J.; DeFronzo, RA.; Fox, PT. & Gao, JH. (1999). Altered hypothalamic response to oral glucose intake in obese humans. *Diabetes*, Vol.48, pp. 1801-1806.

Maynard, LM.; Galuska, DA.; Blanck, HM. & Serdula, MK. (2003). Maternal perceptions of weight status of children. *Pediatrics*, Vol.111, pp. 1226-1231.

McAuley, KA.; Williams, SM.; Mann, JI.; Walker, RJ.; Lewis-Barned, NJ.; Temple, LA. & Duncan, AW. (2001). Diagnosing insulin resistance in the general population. *Diabetes Care*, Vol.24, pp. 460-464.

McBride, D.; Barrett, SP.; Kelly, JT.; Aw, A. & Dagher, A. (2006). Effects of expectancy and abstinence on the neural response to smoking cues in cigarette smokers: an fMRI study. *Neuropsychopharmacology*, Vol.31, No.12, pp. 2728-2738.

McMillen, IC.; Rattanatray, L.; Duffield, JA.; Morrison, JL.; MacLaughlin, SM.; Gentili, S. & Muhlhausler, BS. (2009). The early origins of later obesity: pathways and mechanisms. *Advan Exp Med Biol*, Vol.646, pp. 71-81.

McNeal, JU. & Yeh, C. (1997). Development of consumer behavior patterns among Chinese children. *J Consum Market*, Vol.14, pp. 45-59.

Mi, J.; Cheng, H.; Zhao, XY.; Hou, DQ.; Chen, FF. & Zhang, KL. (2008). Developmental origin of metabolic syndrome: interaction of thinness at birth and overweight during adult life in Chinese population. *Obes Rev*, Vol.9, No.1, pp. 91-94.

Miller, EK. & Cohen, JD. (2001). An integrative theory of prefrontal cortex function. *Annu Rev Neurosci*, Vol.24, pp. 167–202.

Mogenson, GJ. (1982). Studies of the nucleus accumbens and its mesolimbic dopaminergic affects in relation to ingestive behaviors and reward. In: *The Neural Basis of Feeding and Reward,* GB. Hoebel & D. Novin (Eds.), Haer Institute, Brunswick, ME.

Mokdad, AH.; Marks, JS.; Stroup, DF. & Gerberding, JL. (2004). Actual causes of death in the United States, 2000. *JAMA,* Vol.291, No.10, pp. 1238-1245.

Morris, JS. & Dolan, RJ. (2001). Involvement of human amygdala and orbitofrontal cortex in hunger-enhanced memory for food stimuli. *J Neurosci,* Vol.21, pp. 5304–5310.

Murakami, K.; Sasaki, S.; Takahashi, Y.; Okubo, H.; Hosoi, Y.; Horiguchi, H.; Oguma, E. & Kayama, F. (2006). Dietary glycemic index and load in relation to metabolic risk factors in Japanese female farmers with traditional dietary habits. *Am J Clin Nutr,* Vol.83, pp. 1161-1169.

O'Doherty, J.; Rolls, ET.; Francis, S.; Bowtell, R.; McGlone, F.; Kobal, G.; Renner, B. & Ahne, G. (2000). Sensory-specific satiety-related olfactory activation of the human orbitofrontal cortex. *Neuroreport,* Vol.11, No.2, pp. 399-403.

O'Doherty, JP. (2004). Reward representations and reward-related learning in the human brain: insights from neuroimaging. *Curr Opin Neurobiol,* Vol.14, No.6, pp. 769-776.

Ogura, K.; Shinohara, M.; Ohno, K. & Mori, E. (2008). Frontal behavioral syndromes in Prader-Willi syndrome. *Brain Dev,* Vol.30, No.7, pp. 469-476.

Parvanta, SA.; Brown, JD.; Du, S.; Zimmer, CR.; Zhao, X. & Zhai, F. (2010). Television use and snacking behaviors among children and adolescents in China. *J Adolesc Health,* Vol.46, No.4, pp. 339-345.

Petry, NM. (2006). Should the scope of addictive behaviors be broadened to include pathological gambling? *Addiction,* Vol.101, No.1, pp. 152-160.

Pfefferbaum, A.; Sullivan, EV.; Mathalon, DH. & Lim, KO. (1997). Frontal lobe volume loss observed with magnetic resonance imaging in older chronic alcoholics. *Alcohol Clin Exp Res,* Vol.21, pp. 521–529.

Pi-Sunyer, FX. (2002). The medical risks of obesity. *Obesity Surg,* Vol., No.1, pp. 6S–11S.

Popkin, BM. (2001). The nutrition transition and obesity in the developing world. *J Nutr,* Vol.131, pp. 871S-873S.

Popkin, BM.; Paeratakul, S.; Zhai, F. & Ge, K. (1995). A review of dietary and environmental correlates of obesity with emphasis on developing countries. *Obes Res,* Vol.3, No.2, pp. 145s-53s.

Potenza, MN.; Hong, KI.; Lacadie, CM.; Fulbright, RK.; Tuit, KL. & Sinha, R. (2012). Neural correlates of stress-induced and cue-induced drug craving: influences of sex and cocaine dependence. *Am J Psychiatry,* [Epub ahead of print].

Rada, P. & Hoebel, BG. (2005). Acetylcholine in the accumbens is decreased by diazepam and increased by benzodiazepine withdrawal: a possible mechanism for dependency. *Eur J Pharmacol,* Vol.508, pp. 131–138.

Rada, P.; Avena, NM. & Hoebel, BG. (2005). Daily bingeing on sugar repeatedly releases dopamine in the accumbens shell. *Neuroscience,* Vol.134, No.3, pp. 737-744.

Raman, RP. (2002). Obesity and health risks. *Journal of the American College of Nutrition,* Vol.21, pp. 34S–139S.

Rhee, K. (2008). Childhood overweight and the relationship between parent behaviors, parenting style, and family functioning. *Annals Amer Acad Pol Soc Sci,* Vol.615, pp. 11-37.

Robbins, TW. & Everitt, BJ. (1999). Drug addiction: bad habits add up. *Nature*, Vol.398, No.6728, pp. 567-570.

Robinson, TE. & Berridge, KC. (1993). The neural basis of drug craving: an incentive-sensitization theory of addiction, *Brain Research Reviews*, Vol.18, pp. 247–291.

Rolls, ET. (2000). The orbitofrontal cortex and reward. *Cereb Cortex*, Vol.10, No.3, pp. 284-294.

Rosenbaum, M.; Sy, M.; Pavlovich, K.; Leibel, RL. & Hirsch, J. (2008). Leptin reverses weight loss-induced changes in regional neural activity responses to visual food stimuli. *J Clin Invest*, Vol.118, No.7, pp. 2583-2591.

Rosenkranz, JA. & Grace, AA. (2001). Dopamine attenuates prefrontal cortical suppression of sensory inputs to the basolateral amygdala of rats. *J Neurosci*,Vol.21, pp. 4090–4103.

Ross, HE. & Ivis, F. (1999). Binge eating and substance use among male and female adolescents. *International Journal of Eating Disorders*, Vol.26, pp. 245–260.

Ruiz, JR.; Labayen, I.; Ortega, FB.; Legry, V.; Moreno, LA.; Dallongeville, J.; Martínez-Gómez, D.; Bokor, S.; Manios, Y.; Ciarapica, D.; Gottrand, F.; De Henauw, S.; Molnár, D.; Sjöström, M.; Meirhaeghe, A. & HELENA Study Group. (2010). Attenuation of the effect of the FTO rs9939609 polymorphism on total and central body fat by physical activity in adolescents: the HELENA study. *Arch Pediatr Adolesc Med*, Vol.164, pp. 328–333.

Saad, MF.; Khan, A.; Sharma, A.; Michael, R.; Riad-Gabriel, MG.; Boyadjian, R.; Jinagouda, SD.; Steil, GM. & Kamdar, V. (1998). Physiological insulinemia acutely modulates plasma leptin. *Diabetes*, Vol. 47, No.4, pp. 544-549.

Sahu, A. & Kalra, SP. (1993). Neuropeptide regulation of feeding behavior: Neuropeptide Y. *TEM*, Vol.4, No.7, pp. 217–224.

Sato, Y.; Ito, T.; Udaka, N.; Kanisawa, M.; Noguchi, Y.; Cushman, SW. & Satoh, S. (1996). Immunohistochemical localization of facilitated-diffusion glucose transporters in rat pancreatic islets. *Tissue Cell*, Vol.28, No.6, pp. 637-643.

Schoenbaum, G. & Shaham, Y. (2008). The role of orbitofrontal cortex in drug addiction: a review of preclinical studies. *Biol Psychiatry*, Vol.63, No.3, pp. 256-262.

Schroeder, BE.; Binzak, JM. & Kelley, AE. (2001). A common profile of prefrontal cortical activation following exposure to nicotine- or chocolate associated contextual cues. *Neuroscience*, Vol.105, pp. 535–545.

Scuteri, A.; Sanna, S.; Chen, WM.; Uda, M.; Albai, G.; Strait, J.; Najjar, S.; Nagaraja, R.; Orrú, M.; Usala, G.; Dei, M.; Lai, S.; Maschio, A.; Busonero, F.; Mulas, A.; Ehret, GB.; Fink, AA.; Weder, AB.; Cooper, RS.; Galan, P.; Chakravarti, A.; Schlessinger, D.; Cao, A.; Lakatta, E. & Abecasis, GR. (2007). Genome-wide association scan shows genetic variants in the FTO gene are associated with obesity-related traits. *PLoS Genet*, Vol.3, No. e115.

Shapira, NA.; Liu, Y.; He, AG.; Bradley, MM.; Lessig, MC.; James, GA.; Stein, DJ.; Lang, PJ. & Goodman, WK. (2003). Brain activation by disgust-inducing pictures in obsessive- compulsive disorder. *Biol Psychiatry*, Vol.54, No.7, pp. 751–756.

Shi, Z.; Lien, N.; Kumar, BN. & Holmboe-Ottesen, G. (2005). Socio-demographic differences in food habits and preferences of school adolescents in Jiangsu Province, China. *Eur J Clin Nutr*, Vol.59, pp. 1439-1448.

Shi, Z.; Luscombe-Marsh, ND.; Wittert, GA.; Yuan, B.; Dai, Y.; Pan, X. & Taylor, AW. (2010). Monosodium glutamate is not associated with obesity or a greater prevalence of weight gain over 5 years: findings from the Jiangsu Nutrition Study of Chinese adults. *Br J Nutr*, Vol.104, pp. 457-463.

Shi, Z; Lien, N; Kumar, BN. & Holmboe-Ottesen, G. (2007). Perceptions of weight and associated factors of adolescents in Jiangsu Province, China. *Public Health Nutr*, Vol.10, pp. 298-305.

Simmons, WK.; Martin, A. & Barsalou, LW. (2005). Pictures of appetizing foods activate gustatory cortices for taste and reward. *Cerebral Cortex*, Vol.15, pp. 1602-1608.

Singh, NN.; Lancioni, GE.; Singh, AN.; Winton, AS.; Singh, J.; McAleavey, KM. & Adkins, AD. (2008). A mindfulness-based health wellness program for an adolescent with Prader- Willi syndrome. *Behav Modif*, Vol.32, No.2, pp. 167-181.

Small, DM.; Zatorre, RJ.; Dagher, A.; Evans, AC. & Jones-Gotman, M. (2001). Changes in brain activity related to eating chocolate: from pleasure to aversion. *Brain*, Vol.124, No.9, pp. 1720-1733.

Solinas, M. & Goldberg, SR. (2005). Motivational effects of cannabinoids and opioids of food reinforcement depend on simultaneous activation of cannabinoid and opioid systems. *Neuropscyhopharmacology*, Vol.30, No.11, pp. 2035-2045.

Spring, B.; Schneider, K.; Smith, M.; Kendzor, D.; Appelhans, B.; Hedeker, D. & Pagoto, S. (2008). Abuse potential of carbohydrates for overweight carbohydrate cravers. *Psychopharmacology (Berl)*, Vol.197, No.4, pp. 637-647.

Swanson, LW. & Petrovich, GD. (1998). What is the amygdala? *Trends Neurosci*, Vol.21, pp. 323–331.

Tartar, RE.; Ammerman, RT. & Ott, PJ. (1998). Handbook of substance abuse. *Neurobehavioral Pharmacology*. Premium Press, New York, NY.

Tataranni, PA. & DelParigi, A. (2003). Functional neuroimaging: a new generation of human brain studies in obesity research. *Obes Rev*, Vol.4, No.4, pp. 229-238.

Urban, NB. & Martinez, D. (2012). Neurobiology of addiction: insight from neurochemical imaging. *Psychiatr Clin North Am*, Vol.35, No.2, pp.:521-541.

Volkow, ND. & Fowler, JS. (2000). Addiction, a disease of compulsion and drive: involvement of the orbitofrontal cortex. *Cereb Cortex*, Vol. 10, No.3, pp. 318-325.

Volkow, ND. & Wise, RA. (2005). How can drug addiction help us understand obesity? *Nat Neurosci*, Vol.8, No.5, pp. 555-560.

Volkow, ND. & Li, TK. (2004). Science and society: drug addiction: the neurobiology of behaviour gone awry. *Nat. Rev. Neurosci*, Vol. 5, pp. 963–970.

Volkow, ND.; Fowler, JS. & Wang, GJ. (2004). The addicted human brain viewed in the light of imaging studies: brain circuits and treatment strategies. *Neuropharmacology*, Vol.47, No.1, pp. 3-13.

Volkow, ND.; Wang ,GJ.; Fowler, JS.; Logan, J.; Gatley, SJ.; Hitzemann, R.; Chen, AD.; Dewey, SL. & Pappas, N. (1997). Decreased striatal dopaminergic responsiveness in detoxified cocaine-dependent subjects. *Nature*, Vol.386, pp. 830–833.

Volkow, ND.; Wang, GJ.; Fowler, JS. & Telang, F. (2008). Overlapping neuronal circuits in addiction and obesity: evidence of systems pathology. *Philos Trans R Soc Lond B Biol Sci*. Vol.363, No.1507, pp. 3191-3200.

Volkow, ND.; Wang, GJ.; Fowler, JS.; Logan, J.; Jayne, M.; Franceschi, D.; Wong, C.; Gatley, SJ.; Gifford, AN.; Ding, Y-S. & Pappas, N. (2002). "Nonhedonic" food motivation in humans involves dopamine in the dorsal striatum and methylphenidate amplifies this effect. *Synapse*, Vol.44, No.3, pp. 175-180.

von Deneen, KM. & Liu, Y. (2011). Obesity as an addiction: Why do the obese eat more? *Maturitas*, Vol.68, No.4, pp. 342-345.

von Deneen, KM.; Gold, MS. & Liu, Y. (2009). Food addiction and cues in Prader-Willi Syndrome. *J Addict Med*, Vol.3, pp. 19–25.

von Deneen, KM.; Wei, Q.; Tian, J. & Liu, Y. (2011). Obesity in China. What are the causes? *Curr Pharm Des*, Vol.17, No.12, pp. 1132-1139.

Walther, K.; Birdsill, AC.; Glisky, EL. & Ryan, L. (2010). Structural brain differences and cognitive functioning related to body mass index in older females. *Hum Brain Mapp*, Vol.31, pp. 1052-1064.

Wang, GJ.; Volkow, ND.; Logan, J.; Rappas, NR.; Wong, CT.; Zhu, W.; Netusil, N. & Fowler JS. (2001). Brain dopamine and obesity. *Lancet*, Vol.357, No.9253, pp. 354-357.

Wang, GJ.; Volkow, ND.; Telang, F.; Jayne, M.; Ma, J; Rao, M.; Zhu, W.; Wong, CT.; Pappas, NR.; Geliebter, A. & Fowler, JS. (2004). Exposure to appetitive food stimuli markedly activates the human brain. *Neuroimage*, Vol.21, No.4, pp. 1790-1797.

Wang, GJ.; Volkow, ND.; Thanos, PK. & Fowler, JS. (2009). Imaging of brain dopamine pathways: implications for understanding obesity. *J Addict Med*, Vol.3, pp. 8–18.

Wang, K.; Ao, YT.; Zhao, L.; Guo, YY.; Shagedeke; Xu, YS.; Song, T.; Gerli & He, BX. (2006). Analysis on obesity and its risk factors among inhabitants of Bortala prefecture of Xinjiang autonomous region. *Chinese J Public Health*, Vol.22, No.9, pp. 1128-1130.

Wang, Y.; Beydoun, MA.; Liang, L.; Caballero, B. & Kumanyika, SK. (2008a). Will all Americans become overweight or obese? Estimating the progression and cost of the US obesity epidemic. *Obesity*, Vol.16, pp. 2323–2330.

Wang, Z.; Zhai, F.; Du, S. & Popkin, B. (2008b). Dynamic shifts in Chinese eating behaviors. *Asia Pac J Clin Nutr*, Vol.17, pp. 123-130.

Warren, MW. & Gold, MS. (2007). The relationship between obesity and drug use. *Am J Psychiatry*, Vol.164, No.8, pp. 1268-1269.

Wise, RA. (2006). Role of brain dopamine in food reward and reinforcement. *Philos Trans R Soc Lond B Biol Sci*, Vol.361,pp. 1149–1158.

Wurtman, RJ. & Wurtman, JJ. (1995). Brain serotonin, carbohydrate-craving, obesity and depression. *Obes Res*, Vol.3, No.4, pp. 477S-480S.

Xi, B. & Mi, J. (2009). FTO polymorphisms are associated with obesity but not with diabetes in East Asian populations: a meta-analysis. *Biomed Environ Sci*, Vol.22, No.6, pp. 449- 457.

Xu, H.; Song, Y.; You, NC.; Zhang, ZF.; Greenland, S.; Ford, ES.; He, L. & Liu, S. (2010). Prevalence and clustering of metabolic risk factors for type 2 diabetes among Chinese adults in Shanghai, China. *BMC Public Health*, Vol.10, pp. 683.

Zapata, A.; Chefer, VI.; Ator, R.; Shippenberg, TS. & Rocha, BA. (2003). Behavioural sensitization and enhanced dopamine response in the nucleus accumbens after intravenous cocaine self-administration in mice. *Eur J Neurosci*, Vol.17, No.3, pp. 590- 596.

Zemmet, P. (2000). Diabetes and obesity worldwide epidemics in full flight. *60th Scientific Sessions of the American Diabetes Association*, San Antonio, Texas.

Zhai, F.; Wang, H.; Du, S.; He, Y.; Wang, Z.; Ge, K. & Popkin, BM. (2009). Prospective study on nutrition transition in China. *Nutr Rev*, Vol.67, pp. S56-61.

Zhang, Y.; von Deneen, KM.; Tian, J.; Gold, MS. & Liu, Y. (2011). Food addiction and neuroimaging. *Curr Pharm Des*, Vol.17, No.12, pp. 1149-1157.

Zhang, YB. & Harwood, J. (2004). Modernization and tradition in an age of globalization: cultural values in Chinese television commercials. *J Commun*, Vol.54, pp. 156-172.

10

Pathways Involved in the Cardiac Adaptive Changes Observed During Morphine Withdrawal

M.L. Laorden, M. V. Milanés and P. Almela
Department of Pharmacology, University of Murcia, Murcia, Spain

1. Introduction

The development of opioid addiction involves complex adaptive changes in opioid receptors and associated signalling systems, leading to neuronal plasticity in the brain regions projecting to different systems including the cardiovascular system. So, adaptive changes also occur in peripheral tissues and cells expressing opioid receptors, such as in the heart (Pugsley, 2002).

The effects of drugs of abuse, especially cocaine, on the cardiovascular system, have been extensively documented in animal model and in human. There is emerging evidence that drug abuse might trigger a variety of cardiac disorders from arrhythmias to acute myocardial infarction, heart failure and even sudden cardiac death (Lippi et al., 2010). Thus, various types of cardiac arrhythmias have been described in heroin addicts. Moreover, street heroin addicts frequently die suddenly, and there is evidence that this is an arrhythmia-related event (Nerantzis et al., 2011).

The majority of studies dealing with morphine on the field of cardiology are oriented on clinical usage of this drug and current cardiovascular research has been limited to the evaluation of factors or pathways believed to contribute to its physiological actions, such as delta- and kappa-opioid receptors, cyclooxygenase-2, inducible nitric oxide synthase or reactive oxygen species (Huh et al., 2001; Wang et al., 2001; Jiang et al., 2006; Xu et al., 2011).

Given the importance of morphine in clinical practice for the treatment of pain, investigation of its impact on the heart at the molecular levels requires more attention. Therefore, in this chapter we will discuss our recent discoveries about the implication of different molecular pathways in the cardiac adaptive changes that occur during morphine withdrawal.

The noradrenergic pathways and the hypothalamo-pituitary-adrenocortical (HPA) axis, a system largely controlled by corticoticotropin-releasing factor (CRF) in the paraventricular nucleus (PVN) of the hypothalamus, comprise two major adaptation mechanisms to stress. Like stressors, morphine withdrawal activates HPA axis in rats, which results in neuronal activation of stress-related neurosecretory neurons in the parvocellular neurons of the PVN. The PVN is anatomically divided into three magnocellular and five parvocellular subdivisions. The parvocellular subdivisions comprise the dorsal, lateral, medial periventricular and anterior parvocellular subnuclei (fig. 1).

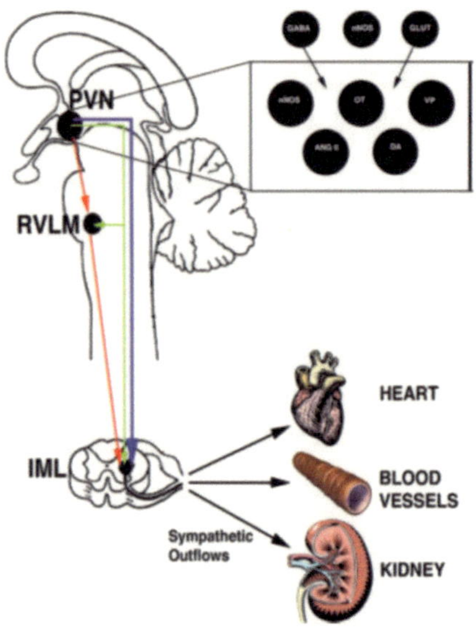

Fig. 1. Schematic illustrating the three main pathways by which the paraventricular nucleus of the hypothalamus (PVN) can influence sympathetic activity. Rostral ventrolateral medulla (RVLM), spinal intermediolateral cell column (IML). (Taken from Pyner, 2009).

These regions project to autonomic nuclei in the brain stem and spinal cord and are responsible for the activation of the sympathetic nervous system including cardiovascular regulation (Sawchenko and Swanson, 1982). In addition, the PVN receives afferent projections from several limbic structures that are implicated in behavioural and cardiovascular control, such as the medial amygdale, the prefrontal cortex and the lateral septum (Ongur et al., 1998; Risold and Swanson, 1997).

2. Hemodynamic variables during chronic morphine treatment and its withdrawal

Previous studies have demonstrated that chronic μ-opiod receptor stimulation decreases muscle sympathetic nerve activity (Kienbaum et al., 2001; 2002), NA plasma concentration (Kienbaum et al., 2001) and dopamine turnover in the heart (Rabadán et al., 1997). According to these data, we have demonstrated that chronic morphine treatment decreases two baseline cardiovascular parameters, mean arterial blood pressure (MAP) and heart rate (HR). However, μ-opioid receptor blockade by naloxone unmasks these effects, resulting in markedly increases in both parameters (fig. 2 and 3). In agreement with these data, naloxone administration to patients with chronic opioid abuse or to morphine dependent rats results in markedly increased muscle sympathetic nerve activity, NA plasma concentrations (Peart and Gross, 2006), NA and dopamine turnover (Almela et al., 2008; Milanés et al., 2000b) and total tyrosine hydroxylase (TH) expression (Almela et al., 2008). Altogether, these results suggest that an up-regulation of TH would be expected to increase the capacity of noradrenergic neurons to synthesize NA, which could contribute to the increase in NA turnover and in the hemodynamic changes seen in the heart during morphine withdrawal.

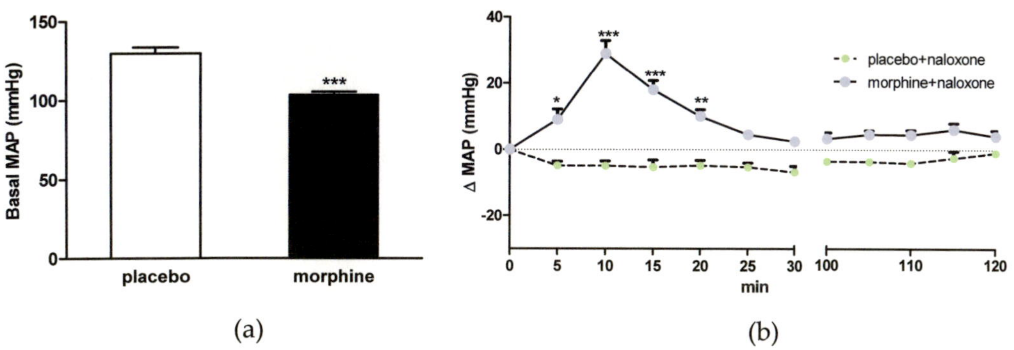

Fig. 2. Baseline mean arterial blood pressure (MAP) (mmHg) (A) in rats implanted with morphine or placebo pellets. Effects of naloxone (2 mg/kg s.c.) on changes in MAP (B). Naloxone was injected at time 0. Data are the mean±S.E.M. (n=5–7). ***P<0.001, **P<0.01, *P<0.05 versus placebo+naloxone.

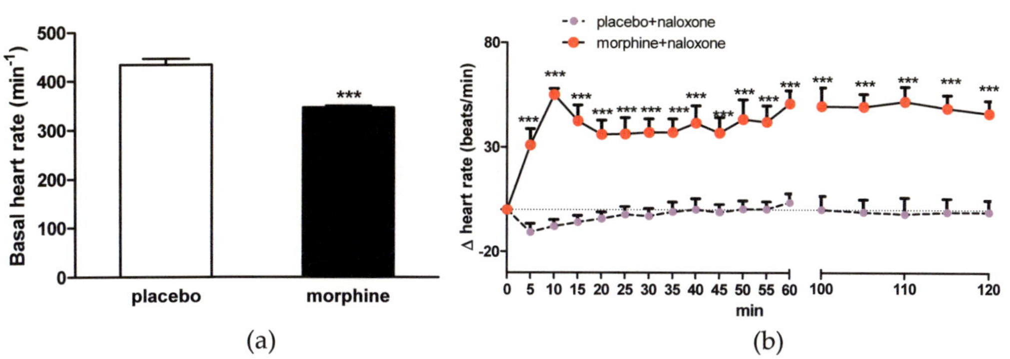

Fig. 3. Baseline heart rate (min−1) (A) in rats implanted with morphine or placebo pellets. Effects of naloxone (2 mg/kg s.c.) on changes in heart rate (B). Naloxone was injected at time 0. Data are the mean±S.E.M. (n=5–7). ***P<0.001, **P<0.01, *P<0.05 versus placebo+naloxone.

3. Evaluation of changes in pERK1/2 during morphine withdrawal

Extracellular signal-regulated kinase (ERK), one member of mitogen-activated extracellular kinase (MAPK) family, transduces a broad range of extracellular stimuli into diverse intracellular responses. ERK signalling pathway could be important as regulator of cardiac function (Michel et al., 2001) and neuronal plasticity (Adams et al., 2002). Recently, several studies have shown that this pathway contributes to naloxone-precipitated withdrawal in morphine dependent rats (Ren et al., 2004; Almela et al., 2007, 2008, 2011).

Our time course study showed that there was a significant elevation of phospho(p)ERK1 and phospho(p)ERK2 levels in the right (fig. 4) and left ventricle 30, 60, 90 or 120 min after naloxone administration to morphine dependent rats. We also studied the distribution of these proteins by immunohistochemical procedures and we observed high levels of pERK1/2 immunoreactivity in the right and left ventricle after naloxone administration to morphine-treated rats (fig. 5). The immunolabelling was mainly present in cytoplasmic compartments, suggesting a local activation of the protein. A nuclear staining was also observed in some myocytes, supporting a nuclear translocation of activated ERK proteins. These immunohistochemical results were consistent with western blot analyses (figure 4).

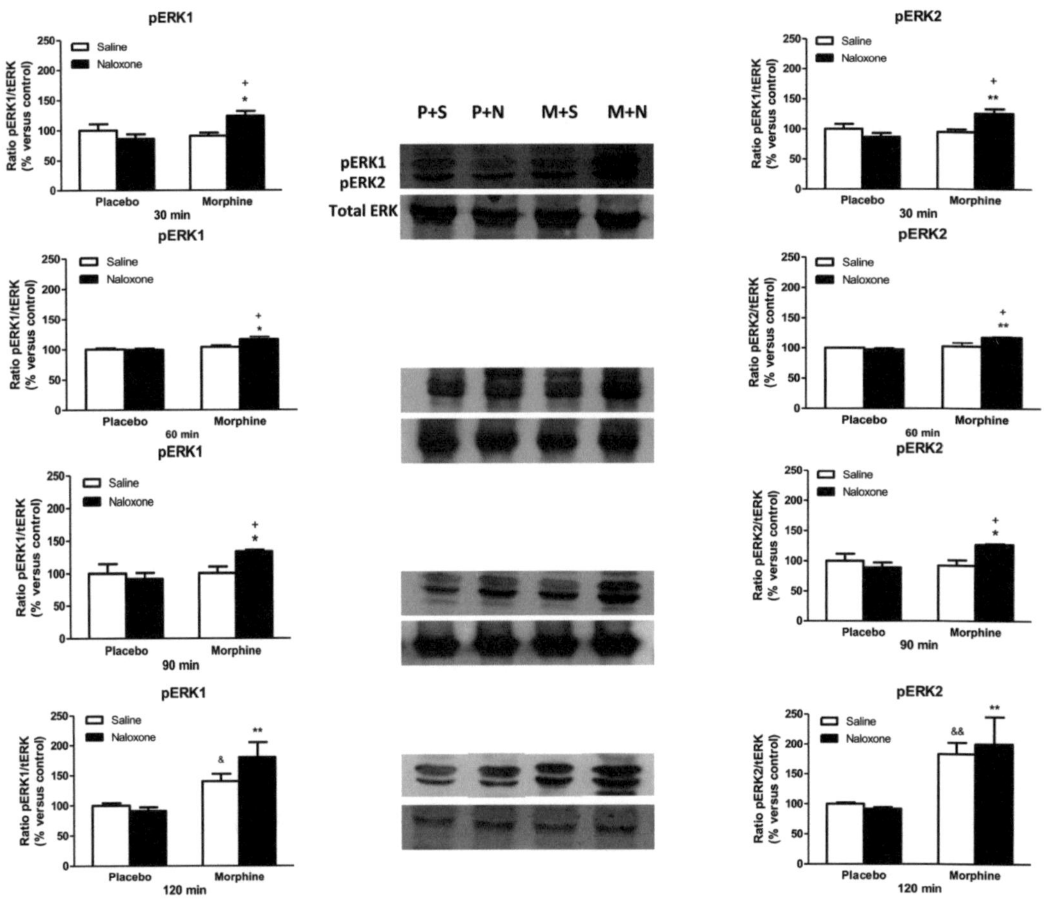

Fig. 4. Western-blotting analysis of phospho(p)ERK1 and phospho(p)ERK2 in the right ventricle 30, 60, 90 and 120 min after saline (S) or naloxone (N) administration to placebo- (P) or morphine- (M) pretreated rats. The immunoreactivity corresponding to pERK1 or pERK2 is expressed as a percentage of that in the control group defined as 100% value. Data are the mean±S.E.M. (n=5–6). **P<0.01, *P<0.05 versus the placebo group injected with naloxone; +P<0.05 versus the dependent group injected with saline instead of naloxone; &&P<0.01, &P<0.05 versus the placebo group receiving saline.

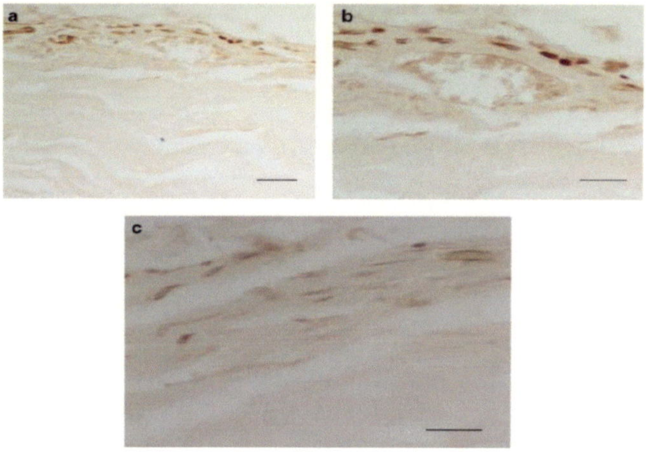

Fig. 5. Immunohistochemical detection of phospho(p)ERK1/2 in the left ventricular wall. Rats were made dependent on morphine for 7 days and on day 8 were injected with naloxone (2 mg/kg s.c.). 90 min after injections, rats were perfused and the right and left ventricle was processed for pERK1/2 immunohistochemistry. Scale bar 30 µm (a), 20 µm (b, c).

4. Tyrosine hydroxylase phosphorylation

TH, the rate limiting enzyme in the synthesis of catecholamines, plays important roles in the regulation of sympathetic nervous system and its impact on cardiac function (Rao et al., 2007). In particular, increases in the phosphorylation of Ser40 and Ser31 accelerate TH activity, thereby stimulating production of neurotransmitter in catecholamines terminals (Kumer and Vrana, 1996; Dunkley et al., 2004). TH expression is subjected to intricate regulation by a number of mechanisms, including transcriptional and post-transcriptional processes (Kumer and Vrana, 1996; Mallet, 1999). Short-term regulation of catecholamine biosynthesis occurs through the modulation of the state of phosphorylation of TH. TH phosphorylation and activation is the primary mechanism responsible for the maintenance of catecholamine levels in tissues after catecholamine secretion. TH can be phosphorylated at serine (Ser) residues 8, 19, 31 and 40 by a variety of PKs (Campbell et al., 1986). PKA and PKC phosphorylate TH only at Ser40 (Roskoski et al., 1987; Funakoshi et al., 1991). ERK1 and ERK2 were shown to phosphorylate Ser31 in situ (Haycock et al., 1992). The phosphorylation of Ser40 increases the enzyme's activity in vitro, in situ and in vivo. Phosphorylation at Ser31 also increases the activity but to a much lesser extent than Ser40 phosphorylation. The phosphorylation of TH at Ser19 or Ser8 has no direct effect on TH activity (Dunkley et al., 2004) (fig. 6).

Previous studies have shown that naloxone-induced morphine withdrawal results in an increased NA turnover at heart level (Milanés et al., 2000a). This enhancement in NA turnover could be due to changes in the state of phosphorylation of TH, which are critically involved in the regulation of catecholamines synthesis and function. Therefore, we have studied the expression and phosphorylation at Ser31 and Ser40 during morphine withdrawal at different time points. Rats withdrawn from morphine presented an increase in total TH expression (fig. 7) and in TH phosphorylated at Ser31 (fig. 8) and Ser40 (fig. 9), together with an enhancement of TH activity (fig. 10). This activation of TH could be responsible for the increase in the hemodynamic parameters described above.

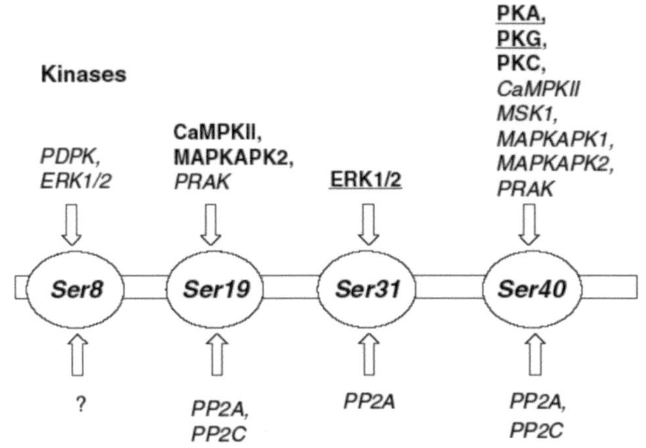

Fig. 6. The protein kinases (PK) and protein phosphatases (PP) capable of modulating tyrosine hydroxylase (TH) phosphorylation in vitro and in situ (Taken from Dunkley et al., 2004).

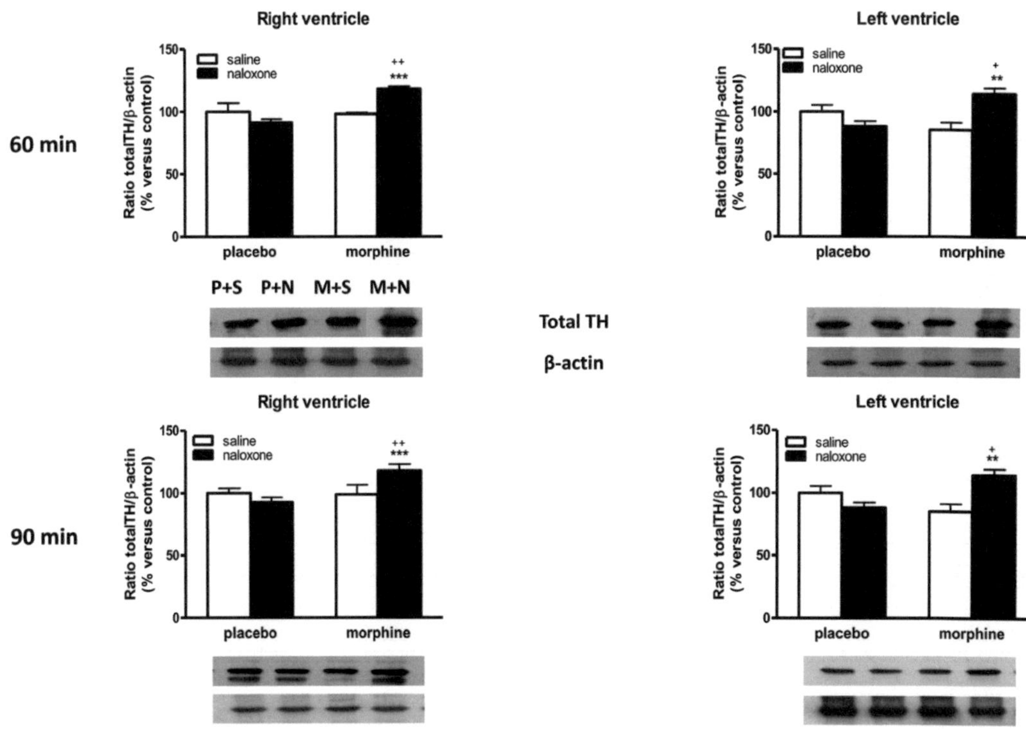

Fig. 7. Western blotting analysis of TH immunoreactivity levels in the right and left ventricle 60 or 90 min after saline (S) or naloxone (N) administration to placebo- (P) or morphine- (M) treated rats. The immunoreactivity corresponding to total TH is expressed as a percentage of that in the control group (P+S; defined as 100%). Data are the mean±S.E.M (n=4–6). $^{**}P<0.01$, $^{***}P<0.001$ versus the group receiving saline instead of naloxone; $^{+}P<0.05$, $^{++}P<0.01$ versus the group pretreated with placebo instead of morphine.

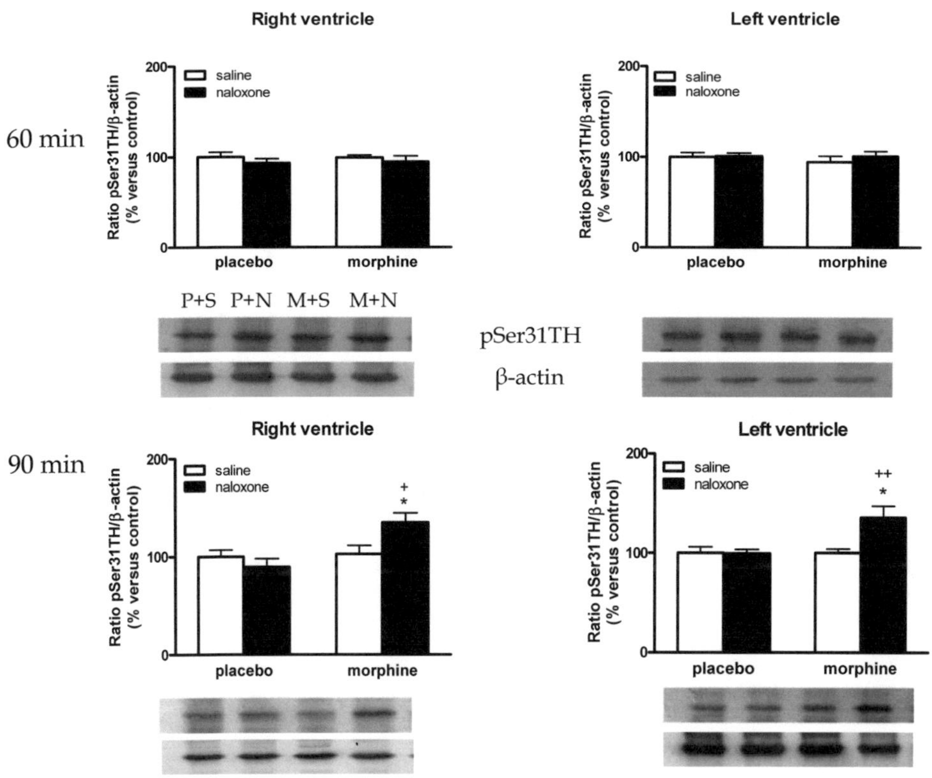

Fig. 8. Western blotting analysis of phospho(p)Ser31TH in the right and left ventricle 60 or 90 min after saline (S) or naloxone (N) administration to placebo- (P) or morphine- (M) treated rats. The immunoreactivity corresponding to pSer31TH is expressed as a percentage of that in the control group (P+S; defined as 100%). Data are the mean±S.E.M. (n=4–6). *P<0.05 versus the group receiving saline instead of naloxone; ++P<0.01, +P<0.05 versus the group pretreated with placebo instead of morphine.

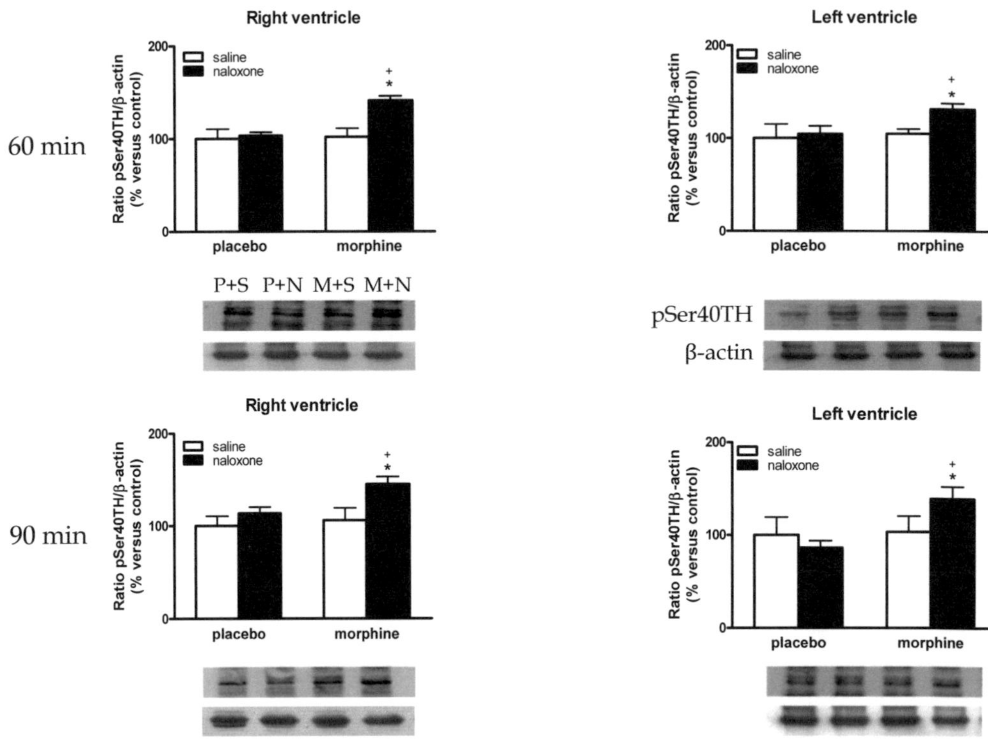

Fig. 9. Western blotting analysis of phospho(p)Ser40 TH in the right and left ventricle 60 or 90 min after saline (S) or naloxone (N) administration to placebo- (P) or morphine- (M) treated rats. The immunoreactivity corresponding to pSer40TH is expressed as a percentage of that in the control group (P+S; defined as 100%). Data are the mean±S.E.M. (n=4–6). *P<0.05 versus the group receiving saline instead of naloxone; +P<0.05 versus the group pretreated with placebo instead of morphine.

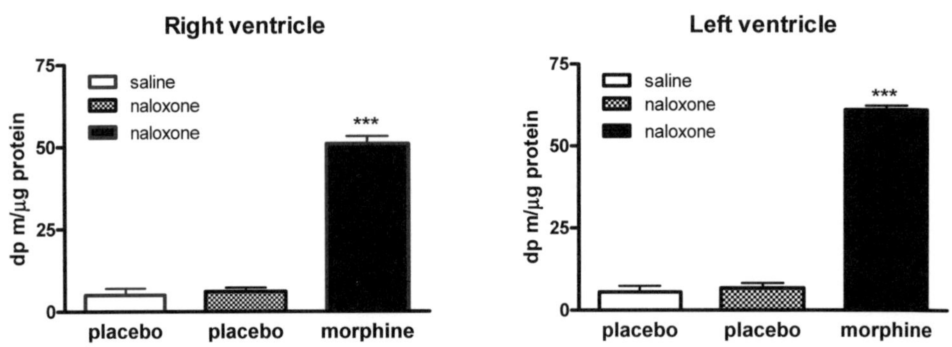

Fig. 10. TH activity in right and left ventricle from placebo or morphine dependent rats 90 min after s.c. administration of saline or naloxone. Data are the mean±S.E.M. (n=4–6). ***P<0.001 versus the group pretreated with placebo instead of morphine.

5. Changes in c-Fos expression

c-Fos immunoreactivity was examined by western blot and immunohistochemistry. Western blot analysis showed that after naloxone injection to rats chronically treated with morphine, there was a significant induction of c-Fos immunoreactivity in the right and left ventricle. Immunohistochemical analysis corroborated these results. Thus, rats dependent on morphine and given naloxone showed a significant induction of c-Fos immunoreactivity in the right ventricle, septum and left ventricle (fig. 11). This increase of c-Fos could contribute to activate TH synthesis through its activity on the AP-1 sequence present in the TH gene promoter region.

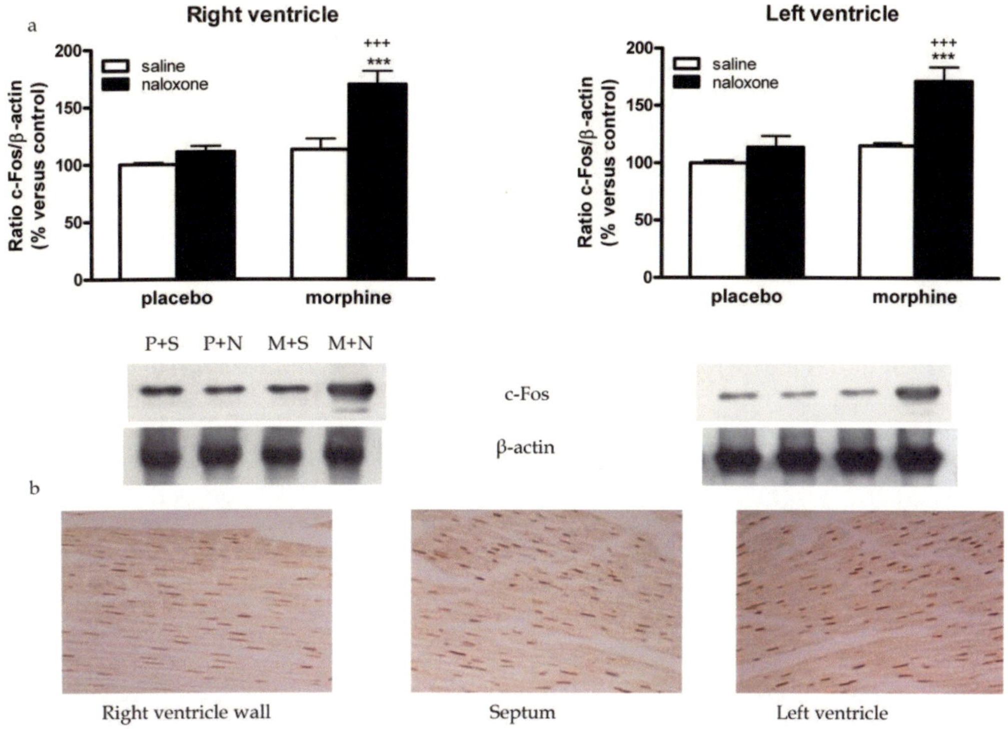

Fig. 11. (a) Representative immunoblots of c-Fos in samples isolated from placebo (P) or morphine (M) dependent rats 90 min after s.c. administration of saline (S) or naloxone (N). For quantification, optical densities of c-Fos immunoreactive bands were measured, normalized to the background values, and expressed as percentage of controls, defined as 100% value. Data are the mean±S.E.M. (n=4–6). $^{+++}$P<0.001 versus M+S; ***P<0.001 versus P+N. (b) Photomicrographs of c-Fos immunoreactvity in the right and left ventricular wall and in the septum, after naloxone-precipitated withdrawal. Scale bar 58 μm.

6. Implication of ERK and PKA in the cardiac adaptive changes observed during morphine withdrawal

To assess the relative contribution of ERK and PKA to the regulation of c-Fos and TH, we examined morphine withdrawal-induced c-Fos expression in animals receiving SL327, a selective ERK inhibitor or HA-1004, a selective PKA inhibitor. SL327 administration before naloxone to rats chronically treated with morphine significantly diminished the increase in c-Fos levels in both ventricles (fig. 12).

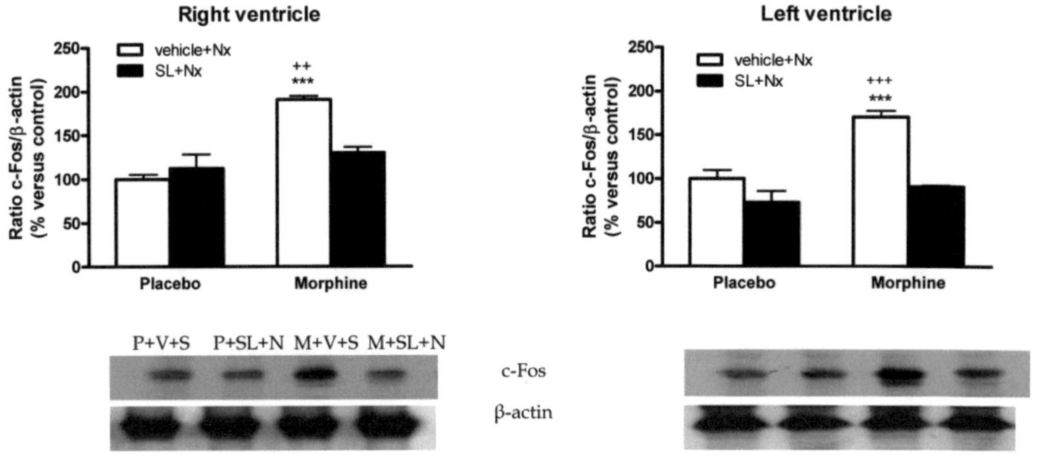

Fig. 12. Morphine withdrawal stimulates c-Fos expression in the right and left ventricle. Representative immunoblots of c-Fos in the right and left ventricle tissue isolated from placebo (P) or morphine (M) dependent rats, 90 min after s.c. administration of naloxone (Nx, N) in the absence (vehicle, veh, V, DMSO) or presence of SL327 (SL, 100 mg/kg) 1 h before naloxone. c-Fos immunoreactive bands were measured, normalized to the background values and expressed as percentages of controls. Data correspond to mean±S.E.M. (n=4). $^{+++}P<0.001$, $^{++}P<0.01$ versus M+SL+N; $^{***}P<0.001$ versus P+V+N.

However, chronic inhibition of PKA concurrently with morphine treatment did not modify c-Fos induction during morphine withdrawal (fig. 13). These results reveal that ERK but not PKA is an important pathway mediating c-Fos induction. However, previous results from our laboratory showed that inhibition of PKC also produced an inhibition of c-Fos expression in the heart (Almela et al., 2006) suggesting that the transcriptional regulation of c-Fos seems to be under a combined control of an ERK-dependent and-independent pathway. On the other hand, the expression of c-Fos, mainly due to phosphorylation of ERK1/2, was not antagonized by propranolol or prazosin (González-Cuello et al., 2004), suggesting that the activation of ERK and c-Fos expression is not due to an indirect mechanism via sympathetic activation.

In addition, our results showed that SL327 blocks the increase in TH phosphorylated at Ser31 observed in the right and left ventricle after the injection of naloxone to morphine dependent rats (fig. 14). The only protein kinase reported to phosphorylate TH at Ser31 in vitro was ERK (Haycock et al., 1992; Lindgren et al., 2002). In situ phosphorylation of TH at Ser31 increases TH activity and catecholamine synthesis (Haycock, 1992). Given that TH is phosphorylated on a specific serine residue (Ser31) by the ERK, it is possible that activation of ERK1/2 in the heart provides a way in which TH is regulated under morphine dependence.

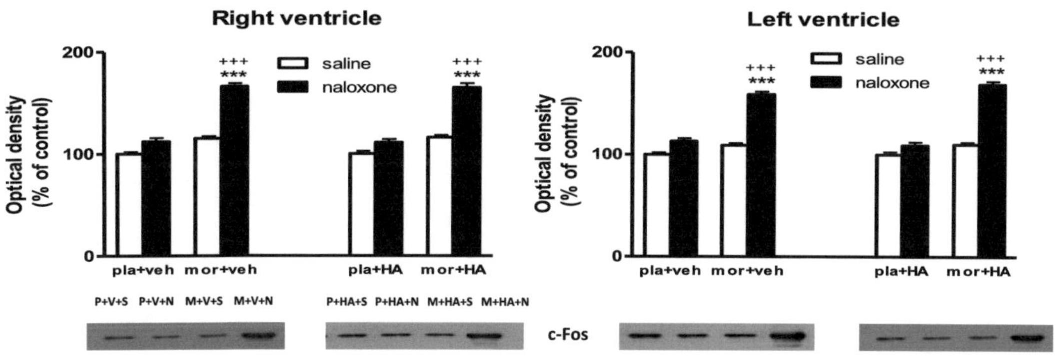

Fig. 13. Western blotting analysis of c-Fos immunoreactivity levels in the right and left ventricle after naloxone-precipitated withdrawal in vehicle- (veh, V) infused rats and in animals chronically administered with HA-1004 (HA). Animals received s.c. implantation of placebo (pla, P) or morphine (mor, M) pellets for 7 days and concomitantly were infused with vehicle or HA-1004 (40 nmol/day). On day 8, rats were injected with saline (S) or naloxone (N, 5 mg/kg, s.c.) and were decapitated 90 min later. The immunoreactivity corresponding to c-Fos is expressed as a percentage of that in the control group (P+V+S; defined as 100% value). Data are the mean±SEM (n=4–6). ***p<0.001 versus the group receiving saline instead of naloxone; $^{+++}$p<0.001 versus the group pretreated with placebo instead of morphine.

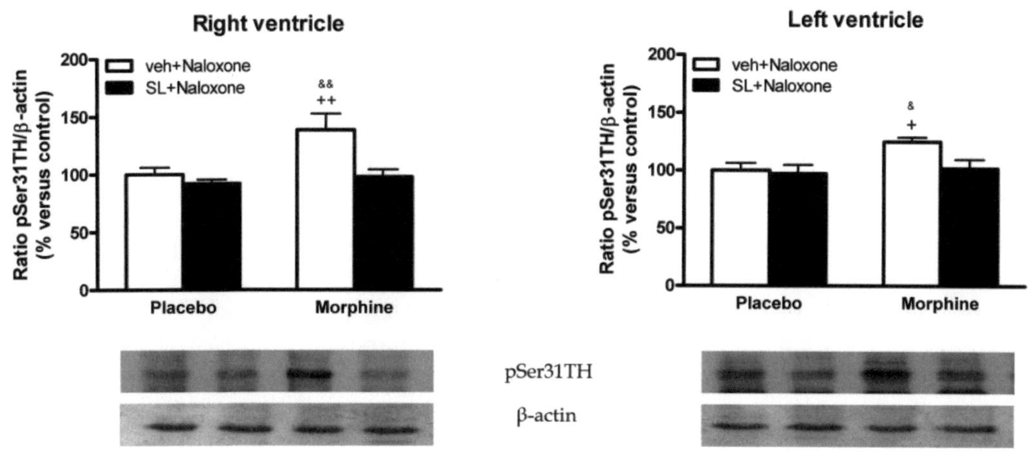

Fig. 14. Phospho(p)Ser31TH immunoblots in right and left ventricle from placebo or morphine dependent rats 90 min after s.c. administration of naloxone in the absence or presence of SL327 (SL, 100 mg/kg, i.p.), 1 h before naloxone. pSer31TH immunoreactive bands were measured, normalized to the background values and expressed as percentage of controls. Data are the mean±S.E.M. (n=4–6). $^{++}$P<0.01 versus the group pretreated with placebo instead of morphine; $^{\&\&}$P<0.01 versus morphine+SL+naloxone.

Similarly, HA-1004 blocked the enhancement of TH phosphorylated at Ser40 in the heart after morphine withdrawal (fig. 15), suggesting that different pathways are implicated in the postranscriptional regulation of TH.

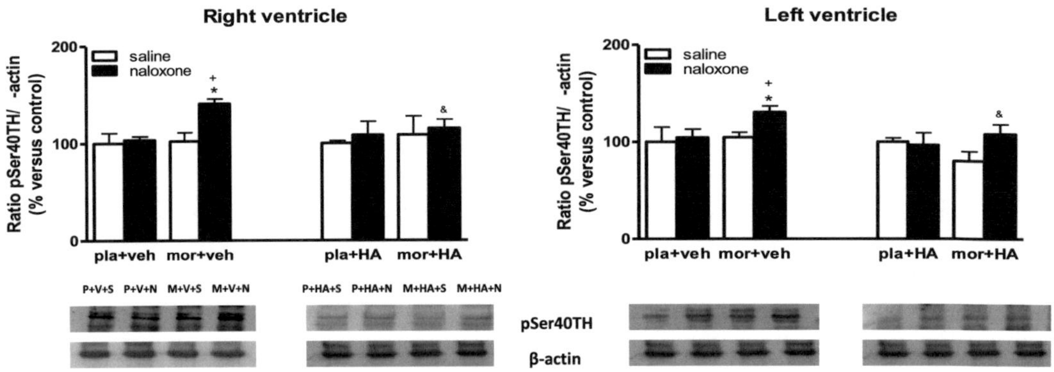

Fig. 15. Western blotting analysis of phospho(p)Ser40TH in the right ventricle 60 min after saline (S) or naloxone (N) administration to placebo- (pla, P) or morphine- (mor, M) treated rats receiving vehicle (veh, V) or HA-1004 (HA). The immunoreactivity corresponding to pSer40TH is expressed as a percentage of that in the control group (P+V+S; defined as 100%). Data are the mean±S.E.M. (n=4–6). *P<0.05 versus the group receiving saline instead of naloxone; +P<0.05 versus the group pretreated with placebo instead of morphine; &P<0.05 versus the group receiving vehicle instead of HA-1004.

7. Crosstalk between PKA and ERK

It is now appreciated that crosstalk among various signal pathways plays an important role in activation of intracellular and intranuclear signal transduction cascades. In our study, chronic treatment with HA-1004 antagonized the increase in ERK1/2 phosphorylation observed during morphine withdrawal in the heart (fig. 16). These results suggest a crosstalk between PKA and ERK pathways.

To assess the contribution of PKA to the regulation of TH, we examined TH phosphorylated at Ser31 during morphine withdrawal in animals receiving the selective inhibitor of PKA HA-1004. This inhibitor prevents the ability of naloxone-precipitated morphine withdrawal to increase TH phosphorylated at Ser31 levels in the right and left ventricle (fig. 17).

Although the mechanism of crosstalk between PKA and ERK pathways has not yet been clarified, it is possible that PKA pathway facilitates MEK1/2 that activates the ERK1/2 pathway (Obama et al., 2007; Stork and Schmitt, 2002). The activated ERK pathway increases the phosphorylation of proteins related to morphine dependence, including TH. Using phosphorylation state-specific antibodies directed toward TH at Ser31, we have shown that HA-1004 blocked the increase in the level of TH phosphorylation at Ser31 induced after naloxone injection to morphine dependent rats in the right and left ventricle. These data suggest that crosstalk between PKA and ERK pathways is a key regulatory design necessary to regulate the Ser31 phosphorylation of TH.

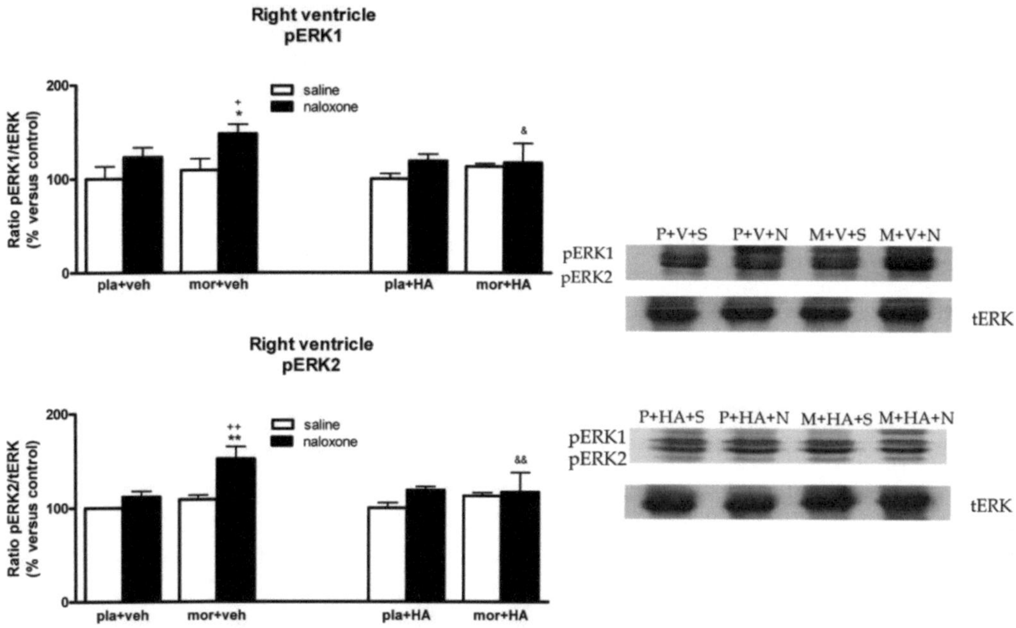

Fig. 16. Western blotting analysis of phospho(p)ERK1 and phospho(p)ERK2 immunoreactivity levels in the right ventricle 60 min after saline (S) or naloxone (N) administration to placebo- (pla, P) or morphine- (mor, M) treated rats receiving vehicle (veh, V) or HA-1004 (HA). The immunoreactivity corresponding to pERK1 or pERK2 is expressed as a percentage of that in the control group (P+V+S; defined as 100% value). Data are the mean±S.E.M. (n=4-6). **P<0.01, *P<0.05 versus the dependent group receiving saline instead of naloxone. ++P<0.01, +P<0.05 versus the group pretreated with placebo instead of morphine injected with naloxone. &&P<0.01, &P<0.05 versus the group receiving vehicle instead of HA.

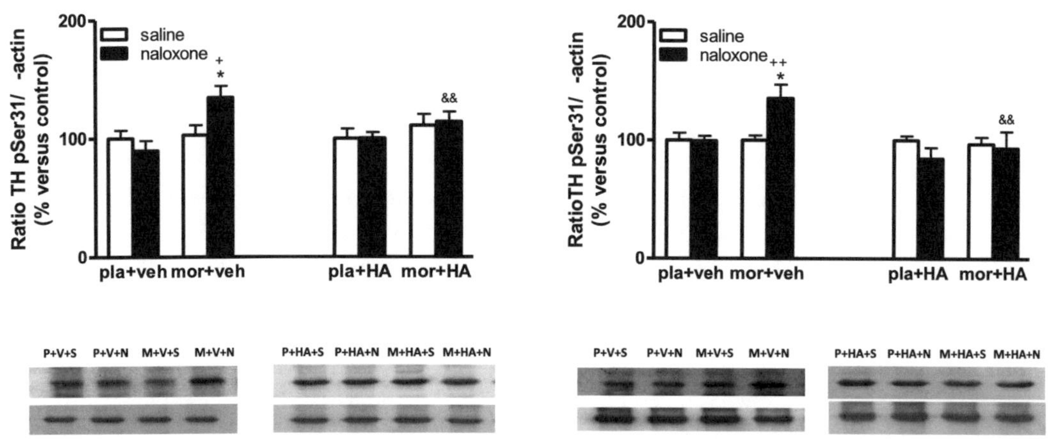

Fig. 17. Western blotting analysis of phospho(p)Ser31TH in the right and left ventricle 90 min after saline (S) or naloxone (N) administration to placebo- (pla, P) or morphine- (mor, M)

treated rats receiving vehicle (veh, V) or HA-1004 (HA). The immunoreactivity corresponding to pSer31TH is expressed as a percentage of that in the control group (P+V+S or P+HA+S; defined as 100% value). Data are the mean±S.E.M. (n=4–6). *p<0.05 versus the dependent group receiving saline instead of naloxone; ++P<0.01, +P<0.05 versus the group pretreated with placebo instead of morphine injected with naloxone. &&P<0.01 versus the group receiving vehicle instead of HA.

8. Conclusion

Naloxone administration after chronic morphine treatment, triggers neurochemical adaptations in the noradrenergic system and enhances PKA and ERK pathways. The functional consequences of this activation include an increase in TH activation and NA turnover and an enhancement in c-Fos expression. Many pathways implicated in the adaptive changes observed during withdrawal are subject to feedback mechanisms that can either amplify or suppress their own signalling and there is considerable signalling from one pathway to another, a phenomenon known as crosstalk. Consequently, the responses that cells mount to specific environmental conditions depend on the sum of the intensity and duration of signals from several pathways and how they interact with each other. Although the mechanism of crosstalk between PKA and ERK pathways has not yet been clarified, it is possible that PKA pathway facilitates MEK1/2 that activates the ERK1/2 pathway (Obama et al., 2007; Stork and Schmitt, 2002). The activated ERK pathway increases the phosphorylation of proteins related to morphine dependence, including TH. Our data suggest that crosstalk between PKA and ERK pathways is a key regulatory design necessary to regulate the phosphorylation of TH. These findings provide a new explanation to understand the complex mechanisms implicated in the adaptive changes observed during morphine withdrawal and could be useful for future treatment strategies.

9. Acknowledgment

This work was supported by Ministerio de Educación y Ciencia (Grants SAF 2010-17907), Fundación Séneca, CARM (15405/PI/10) and Instituto de Salud Carlos III (RETICS: RD06/001/1006).

10. References

Adams, J.P. & Sweatt, J.D. (2002) Molecular psychology: roles for the ERK MAP kinase cascade in memory. *Annu Rev Pharmacol Toxicol,* Vol. 42, pp. 135-163.

Almela, P.; Cerezo, M.; Milanés, M.V. & Laorden, M.L. (2006) Role of PKC in regulating of Fos and TH expression after naloxone induced morphine withdrawal in the heart. *Naunyn-Schmiedeberg's Arch Pharmacol,* Vol. 372, pp. 374-382.

Almela, P.; Milanés, M.V. & Laorden, M.L. (2007) Activation of ERK signaling pathway contributes to the adaptive changes in rat hearts during naloxone-induced morphine withdrawal. *Br J Pharmacol,* Vol. 151, pp. 787-797.

Almela, P.; Milanés, M.V. & Laorden, M.L. (2008) The PKs PKA and ERK 1/2 are involved in phosphorylation of TH at serine 40 and 31 during morphine withdrawal in rat hearts. *Br J Pharmacol,* Vol. 155, pp. 73-83.

Almela P.; Martínez-Laorden E.; Atucha N.M.; Milanés M.V. & Laorden M.L. (2011) Naloxone-precipitated morphine withdrawal evokes phosphorylation of heat shock protein 27 in rat heart through extracellular signal-regulated kinase. *J Mol Cell Cardiol,* Vol. 51, pp. 129-39.

Armour, J.A. (1991) Intrinsic cardiac neurons. *J Cardiovasc Electrophysiol,* Vol. 2, pp. 331–341.

Campbell, D.G.; Hardie, D.G. & Vulliet, P.R. (1986) Identification of four phosphorylation sites in the N-terminal region of tyrosine hydroxylase. *J Biol Chem,* Vol. 261, pp. 10489–10492.

Cerezo, M.; Milanés, M.V. & Laorden, M.L. (2005) Alterations in protein kinase A and different protein kinase C isoforms in the heart during morphine withdrawal. *Eur J Pharmacol,* Vol. 522, pp.9-19.

Childers, S.R. (1991) Opioid receptor-coupled second messengers systems. *Life Sci,* Vol. 48, pp. 1991-2003.

Dunkley, P.; Bobrovskaya, L.; Graham, M.E., von Nagy-Felsobuki, E.I. & Dickson, P.W. (2004) Tyrosine hydroxylase phosphorylation: Regulation and consecuences. *J Neurochem,* Vol. 91, pp. 1025-1043.

Funakoshi, H.; Okuno, S. & Fujisawa, H. (1991). Different effects on activity caused by phophorylation of tyrosine hydroxylase at serine 40 by three multifunctional protein kinases. *J Biol Chem,* Vol. 266, pp. 15614–15620.

González-Cuello, A.; Milanés, M.V.; Avilés, M. & Laorden, M.L. (2004) Changes in c-fos expression in the rat heart during morphine withdrawal. Involvement of alpha$_2$-adrenoceptors. *Naunyn-Schmiedeberg's Arch Pharmacol,* Vol. 370, pp. 17-25.

Haycock, J.W.; Ahn, N.G.; Cobbe, M.H. & Krebs, E.G. (1992) ERK 1 and ERK 2, two microtubule-associated protein 2 kinases, mediate the phosphorylation of tyrosine hydroxylase at serine-31 in situ. *Proc Natl Acad Sci USA,* Vol. 89, pp. 2365-2369.

Huh, J.; Gross, G.J.; Nagase, H. & Liang, B.T. (2001) Protection of cardiac myocytes via delta(1)-opioid receptors, protein kinase C, and mitochondrial K(ATP) channels. *Am J Physiol Heart Circ Physiol,* Vol. 280, pp. H377-383.

Hussain, M.; Drago, G.A.; Bhogal, M.; Colyer, J. & Orchard, C.H. (1999) Effects of the protein kinase A inhibitor H-89 on Ca^{2+} regulation in isolated ferret ventricular myocites. *Pflugers Arch,* Vol. 437, pp. 529-537.

Jiang, X.; Shi, E.; Nakajima, Y. & Sato, S. (2006) COX-2 mediates morphine-induced delayed cardioprotection via an iNOS-dependent mechanism. *Life Sci,* Vol. 78, pp. 2543-2549.

Johnson, S.M. & Fleming, W.W. (1989) Mechanisms of cellular adaptive sensitivity changes: Aplication to opioid tolerance and dependence. *Pharmacol Rev,* Vol. 41, pp. 435-488.

Kamp, T.J. & Hell, J.W. (2000) Regulation of cardiac L-type calcium channels by protein kinase A and protein kinase C. *Circ Res,* Vol. 87, pp. 1095-1102.

Kienbaum, P.; Heuter, T.; Michel, M.C.; Scherbaum, N.; Gastpar, M. & Peters, J. (2001) Chronic μ-opioid receptor stimulation in humans decreases muscle sympathetic nerve activity. *Circulation*, Vol. 103, pp. 850-855.

Kienbaum, P.; Heuter, T.; Scherbaum, N.; Gastpar, M. & Peters, J. (2002) Chronic μ-opioid receptor stimulation alters cardiovascular regulation in humans: differential effects on muscle sympathetic and heart rate responses to arterial hypotension. *J Cardiovasc Pharmacol*, Vol. 40, pp. 363-369.

Koob, G.F. & Bloom, F.E. (1988) Cellular and molecular mechanisms of drug dependence. *Science*, Vol. 242, pp. 715-723.

Kumer, S.C. & Vrana, K.E. (1996) Intricate regulation of tyrosine hydroxylase activity and gene expression. *J Neurochem*, Vol. 67, pp. 443-462.

Lindgren, N.; Goiny, M.; Herera-Marschitz, M.; Haycock, J.W.; Hökfelt, T. & Fisone, G. (2002) Activation of extracellular signals-regulated kinases 1 and 2 by depolarization stimulates tyrosine-hydroxylase phosphorylation and dopamine synthesis in rat brain. *Eur J Neurosci*, Vol. 15, pp. 769-773.

Lippi, G.; Plebani, M. & Cervellin, G. (2010) Cocaine in acute myocardial infarction. *Adv Clin Chem*, Vol. 51, pp. 53-70.

Mallet, J. (1999) Tyrosine hydroxylase from cloning to neuropsychiatric disorders. *Brain Res Bull*, Vol. 50, pp. 381–382.

Michel, M.C.; Li, Y. & Heusch, G. (2001) Mitogen-activated protein kinases in the heart. *Naunyn-Schmiedeberg´s Arch Pharmacol*, Vol. 363, pp. 245-266.

Milanés, M.V.; Fuente, T.; Marín, M.T. & Laorden, M.L. (1999) Catecholaminergic activity and 3´,5´-cyclic adenosine monophosphate concentrations in the right ventricle after acute and chronic morphine administration in the rat. *Br J Anaesth*, Vol. 83, pp. 784-788.

Milanés, M.V.; Fuente, T. & Laorden, M.L. (2000a) Catecholaminergic activity and 3´,5´-cyclic adenosine monophosphate levels in heart right ventricle after naloxone induced withdrawal. *Naunyn-Schmiedeberg´s Arch Pharmacol*, Vol. 361, pp. 61-66.

Milanés, M.V. & Laorden, M.L. (2000b) Changes in catecholaminergic pathways innervating the rat heart ventricle during morphine dependence. Involvement of A1 and A2 adrenoceptors. *Eur J Pharmacol*, Vol. 397, pp. 311-318.

Milanés, M.V.; Martínez, M.D.; González-Cuello, A. & Laorden, M.L. (2001) Evidence for a peripheral mechanism in cardiac opioid withdrawal. *Naunyn-Schmiedeberg's Arch Pharmacol*, Vol. 364, pp. 193–198.

Nerantzis, C.E.; Koulouris, S.N.; Marianou, S.K.; Pastromas, S.C., Koutsaftis, P.N. & Agapitos, E.B. (2011) Histologic findings of the sinus node and the perinodal area in street heroin addicts, victims of sudden unexpected death. *J Forensic Sci*, Vol. 56, pp. 645-648.

Obama, Y.; Horgan, A. & Sork, J.S. (2007) The requirement of Ras and Rap1 for the activation of ERKs by cAMP, PACAP, and KCL in cerebellar granule cells. *J Neurochem*, Vol. 101, pp. 470-482.

Ongur, D.; An, X. & Price, J.L. (1998) Prefrontal cortical projections to the hypothalamus in macaque monkeys. *J Comp Neurol*, Vol. 401, pp. 480-505.

Peart, J.N. & Gross, G.J. (2006) Cardioprotective effects of acute and chronic opioid treatment is mediated via different signalling pathways. *Am J Physiol Heart Circ Physiol*, Vol. 291, pp. H1746-53.

Pugsley, M.K. (2002) The diverse molecular mechanism responsible for the actions of opioids on the cardiovascular system. *Pharmacol Ther,* Vol. 93, pp. 51-75.

Pyner, S. (2009) Neurochemistry of the paraventricular nucleus of the hypothalamus: implications for cardiovascular regulation. *J Chem Neuroanat,* Vol. 38, pp. 197-208.

Rabadán, J.V.; Milanés, M.V. & Laorden, M.L. (1997) Effects of chronic morphine treatment on catecholamines content and mechanical response in the rat heart. *J Pharmacol Exp Ther,* Vol. 280, pp. 32-37.

Rabadán, J.V.; Milanés, M.V. & Laorden, M.L. (1998) Changes in right atrial catecholamine content in naive rats and after naloxone-induced withdrawal. *Br J Anaesth,* Vol. 80, pp. 354-359.

Rao F.; Zhang L.; Wessel J.; Zhang K.; Wen G.; Kennedy B.P.; Rana B.K.; Das M.; Rodriguez-Flores J.L.; Smith D.W.; Cadman P.E.; Salem R.M.; Mahata S.K.; Schork N.J.; Taupenot L.; Ziegler M.G. & O'Connor D.T. (2007) Tyrosine hydroxylase, the rate-limiting enzyme in catecholamine biosynthesis: discovery of common human genetic variants governing transcription, autonomic activity, and blood pressure in vivo. *Circulation,* Vol. 116, pp. 993–1006.

Ren, X.; Noda, Y.; Mamiya, T.; Nagai, T. & Nabeshima, T.A. (2004) Neuroactive steroid, dehydroepiandrosterone sulfate, prevents the development of morphine dependence and tolerance via c-Fos expression linked to the extracellular signal-regulated protein kinase. *Behav Brain Res,* Vol. 152, pp. 243-250.

Risold, P.Y. & Swanson, L.W. (1997) Connections of the rat lateral septal complex. *Brain Res Rev,* Vol. 24, pp. 115-195.

Roskoski, R.J.; Vulliet, P.R. & Glass, B.D. (1987) Phosphorylation of tyrosine hydroxylase by cyclic GMP-dependent protein kinase. *J Neurochem,* Vol. 48, pp. 840–845.

Sawchenko, P.E. & Swanson, L.W. (1982) Immunohistochemical identification of neurons in the paraventricular nucleus of the hypothalamus that project to the medulla or to the spinal cord in the rat. *J Comp Neurol,* Vol. 205, pp. 260-272.

Self, D.W. & Nestler, E.J. (1995) Molecular mechanisms of drug reinforcement and addiction. *Ann Rev Neurosci,* Vol. 18, pp. 463-495.

Stork, P. & Schmitt, J. (2002) Crosstalk between cAMP and MAP kinase signalling in the regulation of cell proliferation. *Trends Cell Biol,* Vol. 12, pp. 258-266.

Sugden, P.H. & Bogoyevitch, M.A. (1995) Intracellular signalling through protein kinases in the heart. *Cardiovasc Res,* Vol. 30, pp. 478-492.

Wang, G.Y.; Wu, S.; Pei, J.M.; Yu, X.C. & Wong, T.M. (2001) Kappa- but not delta-opioid receptors mediate effects of ischemic preconditioning on both infarct and arrhythmia in rats. *Am J Physiol Heart Circ Physiol,* Vol. 280, pp. H384-391.

Xu, J.; Tian, W.; Ma, X.; Guo, J.; Shi, Q.; Jin, Y.; Xi, J. & Xu, Z. (2011) Mechanism underlying morphine-induced Akt activation: Roles of protein phosphatases and reactive oxygen species. *Cell Biochem Biophys*, Vol. 61, pp. 303-311.

Section 3

Addiction Treatment – Pharmacology

11

Medication Development for the Treatment of Cocaine Addiction – Progress at Preclinical and Clinical Levels

Zheng-Xiong Xi
National Institute on Drug Abuse, Intramural Research Program,
National Institutes of Health, Baltimore, MD
USA

1. Introduction

Cocaine addiction continues to be an important public health problem in the United States and other countries. Acute cocaine produces potent rewarding and psychostimulant effects primarily by blocking dopamine (DA) transporters (DAT) in the brain's reward system - the mesocorticolimbic DA system. However, repeated use of cocaine leads to addiction, persistent craving and a high risk of relapse. To date, there are no proven pharmacotherapies for cocaine addiction. Recent progress in the neurobiology of drug dependence in preclinical animal models has lead to the discovery of various novel compounds that appear to be promising for the treatment of drug addiction. Some have been tested in controlled clinical trials and have produced encouraging results in reducing cocaine use and in increasing abstinence from relapse. In this review article, I will focus on those medication strategies that are well-studied in experimental animals and are currently under clinical trials for the treatment of addiction or for other diseases. These strategies include DAT-based agonist therapy, DA receptor-based antagonist therapy, glutamate-based therapy, GABA-based therapy and endocannabinoid-based therapy. For each treatment, I will first review the rationale and the underlying neurochemical mechanisms of the therapy, and then summarize the major findings of the drugs in each category at both preclinical and clinical levels.

2. Dopamine transporter-based agonist therapies

Rationale: The mesocorticolimbic DA system is thought to be critically involved in drug reward and addiction (Wise, 2005; Sulzer, 2011). This system originates from the DA neurons in the ventral tegmental area (VTA) in the midbrain and projects predominantly to the nucleus accumbens (NAc) and prefrontal cortex (PFC) in the forebrain (Figure 1). Almost all addictive drugs, such as cocaine, heroin, nicotine and alcohol, have been shown to increase extracellular DA in the NAc via different mechanisms (Wise, 2005; Sulzer, 2011). For example, cocaine elevates extracellular DA by blockade of DAT, while heroin increases extracellular DA by inhibition of GABA release in the VTA that disinhibits (activates) DA neurons. Such an increase in NAc DA has been thought to underlie the euphoria associated with drug abuse. Based on this DA hypothesis, much attention in medication development for treatment of addiction has been focused on manipulation of DA transmission in the brain reward circuitry. One strategy is to target DAT (agonist therapy), and another is to target brain DA receptors (antagonist therapy) (Figure 2).

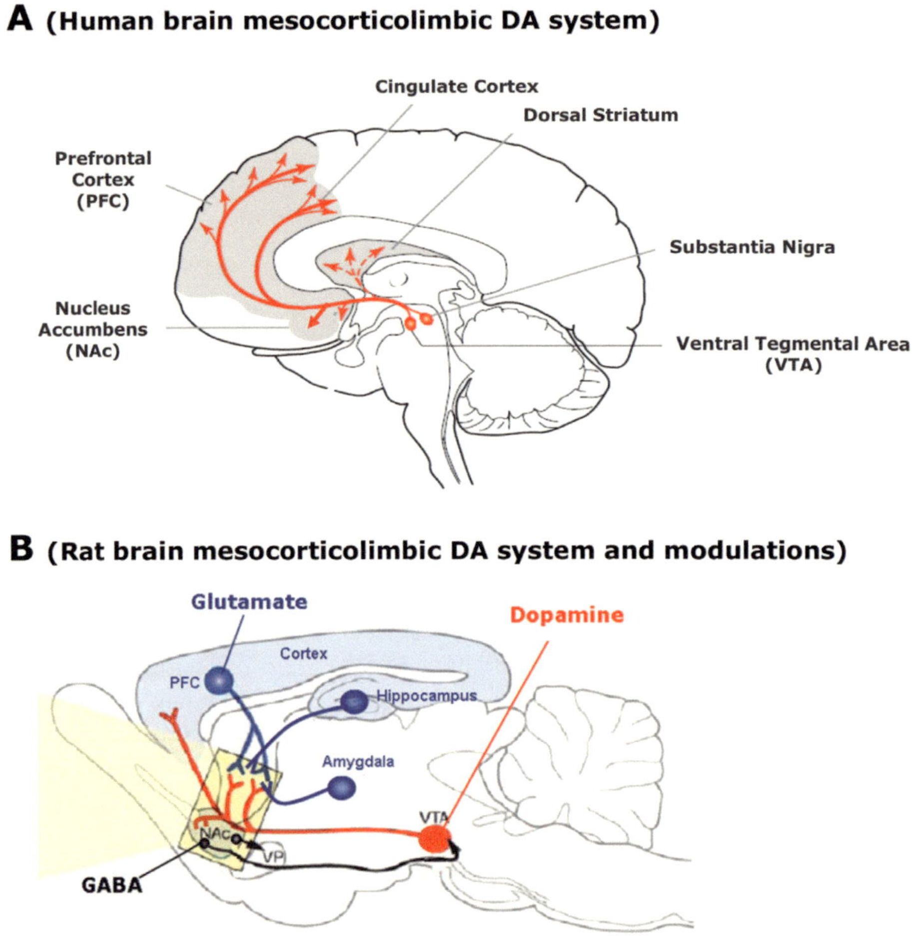

Fig. 1. Schematic diagrams, illustrating the mesocorticolimbic DA reward system in human (A) and rat (B) brains. The mesocorticolimbic DA system originates in the midbrain ventral tegmental area (VTA) and projects predominantly to the nucleus accumbens (NAc) and prefrontal cortex (PFC). Dopaminergic afferents from the VTA and glutamatergic afferents from the PFC, hippocampus and amygdala synapse on NAc medium-spiny (GABAergic) neurons (MSN), which project to the VTA and the ventral pallidum (VP).

Agonist or substitution therapies have been successful in the treatment of opioid (Mattick et al., 2009) and nicotine dependence (Xi et al., 2009; Xi, 2010). As such, drugs that block the DAT, but have lower addictive potential than cocaine, would have potential as 'cocaine-like' agonist therapies for the treatment of cocaine addiction. Indeed, this strategy has been at the forefront of medication development for the treatment of cocaine addiction for more than a decade (Rothman and Baumann, 2006; Howell and Kimmel, 2008). To date, many DAT inhibitors have been developed, and several of them have been tested in human clinical trials (Newman and Kulkarni, 2002; Runyon and Carroll, 2006; Rothman et al., 2006, 2008).

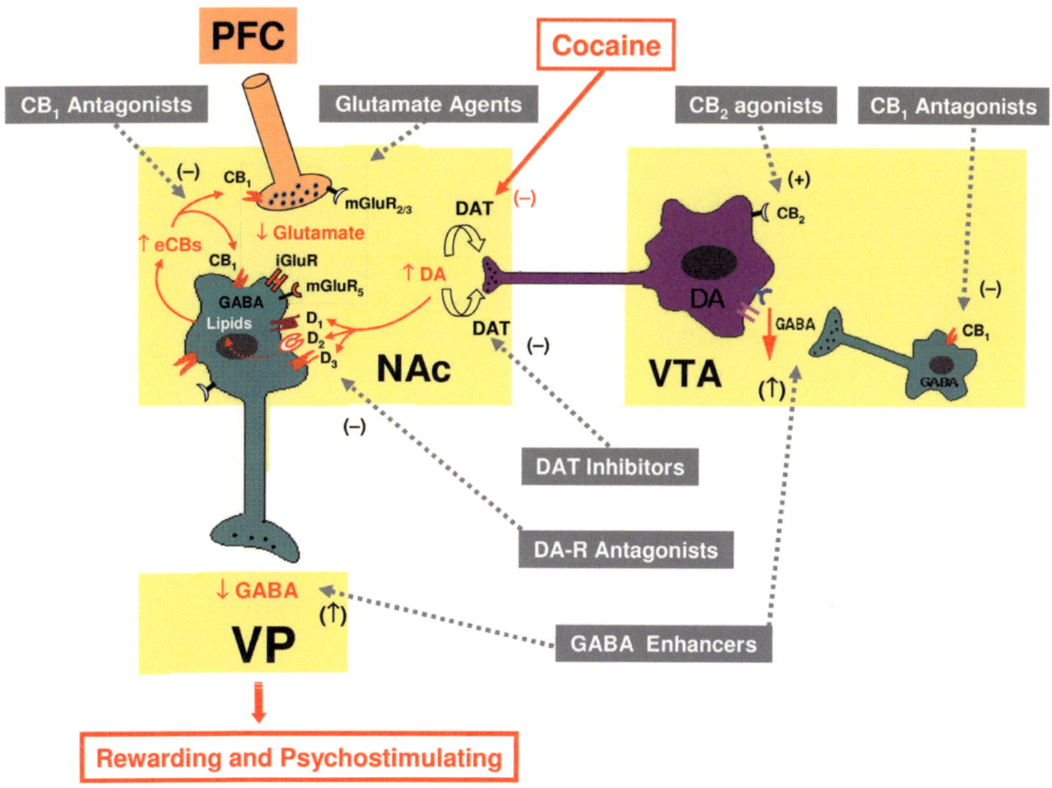

Fig. 2. Schematic diagram of the VTA-NAc-VP reward pathway, illustrating the actions of acute cocaine on extracellular DA, endocannabinoids (eCBs), glutamate and GABA in the NAc and VP, and the sites of action of various mechanism-based pharmacological agents in the brain reward system. Cocaine elevates extracellular DA in the NAc by blocking DAT on presynaptic DA terminals. DA activates postsynaptic DA receptors, in particular D2 and D3 receptors, producing an overall inhibitory effect on NAc medium-spiny (GABAergic) neurons (MSN). In addition, activation of D2 receptors may also increase eCB release from MSNs, which subsequently activates cannabinoid CB1 receptors located on presynaptic glutamatergic terminals and GABAergic MSNs themselves, causing a reduction in glutamate release and in MSN excitability. Thus, increases in NAc DA and eCBs and a reduction in NAc glutamate release lead to a reduction in MSN excitability and GABA release in the VTA (not shown) and VP. Decreased GABA release in the VTA causes an increase in DA neuron activity (via a disinhibition mechanism) and DA release in the NAc. Based upon these neurochemical hypotheses, various pharmacological therapies have been proposed and tested in animal models of drug addiction to interfere with cocaine's action. More details are discussed in the text of this review.

However, none have proven to be successful due to significant abuse liability by those compounds themselves and/or unwanted side-effects. Given the recent finding that rewarding and psychostimulant effects of the drugs are positively correlated with the speed of onset and offset of action on brain DA (Volkow et al., 1995; Kimmel et al., 2007; Xi and Gardner, 2008), it has been proposed that DAT inhibitors (Figure 2), in particular those with a slower-onset longer-acting profile than cocaine, would have lower addictive potential by themselves. In the following sections, we will review several DAT inhibitors with such a slow-onset long-action profile.

2.1 GBR-12909

Preclinical studies: GBR-12909 (Vanoxerine), a phenyl-substituted piperazine derivative, is a relatively slow-onset long-acting DAT inhibitor compared to cocaine (Howell and Wilcox, 2001). To date, it is the most extensively studied DAT inhibitor proposed to be beneficial in the treatment of cocaine addiction (Rothman et al., 2008). GBR-12909 binds at the DAT site with high affinity, and selectively inhibits DA re-uptake. GBR-12909 can also compete with psychostimulants at the DAT site, thus blocking cocaine- or amphetamine-induced increases in extracellular DA. Compared to the same doses of cocaine, GBR-12909-induced increases in striatal DA and locomotion are relatively slow-onset and long-lasting (Baumann et al., 1991, 1994; Kelley and Lang, 1989). Pretreatment with GBR-12909 significantly inhibits cocaine self-administration in rats and nonhuman primates at doses that have little or no effect on food self-administration (Glowa et al., 1995). Repeated treatment with low doses of GBR-12909 sustains the selective suppression of cocaine self-administration *versus* food self-administration (Glowa et al., 1995). Further, a single injection of a slow-release formulation of GBR-12909 produced a prolonged (up to one month) suppression of cocaine self-administration in nonhuman primates (Glowa et al., 1996). These findings support GBR-12909 as a potential candidate for the treatment of cocaine addiction (Rothman et al., 2008).

Clinical trials: GBR-12909 was investigated in clinical trials at NIDA and University of Texas from 2003 to 2008 (Table 1). However, the appearance of cardiovascular side-effects has prevented its further development as an anti-cocaine medicine at NIDA, NIH (Vocci and Elkashef, 2005).

2.2 RTI-336

Preclinical studies: RTI-336 is a novel DAT inhibitor of the 3-phenyltropane class and has a slower-onset (30 min *vs.* < 10 min) longer-acting (4 hrs *vs.* 1-2 hrs) profile than cocaine (Carroll et al., 2006; Kimmel et al., 2007). It has >1000- and >400-fold selectivity for DAT over serotonin transporter (SERT) and norepinepherine transporter (NET), respectively (Carroll et al., 2006). Pretreatment with RTI-336 produced a dose-dependent reduction in cocaine self-administration in both rats and nonhuman primates (Haile et al., 2005; Howell et al., 2007). The ED_{50} dose of RTI-336 for reducing cocaine self-administration resulted in approximately 90% DAT occupancy, suggesting that high levels of DAT occupancy by RTI-336 are required to reduce cocaine self-administration. However, co-administration of the ED_{50} dose of RTI-336 with the SERT inhibitors fluoxetine or citalopram produced more robust reductions in cocaine self-administration in non-human primates than RTI-336 alone (Howell et al., 2007), suggesting that blockade of both DAT and SERT may be more effective in attenuating cocaine's reinforcing effects than selective blockade of DAT alone (Rothman et al., 2007). In addition, at the doses that effectively suppressed cocaine self-administration, RTI-336 also inhibited food-taking behavior (Howell et al., 2007). This differs from GBR-12909, which selectively inhibits cocaine self-administration but not food-taking behavior. RTI-336, like many other DAT inhibitors, reliably maintained self-administration behavior in all non-human primates tested (Howell et al., 2007) and produced locomotor stimulating effects in mice and rats, suggesting abuse potential by itself. However, compared to cocaine, RTI-336 maintained lower rates of responding and lower progressive-ratio (PR) break-points in the self-administration paradigm. It also produced weaker locomotion hyperactivity and drug discriminative stimulus effects, and showed very low sensitization in locomotion (Carroll et al., 2006; Czoty et al., 2010). These data suggest that RTI-336 may have lower abuse potential than cocaine.

Clinical trials: RTI-336 has been investigated in Phase I clinical trials at RTI International (NC, USA) and NIDA (MD, USA) since 2008 (Table 1). It was a double-blind, placebo-controlled Phase I study to evaluate the safety, tolerability, and pharmacokinetics of RTI-336 in healthy, male subjects. The study has been completed, but not yet reported.

Compound	Company	Pharmacology	Indication	Status	Reference
GBR-12909	Antia Lab., China; Others	DAT inhibitor	Safety and PK profiles; Cocaine addiction	Phase I, terminated at NIDA in 2008	http://clinicaltrials.gov
RTI-336	RTI, NC, USA	DAT inhibitor	Safety, tolerability & PK profiles	Phase I,	http://clinicaltrials.gov
Methylphenidate	Shire US, Dublin, Ireland	DAT inhibitor	Substance Abuse (cocaine, methamphetamine)	Phase II	http://clinicaltrials.gov
Modafinil	Cephalon, PA, USA	DAT inhibitor; Glutamate enhancer; GABA inhibitor	Drug Addiction (cocaine, methamphetamine Schizophrenia	Phase II Phase IV	http://clinicaltrials.gov
Disulfiram	LKT Lab., MN, USA	Aldehyde dehydrogenase inhibitor; Dopamine-β-hydroxylase inhibitor	Substance Abuse (cocaine, heroin or methamphetamine) Others	Phase III	http://clinicaltrials.gov

Table 1. DAT- or DA-related drug candidates in clinical trials

2.3 CTDP-31,345

Based upon the above finding that a combination of DAT and SERT inhibitors appears to be more potent and effective than DAT inhibitor alone in attenuation of cocaine self-administration (Howell et al., 2007), we studied slow-onset long-acting monamine transporter

(MAT) inhibitors that have higher affinity for both DAT and SERT over to NET. In addition, our interest in non-selective MAT inhibitors as potential anti-cocaine medications originally stems from the fact that cocaine is also a non-selective MAT inhibitor. Thus, it was hypothesized that a 'cocaine-like' MAT inhibitor with slow-onset and long-acting profiles would be able to substitute for cocaine for the treatment of cocaine dependence (Peng et al., 2010c). CTDP-31,345 is such a MAT inhibitor with slow-onset (30-60 min) long-acting (at least 6 hrs) (Peng et al., 2010c) and with higher selectivity for DAT and SERT over NET (K_i = 18, 23 and 81 for DAT, SERT and NET, respectively) (Froimowitz et al., 2000). The "CTDP" terminology derives from the "Cocaine Treatment Discovery Program" of the NIDA Extramural Program. Structurally, it is a *trans*-aminotetralin derivative (Peng et al., 2010c). It is a prodrug, which is metabolized (*N*-demethylated) to CTDP-31,346, a slow-onset long-acting MAT inhibitor. Pretreatment with a single dose of CTDP-31,345 produced a dose-dependent long-term (24-48 h) reduction in cocaine self-administration in rats (Peng et al., 2010c). CTDP-31,345 itself appears to have lower abuse liability than cocaine because it produces weaker brain-stimulation reward and maintains a lower rate of self-administration than cocaine (Peng et al., 2010c). In addition, systemic administration of CTDP-31,345 produces moderate, but long-lasting, increases in NAc DA, which may translate to decreases in drug craving and relapse by restoring reduced synaptic DA in brain reward circuits (Volkow et al., 1999). CTDP-31,345 is not currently in clinical trials.

2.4 Methylphenidate

Preclinical studies: Methylphenidate is a FDA-approved DAT inhibitor for the treatment of attention deficit hyperactivity disorder (ADHD). It binds to presynaptic DAT and NET, but not to SERT, blocking DA and NE re-uptake and increasing synaptic DA and NE (Leonard et al., 2004). Methylphenidate is self-administered in rodents, and pretreatment with methylphenidate significantly shifts the cocaine self-administration dose-response curve to the left (Hiranita et al., 2009, 2011), suggesting that methylphenidate has cocaine-like abuse potential and produces additive effects in combination with cocaine.

Clinical trials: ADHD has high comorbidity with cocaine-dependent patients as much as 30% in some studies (Schubiner et al., 2000). Because of this, its therapeutic effects for the treatment of cocaine addiction in this population have been recently evaluated in clinical trials (Table 1). Placebo-controlled studies produced mixed results with one study reporting no effect (Schubiner et al., 2002) while three studies demonstrating a significant reduction in both cocaine use and the positive subjective effects of cocaine compared to placebo (Winhusen et al., 2006; Collins et al., 2006; Levin et al., 2007). Because the half-life of methylphenidate is short (2-3 hrs in humans), the drug has been made available in sustained-release formulations in addition to the traditional immediate-release formulation. The sustained-release methylphenidate displayed much lower abuse potential than immediate-release, and appears to be more effective than immediate-release in decreasing cocaine use and the positive subjective effects (Arria and Wish, 2006; White et al., 2006).

2.5 CTDP-32,476

Based on the aforementioned findings of sustained-release methylphenidate in clinical trials, we have recently developed a series of methylphenidate analogs with slow-onset long-acting profiles as medication candidates for the treatment of cocaine addiction. CTDP-32,476 is a representative compound in this drug category. Structurally, CTDP-32,476 is a metabolically stable methylphenidate analog, in which the metabolically unstable ester moiety of methylphenidate is removed from methylphenidate's structure (Froimowitz et al. 2007). *In vitro* binding assays suggest that CTDP-32,476 is a selective DAT inhibitor with ~50-fold and ~350-fold selectivity for DAT over NET and SERT (K_i= 16, 5900 and 840 nM for DAT, SERT and NET, respectively) (Froimowitz et al., 2007). Functional reuptake assays reveal that CTDP-32,476 has IC_{50} values of 8.6, 490 and 120 nM for inhibition of DA, 5-HT and NE reuptake, respectively. In addition, it also displays approximately 30-fold higher affinity for the DAT than cocaine (K_i: 16 *vs.* 500 nM; IC_{50}: 8.6 *vs.* 244 nM) (Froimowitz et al., 2007). Systemic administration of CTDP-32,476 produced a slow-onset (20-60 min) long-term (6-12 hrs) increase in locomotion and extracellular DA in the NAc (Xi et al., 2009). Pretreatment with CTDP-32,476 significantly and dose-dependently inhibited intravenous cocaine self-administration under both FR and PR reinforcement, shifted the cocaine dose-response self-administration curves downward and to the right, and attenuated cocaine-induced increases in locomotion and extracellular DA in the NAc (Xi et al., 2011a). These data suggest that pretreatment with CTDP-32,476 produced functional antagonism of cocaine's action, likely by attenuating cocaine's binding to DAT. CTDP-32,476 itself appears to have much lower addictive potential than cocaine. Drug naïve rats selectively self-administer cocaine, but not CTDP-32,476. In rats trained to self-administer cocaine, CTDP-32,476 maintained significantly lower rates of self-administration and lower PR break-points than cocaine. Taken together, these data suggest that CTDP-32,476 appears to be an excellent agonist therapy for cocaine dependence. CTDP-32,476 has not been tested in human clinical trials.

2.6 Modafinil

Preclinical studies: Modafinil is a wake-promoting drug used in the clinic for the treatment of narcolepsy and idiopathic hypersomnia (Wise et al., 2007). However, the neurochemical mechanisms underlying modafinil's action are not fully understood. It is reported that modafinil increases extracellular levels of glutamate in numerous brain regions including striatum, thalamus, hippocampus, and hypothalamus (Ballon and Feifel, 2006; Wise et al., 2007). In addition, it also inhibits brain GABA release (Ballon and Feifel, 2006). Recent studies suggest that modafinil is a DAT inhibitor in humans and primates (Madras et al., 2006; Volkow et al., 2009). This is further supported by the findings that mice lacking DAT or DA (D1 and D2) receptors do not respond to the wake-promoting effects of modafinil (Qu et al., 2008; Wisor et al., 2001). *In vivo* microdialysis studies demonstrated that modafinil increases extracellular DA (Wisor et al., 2001; Ferraro et al., 1997; Murillo-Rodríguez et al., 2007). Neuroimaging studies in both non-human primates and healthy human subjects demonstrated significant occupancy of DAT (and also NET) by intravenously-administered modafinil (Madras et al., 2006; Volkow et al., 2009). Consistent with these findings, modafinil has been shown to have weak cocaine-like discriminative and reinforcing effects in both rodents and non-human primates (Gold and Balster., 1996; Deroche-Gamonet et al., 2002), and weak stimulant-like subjective effects in humans (Kruszewski, 2006; O'Brien et al., 2006). Based on these recent findings, modafinil is categorized as a DAT-based 'agonist therapy' for cocaine dependence.

Clinical studies: Dackis et al (2003) first reported that modafinil's stimulant-like activity may diminish the symptoms of cocaine withdrawal, including hypersomnia, lethargy, dysphoric mood, cognitive impairment, and increased appetite, thereby reducing the desire to use cocaine. The first randomized, double-blind clinical trial involved 62 cocaine-dependent outpatients who received either a single dose of modafinil or placebo daily for 8 weeks (Dackis et al., 2005). Patients treated with modafinil had significantly less cocaine use than patients treated with placebo (Hart et al., 2008). No significant adverse effects were noted. The therapeutic effects of modafinil in cocaine users have been supported by a recently completed multi-site, placebo-controlled clinical trial involving 210 cocaine-dependent outpatients (Anderson et al., 2009). Currently, more than 10 additional clinical trials are under way to further evaluate the efficacy of modafinil treatment for cocaine addiction (Table 1).

2.7 Disulfiram

Preclinical studies: Although disulfiram is not a DAT inhibitor, I list it under this treatment category because it elevates extracellular DA by inhibiting DA metabolism, producing effects similar to DAT inhibitors. In 1937, disulfiram was first reported as a potential treatment for alcoholism by Williams, a plant physician in a chemical company. Unexpectedly, Williams observed that after exposure to disulfram, his laboratory assistants could not drink alcohol in any form because alcohol produced a series of unwanted effects such as flushing, sweating, headaches, nausea, tachycardia, palpitations, arterial hypotension and hyperventilation (Williams, 1937). Since then, disulfiram has been used in the treatment of alcoholism for more than half a century (Suh et al., 2006; Barth and Malcolm, 2010). Disulfiram is an inhibitor of aldehyde dehydrogenase, the enzyme that transforms acetaldehyde into acetate during alcohol metabolism (Weinshenker, 2010). When a person drinks alcohol while taking disulfiram, the resulting acetylaldehyde accumulation causes an aversive reaction as described above, which discourages further drinking. In addition, disulfiram also inhibits dopamine-β-hydroxylase (DBH) (Weinshenker, 2010), the enzyme that transforms DA into norepinephrine. Such DBH inhibition would increase brain DA levels while decreasing brain NE release. This effect could be therapeutic for cocaine dependence since an increase in brain DA may be helpful in attenuating withdrawal syndromes and craving (Volkow et al., 1999), while a decrease in NE may be helpful in attenuating relapse to drug use (Smith and Aston-Jones, 2008; Weinshenker, 2010). In experimental animals, disulfram stimulates DA release and potentiates cocaine-induced increases in extracellular DA in the prefrontal cortex (Devoto et al., 2011). It also facilitates the development and expression of locomotor sensitization to cocaine in rats (Haile et al., 2003). However, in animal models of relapse, pretreatment with disulfram attenuates cocaine-induced reinstatement of drug-seeking behaviour (Schroeder et al., 2010).

Clinical trials: The initial impetus for the use of disulfiram to treat cocaine dependence was the high rate of comorbidity between cocaine abuse and alcohol abuse (Gossop and Carroll, 2006). Thus, it was hypothesized that a reduction in alcohol use would lead to secondary reduction in cocaine use. Additionally, abstinence from alcohol would prevent formation of cocaethylene, a metabolite formed when alcohol and cocaine are present together. Cocaethylene has pharmacological actions similar to cocaine and increases subjective euphoria and heart rate (Hart et al., 2000). Several short-term clinical trials in outpatients using both cocaine and alcohol showed that disulfiram, along with cognitive behavioural therapy (CBT), significantly reduced cocaine and alcohol use (Carroll et al., 1998; Higgins et al., 1993; Grassi et al., 2007). In one study, the reduction in cocaine use was still present one year after treatment (Carroll et al., 2000). An 11-week, double-blind, placebo-controlled trial evaluated the efficacy of disulfiram, naltrexone and their combined treatment in 208 patients with concurrent cocaine and alcohol dependence. Patients taking disulfiram alone or in combination with naltrexone were more likely to achieve combined abstinence from cocaine and alcohol than placebo-treated patients (Pettinati et al., 2008). In several randomized, placebo-controlled trials, disulfiram seemed to directly reduce cocaine use rather than reducing it indirectly by reducing concurrent alcohol use (George et al., 2000; Petrakis et al., 2000; Carroll et al., 2004). In addition, dilsufiram appears to be effective in attenuating cocaine use in comorbid cocaine- and opioid-dependent individuals (Oliveto et al., 2011). As a caveat, disulfiram is reported to inhibit cocaine metabolism, and therefore increases cocaine plasma levels in humans (Baker et al., 2006). Because of this, it should be used cautiously in comorbid cocaine and alcohol patients with severe cardiovascular diseases (Malcolm et al., 2008).

3. Dopamine receptor-based antagonist therapies

Rationale: Cocaine's action is largely mediated by elevation of extracellular DA that activates postsynaptic DA receptors. Thus, blockade of DA receptors is a plausible therapeutic approach for cocaine addiction (Figure 2). There are five DA receptor subtypes identified in the brain that are classified as D1-like (D1, D5) and D2-like (D2, D3, D4) based on their pharmacological profile (Beaulieu and Gainetdinov, 2011). Although both D1 and D2 receptor subtypes have been shown to play predominant roles in mediating actions of DA, clinical trials with selective D1 or D2 receptor antagonists for the treatment of cocaine addiction have failed due to ineffectiveness and/or unwanted side-effects such as sedation and extra pyramidal locomotor syndromes (see review by Platt et al., 2002; Gorelick et al., 2004). In response, efforts have increased to develop relatively low selective D1/2 receptor antagonists or D3 receptor-based antagonist therapies for cocaine dependence.

3.1 *Levo*-tetrahydropalmatine (*l*-THP)

Preclinical studies: Tetrahydropalmatine (THP) is a tetrahydroprotoberberine (THPB) isoquinoline alkaloid and a primary active constituent of the herbal plant species *Stephania rotunda Lour* and *Corydalis ambigua* (Yanhusuo) (Jin et al., 1987). The levo-isomer of THP (*l*-THP) has been shown to contribute to many of the therapeutic effects of these herbs such as sedative, neuroleptic and analgesic effects (Chu et al., 2008; Jin, 1987). Purified or synthetic *l*-THP has been approved in China as a traditional sedative-analgesic agent for the treatment of chronic pain and anxious insomnia for more than 40 years. Pharmacologically, *l*-THP is a non-selective DA receptor antagonist with roughly 3-fold selectivity for D1 *versus* D2 receptor and 10-fold selectivity for D1 *versus* D3 receptor (K_i = 124, 388, or 1420 nM for D1, D2, or D3 receptors, respectively) (Wang and Mantsch, 2012). In addition, it has moderate binding affinity to alpha (α_1, α_{2A}) adrenergic and 5-HT_{1A} (K_i = 340 nM) receptors. Because cocaine is a non-selective MAT inhibitor, which increases brain DA, NE and 5-HT levels, it was hypothesized that blockade of multiple DA, adrenergic and 5-TH_{1A} receptors by *l*-THP would functionally antagonize cocaine's action (Mantsch et al., 2007; Xi et al., 2007). In support of this hypothesis, *l*-THP was found to significantly inhibit intravenous cocaine self-administration under FR and PR reinforcement schedules (Mantsch et al., 2007, 2010; Xi et al., 2007), cocaine-induced conditioned place preference (CPP) (Luo et al., 2003), cocaine-enhanced electrical brain-stimulation reward (Xi et al., 2007), and cocaine-, cue- or stress-induced reinstatement of drug-seeking behaviour in rats (Mantsch et al., 2007, 2010; Figueroa-Guzman et al., 2011). These anti-cocaine effects are unlikely due to *l*-THP-induced sedation or locomotor impairment, since the effective doses that decrease cocaine's effects are much lower (3-10 fold) than those that produce locomotion inhibition (Xi et al., 2007). These data suggest that *l*-THP may have therapeutic potential for treatment of cocaine addiction in humans.

Clinical studies: A pilot study examined the efficacy of *l*-THP in reducing craving and relapse in 120 heroin addicts (Yang et al., 2008). In this randomized, double-blind, placebo-controlled study, patients received 4 weeks of *l*-THP treatment and three months follow-up after *l*-THP treatment. The results showed that *l*-THP significantly lowered opiate withdrawal symptoms and craving and increased abstinence rate. Another study examined the therapeutic effect of *l*-THP combined with methadone for heroin detoxification (Hu et al., 2006), and found that *l*-THP, combined with methadone, significantly elevated detoxification rate, lowered total amount of methadone and decreased time for the detoxification. *L*-THP is being investigated in human clinical trial for the treatment of cocaine addiction in University of Maryland, Baltimore (Table 2).

Compound	**Company**	**Pharm. Action**	**Indication**	**Status**	**Reference**
L-THP	Best & Wide, Nanning, China	D1/D2/D3 Antagonist	Drug abuse (heroin, cocaine)	Phase I, Phase II	Yang et al., 2008; Wang & Mantsch, 2012
BP-897	Bioproject, Paris, France	D3 Partial Agonist	Safety Study	Phase II	Garcia-Ladona & Cox, 2003
Cariprazine	Gideon Richter, Budapest, Hungary	D3-Partial Agonist	Bipolar disorder; Schizophrenia	Phase III	http://clinicaltrials.gov
ABT-925	Abbott, IL, USA	D3 Antagonist	Schizophrenia	Phase II	http://clinicaltrials.gov
ABT-614	Abbott, IL, USA	D3 Antagonist	PK properties D3R binding by PET	Phase I	http://clinicaltrials.gov
GSK598809	GSK, Uxbridge, UK	D3 Antagonist	Substance abuse (nicotine); Food reward	Phase II	http://clinicaltrials.gov
GSK618334	GSK, Uxbridge, UK	D3 Antagonist	Substance abuse (alcoholism)	Phase I	http://clinicaltrials.gov
S33138	Institut de Recherches Servier, Croissy sur Seine, France	D3-Preferring Antagonist	D3R binging by PET; Safety	Phase I	Thomasson-Perret et al., 2008; Millan et al., 2008

Table 2. DA receptor-based drug candidates in clinical trials

3.2 BP-897

Preclinical studies: BP-897 is the first developed D3-selective partial agonist (Pilla et al., 1999) or antagonist (Wicke and Garcia-Ladona, 2001). A series of studies have assessed the efficacy of BP-897 in animal models of drug addiction (see reviews by Garcia-Ladona and Cox, 2003; Le Foll et al., 2005; Heidbreder et al., 2005). BP-897 produces a dose-dependent decrease in cocaine self-administration under second-order reinforcement, cocaine-induced CPP, cocaine's discriminative stimulus properties, and cocaine- or cue-induced reinstatement of cocaine-seeking behaviour. These data support the potential use of BP-897 in the treatment of cocaine addiction, particularly in relapse to drug-seeking behavior.

Clinical trials: BP-897 entered Phase II clinical studies for the treatment of drug addiction in the early 2000s. However, the detailed results about its safety, pharmacokinetics and therapeutic efficay have not yet been reported.

3.3 Cariprazine

Preclinical studies: Cariprazine (RGH-188) is a novel D3 receptor partial agonist with 10-fold selectivity for D3 over D2 (Gründer, 2010; Kiss et al., 2010). It is also a weak 5-HT_{1A} and 5-HT_{5C} partial agonist. Although limited preclinical data are available, the 'concept-proven' finding with BP-897 suggests that cariprazine might be similarly effective in attenuation of cocaine's actions.

Clinical studies: Cariprazine is currently in Phase III clinical trials for the treatment of schizophrenia and bipolar disorder (Table 2). Data from Phase II trials in patients with schizophrenia and bipolar mania indicate that the drug has antipsychotic and antimanic properties that are superior to placebo. The efficacy of cariprazine for treatment of cocaine addiction has not been evaluated.

3.4 SB-277011A

Preclinical studies: SB-277011A is the most well-characterized D3 receptor antagonist in preclinical animal models of drug addiction to date (Heidebreder et al., 2005; Heidbreder and Newman, 2010). SB-277011A has high affinity for human D3 receptor, and the selectivity for human and rat D3 over D2 receptor is 120 and 80, respectively (Reavill et al., 2000). In experimental animals, SB-277011A significantly and dose-dependently attenuates cocaine-enhanced brain-stimulation reward (Vorel et al., 2002; Spiller et al., 2008), cocaine-induced CPP (Vorel et al., 2002), cocaine self-administration under PR or FR10 (but not FR1 or FR2) reinforcement (Xi et al., 2005), and reinstatement of drug-seeking behavior caused by cocaine priming, cue or footshock stress (Vorel et al., 2002; Xi et al., 2004b; Gilbert et al., 2005). In addition, systemic administration or intracranial microinjections into the NAc or basolateral amygdala significantly and dose-dependently inhibited contextual cue-induced incubation of cocaine craving in rats (Xi et al., 2012). These data suggest that SB-277011A is a promising candidate in medication development for treatment of cocaine addiction.

Clinical trials: Further development of SB-277011A as a medication for treatment of cocaine addiction has been halted by GlaxoSmithKline Pharmaceuticals, due to unexpected poor bioavailability (~2%) and a short half-life (<20 min) in primates (Austin et al., 2001; Remington and Kapue, 2001). Therefore, much effort has been made to develop other D3-

selective antagonists with higher bioavailability and more promising pharmacotherapeutic profiles (Newman et al., 2005).

3.5 GSK598809 and GSK618334

Preclinical studies: Based on the results with SB-277011A, GSK is currently developing other D3 receptor antagonists, such as GSK618334 and GSK598809, for the treatment of substance abuse and addiction. GSK598809 is a novel, potent and selective DA D_3 receptor antagonist (Searle et al., 2010). Functional assays showed that GSK598809 has >100-fold selectivity for D_3 receptors over D_2, histamine H_1, muscarinic M_1, M_2, M_3, M_4, serotonin 5-HT_{1A}, 5-HT_{1B} and 5-HT_{1D} receptors (te Beek et al., 2012). CPP experiments in animal models indicated that GSK598809 significantly reduced nicotine- and cocaine-seeking behaviour in a dose-dependent manner (te Beek et al., 2012). In addition, GSK598809 significantly prevented relapse to nicotine-seeking behaviour, although no effect was observed on reducing alcohol consumption in rats.

Clinical studies: GSK618334 is currently under Phase I and Phase II clinical trials (Table 2). A recent PET imaging study suggests that GSK598809 significantly and dose-dependently inhibits [^{11}C]PHNO binding in D3-rich brain regions such as the ventral striatum, globus pallidus and substantia nigra (Searle et al., 2010). In healthy volunteers, single doses of GSK598809 were generally well tolerated. Plasma concentration of GSK598809 increased rapidly after oral administration (T_{max} 2-3 hrs) and subsequently decreased in an apparent bi-exponential manner (terminal half-life of roughly 20 hrs). The CNS effects of GSK598809 alone were limited to elevation of serum prolactin and a small decrease in adaptive tracking performance (te Beek et al., 2012). GSK598809, at a dose (175 mg) that associated >90% D2/3 receptor occupancy, appeared to have no overall effect on attention bias to food-related cues (as measured behaviorally) (Nathan et al., 2011), on subjective hunger or craving ratings and on brain response to food images (as measured by fMRI) in overweight and obese binge eating individuals (Dodds et al., 2012). These findings are consistent with previous findings in experimental animals demonstrating that SB-277011A or NGB-2904 have no significant effects on food-induced CPP and food-taking behavior (Vorel et al., 2002; Ross et al., 2007; Thanos et al., 2008). Contrary to the promising finding in experimental animals, a recent clinical trial with GSK598809 for the treatment of alcoholism demonstrated that it produces an additive, not an expected inhibitory, effect on alcohol intake (te Beek et al., 2012). GSK598809 is currently under Phase II clinic trial for treatment of nicotine dependence (http://clinicaltrials.gov/). The effects of GSK598809 on cocaine dependence have not yet been evaluated.

3.6 ABT-925

ABT-925, also known as A-437203 or BSF-201640, is a selective D3 receptor antagonist developed by Abbott Laboratories. It has an approximately 100-fold selectivity for D3 versus D2 receptors (Geneste et al., 2006). Although the preclinical data for this compound are currently unavailable, proof-of-concept for D3 receptor antagonists in treatment of schizophrenia and drug abuse has been well-estabolished. In Phase I and Phase II clinical trials (Table 2), ABT-925 was safe and generally well tolerated up to the highest dose levels tested (600 mg single dose, 500 mg once daily for 7 days) (Day et al., 2010; Graff-Guerrero et al., 2010; Redden et al., 2011). However, a recent double-blind, placebo-controlled study for the treatment of acute schizophrenia suggest that ABT-925, at 50-150 mg per day, did not produce statistically significant therapeutic effects compared to placebo (Redden et al., 2011).

3.7 NGB-2904

NGB-2904 is another highly selective D3 receptor antagonist with >150-fold or 800-fold selectivity for primate or rat D3 over D2 receptors and 5000-fold selectivity for D3 over D1, D4, and D5 receptors (Yuan et al., 1998). Based upon its high selectivity for DA D3 receptors, we have recently evaluated the pharmacological effects in animal models of drug addiction. We found that systemic administration of NGB-2904 dose-dependently inhibits cocaine self-administration under PR (but not FR2) reinforcement (Xi et al., 2006b), cocaine-enhanced electrical brain reward function (Xi et al., 2006b; Spiller et al., 2008), and cocaine- and cocaine cue-induced reinstatement of cocaine-seeking behavior (Gilbert et al., 2005; Xi et al., 2006b). NGB-2904 alone neither produces dysphorigenic effects in brain-stimulation reward nor substitutes for cocaine in self-administration, suggesting that NGB-2904 itself has no abuse potential (Xi and Gardner, 2007). NGB-2904 is not currently under clinical trials, and detailed data regarding bioavailability and pharmacokinetic properties are presently unavailable.

3.8 YQA-14

YQA-14 is a novel D3 receptor antagonist developed recently (Song et al., 2012). Structurally, YQA-14 is a NGB-2904 analog. *In vivo* pharmacokinetic assays suggest that YQA-14 has improved oral bioavailability (>40%) and a longer half-life (>6 h in humans) compared to SB-277011A (~20 min in primates). In experimental animals, YQA-14 dose-dependently inhibits cocaine self-administration under both FR2 and PR reinforcement schedules, cocaine-induced CPP, cocaine-enhanced brain-stimulation reward, and cocaine- or cue-induced reinstatement of drug-seeking behavior (Song et al., 2012). Strikingly, at the doses that inhibit cocaine's actions, YQA-14 failed to alter oral sucrose self-administration and locomotor activity. YQA-14 is neither self-administered in drug-naïve rats nor substitutes for cocaine in maintenance of self-administration in rats previously trained for cocaine self-administration, suggesting that YQA-14 itself has no abuse liability. Deletion of DA D3 receptors in D3-knockout mice almost completely abolished the inhibitory effect by YQA-14 of cocaine self-administration, suggesting an effect mediated by blocking DA D3 receptors *in vivo* (Song et al., 2012). YQA-14 is currently not under clinical trials.

3.9 S33138

Preclinical studies: S33138 is a preferential D3 *versus* D2 receptor (~25-fold selectivity) antagonist (Millan et al., 2008). It was hypothesized that blockade of D3 plus partial blockade of D2 receptors may produce additive anti-cocaine therapeutic effects, but have fewer unwanted side-effects such as sedation and extrapyramidal locomotor impairment due to partial blockade of D2 receptors (Peng et al., 2009). In experimental animals, we found that S33138 produced biphasic effects - low doses increase, while high doses inhibit, cocaine self-administration under FR2 reinforcement. We interpret this increase in cocaine self-administration as a compensatory response to a reduction in cocaine's rewarding efficacy at low doses. In addition, S33138 also dose-dependently inhibits cocaine-enhanced brain-stimulation reward and cocaine-induced reinstatement of drug-seeking behavior (Peng et al., 2009). S33138, at low-to-moderate doses, has no effect on brain reward function by itself, while at high doses, produces an aversive-like effect as assessed by electrical brain-stimulation reward experiments, suggesting a D2 receptor-mediated effect at high doses. Further high doses of S33138 also inhibit oral sucrose self-administration, suggesting possible unwanted effects on nature reward at high doses.

Clinical trials: S33138 is currently under clinical trials as an anti-psychotic agent for the treatment of schizophrenia and other psychiatric diseases (Millan and Brocco, 2008; Thomasson-Perret et al., 2008). The efficacy of S33138 for treatment of cocaine addiction has not been evaluated in human clinical trials.

4. Glutamate-based medication strategies

Rationale: L-glutamate is the major excitatory neurotransmitter in the brain and acts through two heterogeneous families of glutamate receptors: ionotropic (iGluR) and metabotropic (mGluR) glutamate receptors. While iGluRs (i.e. NMDA, AMPA and kainite) are ligand-gated ion channels and responsible for fast excitatory neurotransmission, mGluRs ($mGluR_{1-8}$) are G-protein-coupled receptors linked to intracellular second messenger pathways. The eight subtypes of mGluRs have been classified into three groups on the basis of sequence similarities and pharmacological properties. Group I ($mGluR_{1,5}$) receptors activate phospholipase C via G_q proteins, whereas group II ($mGluR_{2,3}$) and group III ($mGluR_{4,6,7,8}$) receptors inhibit adenylate cyclase via $G_{\alpha i/o}$ proteins (see review by Cartmell and Schoepp, 2000).

Although the role of glutamate in mediating cocaine's rewarding effects remains unclear (see review by Xi and Gardner, 2008), growing evidence suggests that glutamate is critically involved in relapse to drug-seeking behavior (Figure 3) (Kalivas, 2009; Bowers et al., 2010). In brief, chronic cocaine produces a reduction in basal levels of extracellular glutamate or glutamate transmission in the NAc during cocaine withdrawal, while cocaine priming or re-exposure to cocaine-associated cues stimulate glutamate release in both the VTA and NAc. These findings suggest that both a reduction in basal glutamate transmission and enhanced glutamate responding to cocaine or cocaine-associated cues may constitute a neurobiological substrate of relapse to drug-seeking behavior (Kalivas, 2009). Based on this hypothesis, a number of pharmacotherapeutic strategies have been proposed. These include, first, normalization (increase) of reduced basal glutamate neurotransmission during abstinence, and second, antagonism of enhanced glutamate responses to cocaine or cocaine-associated cues (Figure 3).

4.1 *N*-acetylcysteine

Preclinical studies: N-acetylcysteine (NAC) is a cystine prodrug. It is approved for the treatment of pulmonary complications of cystic fibrosis and paracetamol (acetaminophen) overdose. By providing a source of extracellular cysteine, which is converted to cystine, NAC can exchange extracellular cystine for intracellular glutamate. This restores (renormalizes) decreased basal levels of extracellular glutamate (Baker et al., 2003). The increased extracellular glutamate may subsequently attenuate cocaine-induced increases in glutamate release by activation of presynaptic mGluR2/3 receptors, and therefore inhibits cocaine- or cocaine cue-induced reinstatement of drug-seeking behaviour (Figure 3). NAC did not decrease cocaine self-administration or acute cocaine-induced hyperactivity, while it decreased repeated cocaine-induced escalation of drug intake and behavioural sensitization (Madayag et al., 2007). In addition, repeated NAC treatments also attenuated cocaine-induced increases in drug seeking in rats (Baker et al., 2003; Amen et al., 2010). Interestingly, NAC is also a prodrug for the synthesis of the endogenous antioxidant glutathione, and that NAC pretreatment protects animals from high dose methamphetamine- or amphetamine-induced DA neurotoxicity and behavioural changes by lowering oxidative stress levels (Fukami et al., 2004; Achat-Mendes et al., 2007).

Clinical trials: NAC is currently under clinical trials (Table 3). In double-blind, placebo-controlled clinic trials, NAC was well tolerated and produced a significant reduction in cocaine-related withdrawal symptoms and/or cravings triggered by exposure to cocaine-related cues or by an experimenter-delivered intravenous injection of cocaine (LaRowe et al., 2006, 2007; Amen et al., 2010). A 4-week open-label clinical trial demonstrated that NAC significantly reduced cocaine use in 16 of 23 human cocaine-dependent subjects (Mardikian et al., 2007). More clinical trials are currently underway (http://clinicaltrials.gov/).

Compound	Company	Pharm. Action	Indication	Status	Reference
N-acetylcysteine (NAC)	TwinLab, NY, USA; Others	Cystine prodrug	Substance abuse (cocaine, nicotine, methamphetamine)	Phase II	http://clinicaltrials.gov
AZD8529	AntraZeneca, London, UK	mGluR2/3 PAM	Schizophrenia	Phase II	http://clinicaltrials.gov
ADX71149	Janssen, USA	mGluR2 PAM	Schizophrenia; Anxiety	Phase II	http://www.addexpharma.com/pipline/
LY214023	Eli Lilly, USA	mGluR2/3 PAM	PK study	Phase I	http://clinicaltrials.gov
LY404039	Eli Lilly, USA	mGluR2/3 PAM	Schizophrenia	Phase II	Patil et al., 2007
LY354740	Eli Lilly, USA	mGluR2 PAM	Schizophrenia; Anxiety	Phase II	Dunayevich et al., 2008
JNJ-40411813	Johnson & Johnson, USA	mGluR2 PAM	Schizophrenia	Phase II	http://clinicaltrials.gov
GPI-5633	Guiford, USA	mGluR3 PAM	Safety & PK profile	Phase I	Van der Post et al., 2005
Fenobam	Enzo Life Sci. USA; Others	mGluR5 NAM	Anxiety; Fragile X syndrome	Phase II	http://clinicaltrials.gov
ADX10059	Addex Switzerland	mGluR5 NAM	Gastro-oesophageal reflux	Phase II	http://clinicaltrials.gov
STX107	Seaside, USA	mGluR5 NAM	Fragile X Syndrome	Phase II	http://clinicaltrials.gov

Table 3. Glutamate-based drug candidates in clinical trials

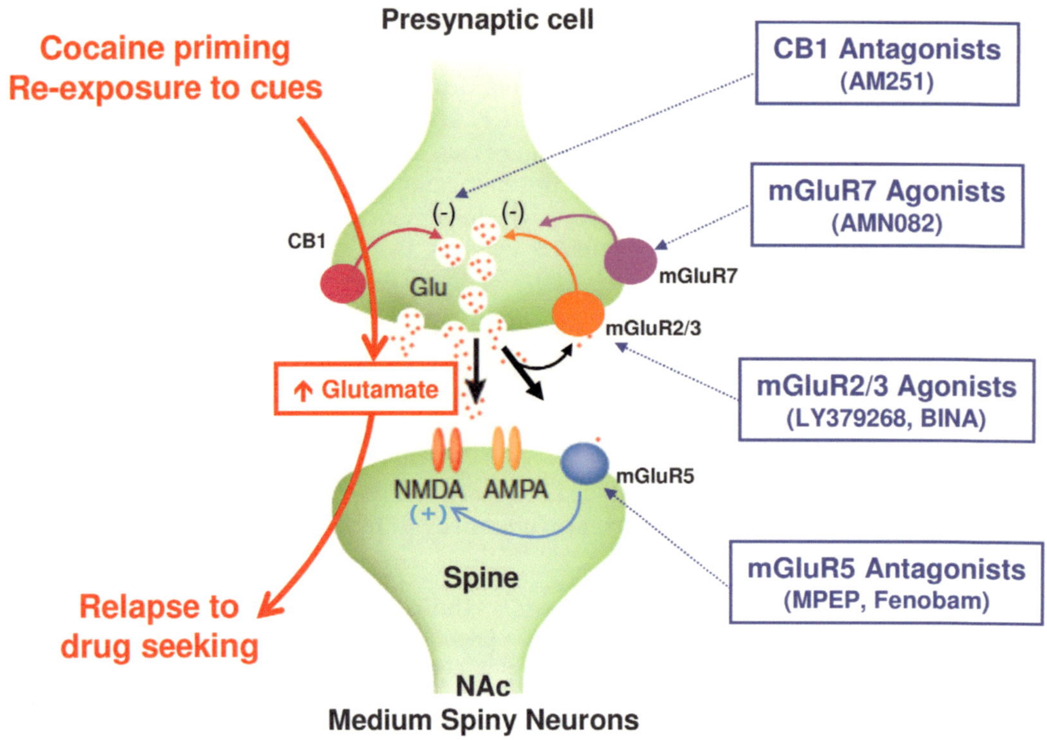

Fig. 3. Schematic diagram of glutamatergic synaptic transmission in the NAc, illustrating that cocaine priming or re-exposuse to cocaine-associated cues evokes an increase in glutamate release and relapse to drug-seeking behaviour in rats. Various compounds that target CB1 and mGluRs may attenuate cocaine- or cue-induced increase in glutamate release or in postsynaptic glutamate receptor signalling, and therefore, inhibit relapse to drug-seeking behaviour.

4.2 MPEP

Preclinical studies: MPEP is a selective $mGluR_5$ negative allosteric modulator (NAM) or antagonist (Gasparini et al., 1999). The first study to examine the role of mGluR5 in drug addiction reported that deletion of mGluR5 subtype abolishes cocaine self-administration in mice, while systemic administration of MPEP significantly inhibited cocaine self-administration in mice (Chiamulera et al., 2001). Since then, a large number of studies suggest that systemic administration of MPEP or its analog MTEP (a more selective mGluR5 NAM) (Lea and Faden, 2006) significantly and dose-dependently inhibits cocaine self-administration in rats (Xi et al., 2004a, 2004c; Tessari et al., 2004; Paterson and Markou, 2005; Kenny et al., 2005; Lee et al., 2005), cocaine-induced CPP (McGeehan and Olive, 2003; Herzig and Schmidt, 2004), cocaine-induced hyperactivity (McGeehan et al., 2004), and cocaine-, cue- or stress-induced reinstatement of cocaine-seeking behaviour (Xi et al., 2004a, 2004c; Lee et al., 2005; Backstrom and Hyytia, 2006; Kumaresan et al., 2009; Martin-Fardon and Weiss, 2011; Wang et al., 2012). These data strongly suggest that mGluR5 antagonists may be promising in the treatment of cocaine addiction.

Clinical trials: MPEP and MTEP have not been tested in clinical trials. Relatively poor selectivity of MPEP for mGluR5 over other targets (NET, NR2B-containing NMDA receptor, monoamine oxidase A and mGluR4) may have prevented its use in human clinical trials.

4.3 Fenobam

Preclinical studies: Fenobam (McN-3377) was originally developed as a nonbenzodiazepine anxiolytic in the 1980s with an unknown molecular target until 2005 when it was reported that fenobam is a selective mGluR5 NAM or antagonist (Porter et al., 2005). Fenobam was reported to have improved mGluR5 selectivity compared to MPEP, as assessed by the use of mGluR5-KO mice, and rapidly penetrate brain-blood barrier to concentrate in the brain (Montana et al., 2009). Systemic administration of fenobam dose-dependently elevates stimulation threshold for brain-stimulation reward in rats, suggesting a reduction in brain reward function (Cleva et al., 2012). In addition, our pilot experimental data also suggest that oral administration of fenobam significantly inhibits cocaine self-administration and cocaine- or cue-, induced cocaine-seeking behaviour.

Clinical trials: Fenobam was investigated in Phase II clinical trials in the 1980s for the treatment of anxiety and depression (Table 3). Earlier single- or double-blind, placebo-controlled clinical trials demonstrated that fenobam was effective in attenuating severe anxiety with good safety profiles (Pecknold et al., 1982; Pecknold et al., 1980; Lapierre and Oyewumi, 1982). However, in another report, it was reported to be inactive and have psychostimulant effects by itself (Friedmann et al., 1980). At the time, fenobam was discontinued from further development as an anxiolytic. In 2006, it was granted orphan drug designation by the FDA for clinical trials in the treatment of Fragile X syndrome, an inherited mental retardation disorder. The efficacy of fenobam in the treatment of cocaine addiction has not yet been evaluated.

4.4 ADX10059

ADX10059 is another novel mGluR5-selective NAM or antagonist with an IC_{50} of 17.1 nM at human mGluR5, showing good selectivity for mGluR5 over > 65 other receptors, transporters, ion channels and enzymes (Marin and Goadsby, 2010). Although limited preclinical data are available, it has been under Phase I and Phase II clinical trials for the treatment of gastro-oesophageal reflux disease (Zerbib et al., 2010, 2011) and migraine (Marin and Goadsby, 2010) (Table 3). To date, ADX10059 has been studied in at least 10 clinical trials. However, Addex Pharmaceuticals announced the discontinuation of development of ADX10059 in December 2009 due to liver enzyme changes. The efficacy of ADX10059 in the treatment of cocaine addiction has not been evaluated.

4.5 LY379268

Preclinical studies: LY379268 is a systemically effective $mGluR_{2/3}$ orthosteric (competitive) agonist (Marek, 2004). The $mGluR_{2/3}$ receptors have become attractive targets in medication development for the treatment of drug addiction because $mGluR_{2/3}$ receptors function as glutamate autoreceptors, modulating presynaptic glutamate release (Xi et al., 2002a) (Figure 3). In addition, $mGluR_{2/3}$ modulates DA and other neurotransmitter release in the NAc. Since cocaine-induced increases in NAc DA and glutamate are critically involved in drug reward and relapse, it was proposed that $mGluR_{2/3}$ agonists might be useful for the treatment of cocaine addiction (Xi et al., 2002a). Systemic administration of LY379268 inhibits cocaine self-administration and cocaine cue-induced reinstatement of drug-seeking behaviour (Baptista et al., 2004; Peters and Kalivas, 2006). Microinjections of LY369268 into the NAc or central amygdala also inhibit cocaine- or food-triggered reinstatement of reward-seeking behaviour (Peters and Kalivas, 2006) or incubation of cocaine craving in rats (Lu et al., 2007). These data suggest that LY369268 may be useful for the treatment of cocaine addiction.

Clinical studies: LY379268 is not currently under clinical trials. This may be related to its intrinsic competitive agonist properties that may produce unwanted side-effects by itself and/or reduce efficacy due to competitive binding inhibition by excessive glutamate release under pathological conditions. In contrast to LY379268, several other mGluR2/3 positive allosteric modulators (PAMs) are being investigated in Phase I and Phase II clinical trials for the treatment of schizophreria and anxiety (Mezler et al., 2010; Patil., et al., 2007). These compounds include AZD8529, LY404039, LY354740, and LY2140023 (Table 3). The potential effects of these mGluR2/3 agonists in treatment of cocaine addiction have not been evaluated.

4.6 BINA

Preclinical studies: Biphenylindanone A (BINA) is a selective mGluR2 PAM or agonist (Johnson et al., 2003; Galici et al., 2006). Recent studies suggest that the pharmacological effects of LY379268 (a competitive mGluR2/3 orthosteric agonist) in animal models relevant to neuropsychiatric diseases could be mediated predominantly by activation of mGluR2, not mGluR3 receptor (Woolley et al., 2008), suggesting that mGluR2-selective agonists may produce similar therapeutic effects but have fewer unwanted effects than LY379268. Recently, Markou and her colleagues have compared the pharmacotherapeutic effects of BINA and LY379268 in animal models of drug addiction. They found that BINA selectively inhibits cocaine self-administration and cue-induced reinstatement of cocaine-seeking behaviour without affecting behaviours motivated by food reinforcement, while LY379268 nonselectively inhibits both cocaine- and food-taking and –seeking behaviour (Jin et al., 2010). These data suggest that selective mGluR2 PAMs (BINA) might have better therapeutic potential than dual mGluR2/3 agonists (LY379268) for the treatment of cocaine addiction.

Clinical trials: BINA is currently not under clinical trials. However, other mGluR2 PAMs such as AZD71149, LY354740 and JNJ-40411813 are currently under clinical trials for safety and *in vivo* binding property in healthy volunteers (Table 3).

4.7 2-PMPA and GPI-5693

Preclinical studies: 2-PMPA and GPI-5693 (also called 2-MPPA) are inhibitors of NAALADase (*N*-acetylated-α-linked acidic dipeptidase, also called glutamate carboxypeptidase II, GCPII), an enzyme that hydrolyzes *N*-acetylaspartate-glutamate (NAAG) to *N*-acetylaspartate (NAA) and glutamate (Neal et al., 2000, 2011). NAAG is an endogenous $mGluR_3$ agonist, which negatively modulates the release of glutamate and other neurotransmitters (Neale et al., 2000, 2011). Given the important role of NAc glutamate in relapse to drug seeking as stated above, it was hypothesized that inhibition of NAALADase by 2-PMPA and GPI-5693 would increase extracellular NAAG and decrease extracellular glutamate levels (due to decreased glutamate release from NAAG degradation), while the increase in NAAG would further inhibit glutamate release from neuronal terminals and/or glial cells by activating mGluR3 receptors (Xi et al., 2002a, 2010b). In addition, NAAG also inhibits DA release by activating mGluR3 receptors located on DA terminals in the NAc (Xi et al., 2010b). Thus, the endogenous NAALADase-NAAG-mGluR3 signal system may constitute a novel important target in medication development for the treatment of cocaine addiction. Earlier studies have shown that systemic administration of 2-PMPA inhibits cocaine-induced CPP (Slusher et al., 2001) and cocaine-induced behavioural sensitization (Shippenberg et al., 2000). Recently, we reported that systemic administration of 2-PMPA or GPI-5693 inhibited cocaine self-administration, cocaine-enhanced brain-stimulation reward, and cocaine-triggered reinstatement of drug-seeking behaviour (Xi et al., 2010a, 2010b; Peng et al., 2010b). This action was blocked by pretreatment with LY341495, a selective mGluR2/3 antagonist. In addition, 2-PMPA dose-dependently attenuated cocaine-induced increases in extracellular DA and glutamate in the NAc (Xi et al., 2010a; 2010b). Taken together, these data suggest that inhibition of NAALADase by 2-PMPA or GPI-5693 produces an inhibitory effect on cocaine-taking and cocaine-seeking behaviour

Clinical trials: GPI-5693 was investigated in a Phase I clinical trial for its safety, pharmacokinetics and efficacy for treatment of neuropathic pain (Table 3) (van der Post et al., 2005). It was reported to be safe and tolerable in healthy subjects.

4.8 AMN082

AMN082 is a novel systemically active mGluR7 PAM or agonist (Mitsukawa et al., 2005). The $mGluR_7$ receptor subtype has attracted much attention in medication development for treatment of addiction for several reasons (Li et al., 2012). First, mGluR7 is the most abundant subtype of the group III mGluR subtypes in reward-related brain regions such as striatum, hippocampus and olfactory tubercles (Ferraguti and Shigemoto, 2006). Second, activation of group III mGluRs (including mGluR7) by L-AP4 inhibits DA and glutamate release in the NAc (Hu et al., 1999; Xi et al., 2003b). Third, it is the most conserved mGluR subtype across different mammalian species (Makoff et al., 1996), suggesting that selective $mGluR_7$ ligands that are effective in experimental animals are more likely to be effective in humans. And fourth, the development of AMN082 has allowed us to explore the role of mGluR7 in drug reward and addiction.

Based on the above, we and others have recently reported that systemic administration of AMN082 inhibits cocaine self-administration behaviour under both FR2 and PR reinforcement, cocaine-enhanced brain reward function, and cocaine-induced reinstatement of drug-seeking behaviour. In addition, AMN082 also decreases, while the selective mGluR7 antagonist MMPIP increases, alcohol intake and preference (Salling et al., 2008; Bahi et al., 2011). Importantly, the same doses of AMN082 neither alters locomotion or sucrose self-administration (Li et al., 2010; Bahi et al., 2011; but see Salling et al., 2008) nor alters brain reward function (Li et al., 2008), suggesting that AMN082 produces therapeutic anti-cocaine effects without significant unwanted effects such as sedation, dysphoria or natural reward depression. Further mechanistic studies suggest that a NAc-VP GABAergic mechanism underlies its antagonism of cocaine reward (Li et al., 2008, 2009), while a glutamate-mGluR2/3 mechanism underlies its antagonism of relapse to drug-seeking behaviour (Li et al., 2008, 2010, 2012). Together, these preclinical data suggest a potential utility of AMN082 in the treatment of cocaine addiction. AMN082 has not yet been tested in clinical trials.

5. GABA-based medication strategies

Rationale: It is well known that the mesolimbic DA system is critically involved in drug reward and addiction. However, it remains unclear how increased NAc DA underlies these actions. Anatomically, the majority of neurons in the striatum are medium-spiny GABAergic output neurons, which receive DA projections from the VTA and glutamatergic projections predominantly from the prefrontal cortex, and project to the dorsal globus pallidus (from the dorsal striatum) and the ventral pallidum (VP) and VTA (from the ventral striatum, i.e. the NAc) (Bennett and Bolam, 1994; Groenewegen et al., 1996). Overall, DA produces a net inhibitory effect on striatal medium-spiny GABAergic neurons (Nicola and Malenka, 1997; Umemiya and Raymond, 1997), predominantly by activation of D2-like DA receptors (Centonze et al., 2002). Similarly, cocaine also produces an overall inhibitory effect on VTA GABAergic neurons (Cameron and Williams, 1994), striatal GABAergic neurons (Uchimura and North, 1990; White et al., 1993; Centonze et al., 2002; Schramm-Sapyta et al., 2006), and GABA release in the VP (Tang et al., 2005; Li et al., 2010). Based on this, the NAc-VP/VTA GABAergic projection constitutes common final pathway underlying drug reward and addiction (Figure 2). Thus, it has been hypothesized that a pharmacological strategy that enhances GABAergic transmission in the VTA and/or the VP would produce an inhibitory effect on cocaine- or DA-induced reductions in GABA release, therefore antagonizing cocaine's rewarding effects. Based on this, several GABAergic compounds have been studied extensively in experimental animals.

5.1 Gamma-vinyl GABA

Preclinical studies: Gamma-vinyl GABA (GVG) (also called vigabatrin) is an irreversible GABA transaminase inhibitor. GABA transaminase is an enzyme that breaks down GABA, causing an increase in brain GABA after GVG administration (Peng et al., 2010a). In the 1990s, Dewey and colleagues first proposed that GVG might be useful for the treatment of drug addiction (Dewey et al., 1998). Since then, many preclinical studies appear to support this hypothesis (Xi and Gardner, 2008). Systemic administration of GVG inhibits cocaine self-administration, cocaine-enhanced brain-stimulation reward, cocaine-induced CPP and behavioural sensitization (see review by Xi and Gardner, 2008). Similarly, it also dose-dependently inhibits cocaine-induced reinstatement of drug-seeking behaviour (Peng et al., 2008). All these data support the use of GVG in the treatment of cocaine addiction.

Clinical trials: GVG is currently under clinical trials for treatment of cocaine addiction (Table 4). In three open-labeled studies, GVG was well-tolerated and produced a significant increase in cocaine abstinence rate (Brodie et al., 2003, 2005; Fechtner et al., 2006). In a more recent randomized, double-blind, placeto-controled trial, short-term GVG treatment significantly increased abstinence rate compared to placebo (Brodie et al., 2009). However, in another clinical trial for the treatment of methamphetamine dependence, GVG was not effective (De La Garza et al., 2009). GVG is not marketed in the USA because of concerns over ophthalmological side-effects, but none were observed during these short-term studies (Fechtner et al., 2006). More studies are underway to confirm its efficacy for cocaine dependence (http://clinicaltrials.gov).

Compound	Company	Pharm. Action	Indication	Status	Reference
GVG	Aventis, Quebec, Canada	GABA transaminase inhibitor	Substance abuse (cocaine, methamphetamine)	Phase II	http://clinicaltrials.gov
Topiramate	Meliapharm, Montreal, Canada VIVUS, CA, USA	$GABA_A$ PAM	Substance abuse (cocaine)	Phase II	http://clinicaltrials.gov
Tiagabine	Cephalon, PA, USA	GABA transporter inhibitor	Substance abuse (cocaine); Anxiety Schizophrenia	Phase II Phase III	http://clinicaltrials.gov
Baclofen	Remedy Repack, PA, USA	$GABA_B$ receptor agonist	Substance abuse (cocaine, nicotine, alcohol)	Phase II	http://clinicaltrials.gov
Gabapentin	Meliapharm, Montreal, Canada	GABA enhancer, Alpha2delta-Ca^{++} channel blocker	Substance abuse (cocaine, nicotine, alcohol)	Phase II	http://clinicaltrials.gov

Table 4. GABA receptor-based drug candidates in clinical trials

5.2 Tiagabine

Preclinical studies: Tiagabine is a selective type 1 GABA transporter (GAT1) inhibitor, which increases extracellular GABA levels (Eriksson et al., 1999). It has been approved as an antiepileptic medication (Schousboe et al., 2011). Preclinical studies suggest that tiagabine inhibited intravenous cocaine self-administration in rats (Filip et al., 2007) or baboons (Weerts et al., 2005), but had no significant effect on cocaine-induced reinstatement of drug-seeking behaviour (Filip et al., 2007; Weerts et al., 2007). Our experimental data suggest that tiagabine, at much higher doses (10-20 mg/kg) than those used in the above-cited studies, selectively inhibited cocaine self-administration, but had no effect on cocaine-induced reinstatement of drug-seeking behaviour in rats (Yang et al., 2012).

Clinical trials: The results of clinical trials with tiagabine are mixed. Two small-scale (45 and 76 subjects, respectively) placebo-controlled clinical trials indicated that tiagabine produced a moderate reduction (~30%) in cocaine use in methadone-treated cocaine addicts (González et al., 2003, 2007), while other studies demonstrated that the same doses of tiagabine neither altered the acute effects of cocaine (Lile et al., 2004), nor lowered cocaine use in cocaine addicts (Winhusen et al., 2005; 2007).

5.3 Topiramate

Preclinical studies: Topiramate is a positive modulator of $GABA_A$ receptors (acting at non-benzodiazepine sites) and a licensed antiepileptic drug (Czuczwar and Patsalos, 2001). In addition, topiramate has other pharmacological actions, including antagonism of AMPA/kainate glutamate receptors, inhibition of voltage-gated sodium and calcium channels and inhibition of carbonic anhydrase (Johnson, 2005). In animal studies, topiramate was reported to inhibit cocaine self-administration and attenuate NAc DA response to cocaine or cocaine-associated cues (Johnson, 2005).

Clinical studies: In a double-blind, placebo-controlled clinical trial (40 subjects), topiramate significantly increased abstinence rates compared to placebo (Kampman et al., 2004). A recent 12-week, open-label pilot study showed a significant reduction in craving intensity and duration in 25% of the sample group (Reis et al., 2008). Evidence for a beneficial role of topiramate in the treatment of cocaine dependence is promising but is limited by small sample sizes (Cubells, 2006; Minozzi et al., 2008). More studies are currently underway (Table 4).

5.4 Baclofen

Preclinical studies: Baclofen is a selective $GABA_B$ receptor agonist, licensed as an antispasmodic for patients with spinal cord injuries or multiple sclerosis. In rodents, pretreatment with baclofen dose-dependently attenuates cocaine self-administration under FR and PR reinforcement (Roberts et al., 1996; Brebner et al., 2000), cocaine-enhanced brain-stimulation reward (Slattery et al., 2005), and cocaine-induced increases in NAc DA (Fadda et al., 2003). It also inhibited cocaine- or cue-induced cocaine-taking and cocaine-seeking behaviour (Di Ciano and Everitt, 2003; Campbell et al., 1999; Weerts et al., 2007).

Clinical trials: In an initial open-label clinical trial, baclofen reduced self-reports of craving and cocaine use in 10 cocaine abusers (Ling et al., 1998). In a subsequent 16-week double-blind study in 35 cocaine-dependent subjects, baclofen reduced cocaine use and increased the number of cocaine-free urines (Shoptaw et al., 2003), but did not alter cocaine craving. In a recent placebo-controlled, double-blind study, baclofen lowered cocaine intake, decreased cocaine craving, and attenuated cocaine's cardiovascular effects in both cocaine- and opioid-dependent subjects (Haney et al., 2006). However, a more recent large scale (160 cocaine addicts), double-blind, placebo-controlled clinical trial demonstrated that baclofen was not effective in attenuating cocaine use (Kahn et al., 2009). Thus, more studies are required to determine its efficacy in relapse prevention.

5.5 Gabapentin

Preclinical studies: Gabapentin is structurally analogous to GABA but, unlike the latter, it crosses the blood-brain barrier and can be administered systemically. Pharmacologically, gabapentin is a GABAmimetic drug that increases extracellular GABA levels, possibly by increasing the synthesis and nonvesicular release of GABA as well as by preventing GABA catabolism (Taylor et al., 1998). In addition, gabapentin also inhibits alpha2delta subunit-composed voltage-dependent Ca^{++} channels (Gee et al., 1996). Early studies suggest that gabapentin (1-30 mg/kg, i.p.) significantly inhibited cocaine-induced hyperactivity and locomotor sensitization (Filip et al., 2006; but see Itzhak and Martin, 2000). However, other studies demonstrate that gabapentin, at a broad dose range (10-200 mg/kg i.p.), neither inhibited cocaine self-administration nor altered cocaine-induced reinstatement of drug-seeking behaviour in rats (Filip et al., 2007; Peng et al., 2008b). *In vivo* microdialysis studies demonstrate that gabapentin, at 100-200 mg/kg, produced a significant increase (~50 %) in extracellular GABA in the NAc, but failed to alter either basal or cocaine-enhanced NAc DA (Peng et al., 2008b). These data suggest that gabapentin is a weak GABA enhancer and may have limited potential in the treatment of cocaine addiction.

Clinical trials: Early clinical studies and small-scale, open-label outpatient trials demonstrated that gabapentin reduced cocaine craving and use (Raby and Coomaraswamy, 2004; Myrick et al., 2001; Hart et al., 2004, 2005). However, this finding was not repeated by larger-scale, double-blind, placebo-controlled clinical trials demonstrating that gabapentin, at doses up to 2400-3200 mg/day for 6-12 weeks, had no effect on abstinence rate, craving or subjective effects of cocaine (Bisaga et al., 2006; Berger et al., 2005; González et al., 2007; Hart et al., 2007). More clinical trials are currently under way to evaluate the effects of gabapentin or gabapentin combined with the antidepressant sertraline on cocaine or other addictive drug dependence (Table 4).

6. Cannabinoid-based medication strategies

Rationale: Marijuana is the most widely used illicit drug in the United States. Δ^9-tetrahydrocannabinol (Δ^9-THC) is the major psychoactive ingredient in marijuana. Two major types of cannabinoid receptors, CB_1 and CB_2, have been cloned. Since CB_1 receptors are found in both brain and peripheral tissues, whereas CB_2 receptors are found predominantly in peripheral immune system, it is generally belived that the psychoactive effects of Δ^9-THC or marijuana are mediated by activation of brain CB1, not CB2, receptors (Tanda and Goldberg, 2003). However, growing evidence suggests that functional CB_2 receptors are also found in the brain (Van Sickle et al., 2005; Gong et al., 2006; Xi et al., 2011), suggesting that brain CB_2 receptors may be also involved in marijuana's actions.

As stated above, the mesolimbic DA and the downstream NAc-VP GABAergic transmission have been thought to underlie cocaine reward and addiction. Growing evidence suggests that similar mechanisms may also underlie the action produced by Δ^9-THC or marijuana. It was reported that Δ^9-THC elevates extracellular DA in the NAc (Chen et al., 1990; Tanda et al., 1997). This action could be mediated by a GABAergic mechanism, i.e., Δ^9-THC may initially activate CB1 receptors located on VTA GABAergic interneurons and produce a decrease in GABA release, which subsequently disinhibits (or activates) VTA DA neurons (Figure 2) (Fernandez-Ruiz et al., 2010). In addition, CB_1 receptors are also highly expressed on presynaptic glutamatergic terminals in the NAc (Lupica et al., 2004). Thus, activation of CB1 receptors located on glutamatergic terminals decreases glutamate inputs onto medium-spiny GABAergic neurons in the NAc and decrease GABA release in their projection areas – the VP and VTA. Further, CB1 receptors are also expressed on striatal GABAergic neurons, and activation of the CB1 receptors produces a direct inhibitory effect on medium-spiny GABAergic neurons and decreases GABA release in the VP and the VTA (Maldonado et al., 2011). Lastly, cocaine or DA has been shown to increase endocannabinoid release in the striatum (Giuffrida et al., 1999; Centonze et al., 2004; Caille et al., 2007), which subsequently increases endocannabinoid binding to CB1 receptors located on presynaptic glutamatergic terminals and postsynaptic GABAergic neurons (Figure 2). Taken together, activation of

CB1 receptors located on both GABAergic and glutamatergic neurons causes an increase in NAc DA and a decrease in GABA release in both the VTA and VP. This decrease in NAc-VP GABAergic transmission constitutes a final common pathway underlying drug reward and addiction. Accordingly, blockade of CB_1 receptors in both the VTA and NAc would attenuate the actions of cocaine on NAc DA and VP GABA release, and therefore attenuate cocaine reward and addiction.

6.1 SR141716A

Preclinical studies: SR141716A (also called rimonabant) is the first developed CB_1 receptor antagonist (also an inverse agonist) (Rinaldi-Carmona et al., 1994). SR141716A was reported to inhibit cocaine self-administration under PR reinforcement (Soria et al., 2005; Xi et al., 2008), decrease cocaine-enhanced NAc DA (Cheer et al., 2007; Soria et al., 2005), and inhibit cocaine- and cue-induced reinstatement of drug-seeking behaviour (De Vries et al., 2001), while other studies suggest that it has no effect on cocaine self-administration under low FR reinforcement, cocaine-induced CPP, or cocaine-induced behavioural sensitization (Arnold, 2005). These data suggest that SR141716A may have therapeutic effects in attenuating relapse to drug-seeking behaviour, but is limited in terms of attenuating cocaine's acute rewarding effects (Beardsley and Thomas, 2005; Xi and Gardner, 2008).

Clinical trials: SR141716A was the first CB1 receptor antagonist to be approved for clinical trials for the treatment of obesity and cigarette smoking. However, there are some safety concerns with rimonabant - increased risk of anxiety, depression, and suicide tendency, which had led it to being withdrawn from the market in Europe and North America in 2008. Since then, many pharmaceutical companies (Sanofi-Aventis, Merck, Pfizer, Solvay) have announced that they will stop further clinical research on this class of drug.

6.2 AM251

Preclinical studies: AM251 is a more potent and selective CB_1 receptor antagonist than SR141716A (Krishnamurthy et al., 2004). In animal models of drug addiction, AM251 appears to be more potent and effective than SR141716A in attenuating cocaine's action (Xi et al., 2006, 2008). For example, AM251 significantly and dose-dependently inhibited cocaine self-administration (under PR, but not FR reinforcement) (Xi et al., 2008), cocaine-enhanced brain-stimulation reward (Xi et al., 2008), and cocaine-induced behavioural sensitization (Corbille et al., 2007), as well as cocaine-triggered reinstatement of drug-seeking behaviour (Xi et al., 2006). Further, a glutamate-mGluR2/3 mechanism has been shown to underlie the antagonism of reinstatement of drug seeking (Xi et al., 2006). That is, blockade of CB1 receptors by AM251 elevates extracellular glutamate in the NAc, which subsequently increased glutamate binding to presynaptic mGluR2/3 receptors, inhibiting cocaine-induced increases in glutamate release and relapse to drug-seeking behaviour (Xi et al., 2006) (Figure 3). These findings suggest that AM251 may be more potent and effective than SR141716A for treatment of cocaine addiction.

Clinical trials: Since the above mentioned side-effects of SR141716A have been linked to its inverse agonist property, it is generally believed that AM251, a CB1 receptor antagonist with similar inverse agonist property might have the same unwanted side-effects. It is not under clinical trials.

6.3 JWH133

Preclinical studies: In addition to CB1 receptors, recent breakthrough findings suggest that brain CB_2 receptors are also involved in drug reward and addiction (Onaivi et al., 2008; Xi et al., 2011; Aracil-Fernández, et al., 2012). JWH133 and GW405833 are highly selective CB2 receptor agonists. We have recently reported that systemic, intranasal or intra-NAc administration of JWH133 or GW405833 significantly and dose-dependently inhibits cocaine self-administration, cocaine-induced increases in locomotion and extracellular DA in wild-type and CB1-KO mice, but not in CB2-KO mice. Similarly, overexpression of CB2 receptors in mouse brain decreases intravenous cocaine self-administration and cocaine-induced locomotor sensitization (Aracil-Fernández, et al., 2012). These data suggest that CB2 receptor agonists may have therapeutic potential for the treatment of cocaine addiction (Figure 2) (Xi et al., 2011).

Clinical trials: JWH133 and GW405833 are currently not under clinical trials. However, many other selective CB2 receptor agonists, such as cannabinor, GW842166, GRC-10693, LY-2828360, ABT-521, and KHK-6188, are currently under Phase I and Phase II clinical trials for the treatment of pain or other diseases (Table 5). In addition, several dual CB1/CB2

Compound	Company	Pharm. Action	Indication	Status	Reference
Cannabinor	Pharmos, NJ, USA	CB2 agonist	Pain	Phase II	http://www.pharmoscorp.com/development/cannabinor.html
GW842166	GSK, London, UK	CB2 agonist	Pain	Phase II	http://clinicaltrials.gov
GRC 10693	Glenmark, Munbai, India	CB2 agonist	Pain	Phase I	http://www.evaluatepharma.com/Universal/View.aspx?type=Story&id=183092
LY-2828360	Eli Lilly, USA	CB2 agonist	Pain	Phase II	http://clinicaltrials.gov
ABT-521	Abbott, USA	CB2 agonist	Pain	Phase I	http://www.pharmalive.com/special_reports/sample.cfm?reportID=283
KHK-6188	Kyowa Hakka Kirin, Japan	CB2 agonist	Pain	Phase I	http://clinicaltrials.gov
Nabilone (Cesamet): Δ^9-THC analog	NEMA Research, USA	CB1/CB2 agonist	Cannabis addiction; Pain	Phase III Phase IV	http://clinicaltrials.gov
Marinol (Dronabinol): Δ^9-THC	UNIMED, USA	CB1/CB2 agonist	Substance abuse (opioid, marijuana, alcohol), PTSD	Phase II Phase IV	http://clinicaltrials.gov
Sativex: Δ^9-THC + Cannabidiol	GW, London, UK	CB1/CB2 agonist	Cannabis abuse, Pain	Phase II	http://clinicaltrials.gov

Table 5. Cannabinoid-based drug candidates in clinical trials

receptor agonists such as Nabilone (a Δ^9-THC analog), Marinol (Δ^9-THC), Sativex (a mixture of THC and cannabidiol) have been approved for the treatment of pain and chemotherapy-induced nausea and vomiting (Table 5). Based upon the recent findings that activation of CB2 receptors in primary afferents and spinal cord produces analgesic effects (Anand et al., 2009; Beltramo, 2009), and that activation of CB2 receptors in the brainstem inhibits morphine-6-glucuronide-induced emesis (vomiting) (Van Sickle et al., 2005), it is likely that the therapeutic effects of these dual CB1/CB2 receptor agonists may at least in part be mediated by activation of brain CB2 receptors.

7. Conclusion

In this review article, I first briefly reviewed the neurochemical mechanisms underlying cocaine reward and addiction, and then provided the rationale for development of various pharmacological therapies for the treatment of cocaine addiction. Lastly, I summarized the major findings of multiple pharmacological agents in each drug catagory in animal models of drug addiction and the current status in clinical trials for the treatment of drug addiction and/or other neuropsychiatric diseases. In summary, the VTA-NAc-VP pathway, including the mesolimbic DA and the NAc-VP GABAergic transimission, appears to play a critical role in mediating cocaine's rewarding effects (Figure 2), while a NAc glutamate-mGluR2/3 mechanism plays an important role in controlling relapse to drug-seeking behaviour (Figure 3). Accordingly, various pharmacological agents have been proposed and tested in animal models of drug addiction to interfere with the pharmacological actions produced by cocaine. Among those compounds discussed above, the DAT inhibitors (modafinil, RTI-335, CTDP31,345, CTDP-32,476), the DA receptor antagonists (*l*-THP, S33138, GSK598809, YQA-14) and the glutamatergic ligands (NAC, MPEP, LY369268, 2-PMPA) appear to be promising in preclinical animal models of drug addiction. In addition, several compounds (such as modafinil, disulfram, topiramate) were initially found to be effective in humans with unknown mechanisms, while subsequent preclinical studies helped to uncover the mechanisms of the actions. Although many compounds are currently or at some point were, under clinical trials, most of them have been used to evaluate their safety and efficacy for other neuropsychiatric diseases such schizophrenia, anxiety, obesity or smoking, rather than for cocaine addiction. Clearly, more translational studies from preclinical research to human clinical trials are required to promote the medication discovery for the treatment of cocaine dependence.

8. Acknowledgements

This research was supported by the NIDA/IRP, National Institutes of Health. I thank Jennifer Bossert and Tomas Keck of the NIDA/IRP for their proof-reading of on this manuscript.

9. References

Achat-Mendes C, Anderson KL, Itzhak Y. Impairment in consolidation of learned place preference following dopaminergic neurotoxicity in mice is ameliorated by N-acetylcysteine but not D1 and D2 dopamine receptor agonists. Neuropsychopharmacology 2007; 32: 531-41.

Amen SL, Piacentine LB, Ahmad ME, et al., Repeated N-acetyl cysteine reduces cocaine seeking in rodents and craving in cocaine-dependent humans. Neuropsychopharmacology 2010; 36:871-8.

Anand P, Whiteside G, Fowler CJ, Hohmann AG. Targeting CB2 receptors and the endocannabinoid system for the treatment of pain. Brain Res Rev. 2009; 60:255-66.

Anderson AL, Reid MS, Li SH, et al. Modafinil for the treatment of cocaine dependence. Drug Alcohol Depend. 2009; 104:133-9.

Aracil-Fernández A, Trigo JM, García-Gutiérrez MS, et al.,. Decreased cocaine motor sensitization and self-administration in mice overexpressing cannabinoid CB(2) receptors. Neuropsychopharmacology. 2012 37:1749-63.

Arnold JC. The role of endocannabinoid transmission in cocaine addiction. Pharmacol Biochem Behav 2005; 81: 396-406.

Arria, AM, Wish, ED. Nonmedical use of prescription stimulants among students. Pediatric Annals 2006; 35: 565–571.

Austin NE, Baldwin SJ, Cutler L, et al. Pharmacokinetics of the novel, high-affinity and selective dopamine D3 receptor antagonist SB-277011 in rat, dog and monkey: in vitro/in vivo correlation and the role of aldehyde oxidase. Xenobiotica 2001; 31: 677-86.

Backstrom P, Hyytia P. Ionotropic and metabotropic glutamate receptor antagonism attenuates cue-induced cocaine seeking. Neuropsychopharmacology 2006; 31: 778-86.

Bahi A, Fizia K, Dietz M, Gasparini F, Flor PJ. Pharmacological modulation of mGluR7 with AMN082 and MMPIP exerts specific influences on alcohol consumption and preference in rats. Addict Biol. 2012; 17:235-47.

Baker DA, McFarland K, Lake RW, Shen H, Tang XC, Toda S, Kalivas PW. Neuroadaptations in cystine-glutamate exchange underlie cocaine relapse. Nat Neurosci 2003; 6: 743-49.

Baker, JR, Jatlow, P, McCance-Katz, EF. Disulfiram effects on responses to intravenous cocaine administration. Drug and Alcohol Dependence 2006; 87: 202–209

Ballon JS, Feifel D. A systematic review of modafinil: Potential clinical uses and mechanisms of action. J Clin Psychiatry 2006; 67:554-566.

Baptista MA, Martin-Fardon R, Weiss F. Preferential effects of the metabotropic glutamate 2/3 receptor agonist LY379268 on conditioned reinstatement versus primary reinforcement: comparison between cocaine and a potent conventional reinforcer. J Neurosci 2004; 24: 4723-7.

Barth KS, Malcolm RJ. Disulfiram: an old therapeutic with new applications. CNS Neurol Disord Drug Targets 2010; 9:5-12

Baumann MH, Char GU, de Costa BR, Rice KC, Rothman RB. GBR 12909 attenuates cocaine-induced activation of mesolimbic dopamine neurons in the rat. J Pharmacol Exp Ther 1994; 271: 1216-22.

Beardsley PM, Thomas BF. Current evidence supporting a role of cannabinoid CB1 receptor (CB1R) antagonists as potential pharmacotherapies for drug abuse disorders. Behav Pharmacol 2005; 16: 275-96.

Beaulieu JM, Gainetdinov RR. The physiology, signaling, and pharmacology of dopamine receptors. Pharmacol Rev. 2011; 63:182-217.

Beltramo M. Cannabinoid type 2 receptor as a target for chronic - pain. Mini Rev Med Chem. 2009; 9:11-25.

Bennett BD, Bolam JP. Synaptic input and output of parvalbumin-immunoreactive neurons in the neostriatum of the rat. Neuroscience 1994; 62:707-19.

Berger SP, Winhusen TM, Somoza EC, et al. A medication screening trial evaluation of reserpine, gabapentin and lamotrigine pharmacotherapy of cocaine dependence. Addiction 2005; 100 (Suppl 1): 58-67.

Berger UV, Luthi-Carter R, Passani LA, Elkabes S, Black I, Konradi C, Coyle JT. Glutamate carboxypeptidase II is expressed by astrocytes in the adult rat nervous system. J Comp Neurol 1999; 415: 52-64.

Bisaga A, Aharonovich E, Garawi F, Levin FR, Rubin E, Raby WN, Nunes EV. A randomized placebo-controlled trial of gabapentin for cocaine dependence. Drug Alcohol Depend 2006; 81: 267-74.

Bowers MS, Chen BT, Bonci A. AMPA receptor synaptic plasticity induced by psychostimulants: the past, present, and therapeutic future. Neuron. 2010;67:11-24.

Brebner K, Phelan R, Roberts DC. Effect of baclofen on cocaine self-administration in rats reinforced under fixed-ratio 1 and progressive-ratio schedules. Psychopharmacology 2000; 148: 314-21.

Brodie JD, Case BG, Figueroa E, et al., Randomized, double-blind, placebo-controlled trial of vigabatrin for the treatment of cocaine dependence in Mexican parolees. Am J Psychiatry 2009; 166:1269-77.

Brodie JD, Figueroa E, Dewey SL. Treating cocaine addiction: from preclinical to clinical trial experience with γ-vinyl GABA. Synapse 2003; 50: 261-5.

Brodie JD, Figueroa E, Laska EM, Dewey SL. Safety and efficacy of γ-vinyl GABA (GVG) for the treatment of methamphetamine and/or cocaine addiction. Synapse 2005; 55: 122-5.

Caille S, Alvarez-Jaimes L, et al. Specific alterations of extracellular endocannabinoid levels in the nucleus accumbens by ethanol, heroin, and cocaine self-administration. J Neurosci 2007; 27: 3695-702.

Cameron DL, Williams JT. Cocaine inhibits GABA release in the VTA through endogenous 5-HT. J Neurosci 1994; 14: 6763-7.

Campbell UC, Lac ST, Carroll ME. Effects of baclofen on maintenance and reinstatement of intravenous cocaine self-administration in rats. Psychopharmacology 1999; 143: 209-14.

Carroll FI, Howard JL, Howell LL, Fox BS, Kuhar MJ. Development of the dopamine transporter selective RTI-336 as a pharmacotherapy for cocaine abuse. AAPS J 2006; 8:E196-203.

Carroll, KM, Fenton, LR, Ball, SA, et al. Efficacy of disulfiram and cognitive behavior therapy in cocaine-dependent outpatients: a randomized placebo-controlled trial. Arch Gen Psychiatry 2004; 61: 264–272.

Carroll, KM, Nich, C, Ball, SA, et al. One-year follow-up of disulfiram and psychotherapy for cocaine-alcohol users: sustained effects of treatment. Addiction 2000; 95: 1335–1349.

Carroll, KM, Nich, C, Ball, SA, McCance, E, Rounsavile, BJ. Treatment of cocaine and alcohol dependence with psychotherapy and disulfiram. Addiction 1998; 93: 713–727.

Cartmell J, Schoepp DD. Regulation of neurotransmitter release by metabotropic glutamate receptors. J Neurochem 2000; 75: 889-907.

Centonze D, Battista N, Rossi S, et al. A critical interaction between dopamine D2 receptors and endocannabinoids mediates the effects of cocaine on striatal GABAergic transmission. Neuropsychopharmacology 2004; 29: 1488-97.

Centonze D, Picconi B, Baunez C. Cocaine and amphetamine depress striatal GABAergic synaptic transmission through D2 dopamine receptors. Neuropsychopharmacology 2002; 26: 164-75.

Cheer JF, Wassum KM, Sombers LA, et al. Phasic dopamine release evoked by abused substances requires cannabinoid receptor activation. J Neurosci 2007; 27: 791-5.

Chen J, Paredes W, Li J, Smith D, Lowinson J, Gardner EL. Δ9-Tetrahydrocannabinol produces naloxone-blockable enhancement of presynaptic basal dopamine efflux in nucleus accumbens of conscious, freely-moving rats as measured by intracerebral microdialysis. Psychopharmacology 1990; 102: 156-62.

Chiamulera C, Epping-Jordan MP, Zocchi A, et al. Reinforcing and locomotor stimulant effects of cocaine are absent in mGluR5 null mutant mice. Nat Neurosci 2001; 4: 873-4.

Chu H, Jin G, Friedman E, Zhen X. Recent development in studies of tetrahydroprotoberberines: mechanism in antinociception and drug addiction. Cell Mol Neurobiol. 2008; 28:491-9.

Cleva RM, Watterson LR, Johnson MA, Olive MF. Differential Modulation of Thresholds for Intracranial Self-Stimulation by mGlu5 Positive and Negative Allosteric Modulators: Implications for Effects on Drug Self-Administration. Front Pharmacol. 2012; 2:93.

Collins, SL, Levin, FR, Foltin, RW, et al. Response to cocaine, alone and in combination with methylphenidate, in cocaine abusers with ADHD. Drug and Alcohol Dependence 2006; 82: 158–167.

Corbille AG, Valjent E, Marsicano G, et al. Role of cannabinoid type 1 receptors in locomotor activity and striatal signaling in response to psychostimulants. J Neurosci 2007; 27: 6937-47.

Cubells JF. Topiramate for cocaine dependence. Curr Psychiatry Rep 2006; 8: 130-1.

Czoty PW, Martelle JL, Carroll FI, Nader MA. Lower reinforcing strength of the phenyltropane cocaine analogs RTI-336 and RTI-177 compared to cocaine in nonhuman primates. Pharmacol Biochem Behav. 2010; 96:274-8.

Czuczwar SJ, Patsalos PN. The new generation of GABA enhancers. Potential in the treatment of epilepsy. CNS Drugs. 2001; 15:339-50.

Dackis CA, Kampman KM, Lynch KG, Pettinati HM, O'Brien CP. A double-blind, placebo-controlled trial of modafinil for cocaine dependence. Neuropsychopharmacology 2005; 30:205-211.

Dackis CA, Lynch KG, Yu E, et al. Modafinil and cocaine: a double-blind, placebo-controlled drug interaction study. Drug Alcohol Depend 2003; 70:29-37.

Day M, Bain E, Marek G, Saltarelli M, Fox GB. D3 receptor target engagement in humans with ABT-925 using [11C](+)-PHNO PET. Int J Neuropsychopharmacol. 2010; 13:291-2.

De La Garza R 2nd, Zorick T, Heinzerling KG, et al. The cardiovascular and subjective effects of methamphetamine combined with gamma-vinyl-gamma-aminobutyric acid (GVG) in non-treatment seeking methamphetamine-dependent volunteers. Pharmacol Biochem Behav. 2009; 94:186-93.

De Vries TJ, Shaham Y, Homberg JR, et al. A cannabinoid mechanism in relapse to cocaine seeking. Nat Med 2001; 7: 1151-4.

Deroche-Gamonet V, Darnaudéry M, Bruins-Slot L, et al. Study of the addictive potential of modafinil in naive and cocaine-experienced rats. Psychopharmacology 2002; 161:387-395.

Devoto P, Flore G, Saba P, Cadeddu R, Gessa GL. Disulfiram stimulates dopamine release from noradrenergic terminals and potentiates cocaine-induced dopamine release in the prefrontal cortex. Psychopharmacology 2012; 219(4):1153-64.

Dewey SL, Morgan AE, Ashby CR Jr, et al. Brodie JD. A novel strategy for the treatment of cocaine addiction. Synapse 1998; 30: 119-29.

Di Ciano P, Everitt BJ. The GABA(B) receptor agonist baclofen attenuates cocaine- and heroin-seeking behavior by rats. Neuropsychopharmacology 2003a; 28: 510-8.

Dodds CM, O'Neill B, Beaver J, et al. Effect of the dopamine D(3) receptor antagonist GSK598809 on brain responses to rewarding food images in overweight and obese binge eaters. Appetite. 2012 Mar 21. [Epub ahead of print]

Eriksson IS, Allard P, Marcusson J. [3H]tiagabine binding to GABA uptake sites in human brain. Brain Res 1999; 851:183-8.

Fadda P, Scherma M, Fresu A, Collu M, Fratta W. Baclofen antagonizes nicotine-, cocaine-, and morphine-induced dopamine release in the nucleus accumbens of rat. Synapse 2003; 50:1-6.

Fechtner RD, Khouri AS, Figueroa E, et al. Short-term treatment of cocaine and/or methamphetamine abuse with vigabatrin: ocular safety pilot results. Arch Ophthalmol. 2006; 124:1257-62.

Fernández-Ruiz J, Hernández M, Ramos JA. Cannabinoid-dopamine interaction in the pathophysiology and treatment of CNS disorders. CNS Neurosci Ther. 2010; 16:e72-91.

Ferraro L, Antonelli T, O'Connor WT, et al. Modafinil: an antinarcoleptic drug with a different neurochemical profile to d-amphetamine and dopamine uptake blockers. Biol Psychiatry 1997; 42:1181–1183.

Figueroa-Guzman Y, Mueller C, Vranjkovic O, et al. Oral administration of levo-tetrahydropalmatine attenuates reinstatement of extinguished cocaine seeking by cocaine, stress or drug-associated cues in rats. Drug Alcohol Depend 2011; 116:72-9.

Filip M, Frankowska M, Golda A, et al. Various GABA-mimetic drugs differently affect cocaine-evoked hyperlocomotion and sensitization. Eur J Pharmacol 2006; 541: 163-70.

Filip M, Frankowska M, Zaniewska M, et al. Diverse effects of GABA-mimetic drugs on cocaine-evoked self-administration and discriminative stimulus effects in rats. Psychopharmacology 2007; 192: 17-26.

Friedmann CTH, Davis LJ, Ciccone PE, and Rubin RT. Phase II double blind controlled study of a new anxiolytic, fenobam (McN-3377) vs placebo. Curr Ther Res 1980; 27: 144-151.

Froimowitz M, Gu Y, Dakin LA, et al. Slow-onset, long-duration, alkyl analogues of methylphenidate with enhanced selectivity for the dopamine transporter. J Med Chem. 2007; 50:219-32.

Froimowitz M, Wu KM, Moussa A, et al. Slow-onset, long-duration 3-(3',4'-dichlorophenyl)-1-indanamine monoamine reuptake blockers as potential medications to treat cocaine abuse. J Med Chem 2000; 43: 4981-92.

Fukami G, Hashimoto K, Koike K, et al. Effect of antioxidant N-acetyl-L-cysteine on behavioral changes and neurotoxicity in rats after administration of methamphetamine. Brain Res 2004; 1016: 90-5.

Galici R, Jones CK, Hemstapat K, et al. Biphenyl-indanone A, a positive allosteric modulator of the metabotropic glutamate receptor subtype 2, has antipsychotic- and anxiolytic-like effects in mice. J Pharmacol Exp Ther 2006; 318:173-85.

Garcia-Ladona FJ, Cox BF. BP 897, a selective dopamine D3 receptor ligand with therapeutic potential for the treatment of cocaine-addiction. CNS Drug Rev 2003; 9: 141-58.

Gasparini F, Lingenhöhl K, Stoehr N, , et al. 2-Methyl-6-(phenylethynyl)-pyridine (MPEP), a potent, selective and systemically active mGlu5 receptor antagonist. Neuropharmacology 1999; 38:1493-503.

Gee NS, Brown JP, Dissanayake VU, et al. The novel anticonvulsant drug, gabapentin (Neurontin), binds to the alpha2delta subunit of a calcium channel. J Biol Chem 1996; 271: 5768-76.

Geneste H, Amberg W, Backfisch G, et al. (2006). Synthesis and SAR of highly potent and selective dopamine D3-receptor antagonists : variations on the 1H-pyrimidin-2-one theme. Bioorganic & Medicinal Chemistry Letters 2006; 16: 1934–1937.

George, TP, Chawarski, MC, Pakes, J, et al. Disulfiram versus placebo for cocaine dependence in buprenorphine-maintained subjects: a preliminary trial. Biological Psychiatry 2000; 47: 1080–1086.

Gilbert JG, Newman AH, Gardner EL, Ashby CR Jr, Heidbreder CA, Pak AC, Peng XQ, Xi ZX. Acute administration of SB-277011A, NGB 2904, or BP 897 inhibits cocaine cue-induced reinstatement of drug-seeking behavior in rats: role of dopamine D3 receptors. Synapse 2005; 57: 17-28.

Giuffrida A, Parsons LH, Kerr TM, et al. Dopamine activation of endogenous cannabinoid signaling in dorsal striatum. Nat Neurosci 1999; 2: 358-363.

Glowa JR, Fantegrossi WF, Lewis DB, et al. Sustained decrease in cocaine-maintained responding in rhesus monkeys with 1-[2-[bis(4-fluorophenyl)methyoxy]ethyl]-4-(3-hydroxy-3-phenylpropyl)piperazinyl decanoate, a long-acting ester derivative of GBR 12909. J Med Chem 1996; 39: 4689-91.

Glowa JR, Wojnicki FHE, Matecka D, et al. Effects of dopamine reuptake inhibitors on food- and cocaine-maintained responding: I. Dependence on unit dose of cocaine. Exp Clin Psychopharmacol 1995; 3: 219-31.

Gold LH, Balster RL. Evaluation of the cocaine-like discriminative stimulus effects and reinforcing effects of modafinil. Psychopharmacology 1996; 126:286-292.

Gong JP, Onaivi ES, Ishiguro H, Liu QR, Tagliaferro PA, Brusco A, Uhl GR. Cannabinoid CB2 receptors: immunohistochemical localization in rat brain. Brain Res. 2006;1071:10-23.

González G, Desai R, Sofuoglu M, et al. Clinical efficacy of gabapentin versus tiagabine for reducing cocaine use among cocaine dependent methadone-treated patients. Drug Alcohol Depend 2007; 87: 1-9.

González G, Sevarino K, Sofuoglu M, et al. Tiagabine increases cocaine-free urines in cocaine-dependent methadone-treated patients: results of a randomized pilot study. Addiction 2003; 98: 1625-32.

Gorelick DA, Gardner EL, Xi ZX. Agents in development for the management of cocaine abuse. Drugs 2004, 64:1547-73.

Gossop M, Carroll KM. Disulfiram, cocaine, and alcohol: two outcomes for the price of one? Alcohol Alcohol 2006; 41: 119-20.

Graff-Guerrero A, Redden L, Abi-Saab W, et al. Blockade of [11C](+)-PHNO binding in human subjects by the dopamine D3 receptor antagonist ABT-925. Int J Neuropsychopharmacol. 2010; 13:273-87.

Grassi, MC, Cioce, AM, Giudici, FD, Antonilli, L, Nencini, P. Short-term efficacy of Disulfiram or Naltrexone in reducing positive urinalysis for both cocaine and cocaethylene in cocaine abusers: a pilot study. Pharmacology Research 2007; 55: 117–121.

Groenewegen HJ, Wright CI, Beijer AV. The nucleus accumbens: gateway for limbic structures to reach the motor system? Prog Brain Res 1996; 107: 485-511.

Gründer G. Cariprazine, an orally active D2/D3 receptor antagonist, for the potential treatment of schizophrenia, bipolar mania and depression. Curr Opin Investig Drugs. 2010; 11:823-32.

Haile CN, During MJ, Jatlow PI, Kosten TR, Kosten TA. Disulfiram facilitates the development and expression of locomotor sensitization to cocaine in rats. Biol Psychiatry. 2003; 54:915-21.

Haile CN, Zhang XY, Carroll FI, Kosten TA. Cocaine self-administration and locomotor activity are altered in Lewis and F344 inbred rats by RTI 336, a 3-phenyltropane analog that binds to the dopamine transporter. Brain Res 2005; 1055:186-195.

Haney M, Hart C, Collins ED, Foltin RW. Smoked cocaine discrimination in humans: effects of gabapentin. Drug Alcohol Depend 2005; 80: 53-61.

Haney M, Hart CL, Foltin RW. Effects of baclofen on cocaine self-administration: opioid- and nonopioid-dependent volunteers. Neuropsychopharmacology 2006; 31: 1814-21.

Hart C, Jatlow P, Sevarino K, Cance-Katz E. Comparison of intravenous cocaethylene and cocaine in humans. . Psychopharmacology 2000; 149: 153-62.

Hart CL, Haney M, Collins ED, Rubin E, Foltin RW. Smoked cocaine self-administration by humans is not reduced by large gabapentin maintenance doses. Drug Alcohol Depend 2007; 86: 274-7.

Hart CL, Haney M, Vosburg SK, Rubin E, Foltin RW. Smoked cocaine self-administration is decreased by modafinil. Neuropsychopharmacology 2008; 33:761-768.

Hart CL, Ward AS, Collins ED, Haney M, Foltin RW. Gabapentin maintenance decreases smoked cocaine-related subjective effects, but not self-administration by humans. Drug Alcohol Depend 2004; 73: 279-87.

Heidbreder CA, Gardner EL, Xi ZX, et al. The role of central dopamine D3 receptors in drug addiction: a review of pharmacological evidence. Brain Res Rev 2005; 49: 77-105.

Heidbreder CA, Newman AH. Current perspectives on selective dopamine D(3) receptor antagonists as pharmacotherapeutics for addictions and related disorders. Ann N Y Acad Sci. 2010; 1187:4-34.

Herzig V, Schmidt WJ. Effects of MPEP on locomotion, sensitization and conditioned reward induced by cocaine or morphine. Neuropharmacology 2004; 47: 973-84.

Higgins, ST, Budney, AJ, Bickel, WK, Hughes, JR, Foerg, F. Disulfiram therapy in patients abusing cocaine and alcohol. American Journal of Psychiatry 1993; 150: 675–676.

Hiranita T, Soto PL, Kohut SJ, et al. Decreases in Cocaine Self Administration with Dual Inhibition of Dopamine Transporter and {sigma} Receptors. J Pharmacol Exp Ther 2011; 339:662-77.

Hiranita T, Soto PL, Newman AH, Katz JL. Assessment of reinforcing effects of benztropine analogs and their effects on cocaine self-administration in rats: comparisons with monoamine uptake inhibitors. J Pharmacol Exp Ther 2009; 329:677-86.

Howell LL, Carroll FI, Votaw JR, Goodman MM, Kimmel HL. Effects of combined dopamine and serotonin transporter inhibitors on cocaine self-administration in rhesus monkeys. J Pharmacol Exp Ther 2007; 320:757-765.

Howell LL, Kimmel HL. Monoamine transporters and psychostimulant addiction. Biochem Pharmacol 2008; 75: 196-217.

Howell LL, Wilcox KM. The dopamine transporter and cocaine medication development: drug self-administration in nonhuman primates. J Pharmacol Exp Ther 2001; 298: 1-6.

Hu G, Duffy P, Swanson C, Ghasemzadeh MB, Kalivas PW. The regulation of dopamine transmission by metabotropic glutamate receptors. J Pharmacol Exp Ther 1999; 289: 412-6.

Hu Y, Qiu Y, Zhong Y, He H. Therapeutic effects of rotundine combined with methadone in treatment of heroin dependence. Chinese Journal of Drug Abuse Prevention and Treatment. 2006; 12:270-271.

Itzhak Y, Martin JL. Effect of riluzole and gabapentin on cocaine- and methamphetamine-induced behavioral sensitization in mice. Psychopharmacology 2000; 151: 226-233.

Jin G-Z. (-)-Tetrahydropalmatine and its analogues as new dopamine receptor antagonists. Trends Pharmacol Sci 1987; 8: 81–82.

Jin X, Semenova S, Yang L, Ardecky R, et al. The mGluR2 positive allosteric modulator BINA decreases cocaine self-administration and cue-induced cocaine-seeking and counteracts cocaine-induced enhancement of brain reward function in rats. Neuropsychopharmacology 2010; 35:2021-36.

Johnson BA. Recent advances in the development of treatments for alcohol and cocaine dependence: focus on topiramate and other modulators of GABA or glutamate function. CNS Drugs 2005; 19: 873-96.

Johnson MP, Baez M, Jagdmann Jr GE, et al. Discovery of allosteric potentiators for the metabotropic glutamate 2 receptor: synthesis and subtype selectivity of N-(4-(2-methoxyphenoxy)phenyl)-N-(2,2,2-trifluoroethylsulfonyl)pyrid-3-ylmethylamine. J Med Chem 2003; 46: 3189–3192.

Kahn R, Biswas K, Childress AR, Shoptaw S, Fudala PJ, Gorgon L, et al. Multi-center trial of baclofen for abstinence initiation in severe cocaine-dependent individuals. Drug Alcohol Depend 2009; 103:59-64.

Kalivas PW. The glutamate homeostasis hypothesis of addiction. Nat Rev Neurosci. 2009; 10:561-72.

Kampman KM, Pettinati H, Lynch KG, et al. A pilot trial of topiramate for the treatment of cocaine dependence. Drug Alcohol Depend 2004; 75: 233-240.

Kelley AE, Lang CG. Effects of GBR 12909, a selective dopamine uptake inhibitor, on motor activity and operant behavior in the rat. Eur J Pharmacol 1989; 167: 385-95.

Kenny PJ, Boutrel B, Gasparini F, Koob GF, Markou A. Metabotropic glutamate 5 receptor blockade may attenuate cocaine self-administration by decreasing brain reward function in rats. Psychopharmacology 2005; 179: 247-54.

Kimmel HL, O'Connor JA, Carroll FI, Howell LL Faster onset and dopamine transporter selectivity predict stimulant and reinforcing effects of cocaine analogs in squirrel monkeys. Pharmacol Biochem Behav 2007; 86:45-54.

Kiss B, Horváth A, Némethy Z, Schmidt E, Laszlovszky I, et al. Cariprazine (RGH-188), a dopamine D(3) receptor-preferring, D(3)/D(2) dopamine receptor antagonist-partial agonist antipsychotic candidate: in vitro and neurochemical profile. J Pharmacol Exp Ther. 2010; 333:328-40.

Krishnamurthy M, Li W, Moore BM 2nd. Synthesis, biological evaluation, and structural studies on N1 and C5 substituted cycloalkyl analogues of the pyrazole class of CB1 and CB2 ligands. Bioorg Med Chem 2004; 12: 393-404.

Kruszewski SP. Euphorigenic and abusive properties of modafinil. Am J Psychiatry. 2006; 163:549.

Kumaresan V, Yuan M, Yee J, Famous KR, et al. Metabotropic glutamate receptor 5 (mGluR5) antagonists attenuate cocaine priming- and cue-induced reinstatement of cocaine seeking. Behav Brain Res. 2009; 202:238-44.

Lapierre YD and Oyewumi LK. Fenobam: another anxiolytic? Curr Ther Res 1982; 31: 95-101.

LaRowe SD, Mardikian P, Malcolm R, et al. Safety and tolerability of N-acetylcysteine in cocaine-dependent individuals. Am J Addict 2006; 15: 105-10.

LaRowe SD, Myrick H, Hedden S, et al. Is cocaine desire reduced by N-acetylcysteine? Am J Psychiatry 2007; 164: 1115-7.

Le Foll B, Goldberg SR, Sokoloff P. The dopamine D3 receptor and drug dependence: effects on reward or beyond? Neuropharmacology 2005; 49: 525-41.

Lea PM 4th, Faden AI. Metabotropic glutamate receptor subtype 5 antagonists MPEP and MTEP. CNS Drug Rev 2006; 12: 149-66.

Lee B, Platt DM, Rowlett JK, Adewale AS, Spealman RD. Attenuation of behavioral effects of cocaine by the Metabotropic Glutamate Receptor 5 Antagonist 2-Methyl-6-(phenylethynyl)-pyridine in squirrel monkeys: comparison with dizocilpine. J Pharmacol Exp Ther 2005; 312: 1232-40.

Leonard BE, McCartan D, White J, King DJ. Methylphenidate: a review of its neuropharmacological, neuropsychological and adverse clinical effects. Hum Psychopharmacol. 2004; 19:151-80.

Levin, FR, Evans, SM, Brooks, DJ, Garawi, F. Treatment of cocaine dependent treatment seekers with adult ADHD: double-blind comparison of methylphenidate and placebo. Drug and Alcohol Dependence 2007; 87: 20–29.

Li X, Gardner EL, Xi ZX. The metabotropic glutamate receptor 7 (mGluR7) allosteric agonist AMN082 modulates nucleus accumbens GABA and glutamate, but not dopamine, in rats. Neuropharmacology 2008; 54: 542-551.

Li X, Li J, Gardner EL, Xi ZX. Activation of mGluR7s inhibits cocaine-induced reinstatement of drug-seeking behavior by a nucleus accumbens glutamate-mGluR2/3 mechanism in rats. J Neurochem 2010; 114:1368-1380.

Li X, Li J, Peng XQ, Spiller K, Gardner EL, Xi ZX. Metabotropic glutamate receptor 7 modulates the rewarding effects of cocaine in rats: involvement of a ventral pallidal GABAergic mechanism. Neuropsychopharmacology 2009; 34:1783-1796.

Li X, Xi ZX, Markou A. Metabotropic glutamate receptor 7 (mGluR7): A new target in medication development for treatment of cocaine addiction. Neuropharmacology, 2012, Apr 21. [Epub ahead of print].

Lile JA, Stoops WW, Glaser PE, Hays LR, Rush CR. Acute administration of the GABA reuptake inhibitor tiagabine does not alter the effects of oral cocaine in humans. Drug Alcohol Depend 2004; 76: 81-91.

Ling W, Shoptaw S, Majewska D. Baclofen as a cocaine anti-craving medication: a preliminary clinical study. Neuropsychopharmacology 1998; 18: 403-4.

Lu L, Uejima JL, Gray SM, Bossert JM, Shaham Y. Systemic and central amygdala injections of the mGluR(2/3) agonist LY379268 attenuate the expression of incubation of cocaine craving. Biol Psychiatry 2007; 61: 591-8.

Luo J-Y, Ren Y-H, Zhu R, Lin D-Q, Zheng J-W. The effect of l-tetrahydropalmatine on cocaine induced conditioned place preference, Chin J Drug Depend 2003; 12: 177-9.

Lupica CR, Riegel AC, Hoffman AF. Marijuana and cannabinoid regulation of brain reward circuits. Br J Pharmacol 2004; 143:227-34.

Madayag A, Lobner D, Kau KS, Mantsch JR, et al. Repeated N-acetylcysteine administration alters plasticity-dependent effects of cocaine. J Neurosci. 2007; 27:13968-76.

Madras BK, Xie Z, Lin Z, Jassen A, Panas H, et al. Modafinil occupies dopamine and norepinephrine transporters in vivo and modulates the transporters and trace amine activity in vitro. J Pharmacol Exp Ther 2006; 319:561-569.

Makoff A, Pilling C, Harrington K, Emson P. Human metabotropic glutamate receptor type 7: molecular cloning and mRNA distribution in the CNS. Mol Brain Re. 1996; 40: 165-70.

Malcolm R, Olive MF, Lechner W. The safety of disulfiram for the treatment of alcohol and cocaine dependence in randomized clinical trials: guidance for clinical practice. Expert Opin Drug Saf 2008; 7: 459-72.

Maldonado R, Berrendero F, Ozaita A, Robledo P. Neurochemical basis of cannabis addiction. Neuroscience. 2011; 181:1-17.

Mantsch JR, Li SJ, Risinger R, et al. Levo-tetrahydropalmatine attenuates cocaine self-administration and cocaine-induced reinstatement in rats. Psychopharmacology 2007; 192: 581-91.

Mantsch JR, Wisniewski S, Vranjkovic O, et al. Levo-tetrahydropalmatine attenuates cocaine self-administration under a progressive-ratio schedule and cocaine discrimination in rats. Pharmacol Biochem Behav. 2010; 97:310-6.

Mardikian PN, LaRowe SD, Hedden S, et al. An open-label trial of N-acetylcysteine for the treatment of cocaine dependence: a pilot study. Prog Neuropsychopharmacol Biol Psychiatry 2007; 31: 389-94.

Marek GJ. Metabotropic glutamate 2/3 receptors as drug targets. Curr Opin Pharmacol 2004; 4: 18-22.

Marin JC, Goadsby PJ. Glutamatergic fine tuning with ADX-10059: a novel therapeutic approach for migraine? Expert Opin Investig Drugs. 2010; 19:555-61.

Martin-Fardon R, Weiss F. (-)-2-oxa-4-aminobicylco[3.1.0]hexane-4,6-dicarboxylic acid (LY379268) and 3-[(2-methyl-1,3-thiazol-4-yl)ethynyl]piperidine (MTEP) similarly attenuate stress-induced reinstatement of cocaine seeking. Addict Biol. 2012; 17:557-64.

Mattick RP, Breen C, Kimber J, Davoli M. Methadone maintenance therapy versus no opioid replacement therapy for opioid dependence. Cochrane Database Syst Rev 2009:CD002209.

McGeehan AJ, Janak PH, Olive MF. Effect of the mGluR5 antagonist 6-methyl-2-(phenylethynyl)pyridine (MPEP) on the acute locomotor stimulant properties of cocaine, D-amphetamine, and the dopamine reuptake inhibitor GBR12909 in mice. Psychopharmacology 2004; 174: 266-73.

McGeehan AJ, Olive MF. The mGluR5 antagonist MPEP reduces the conditioned rewarding effects of cocaine but not other drugs of abuse. Synapse 2003; 47: 240-2.

Mezler M, Geneste H, Gault L, Marek GJ. LY-2140023, a prodrug of the group II metabotropic glutamate receptor agonist LY-404039 for the potential treatment of schizophrenia. Curr Opin Investig Drugs 2010; 11:833-45.

Millan MJ, Brocco M. Cognitive impairment in schizophrenia: a review of developmental and genetic models, and pro-cognitive profile of the optimised D(3) > D(2) antagonist, S33138. Therapie. 2008; 63:187-229.

Millan MJ, Mannoury la Cour C, et al. S33138 [N-[4-[2-[(3aS,9bR)-8-cyano-1,3a,4,9b-tetrahydro[1]-benzopyrano[3,4-c]pyrrol-2(3H)-yl)-ethyl]phenylacetamide], a preferential dopamine D3 versus D2 receptor antagonist and potential antipsychotic agent: I. Receptor-binding profile and functional actions at G-protein-coupled receptors. J Pharmacol Exp Ther 2008; 324:587-99.

Minozzi S, Amato L, Davoli M, et al. Anticonvulsants for cocaine dependence. Cochrane Database Syst Rev. 2008; (2):CD006754.

Mitsukawa K, Yamamoto R, Ofner S, et al. A selective metabotropic glutamate receptor 7 agonist: activation of receptor signaling via an allosteric site modulates stress parameters in vivo. Proc Natl Acad Sci USA 2005; 102: 18712-7.

Montana MC, Cavallone LF, Stubbert KK, et al. The metabotropic glutamate receptor subtype 5 antagonist fenobam is analgesic and has improved in vivo selectivity compared with the prototypical antagonist 2-methyl-6-(phenylethynyl)-pyridine. J Pharmacol Exp Ther. 2009; 330:834-43.

Murillo-Rodríguez E, Haro R, Palomero-Rivero M, et al. Modafinil enhances extracellular levels of dopamine in the nucleus accumbens and increases wakefulness in rats. Behav Brain Res. 2007; 176:353–357.

Myrick H, Henderson S, Brady KT, Malcolm R. Gabapentin in the treatment of cocaine dependence: a case series. J Clin Psychiatry 2001; 62: 19-23.

Nathan PJ, O'Neill BV, Mogg K, et al. The effects of the dopamine D3 receptor antagonist GSK598809 on attentional bias to palatable food cues in overweight and obese subjects. Int J Neuropsychopharmacol. 2011; 12:1-13.

Neale JH, Bzdega T, Wroblewska B. N-Acetylaspartylglutamate: the most abundant peptide neurotransmitter in the mammalian central nervous system. J Neurochem 2000; 75: 443-52.

Neale JH, Olszewski RT, Zuo D, et al. Advances in understanding the peptide neurotransmitter NAAG and appearance of a new member of the NAAG neuropeptide family. J Neurochem. 2011; 118:490-8.

Newman AH, Grundt P, Nader MA. Dopamine D3 receptor partial agonists and antagonists as potential drug abuse therapeutic agents. J Med Chem 2005; 48: 3663-79.

Newman AH, Kulkarni S. Probes for the dopamine transporter: new leads toward a cocaine-abuse therapeutic--A focus on analogues of benztropine and rimcazole. Med Res Rev 2002; 22:429-464.

Nicola SM, Malenka RC. Dopamine depresses excitatory and inhibitory synaptic transmission by distinct mechanisms in the nucleus accumbens. J Neurosci 1997; 17: 5697-710.

O'Brien CP, Dackis CA, Kampman K. Does modafinil produce euphoria? Am J Psychiatry 2006; 163:1109.

Oliveto A, Poling J, Mancino MJ, et al. Randomized, double blind, placebo-controlled trial of disulfiram for the treatment of cocaine dependence in methadone-stabilized patients. Drug Alcohol Depend. 2011; 113:184-91.

Onaivi ES, Ishiguro H, Gong JP, et al. Functional expression of brain neuronal CB2 cannabinoid receptors are involved in the effects of drugs of abuse and in depression. Ann N Y Acad Sci. 2008; 1139:434-49.

Paterson NE, Markou A. The metabotropic glutamate receptor 5 antagonist MPEP decreased break points for nicotine, cocaine and food in rats. Psychopharmacology 2005; 179: 255-61.

Patil ST, Zhang L, Martenyi F, et al. Activation of mGlu2/3 receptors as a new approach to treat schizophrenia: a randomized Phase 2 clinical trial. Nat Med. 2007; 13:1102-7.

Pecknold JC, McClure DJ, and Appeltauer L. Fenobam in anxious outpatients. Curr Ther Res 1980; 27:119-123.

Pecknold JC, McClure DJ, Appeltauer L, Wrzesinski L, Allan T. Treatment of anxiety using fenobam (a nonbenzodiazepine) in a double-blind standard (diazepam) placebo-controlled study. J Clin Psychopharmacol. 1982; 2:129-33.

Peng XQ, Ashby CR, Jr., Spiller K, Li X, Li J, Thomasson N, Millan MJ, Mocaer E, Munoz C, Gardner EL, Xi ZX. The preferential dopamine D3 receptor antagonist S33138 inhibits cocaine reward and cocaine-triggered relapse to drug-seeking behavior in rats. Neuropharmacology 2009; 56:752-760.

Peng XQ, Gardner EL, Xi ZX. Gamma-vinyl GABA increases nonvesicular release of GABA and glutamate in the nucleus accumbens in rats via action on anion channels and GABA transporters. Psychopharmacology 2010a; 208:511-519.

Peng XQ, Li J, Gardner EL, Ashby CR, Jr., Thomas A, Wozniak K, Slusher BS, Xi ZX. Oral administration of the NAALADase inhibitor GPI-5693 attenuates cocaine-induced reinstatement of drug-seeking behavior in rats. Eur J Pharmacol 2010b; 627:156-161.

Peng XQ, Li X, Gilbert JG, Pak AC, Ashby CR, Jr., Brodie JD, Dewey SL, Gardner EL, Xi ZX. Gamma-vinyl GABA inhibits cocaine-triggered reinstatement of drug-seeking behavior in rats by a non-dopaminergic mechanism. Drug Alcohol Depend 2008a; 97:216-225.

Peng XQ, Li X, Li J, Ramachandran PV, Gagare PD, Pratihar D, Ashby CR, Jr., Gardner EL, Xi ZX (2008b) Effects of gabapentin on cocaine self-administration, cocaine-triggered relapse and cocaine-enhanced nucleus accumbens dopamine in rats. Drug Alcohol Depend 2008b; 97:207-215.

Peng XQ, Xi ZX, Li X, Spiller K, Li J, Chun L, Wu KM, Froimowitz M, Gardner EL. Is slow-onset long-acting monoamine transport blockade to cocaine as methadone is to heroin? Implication for anti-addiction medications. Neuropsychopharmacology 2010c; 35:2564-2578.

Peters J, Kalivas PW. The group II metabotropic glutamate receptor agonist, LY379268, inhibits both cocaine- and food-seeking behavior in rats. Psychopharmacology 2006; 186: 143-9.

Petrakis, IL, Carroll, KM, Nich, C, et al. Disulfiram treatment for cocaine dependence in methadone-maintained opioid addicts. Addiction 2000; 95: 219–228.

Pettinati HM, Kampman KM, Lynch KG, et al. A double blind, placebo-controlled trial that combines disulfiram and naltrexone for treating co-occurring cocaine and alcohol dependence. Addict Behav. 2008; 33:651-67.

Pilla M, Perachon S, Sautel F, et al. Selective inhibition of cocaine-seeking behaviour by a partial dopamine D3 receptor agonist. Nature 1999; 400:371-5.

Platt DM, Rowlett JK, Spealman RD. Behavioral effects of cocaine and dopaminergic strategies for preclinical medication development. Psychopharmacology 2002; 163: 265-82.

Porter RH, Jaeschke G, Spooren W, et al. Fenobam: a clinically validated nonbenzodiazepine anxiolytic is a potent, selective, and noncompetitive mGlu5 receptor antagonist with inverse agonist activity. J Pharmacol Exp Ther. 2005; 315:711-21.

Qu WM, Huang ZL, Xu XH, Matsumoto N, Urade Y. Dopaminergic D1 and D2 receptors are essential for the arousal effect of modafinil. J Neurosci. 2008; 28:8462–8469.

Raby WN, Coomaraswamy S. Gabapentin reduces cocaine use among addicts from a community clinic sample. J Clin Psychiatry 2004; 65: 84-86.

Reavill C, Taylor SG, Wood MD, et al. Pharmacological actions of a novel, high-affinity, and selective human dopamine D3 receptor antagonist, SB-277011-A. J Pharmacol Exp Ther 2000; 294: 1154-65.

Redden L, Rendenbach-Mueller B, Abi-Saab WM, et al. A double-blind, randomized, placebo-controlled study of the dopamine D_3 receptor antagonist ABT-925 in patients with acute schizophrenia. J Clin Psychopharmacol. 2011; 31:221-5.

Reis AD, Castro LA, Faria R, Laranjeira R. Craving decrease with topiramate in outpatient treatment for cocaine dependence: an open label trial. Rev Bras Psiquiatr 2008; 30: 132-5.

Remington G, Kapur S. SB-277011 GlaxoSmithKline. Curr Opin Investig Drugs 2001; 2:946-9.

Rinaldi-Carmona M, Barth F, Heaulme M, et al. SR141716A, a potent and selective antagonist of the brain cannabinoid receptor. FEBS Lett 1994; 350: 240-4.

Roberts DC, Andrews MM, Vickers GJ. Baclofen attenuates the reinforcing effects of cocaine in rats. Neuropsychopharmacology 1996; 15: 417-23.

Ross JT, Corrigall WA, Heidbreder CA, LeSage MG. Effects of the selective dopamine D3 receptor antagonist SB-277011A on the reinforcing effects of nicotine as measured by a progressive-ratio schedule in rats. Eur J Pharmacol. 2007; 559:173-9.

Rothman RB, Baumann MH, Prisinzano TE, Newman AH. Dopamine transport inhibitors based on GBR12909 and benztropine as potential medications to treat cocaine addiction. Biochem Pharmacol 2008; 75: 2-16.

Rothman RB, Baumann MH. Therapeutic potential of monoamine transporter substrates. Curr Top Med Chem 2006; 6:1845-1859.

Rothman RB, Blough BE, Baumann MH. Dual dopamine/serotonin releasers as potential medications for stimulant and alcohol addictions. AAPS J 2007; 9:E1-10.

Rothman RB, Mele A, Reid AA, et al. GBR 12909 antagonizes the ability of cocaine to elevate extracellular levels of dopamine. Pharmacol Biochem Behav 1991; 40: 387-97.

Runyon SP, Carroll FI. Dopamine transporter ligands: recent developments and therapeutic potential. Curr Top Med Chem 2006; 6:1825-1843.

Salling MC, Faccidomo S, Hodge CW. Nonselective suppression of operant ethanol and sucrose self-administration by the mGluR7 positive allosteric modulator AMN082. Pharmacol Biochem Behav 2008; 91(1):14-20.

Schousboe A, Madsen KK, White HS. GABA transport inhibitors and seizure protection: the past and future. Future Med Chem. 2011; 3:183-7.

Schramm-Sapyta NL, Olsen CM, Winder DG. Cocaine self-administration reduces excitatory responses in the mouse nucleus accumbens shell. Neuropsychopharmacology 2006; 31: 1444-51.

Schroeder JP, Cooper DA, Schank JR, et al. Disulfiram attenuates drug-primed reinstatement of cocaine seeking via inhibition of dopamine β-hydroxylase. Neuropsychopharmacology. 2010; 35:2440-9.

Schubiner H, Saules KK, Arfken CL, et al. Double-blind placebo-controlled trial of methylphenidate in the treatment of adult ADHD patients with comorbid cocaine dependence. Exp Clin Psychopharmacol. 2002; 10:286-94.

Schubiner H, Tzelepis A, Milberger S, Lockhart N, Kruger M, Kelley BJ, Schoener EP. Prevalence of attention-deficit/hyperactivity disorder and conduct disorder among substance abusers. J Clin Psychiatry 2000; 61:244-51.

Searle G, Beaver JD, Comley RA, et al. Imaging dopamine D3 receptors in the human brain with positron emission tomography, [11C]PHNO, and a selective D3 receptor antagonist. Biol Psychiatry 2010; 68:392-9.

Shippenberg TS, Rea W, Slusher BS. Modulation of behavioral sensitization to cocaine by NAALADase inhibition. Synapse 2000; 38: 161-6.

Shoptaw S, Yang X, Rotheram-Fuller EJ, et al. Randomized placebo-controlled trial of baclofen for cocaine dependence: preliminary effects for individuals with chronic patterns of cocaine use. J Clin Psychiatry 2003; 64: 1440-8.

Slattery DA, Markou A, Froestl W, Cryan JF. The GABAB receptor-positive modulator GS39783 and the GABAB receptor agonist baclofen attenuate the reward-facilitating effects of cocaine: intracranial self-stimulation studies in the rat. Neuropsychopharmacology 2005; 30: 2065-72.

Slusher BS, Thomas A, Paul M, Schad CA, Ashby CR Jr. Expression and acquisition of the conditioned place preference response to cocaine in rats is blocked by selective inhibitors of the enzyme N-acetylated-alpha-linked-acidic dipeptidase (NAALADASE). Synapse 2001; 41: 22-8.

Smith RJ, Aston-Jones G. Noradrenergic transmission in the extended amygdala: role in increased drug-seeking and relapse during protracted drug abstinence. Brain Struct Funct. 2008; 213:43-61.

Song R, Yang RF, Wu N, Su RB, Li J, Peng XQ, Li X, Gaál J, Xi ZX, Gardner EL. YQA14: a novel dopamine D(3) receptor antagonist that inhibits cocaine self-administration in rats and mice, but not in D(3) receptor-knockout mice. Addict Biol. 2012; 17:259-73.

Soria G, Mendizabal V, Tourino C, et al. Lack of CB1 cannabinoid receptor impairs cocaine self-administration. Neuropsychopharmacology 2005; 30: 1670-80.

Spiller K, Xi ZX, Peng XQ, et al. The putative dopamine D3 receptor antagonists SB-277011A, NGB 2904 or BP 897 inhibit methamphetamine-enhanced brain stimulation reward in rats. Psychopharmacology 2008; 196:533-542.

Suh JJ, Pettinati HM, Kampman KM, O'Brien CP. The status of disulfiram: a half of a century later. J Clin Psychopharmacol 2006; 26: 290-302.

Sulzer D (2011) How addictive drugs disrupt presynaptic dopamine neurotransmission. Neuron 69:628-649.

Tanda G and Goldberg SR. Cannabinoids: reward, dependence, and underlying neurochemical mechanisms - a review of recent preclinical data. Psychopharmacology 2003; 169: 115-134.

Tanda G, Pontieri FE, Di Chiara G. Cannabinoid and heroin activation of mesolimbic dopamine transmission by a common μ1 opioid receptor mechanism. Science 1997; 276: 2048-50.

Tang X-C, McFarland K, Cagle S, Kalivas PW. Cocaine-induced reinstatement requires endogenous stimulation of μ-opioid receptors in the ventral pallidum. J Neurosci 2005; 25: 4512-20.

Taylor CP, Gee NS, Su T-Z, et al. Summary of mechanistic hypotheses of gabapentin pharmacology. Epilepsy Res 1998; 29: 233-49.

te Beek ET, Zoethout RW, Bani MS, et al. Pharmacokinetics and central nervous system effects of the novel dopamine D3 receptor antagonist GSK598809 and intravenous alcohol infusion at pseudo-steady state. J Psychopharmacol. 2012 26:303-14.

Tella SR. Effects of monoamine reuptake inhibitors on cocaine self-administration in rats. Pharmacol Biochem Behav 1995; 51: 687-92.

Tessari M, Pilla M, Andreoli M, Hutcheson DM, Heidbreder CA. Antagonism at metabotropic glutamate 5 receptors inhibits nicotine- and cocaine-taking behaviours and prevents nicotine-triggered relapse to nicotine-seeking. Eur J Pharmacol. 2004; 499: 121-33.

Thanos PK, Michaelides M, Ho CW, et al. The effects of two highly selective dopamine D3 receptor antagonists (SB-277011A and NGB-2904) on food self-administration in a rodent model of obesity. Pharmacol Biochem Behav 2008; 89:499-507.

Thomasson-Perret N, Pénélaud PF, Théron D, Gouttefangeas S, Mocaër E. Markers of D(2) and D(3) receptor activity in vivo: PET scan and prolactin. Therapie 2008; 63:237-42

Uchimura N, North RA. Actions of cocaine on rat nucleus accumbens neurones in vitro. Br J Pharmacol 1990; 99: 736-40.

Umemiya M, Raymond LA. Dopaminergic modulation of excitatory postsynaptic currents in rat neostriatal neurons. J Neurophysiol 1997; 78: 1248-55.

van der Post JP, de Visser SJ, de Kam ML, et al. The central nervous system effects, pharmacokinetics and safety of the NAALADase-inhibitor GPI 5693. Br J Clin Pharmacol. 2005; 60:128-36.

Van Sickle MD, Duncan M, Kingsley PJ et al. Identification and functional characterization of brainstem cannabinoid CB2 receptors. Science 2005; 310:329-32.

Vocci FJ, Elkashef A. Pharmacotherapy and other treatments for cocaine abuse and dependence. Curr Opin Psychiatry 2005; 18: 265-70.

Volkow ND, Ding Y-S, Fowler JS, et al. Is methylphenidate like cocaine? Studies on their pharmacokinetics and distribution in the human brain. Arch Gen Psychiatry 1995; 52: 456-63

Volkow ND, Fowler JS, Logan J, et al. Effects of modafinil on dopamine and dopamine transporters in the male human brain: clinical implications. JAMA. 2009; 301:1148-54.

Volkow ND, Fowler JS, Wang G-J. Imaging studies on the role of dopamine in cocaine reinforcement and addiction in humans. J Psychopharmacol 1999; 13: 337-45.

Vorel SR, Ashby CR Jr, Paul M, et al. Dopamine D3 receptor antagonism inhibits cocaine-seeking and cocaine-enhanced brain reward in rats. J Neurosci 2002; 22: 9595-603.

Wang JB, Mantsch JR. L-tetrahydropalamatine: a potential new medication for the treatment of cocaine addiction. Future Med Chem. 2012; 4:177-86.

Wang X, Moussawi K, Knackstedt L, Shen H, Kalivas PW. Role of mGluR5 neurotransmission in reinstated cocaine-seeking. Addict Biol. 2012 Feb 17. [Epub ahead of print].

Weerts EM, Froestl W, Griffiths RR. Effects of GABAergic modulators on food and cocaine self-administration in baboons. Drug Alcohol Depend 2005; 80: 369-76.

Weerts EM, Froestl W, Kaminski BJ, Griffiths RR. Attenuation of cocaine-seeking by GABAB receptor agonists baclofen and CGP44532 but not the GABA reuptake inhibitor tiagabine in baboons. Drug Alcohol Depend 2007; 89: 206-13.

Weinshenker D. Cocaine sobers up. Nat Med. 2010; 16:969-70.

White FJ, Hu X-T, Henry DJ. Electrophysiological effects of cocaine in the rat nucleus accumbens: microiontophoretic studies. J Pharmacol Exp Ther 1993; 266: 1075-84.

White, BP, Becker-Blease, KA, Grace-Bishop, K. Stimulant medication use, misuse, and abuse in an undergraduate and graduate student sample. Journal of American College Health 2006; 54, 261–268.

Wicke K, Garcia-Ladona J. The dopamine D3 receptor partial agonist, BP-897, is an antagonist at human dopamine D3 receptors and at rat somatodendritic dopamine D3 receptors. Eur J Pharmacol 2001; 424: 85-90.

Williams E. Effects of alcohol on workers with carbon disulfide JAMA 1937; 109: 1472-3.

Winhusen T, Somoza E, Ciraulo DA, et al. A double-blind, placebo-controlled trial of tiagabine for the treatment of cocaine dependence. Drug Alcohol Depend 2007; 91:141-148.

Winhusen TM, Somoza EC, Harrer JM, et al. A placebo-controlled screening trial of tiagabine, sertraline and donepezil as cocaine dependence treatments. Addiction 2005; 100: 68-77.

Winhusen, T, Somoza, E, Singal, BM, Harrer, J, Apparaju, S, Mezinskis, J, Desai, P, Elkashef, A, Chiang, CN, Horn, P. Methylphenidate and cocaine: a placebo-controlled drug interaction study. Pharmacology, Biochemistry and Behavior 2006; 85: 29–38.

Wise MS, Arand DL, Auger RR, Brooks SN, Watson NF; American Academy of Sleep Medicine. Treatment of narcolepsy and other hypersomnias of central origin. Sleep 2007; 30:1712-1727.

Wise RA. Forebrain substrates of reward and motivation. J Comp Neurol 2005; 493: 115-21.

Wisor JP, Nishino S, Sora I, et al. Dopaminergic role in stimulant-induced wakefulness. J Neurosci. 2001; 21:1787-94.

Woolley ML, Pemberton DJ, Bate S, Corti C, Jones DN. The mGlu2 but not the mGlu3 receptor mediates the actions of the mGluR2/3 agonist, LY379268, in mouse models predictive of antipsychotic activity. Psychopharmacology 2008; 196: 431–440.

Xi Z-X, Baker DA, Shen H, Kalivas PW. Group II metabotropic glutamate receptors modulate glutamate release in the nucleus accumbens. J Pharmacol Exp Ther 2002a; 300: 162-72.

Xi ZX, Gardner EL. Hypothesis-driven medication discovery for the treatment of psychostimulant addiction. Curr Drug Abuse Rev 2008; 1:303-327.

Xi ZX, Gardner EL. Pharmacological actions of NGB 2904, a selective dopamine D3 receptor antagonist, in animal models of drug addiction. CNS Drug Reviews 2007; 13:240-259.

Xi Z-X, Gilbert J, Campos A, Ashby CR Jr, Gardner EL. The metabotropic glutamate receptor 5 antagonist MPEP blocks reinstatement of drug-seeking triggered by cocaine, but not by stress or cues. Abstract at the 66th Annual Meetings of the College on Problems of Drug Dependence, San Juan, Puerto Rico, June 2004a.

Xi Z-X, Gilbert J, Campos AC, Kline N, et al. Blockade of mesolimbic dopamine D3 receptors inhibits stress-induced reinstatement of cocaine-seeking in rats. Psychopharmacology 2004b; 176: 57-65.

Xi Z-X, Gilbert J, Campos AC, Peng X-Q, Ashby CR Jr, Gardner EL. The mGluR5 antagonist MPEP lowers the progressive-ratio break-point for cocaine self-administration, and inhibits reinstatement of drug-seeking triggered by cocaine but not by stress or cues. Abstract at the 34th Annual Meeting of the Society for Neuroscience, San Diego, CA, Oct 23-27, 2004c, Abstract# 691.9.

Xi Z-X, Gilbert JG, Pak AC, Ashby CR Jr, Heidbreder CA, Gardner EL. Selective dopamine D3 receptor antagonism by SB-277011A attenuates cocaine reinforcement as assessed by progressive-ratio and variable-cost--variable-payoff fixed-ratio cocaine self-administration in rats. Eur J Neurosci 2005; 21: 3427-38.

Xi Z-X, Gilbert JG, Peng XQ, Pak AC, Li X, Gardner EL. Cannabinoid CB1 receptor antagonist AM251 inhibits cocaine-primed relapse in rats: role of glutamate in the nucleus accumbens. J Neurosci 2006a; 26: 8531-6.

Xi ZX, Kiyatkin M, Li X, Peng XQ, Wiggins A, Spiller K, Li J, Gardner EL. N-acetylaspartylglutamate (NAAG) inhibits intravenous cocaine self-administration and cocaine-enhanced brain-stimulation reward in rats. Neuropharmacology 2010a; 58:304-313.

Xi ZX, Li X, Li J, Peng XQ, Froimowitz M, Gardner EL. CTDP 32,476: a low addictive slow-onset long-acting dopamine transporter inhibitor that may act as a methadone-like agonist therapy for cocaine addiction. Abstract, 41st Annual Meeting of the Society for Neuroscience, Washington D.C., Nov. 11-16, 2011a;

Xi ZX, Li X, Li J, Peng XQ, Song R, Gardner EL. Dopamine D3 receptors in the nucleus accumbens and central amygdala underlie incubation of cocaine craving in rats. Addiction Biology. 2012; in press.

Xi ZX, Li X, Peng XQ, Gardner EL. Potential use of slow-onset long-acting dopamine transporter inhibitors in the treatment of cocaine addiction. Chinese Journal Drug Depend 2009; 18:268-270.

Xi ZX, Li X, Peng XQ, Li J, Chun L, Gardner EL, Thomas AG, Slusher BS, Ashby CR, Jr. Inhibition of NAALADase by 2-PMPA attenuates cocaine-induced relapse in rats: a NAAG-mGluR2/3-mediated mechanism. J Neurochem 2010b; 112:564-576.

Xi Z-X, Newman AH, Gilbert JG, Pak AC, Peng X-Q, Ashby CR Jr, Gitajn L, Gardner EL. The novel dopamine D3 receptor antagonist NGB 2904 inhibits cocaine's rewarding effects and cocaine-induced reinstatement of drug-seeking behavior in rats. Neuropsychopharmacology 2006b; 31: 1393-405.

Xi ZX, Peng XQ, Li X, Song R, Zhang HY, Liu QR, Yang HJ, Bi GH, Li J, Gardner EL. Brain cannabinoid CB2 receptors modulate cocaine's actions in mice. Nat Neurosci 2011; 14:1160-1166.

Xi ZX, Shen H, Baker DA, Kalivas PW. Inhibition of non-vesicular glutamate release by group III metabotropic glutamate receptors in the nucleus accumbens. J Neurochem 2003b; 87:1204-12.

Xi ZX, Spiller K, Gardner EL. Mechanism-based medication development for the treatment of nicotine dependence. Acta Pharmacol Sin. 2009; 30:723-39.

Xi ZX, Spiller K, Pak AC, Gilbert J, Dillon C, Li X, Peng XQ, Gardner EL. Cannabinoid CB1 receptor antagonists attenuate cocaine's rewarding effects: Experiments with self-administration and brain-stimulation reward in rats. Neuropsychopharmacology 2008; 33:1735-45.

Xi ZX, Yang Z, Li SJ, Li X, Dillon C, Peng XQ, Spiller K, Gardner EL. Levo-tetrahydropalmatine inhibits cocaine's rewarding effects: experiments with self-administration and brain-stimulation reward in rats. Neuropharmacology 2007; 53:771-782.

Xi ZX. Preclinical Pharmacology, Efficacy and Safety of Varenicline in Smoking Cessation and Clinical Utility in High Risk Patients. Drug Health Patient Saf 2010: 39-48.

Yang Z, Shao YC, Li SJ, Qi JL, Zhang MJ, Hao W, Jin GZ. Medication of l-tetrahydropalmatine significantly ameliorates opiate craving and increases the abstinence rate in heroin users: a pilot study. Acta Pharmacol Sin. 2008; 29:781-8.

Yang HJ, Gardner EL, Xi ZX. Tiagabine inhibits cocaine taking, but not cocaine-seeking in rats. Neurosci Lett 2012, in press.

Yuan J, Chen X, Brodbeck R, et al. Highly selective dopamine D3 receptor antagonists. Bioorg Med Chem Lett 1998; 8: 2715-8.

Zerbib F, Bruley des Varannes S, et al. Randomised clinical trial: effects of monotherapy with ADX10059, a mGluR5 inhibitor, on symptoms and reflux events in patients with gastro-oesophageal reflux disease. Aliment Pharmacol Ther 2011; 33:911-21.

Zerbib F, Keywood C, Strabach G. Efficacy, tolerability and pharmacokinetics of a modified release formulation of ADX10059, a negative allosteric modulator of metabotropic glutamate receptor 5: an esophageal pH-impedance study in healthy subjects. Neurogastroenterol Motil 2010; 22: 859-6.

12

N-Acetylcysteine as a Treatment for Addiction

Jennifer E. Murray[1,2,*], Jérôme Lacoste[3] and David Belin[2,4]
[1]*Department of Experimental Psychology, University of Cambridge, Cambridge,*
[2]*INSERM European Associated Laboratory, Psychobiology of Compulsive Habits,*
[3]*Unité de Recherche Clinique Intersectorielle,*
Centre Hospitalier Henri-Laborit, Poitiers,
[4]*INSERM U1084 - LNEC & Université de Poitiers,*
AVENIR Team Psychobiology of Compulsive Disorders, Poitiers,
[1,2]*UK*
[2,3,4]*France*

1. Introduction

Drug addiction is a chronic relapsing disorder characterized by compulsive use despite negative consequences and relapses even after years of abstinence (Leshner, 1997). Criteria put forth by the American Psychiatric Association (2000) for diagnosing drug addiction require at least three of the following symptoms associated with drug use: tolerance; withdrawal; a loss of control over drug intake; unsuccessful attempts to reduce intake; a significant amount of time spent acquiring, using, or recovering from the substance; reduced interest in social or work activities; and continued use despite awareness of adverse physical and psychological consequences (American Psychiatric Association, 2000). In the United States, 22.5 million people, or 8.9% of the population meets the criteria for substance dependence or abuse (Substance Abuse and Mental Health Services Administration, 2010), and in Europe, drug, and especially cocaine, use has been increasing over the last ten years in the general population, with a more pronounced trend in young individuals (EMCDDA, 2009), suggesting that cocaine addiction may continue to spread in western countries. Worldwide estimates suggest more than 8% of the population have an alcohol use disorder and more than 2% have an illicit drug use disorder (World Health Organization, 2010).

The prevalence of drug use despite obvious health and financial consequences is a testament to the tenacity of addiction as a brain disease affecting cognition, motivation and memory (Leshner, 1997). At the psychobiological level, addiction has been hypothesised to reflect the development of loss of executive control over aberrant incentive habits (Belin et al., 2009a, Belin & Everitt, 2010), resulting from drug-induced neuroplasticity processes in vulnerable subjects. These plasticity processes have been suggested to stem from the impact of drug action on the mesolimbic dopamine system, through which drug use can induce a host of changes in the brain resulting in significant neural reorganization (see Lüscher & Malenka, 2011; Russo et al., 2010). Much of this reorganization is due to long term potentiation, or strengthening, of excitatory synapses as a result of drug use. As recently reviewed, the

* Corresponding Author

dopamine signals from neurons originating in the ventral tegmental area (VTA) targeting the nucleus accumbens (NAc) in the ventral striatum modulate glutamate synaptic plasticity and are believed to be critically involved in the pathophysiology of addiction (Chen et al., 2010).

In animal models using passive drug exposure, these neurons show an N-methyl-D-aspartate (NMDA) receptor-dependent strengthening of excitatory synapses (long term potentiation) 24 hrs following an acute experimenter-administered injection of cocaine, amphetamine, nicotine, ethanol, and morphine (Saal et al., 2003; Ungless et al., 2001). Interestingly, this strengthening was not found with the non-abused psychoactive drugs, fluoxetine or carbamazepine, suggesting the role this plasticity may play in determining whether a drug is abused or not.

Although of interest, these data capture neither the volitional aspect of drug use nor the instrumental nature of drug seeking and taking, thereby greatly limiting their translation to the pathophysiology of addiction (Belin et al., 2009b, Belin & Dalley, 2012). Therefore, in preclinical models, a more valid approach to the human drug administration situation is the self-administration paradigm in which - akin to the human experience - an animal, rather than the experimenter, voluntarily administers the drug through instrumental conditioning (see later).

Following two weeks of cocaine self-administration, long term potentiation of glutamate function in DAergic VTA neurons is maintained even after 90 days of abstinence - an effect not found in a yoked, non-contingent control group receiving the same cocaine exposure (Chen et al., 2008). Similarly, measurements in the core of the NAc (NAcC) - where VTA projections are now known to co-release glutamate along with DA (Stuber et al., 2010) - following at least two weeks of cocaine self-administration, showed long-lasting resistance to the induction of long-term synaptic depression compared to yoked controls or controls lever pressing for food reinforcement. Finally, cocaine self-administration followed by either a 3-week abstinence period or 3 weeks of extinction training induced a state of long-term potentiation of glutamate synapses that was resistant to further potentiation (Moussawi et al., 2009). The resistance to further potentiation has been attributed to the prolonged expression of AMPA receptors that had been trafficked to the cell membranes during the drug exposure (Chen et al., 2010) and is indicative of long-lasting neural reorganization brought about by drug abuse. Combined, these data indicate that volitional administration of cocaine results in prolonged changes in NMDA receptor-dependent synaptic plasticity within the nucleus accumbens (Martin et al., 2006).

This long-term strengthening of glutamatergic synapses within the brain reward circuitry as a result of chronic voluntary drug use is also related to dysregulation of glutamate homeostasis (for a review see Kalivas, 2009). Glutamate homeostasis refers to the balance between synaptic glutamate levels and extracellular, extrasynaptic glutamate levels that regulate stable neurotransmission (see Figure 1). If synaptic glutamate release is the key component of glutamate-induced excitatory synaptic transmission, extrasynaptic glutamate is vital for the negative feedback of glutamatergic transmission. This negative feedback is necessary for modulating and inhibiting further excitatory stimulation. Such feedback is supported by activation of extrasynaptically-localized Group II metabotropic glutamate autoreceptors (mGluR2/3 receptors) which results in a regulated reduction of vesicular neurotransmitter release whereby synaptic glutamate concentration is greatly decreased (Dietrich et al, 2002; Manzoni et al., 1997).

Extrasynaptic glutamate availability is primarily provided by the cystine/glutamate exchanger antiporter (system xc-) found on brain glial cell membranes (Baker et al., 2002). System xc- transports the extracellular cystine dimer into the astrocytes and intracellular glutamate out of the astrocytes and into the extracellular space in a 1:1 ratio, thereby enhancing extrasynaptic glutamate levels (Bannai, 1986). Glutamate availability inside the astrocytes is provided by the primary glial glutamate transporter, GLT-1 (Haugeto et al., 1996), and these two systems work in concert to maintain homeostatic glutamate levels. Seven days of cocaine exposure (experimenter administered 15-30 mg/kg daily) followed by three weeks of abstinence, or self-administration (0.25 mg/kg in 2-hr sessions until responding stabilized to <10% variation) followed by extinction (until active lever pressing declined to at least 10% of self-administration levels) decrease basal levels of extracellular glutamate by ~50% within the NAcC. Extracellular glutamate levels are then elevated again into a range between about 160-600% of the withdrawal baseline following cocaine re-exposure (e.g., Baker et al., 2003a; Baker et al., 2003b; McFarland et al., 2003; Pierce et al., 1996). This dysregulation of glutamate homeostasis as a result of drug withdrawal has been suggested to be caused by an overall downregulation of system xc- and is in fact mimicked by blocking system xc- in the NAc (Baker et al., 2003b). Indeed, following chronic cocaine or nicotine self-administration, there is reduced NAc expression of both xCT, the light chain and catalytic subunit of the system xc- antiporter heterodimers, and GLT-1 (Knackstedt et al., 2009; 2010a), indicating these mechanisms are involved in the dysregulation of glutamate homeostasis and may impact the development and trajectory of addiction.

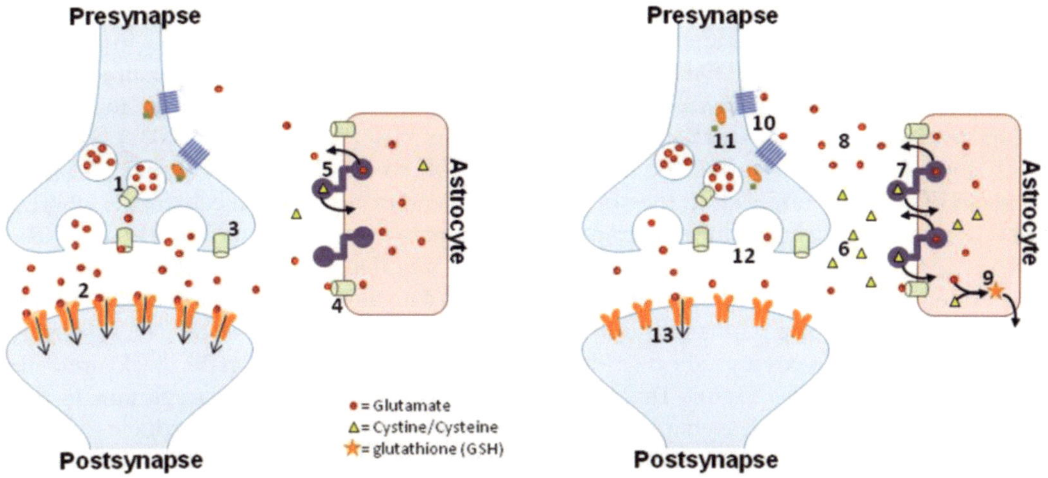

Fig. 1. Actions of N-acetylcysteine on the cystine/glutamate exchanger (system xc-). Glutamate is packaged into presynaptic vesicles by vesicular glutamate transporters (vGluTs) [1]. Following release of glutamate into the synaptic cleft, glutamate binds to postsynaptic localized ionotropic receptors (iGluRs) such as the α-amino-3-hydroxy-5-methylisoxazole-4 propionic acid (AMPA), N-methyl-D-aspartate (NMDA), and kainate receptors [2]. Excitatory amino acid transporters (EAATs) clear extracellular glutamate by taking it back up into cells. These transporters are localized on the presynaptic terminal [3] protecting extrasynaptic receptors from synaptic glutamate and synaptic receptors from extrasynaptic glutamate, and allow for re-packaging glutamate into vesicles. These transporters are also localized on astrocytes [4]. Once in the glial cell, glutamate can be transported into the extrasynaptic

environment by the cystine/glutamate exchanger (system xc-) in a 1:1 ratio [5]. Administration of NAC provides extra synaptic cysteine that is oxidized extracellularly into the cystine [6] required to enhance activation of the cystine/glutamate exchanger [7]. The enhanced xc- activation results in increased glutamate concentration in the extracellular space [8]. Intracellular cystine is rapidly reduced to cysteine where it is combined with intracellular glutamate (and glycine) in the synthesis of glutathione (GSH) which is then released from the astrocyte [9]. Extrasynaptic glutamate binds to and activates mGluR2/3 receptors [10] which negatively regulate adenylyl cyclase [11] thereby suppressing presynaptic glutamate release [12] and reducing postsynaptic iGluR activation [13].

2. Mechanisms of N-acetylcysteine action

The cysteine prodrug and antioxidant precursor, N-acetylcysteine (NAC), has been in use in humans for many years, primarily as a treatment for acetaminophen/paracetamol overdose (Prescott et al., 1977; Scalley & Conner, 1978) and more recently as a mucolytic agent effective in chronic obstructive pulmonary disease (Decramer & Janssens, 2010; Kory et al., 1968) and cystic fibrosis (Dauletbaev et al., 2009; Stamm & Docter, 1965). Further, an evaluation of the potential therapeutic use of NAC in a variety of psychiatric disorders has been recently reviewed (Dean et al., 2011). The aforementioned nature of the neurophysiological changes induced by drug use has also indicated a potential use for NAC treatment in addictions, prompting the initiation of thorough research into NAC as a treatment for addiction in both preclincal models of addiction and drug addicts

In preclinical models of addiction, NAC appears to regulate the systems involved in glutamate homeostasis in the brain. Following 7 days of cocaine exposure and 21 subsequent days of withdrawal, decreased basal extracellular glutamate levels in the NAc are recovered following an IP injection of NAC in rats (Baker et al., 2003a). Notably, inhibition of system xc- prevented the NAC-induced recovery of extracellular glutamate levels in this region, implicating the xc- system in the neurobiological mechanisms whereby NAC normalises cocaine-induced extracellular glutamate dysregulation (Baker et al., 2003a). Thus, NAC may induce a recovery of the downregulated xCT and GLT-1 function (Knackstedt et al., 2009; 2010a). Indeed, the recovery of an altered GLT-1 function allows for increased transport of glutamate into the astrocyte while the recovery of altered system xc- function by xCT recovery allows for increased export of glutamate back into the extrasynaptic space (see Figure 1). The resulting increase in extracellular glutamate then facilitates activation of extrasynaptic mGluR2/3 autoreceptors, ultimately reducing evoked synaptic glutamate release (Moran et al., 2005). This decrease in synaptic glutamate release as a downstream result of NAC administration is the mechanism by which NAC also restores the capacity to induce further long-term potentiation, since blockade of mGluR2/3 receptors prevented this restoration (Moussawi et al., 2009).

NAC is also a known precursor of the endogenous antioxidant, glutathione (GSH), the synthesis of which depends upon the rate-limiting activity of the xc- system. GSH is primarily produced within astrocytes using glutamate and cystine as substrates to generate γ-glutamylcysteine, which is then combined with glycine to create GSH (see Dringen & Hirrlinger, 2003). GSH is released from astrocytes into the extracellular space, where it is broken down by γ-glutamyltranspeptidase into glutamate and a cysteine-glycine dipeptide that is further hydrolyzed into the individual peptides. This reaction is the mechanism by which astrocytes provide the precursors necessary for neuronal GSH production (Dringen & Hirrlinger, 2003). In addition to protecting brain cells from the oxidative stress, GSH has been shown to enhance responsivity of NMDA receptors to glutamatergic stimulation (see Janáky et al., 1999), suggesting some direct modulation of glutamatergic signalling as a result of NAC administration. The role of GSH in addiction has yet to be determined, and thus far, the effects of NAC as a pharmacotherapy for drug dependence appear to be primarily mediated via its actions on system xc- and GLT-1 (Knackstedt et al., 2009; Knackstedt et al., 2010a).

3. N-acetylcysteine in animal models of self-administration, reinstatement, and relapse

The study of the addictive properties of drugs in animals is largely based on variations of the self-administration procedure developed in rats by Weeks (1962; see Belin & Dalley 2012; Panlilio & Goldberg, 2007). Although now conducted with many species, in its simplest and most common form, rats (or mice) are prepared with indwelling intravenous catheters that exit through a backmount to be attached to a tether hanging within a conditioning chamber. Tubing connecting the catheter to a syringe outside the chamber runs through the tether and provides the route by which drugs can be administered directly into the blood stream (see Figure 2).

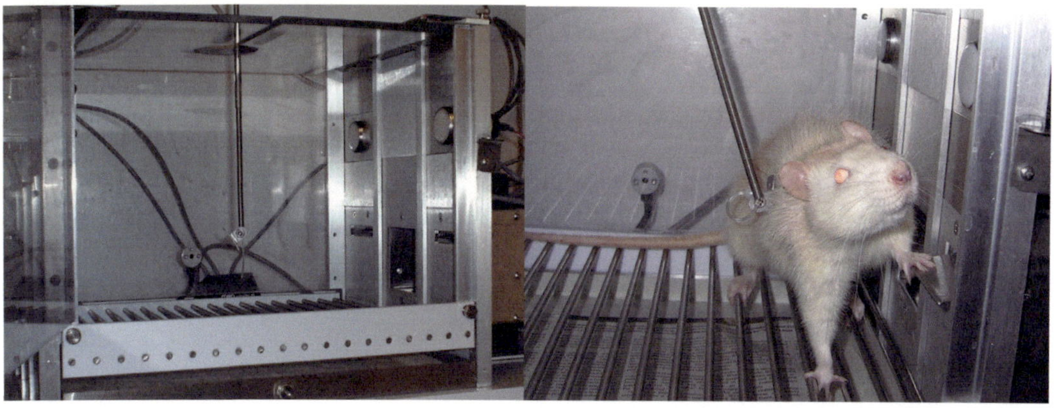

Fig. 2. Operant drug self-administration chamber and procedure. Operant chambers are typically equipped with two retractable levers (assigned as either 'active' or 'inactive') with a cue light above each. When a rat presses the active lever under an FR1 schedule, the resulting drug infusion is accompanied by the onset of the cue light associated with the active lever.

When in the self-administration chamber, two levers are typically available - an 'active' and an 'inactive' lever. Under the most basic Fixed Ratio 1 (FR1) schedule of reinforcement, also called continuous reinforcement, a single press on the active lever results in a drug infusion often paired with a non-drug stimulus, such as a brief presentation of a light. The drug delivery reinforces the behavior, making it more likely the rat will press the active lever again (cf. Hall, 2002). Presses on the inactive lever have no consequence and are used as an index of general activity. This self-administration procedure is particularly useful in determining the abuse liability of psychoactive substances (for a review see O'Connor et al.,

2011). The ability to self administer drugs for short periods of time daily (1-2 hrs per session) results in a stable drug intake over time, a so-called titration process that is suggested to reflect individual control of intake responding to optimal dosing (Wilson et al., 1971; Zimmer et al., 2011) around which blood levels fluctuate in the course of the self-administration session.

Pharmacological challenges during ongoing self-administration, following extinction or abstinence, or before relapse or reinstatement of self-administration (see later) have been useful in identifying potential targets for the development of pharmacotherapies for various forms of addictions (e.g., Schindler et al., 2011; Steensland et al., 2007). Such an approach is based on the common psychodynamic view of the addiction process of which the stages, namely development, maintenance, and relapse/reinstatement, are modelled in Figure 3.

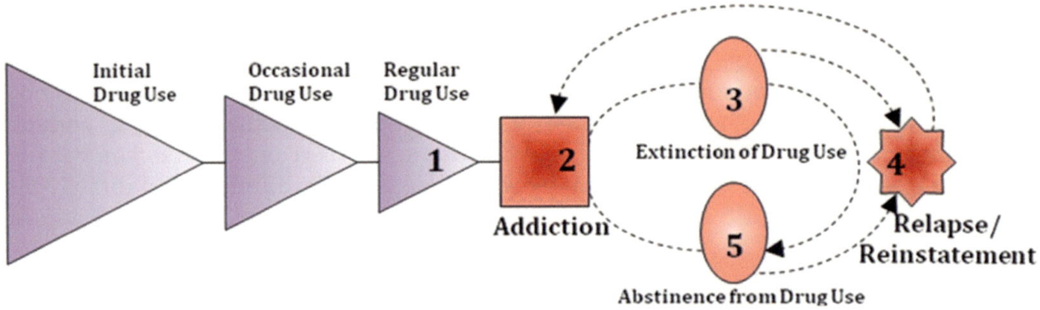

Fig. 3. Stages of the development and maintenance of addiction in humans and animal models. Stages of the addiction cycle that have been targeted with NAC treatment are regular drug use before the development of addiction as defined by the DSM-IV [1], thereby aiming at preventing the transition from controlled to compulsive drug use, the addiction stage (in animal models, when intake has escalated or become habitual) [2], following behavioral extinction of drug seeking predominately seen in animal models - human addicts rarely engage in extinction [3], at the time drug or a drug-associated cue is re-introduced causing reinstatement [4], following short- or long-term abstinence from drug more typical for human addicts and increasingly modelled in animals [5], and at the return to the drug-seeking/taking context, resulting in relapse [4].

A reasonable time point for targeting addiction is when the individual is still regularly engaged in drug use with the intended outcome of reducing intake and eventually stopping use altogether. Therefore, it is of interest to assess potential pharmacotherapies during the self-administration phase. In a standard self-administration task, that is thought to model the stage in which humans engage in regular use but are not necessarily addicted (Figure 3, Stage 1), rats that had access to cocaine for 2 hrs under an FR1 schedule of reinforcement, and administered 60 mg/kg NAC before each daily training session displayed no differential intake as compared with vehicle-treated controls (Amen et al., 2011; Madayag et al., 2007).

The efficacy of NAC on ongoing cocaine intake changes however, with increasing access to cocaine. Indeed, with long (e.g., ≥6 hrs) rather than short (e.g., 2 hrs) daily access to cocaine self-administration, rats no longer titrate intake, but instead tend to increase, or escalate, their intake across days (cf. Ahmed & Koob, 1998). This escalation of drug intake over time, associated with dysregulation of neural networks governing reward (for a review see Koob

& Kreek, 2007), has been suggested to reflect the loss of control over intake that characterises human drug addicts (Figure 3, Stage 2). In an experiment assessing the effects of NAC on cocaine escalation (Madayag et al., 2007), rats initially acquired cocaine (0.5 mg/kg) self-administration in 2-hr sessions under an FR1 schedule of reinforcement until intake stabilized (<10% variation across ≥3 sessions). They were then shifted to 6-hr daily sessions for 11 days in which they were able to self-administer a higher dose of cocaine (1.0 mg/kg) and subsequently given either 60 mg/kg NAC or vehicle pre-treatment. Whereas saline-pre-treated rats displayed typical escalation of their cocaine intake across sessions, NAC-pretreated rats maintained a stable drug intake across days (Madayag et al., 2007). In a similar study, daily pretreatment with the higher dose of 90 mg/kg NAC appeared to reduce cocaine intake across the 12 sessions of long-access cocaine self-administration compared to saline pretreatment (Kau et al., 2008). Combined, the findings that NAC impacts escalation without affecting typical short-access drug self-administration suggests that loss of control over drug intake may be better reflective of dysregulated glutamate homeostasis.

3.1 Treatment during reinstatement of drug seeking

The ultimate goal of any addiction therapy is to achieve and maintain drug abstinence. This therapeutic goal is especially challenging due to the strong associations formed between the interoceptive drug experience and surrounding cues. Re-experiencing a drug or drug cue following a successful quit attempt can evoke and enhance drug craving (e.g., Niaura et al., 1988; O'Brien et al., 1992), thus increasing the likelihood of reinstatement of drug use, often resulting in relapse. As such, finding effective techniques that target the motivational impact of a 'lapse' in drug use (drug-induced reinstatement) or drug-related paraphernalia (cue-induced reinstatement) is of high therapeutic value for maintaining drug abstinence.

From an experimental standpoint, when operant behavior no longer results in the delivery of the reinforcing outcome, extinction occurs, so that instrumental performance declines (Figure 3, Stage 3). Extinction of a behavior is a new learning process that exists alongside the old, previously learned, association (for a review see Bouton, 2002). This new learning is largely dependent on continued absence of the primary reinforcer while the manipulanda (i.e., levers) are still available to press. In humans, these sort of explicit extinction sessions are generally only provided within the context of cue-exposure therapy which aims at presenting inpatients with drug use paraphernalia in the absence of the drug (see Monti & MacKillop, 2007; Siegel & Ramos, 2002). Reinstatement of the previously extinguished behavior can therefore be evoked by presentation of the reinforcer (i.e., drug-induced reinstatement) or a conditioned stimulus (CS) associated with the reinforcer that had not presented during the extinction phase (i.e., cue-induced reinstatement; Figure 3, Stage 4; de Wit & Stewart, 1981).

When an addict 'lapses', or uses once, following abstinence, he is at a much higher risk for re-engaging in regular use. Attenuating the effects of this drug-induced reinstatement may help prevent a 'lapse' in drug abstinence from turning into a full-blown relapse of addiction (e.g., Shadel et al., 2011; Witkiewitz & Masyn, 2008). In rats, cocaine exposure following extinction of self-administration is associated with a glutamate release from prefrontal projections into the NAcC (McFarland et al., 2003), and this release may provide the mechanism that triggers reinstatement of drug seeking. Acute treatment with NAC has been shown to attenuate drug-induced reinstatement. In some of these experiments, rats were trained to self-administer cocaine in 2-hr or 6-hr daily sessions. During the subsequent extinction phase, instrumental responses were reinforced only with contingent presentations of the drug-associated light, and no cocaine was infused, so lever pressing progressively declined. For the drug-induced reinstatement test, rats were injected with a priming dose of cocaine, this pharmacological challenge resulted in a marked increased in the previously extinguished instrumental response, i.e., lever pressing. Pretreatment with 30, 60, or 600 mg/kg NAC before cocaine re-exposure prevented reinstatement of cocaine-seeking behavior (Baker et al., 2003a; Baker et al., 2003b; Kau et al., 2008; Moran et al., 2005). Concurrent blockade of system xc- using (S)-4-carboxyphenylglycine (CPG) during the reinstatement test blocked the reinstatement-attenuating effects of NAC (Kau et al., 2008), thereby suggesting that NAC effects on cocaine-induced reinstatement are mediated through system xc-. Additionally, as measured by in vivo microdialysis during the reinstatement test, NAC administration restored the reduced extracellular glutamate levels that resulted from cocaine self-administration and withdrawal (Baker et al., 2003b). Further, concurrent blockade of mGluR2/3 autoreceptors also prevented the attenuating effects of NAC on cocaine-induced reinstatement (Moran et al., 2005) demonstrating that the effect of NAC restoration of extracellular glutamate on reinstatement may depend upon activation of the mGluR2/3 autoreceptors.

The effects of NAC on drug-induced reinstatement have also been shown when NAC is administered prior to, but not explicitly during, the reinstatement test. In one such experiment, rats were trained to self-administer cocaine under short-access conditions and then underwent extinction followed by cocaine-primed reinstatement (Amen et al., 2011). Following the first test in which cocaine seeking was reinstated, rats were treated with 60 mg/kg NAC for 7 days. The day following the seventh NAC treatment, rats were subjected to a second cocaine-primed reinstatement test. Rats that had received NAC treatment showed significantly reduced cocaine seeking compared to the rats that had received saline treatment during those 7 days (Amen et al., 2011). Although daily treatment with 60 mg/kg NAC before 2-hr cocaine self-administration sessions (see above) had no effect on amount of cocaine taken or subsequent extinction (without NAC pretreatment), cocaine-primed reinstatement was significantly reduced, even though it had been 2-3 weeks since last NAC treatment (Madayag et al., 2007). Similarly, 90 mg/kg NAC pretreatment throughout long-access cocaine self-administration resulted in attenuated cocaine-primed reinstatement that was reversed by inhibition of system xc- following an extinction phase without NAC (Kau et al., 2008). These effects are indicative of the long-lasting protection of glutamate homeostasis as a result of NAC treatment. Indeed, concurrent microdialysis in the NAc immediately prior to the reinstatement test showed that there were lower extracellular basal glutamate levels in rats that had been pretreated with saline during the self-administration stage than in those that had been pretreated with NAC (Madayag et al., 2007). Once cocaine had been administered to induce reinstatement, the saline-pretreated group reached the level of extracellular glutamate that was shown at baseline by the NAC-pretreated group. These findings suggest that NAC administration during self-administration provided protection against the withdrawal-induced downregulation of extracellular glutamate in the NAc and subsequent cocaine-induced reinstatement.

3.2 Treatment during extinction and reinstatement

The effect of chronic NAC treatment during both extinction and subsequent reinstatement tests has also been evaluated (Figure 3, Stages 3 and 4). In one such study (Reichel et al., 2011), rats were trained to self-administer cocaine (50 µg/infusion) under an FR1 schedule until they reached >10 infusions in two hours for twelve consecutive sessions. During the following twelve sessions, lever presses had no programmed consequences (i.e., extinction), and rats were given daily injections of 0, 60 or 100 mg/kg NAC. There was no effect of the lower 60 mg/kg dose of NAC on extinction responding. However, there was a significant enhancement of extinction (i.e., less active lever pressing) when rats were treated daily with 100 mg/kg NAC (Moussawi et al., 2011; Reichel et al., 2011). This effect was also found during extinction of heroin self-administration for which daily administration of 100 mg/kg NAC resulted in enhanced extinction rate (Zhou & Kalivas, 2008). Although NAC treatment was ineffective when applied during acquisition of self-administration, it enhanced extinction learning.

In each of these studies, two tests of reinstatement were then conducted: cue-induced reinstatement and cue+drug- or drug-induced reinstatement. Human addicts are particularly sensitive to cues that had previously been associated with drug use, and exposure to these cues following drug abstinence can reinstate drug seeking and taking behavior, resulting in relapse (see O'Brien et al., 1992; Taylor et al., 2009). Similarly, rats are also quite sensitive to the effects of re-presentation of these drug-associated CSs. As such, the impact of NAC treatment on cue-induced reinstatement of instrumental responding has recently begun to be assessed. For the cocaine self-administration group treated with the lower, 60 mg/kg, dose of NAC, there was a significant reduction in cue-induced reinstatement compared to saline controls, but no effect on cue+drug-induced reinstatement (Reichel et al., 2011). However, when NAC (100 mg/kg) was administered during extinction following either cocaine or heroin self administration, there was a significant reduction in both cue- and cue+drug- or drug-induced reinstatement. These results suggest that, compared to a conditioned stimulus, a higher treatment dose was necessary to disrupt the ability of an unconditioned drug stimulus+drug-associated CS compound to reinstate drug-taking behavior (Moussawi et al., 2011; Reichel et al., 2011; Zhou & Kalivas, 2008). Notably, these effects on reinstatement lasted from two weeks (Moussawi et al., 2011; Reichel et al., 2011) to 40 days (Zhou & Kalivas, 2008) following the last 100 mg/kg NAC treatment, indicating a long-term restoration of glutamate homeostasis in the NAcC brought about by the re-regulation induced by chronic NAC exposure (Moussawi et al., 2011). At the neurophysiological level, rats trained to self-administer cocaine that received saline (rather than NAC) during extinction showed reduced extrasynaptic glutamate levels in the NAcC compared to saline-yoked controls. In rats that received NAC during extinction, there was full recovery of the extrasynaptic glutamate levels two weeks following the last NAC injection – a time period corresponding to the behavioral effect on cue- and cue+drug-induced reinstatement (Moussawi et al., 2011). Furthermore, administration of the mGluR2/3 antagonist, LY341495, into the NAcC prevented the attenuating effects of NAC on cue- and cue+drug-induced reinstatement of cocaine-seeking, again indicating the importance of presynaptic autoreceptors in maintaining glutamate homeostasis (Moussawi et al., 2011).

3.3 Treatment during abstinence

A key concern with the translational potential of the extinction-reinstatement model of drug dependence is that human users are not typically subjected to extinction of responding during presentation of drug-related cues unless they are patients in an explicit cue-exposure therapy session (cf. Monti & MacKillop, 2007). Rather, addicts undergo abstinence - a period in which they either voluntarily (i.e., independently, or by checking into a rehabilitation clinic) or forcibly (e.g., incarceration) abstain from drug use outside the drug-taking environment (Figure 3, Stage 5; Reichel & Bevins, 2009). Following the abstinence period, a person returns home where the associative strength of all the drug-associated cues is still fully intact, and no behavior has been extinguished, and 'relapse' of the addictive behavior often resumes.

A rat model of 'forced abstinence' operationally uses the same drug self-administration protocols as the extinction-reinstatement model, but rather than undergoing an extinction phase in which responding diminishes with repeated non-reinforced lever pressing, the animal is typically left in its home cage for a specified period of time (e.g., 2 weeks) where it can undergo a treatment protocol before returning to the drug-associated conditioning chamber. Notably, extinction and abstinence following cocaine self-administration produce different patterns of protein expression in the NAc (Knackstedt et al., 2010b), warranting further investigation into the efficacy of potential pharmacotherapies in each model of addiction.

The abstinence model has recently been used to assess the efficacy of NAC treatment following cocaine self-administration (Reichel et al., 2011). Rats were trained to self-administer cocaine under an FR1 schedule until they reached >10 infusions in two hours for twelve consecutive sessions. During the subsequent two-week abstinence period, rats were given daily injections of 60 or 100 mg/kg NAC or saline. They were then tested for relapse to cocaine seeking by returning them to the self-administration environment and recording non-reinforced lever presses. Treatment with the lower, 60 mg/kg, dose of NAC during abstinence had no effect on relapse compared to saline, however, treatment with the higher 100 mg/kg dose of NAC during abstinence significantly reduced cocaine-seeking during the relapse test (Reichel et al, 2011). During subsequent tests in which the drug-paired cue, and then the drug+cue, was presented, 100 mg/kg NAC treatment during abstinence maintained a significant effect on drug seeking. Finally, following a second phase of abstinence in which no NAC was administered, there was still a significant attenuation of drug seeking when rats were presented with the drug+cue in the self-administration chamber, again indicative of the long-term re-regulation of glutamate homeostasis provided by NAC administration.

3.4 Treatment during habitual drug seeking

Regular daily drug use is not limited to the taking of the drug. Rather, addicted individuals can invest countless hours 'foraging' for their next high. This foraging takes a person through multiple exposures to stimuli that are predictive of the impending drug experience. As such, not only can these drug-associated CSs reinstate drug-seeking behavior when presented following behavioral extinction but they can also serve as powerful conditioned reinforcers that drive and maintain continued drug foraging over long periods of time when presented contingently. This foraging can continue to persist even after the explicit drug-taking behavior has been extinguished (Olmstead et al., 2001; Zapata et al., 2010), indicating a habitization of the drug-seeking behavior which may be a key characteristic in the transition from casual drug use to addiction (e.g., O'Brien et al., 1998, Everitt & Robbins 2005, Belin et al., 2009a).

Cocaine seeking (see Chapter 2) as opposed to mere cocaine taking, or self-administration, has been operationalized in primates (Goldberg, 1973) and then in rats (Arroyo et al., 1998) and humans (Panlilio et al., 2005) in the so-called second-order schedule of reinforcement. In this specialized model of self-administration, drug seeking is separated from the unconditioned effects of the drug. Cues associated with drug reinforcement function as conditioned reinforcers that maintain persistent, habitual, seeking responses across protracted periods of time without primary drug reinforcement (Everitt & Robbins, 2000; Schindler et al., 2002).

In this procedure, rats are initially trained to self-administer drug under the FR1 schedule of reinforcement with a single lever press resulting in a drug infusion associated contingently with a 20-second cue light presentation. Following stabilization of responding, the response requirement is shifted across days to gradually move the behavior of the rat to what is known as a second-order schedule of reinforcement. There are several ways of increasing the response requirement (cf. Economidou et al., 2011; Vanderschuren et al., 2005, Belin & Everitt 2008), either by introducing ratio / ratio increments or fixed interval schedules with increasing interval durations across days. In the experiment in which NAC effect was measured on early and well-established cue-controlled cocaine seeking (Murray et al., 2012), rats were moved up through the following schedules: FR3; FR5(FR2:S); FR10(FR2:S); FR10(FR4:S); FR10(FR6:S); FR10(FR10:S); FI15(FR10:S). Under each of these schedules of cocaine reinforcement, completion of each unit schedule (given within the parentheses) resulted in a 1-second cue light presentation; cocaine infusions were delivered only upon completion of the first unit schedule according to the schedule outside the parentheses. Therefore, during the final second-order training schedule [i.e., FI15(FR10:S)], cocaine and the 20-second cue light were given on completion of the first FR10:S unit after the Fixed Interval 15-minute period had timed out. In these conditions instrumental responding is no longer under the control of the goal, from which it is now temporally distal, but instead becomes highly dependent upon contingent presentations of conditioned CSs, acting as conditioned reinforcers (cf. Arroyo et al., 1998). As shown in Figure 4, following acquisition of the second-order schedule, removal of CSs (i.e., 1-second light presentations provided under a FR10 schedule of reinforcement are removed, returning the animal to a strict FI15 schedule of reinforcement) results in a decline in lever pressing across sessions in the first 15-minute interval that is reversed when the unit schedule is returned (i.e., 1-second light presentations under FR10). By the time behavior has reached this stage of training, drug seeking during the first 15-min drug-free interval is maintained at very high rates and is thought to reflect cue-controlled habitual cocaine seeking which, at the neurobiological level, has been hypothesised to result of a gradual recruitment of dorsolateral striatal dopamine circuitry (Belin & Everitt, 2008; Ito et al., 2002; Murray et al., in press; Vanderschuren et al., 2005).

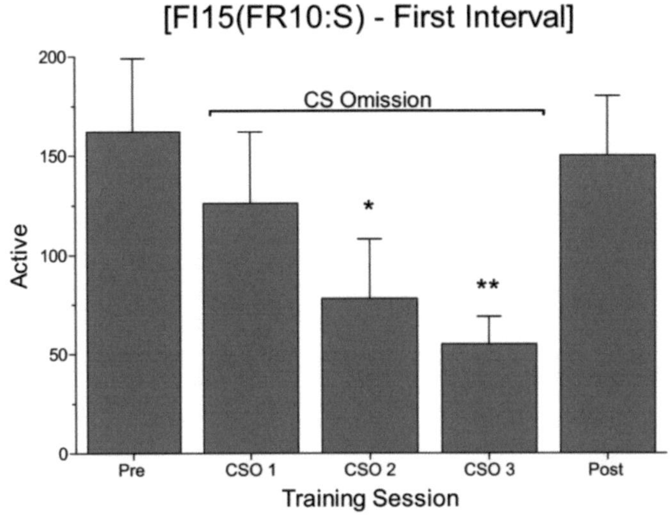

Fig. 4. Control of cocaine seeking by contingent presentations of conditioned reinforcers. Three consecutive days of conditioned reinforcer (1-s cocaine-associated light presentations) omission (CSO 1-3) are compared with performance on the session before conditioned reinforcer omission (Pre) and performance on the session when the reinforcer is returned (Post). * indicates significant difference from Pre, $p<.05$, ** $p<.01$. Adapted from Arroyo et al (1998) with permission from Springer.

Assessment of drug seeking before actual drug reinforcement can be conducted at both an early stage of acquisition and at a later, well-established stage. To assess drug seeking in the early stage when the behavior had only ever been reinforced under an FR1 schedule of reinforcement by the unconditioned drug stimulus with concurrent CS presentations, a switch in the contingency was instituted for a 15-min test session. This testing procedure allowed for measurement of drug seeking now reinforced by 1-sec cue light presentations. Cocaine was delivered only on the first lever press following the 15-min interval, and each test was immediately followed by an FR1 training session. The effects of acute NAC treatment on cocaine seeking during the early-stage tests are shown in Figure 5A. Drug seeking before the experience of unconditioned cocaine effects was reduced with 60 and 90 mg/kg NAC treatment.

After increasing the response requirements and at least 15 sessions of FI15(FR10:S) training, so that cocaine seeking maintained by regular contingent presentations of the drug-associated conditioned reinforcer was well-established, conditions known to be associated with a shift in the locus of control over behavior from the ventral to the dorsolateral striatum (Vanderschuren et al., 2005; Belin & Everitt, 2008), the effect of NAC pre-treatment on cocaine seeking was measured once again (Figure 5B). At this stage, drug seeking was more sensitive to NAC treatment, with 30, 60, and 90 mg/kg disrupting the conditioned reinforcing effects of the cocaine-associated stimulus. The results of this experiment demonstrate that acute NAC treatment dose-dependently reduced cocaine seeking maintained by conditioned reinforcers both at an early stage of acquisition when drug seeking is considered to be goal-directed and following extensive training on the second-order schedule, when drug seeking is considered to be habitual (Murray et al., 2012). These findings demonstrate that NAC pretreatment may be an aid to establish abstinence by reducing cocaine seeking in individuals that actively seek cocaine on a daily basis, rather than only during relapse following an extinction or abstinence period.

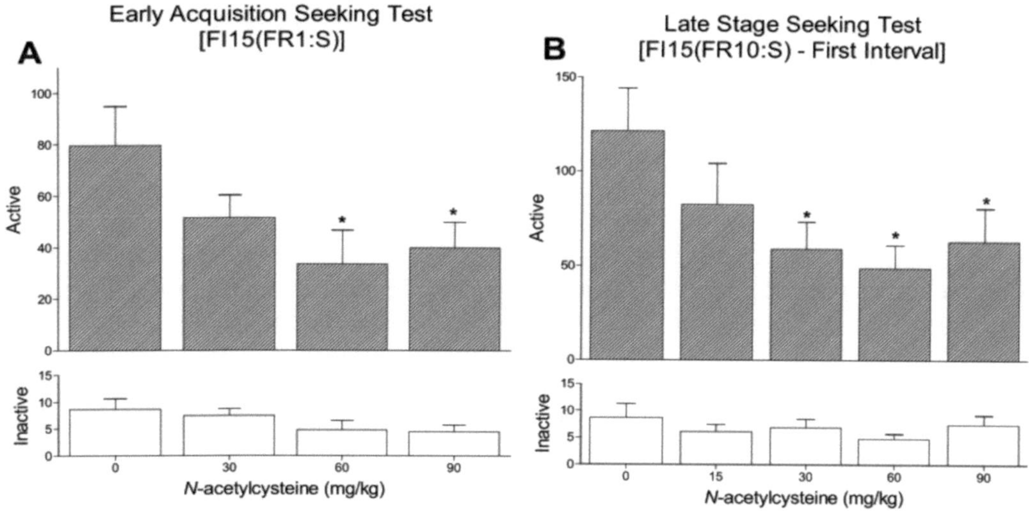

Fig. 5. Effects of NAC on cocaine seeking. Panel A depicts active (top) and inactive (bottom) lever presses during acute NAC treatment in the 15-min cocaine seeking test with contingent conditioned reinforcer presentations (FR1) at an early stage of self-administration. Panel B depicts active (top) and inactive (bottom) lever presses during acute NAC treatment in the first 15-min cocaine seeking interval with contingent conditioned reinforcer presentations (FR10) during the late stage of cocaine self-administration. For both panels, * indicates significant difference from 0 mg/kg NAC, $p<.05$. Adapted from Murray et al. (2012) with permission from Wiley.

4. N-acetylcysteine in humans: From acetaminophen overdose antidote to addictive and impulsive-compulsive spectrum disorders

NAC, as an antioxidant and gluthatione precursor, has been used for more than 30 years in intravenous or oral protocols as an acetaminophen poisoning antidote. Within this framework, NAC has been shown to have low rates of adverse reactions which nevertheless include nausea, vomiting, as well as cutaneous and systemic anaphylactoid reactions. ECG abnormalities, status epilepticus and fatal reaction due to NAC overdose are rare, the latter having been observed only at doses 10 times greater than the recommended antidote dose (for review see Sandilands & Bateman, 2009). Atopy and asthma are major risk factors for developing adverse and anaphylactoid reactions to NAC (Schmidt & Dalhoff, 2001).

Thanks to its antioxidant effect, NAC has dose-dependent protective effects against contrast-induced nephrotoxicity (Briguori et al., 2011). NAC can also be used as both a chelating agent for methylmercury (for review see Dodd et al., 2008) and a mucolytic and anti-inflammatory agent, with controversial efficacy in patients with exacerbations of chronic obstructive pulmonary disease (Decramer et al., 2005). Unlike orally-administered gluthatione and L-cysteine, NAC successfully crosses the blood-brain barrier, and permits restoration of glial and neuronal gluthatione levels, playing a role in the oxidative homeostasis in the brain, protecting neurons against oxidative stress. In addition, NAC treatment reduces levels of some pro-inflammatory cytokines (IL-6, IL-1β, and TNF-α) shown to be implicated in several psychiatric disorders, notably in depressive and bipolar disorders as well as in schizophrenia. NAC has been used to target the prefrontal glutamatergic dysfunction implicated in schizophrenia and impulsive-compulsive behaviors (for reviews see Dean et al., 2011; Sansone & Sansone, 2011). One of the first uses of NAC in psychiatry was a case-report of the amelioration of self-injurious behaviors and craving in a female patient suffering from Post-traumatic Stress Disorder and borderline personality disorder (Pittenger et al., 2005). There are to date very few rigorous studies assessing the efficacy of NAC in the treatment of addiction and impulsive-compulsive spectrum disorders (including behavioral addictions, impulse-control disorders and obsessive-compulsive and related disorders). Those available, despite limited statistical evidence (randomized studies with small size samples, non-randomized cohorts, or case reports), have provided consistent results, in that NAC was always reported to reduce drug use, craving or withdrawal symptoms during the treatment period, sometimes even resulting in a persistent effect on relapse after the end of the trials (Olive et al., 2012).

4.1 NAC and cocaine dependence

NAC treatment for addiction has been primarily studied in cocaine dependent patients, alongside the aforementioned publication of preclinical studies initiated by Kalivas' team (Baker et al., 2003a; Baker et al., 2003b). In one such study, the safety and tolerability of NAC have been assessed in 13 otherwise-healthy, non-treatment-seeking, cocaine-dependent patients with a mean age of 37.1 ± 7.6. During the first hospitalization of the experiment, patients received either four treatments of NAC (600 mg per treatment; 2400 mg total) or placebo spaced 12 h apart. In a cross-over design, the opposite treatment (i.e., NAC or placebo) was given during a hospitalization during the second week. NAC treatment resulted in a significant reduction of withdrawal symptoms (assessed with the Cocaine Selective Severity Assessment, CSSA, a measure of cocaine abstinence signs and symptoms; Kampman et al., 1998) while placebo had no effect. The effect of NAC treatment was not restricted to withdrawal symptoms since it was also accompanied by an overall reduction in self-reported craving (five items, including desire to use, level of craving and other similar constructs, rated on ten-point Likert scales). In this study NAC was well tolerated during the treatment periods, with neither significant adverse effects nor with effects on primary biological parameters (renal and liver functions, complete blood count) between groups. In addition, at completion of the two-week follow-up period patients displayed a marked decrease both in days of cocaine use from 41% ± 7 (in the ninety days before study) to 27% ± 7, and average daily dollar expenditure for cocaine from $30.31 ± 3.44 (in the ninety days before study) to $8.77 ± 2.52, suggesting that a brief NAC treatment, perhaps through promotion of reduced withdrawal symptoms and subjective craving, may have a prolonged efficacy even weeks after the end of the treatment (LaRowe et al., 2006).

In addition to this clinical evaluation, at the end of the treatment period, the same patients were exposed to a cue-reactivity procedure to assess cocaine desire. During two sessions, patients were semi-randomly presented cocaine-related, neutral, and affective (pleasant and unpleasant) slides. Cocaine-related slides produced greater skin conductance than either neutral or pleasant slides. NAC treatment did not modify physiological reactions to any of the slides viewed (i.e., skin conductance and heart rate measures). Cocaine slides evoked higher ratings of craving for, desire to use, and interest in, cocaine, as well as longer viewing times relative to neutral slides. NAC treatment resulted in lower motivation to use cocaine in comparison with placebo when viewing cocaine slides, characterized by a reduced desire to use, a reduced interest in cocaine, and less time viewing cocaine slides. Craving for cocaine was also reported to be lower in NAC- than in placebo-treated participants even though this difference did not reach statistical significance (LaRowe et al., 2007).

In an independent laboratory study in 6 cocaine-dependent patients, with a mean age of 41.8 ± 7.4 and a mean age of drug-use onset of 18.3 ± 4.0, subjective 'high', 'rush', and craving for cocaine were assessed using a computerized version of a ten-point Likert scale. The patient had to use a joystick and move a tab along a horizontal bar with the anchors 'Least Ever' and 'Most Ever' at each extreme end, then push a button at the desired rating after viewing either a neutral or a cocaine video and after a 20 mg/kg IV cocaine infusion. This assessment was conducted the day before and after 3 days of NAC treatment (1200 mg or 2400 mg daily, TID). NAC treatment significantly reduced subjective craving induced by cocaine infusion, as measured before and after treatment. By contrast, NAC affected none of the subjective measures induced by cocaine videos, nor did it affect subjective feelings of high and rush induced by the cocaine infusion (Amen et al., 2011).

Finally, in an open-label study, 23 cocaine-dependent patients, with a mean age of 40 ± 1.4 and a mean lifetime of cocaine use of 13.3 ± 1.5 years, were treated for 4 weeks with three different doses of NAC (1200, 2400 or 3600 mg/day). In a subjective evaluation, the three doses of NAC decreased the mean number of days of use (from 8.3 ± 1.3 to 1.1 ± 1.4) and the dollar amount spent (from $1292.8 ± 508.6 to $52.2 ± 25.9) across the 28 days of treatment. This was in agreement with an objective evaluation revealing that urine drug screens were negative in two-thirds of the sample during treatment (without comparison with baseline due to a lack of significant sampling during this period). Cocaine abstinence symptoms (assessed with the CSSA) decreased during the treatment period. Retention in treatment was significantly better in the 2400 mg and the 3600 mg groups than in the 1200 mg group (88.9% and 83% respectively, vs. 37.5%). Adverse events were mild to moderate, including headache, pruritus and elevated blood pressure, but did not significantly differ among the treatment groups (Mardikian et al., 2007).

These results indicate that administration of NAC (at daily doses of 2400 and 3600 mg) can be an effective treatment for relapse prevention in cocaine-dependent patients, due to its ability to decrease withdrawal symptoms and craving severity. The severity of the cocaine withdrawal symptomatology at treatment entry is negatively correlated with the treatment outcome and the duration of continuous abstinence from cocaine (Kampman et al., 2002). Furthermore, subjective and objective feelings of craving, even during experimental cue-induced and cocaine-infusion procedures, which are predictors of early drug-use outcomes and rapid treatment attrition (Rohsenow et al., 2007), are reduced by NAC, a treatment that results in few mild-to-moderate side effects. Further studies with high-level evidence (i.e., randomized, double-blind, placebo-controlled, long-term studies) must be conducted in cocaine-dependent patients to determine the effective dosing ranges, the optimal duration of treatment, and the indications of NAC as a treatment for cocaine withdrawal or as an anti-addiction drug (used as an adjunct to psychotherapy to help patients in maintain abstinence).

4.2 NAC and marijuana dependence

In an open-label study, 24 cannabis-dependent subjects aged 18-21 were treated for 4 weeks with 1200 mg NAC twice daily (Gray et al., 2010). During the trial, the medication adherence was good (82.6% of scheduled doses), and adverse events were mild-to-moderate - none leading to discontinuation of the treatment. In a subjective evaluation at the fourth week of treatment, NAC significantly decreased the number of days per week cannabis was used, and showed a tendency to reduce the quantity of self-reported marijuana used per day (15.9 ± 2.4 vs. 11.9 ± 2.1 potency-adjusted 'hits'). In an objective evaluation, the cannabinoid content of urine samples was not affected, but craving for marijuana, measured by the Marijuana Craving Questionnaire, was significantly reduced. These results show the potential promise for NAC treatment of cannabis abuse and dependence, especially provided that no effective treatments are available for this particularly vulnerable population. A double-blind placebo-controlled study evaluating the efficacy of NAC (1200 mg twice daily for 8 weeks) combined with Contingency Management on marijuana use in a younger population (ages 13-21) is currently recruiting (NCT01005810).

4.3 NAC and methamphetamine dependence

In a small double-blind placebo-controlled study (Grant et al., 2010), 31 methamphetamine-dependent patients, with a mean age of 36.8 ± 7.12 and a mean age of onset of drug use of 24.3, were treated during 8 weeks with NAC (increased dose from 600 mg daily to 2400 mg daily every 2 weeks) and naltrexone (increased dose from 50 mg daily to 200 mg daily every 2 weeks) or placebo. In a subjective evaluation, at the end of the study, NAC+naltrexone treatment decreased the mean number of days of use every two weeks from 8.1 ± 4.9 to 1.9 ± 1.8 days in comparison with placebo (from 6.3 ± 4.6 to 2.3 ± 3.5 days). In an objective evaluation given at the end of the study however, positive urine drug screens did not differ between groups (46.2% vs. 35.3%). Concerning methamphetamine craving (assessed with the Penn Craving Scale: a self-report measure of frequency, intensity, and duration of craving, ability to resist taking drug, and an overall rating of craving for methamphetamine), NAC+naltrexone treatment did not result in significant improvement since there was no difference between the two groups in their decrease in total score at the end of the study (-43.6% vs. -37.7% for treated and placebo patients, respectively). Rates of adverse events (including nausea and lethargy) did not significantly differ between groups (57.1% vs. 41.2%). This preliminary 8-week study suggested that NAC+naltrexone treatment effectively reduced reported frequency of methamphetamine use even without affecting overall craving for the drug.

4.4 NAC and nicotine dependence

In a double-blind placebo-controlled study, 26 nicotine-dependent patients, with a mean age of 50, who had been smoking for an average of 33 years, were treated for 4 weeks with NAC (2400 mg daily) or placebo (Knackstedt et al., 2009). NAC treatment did not affect the objective measures related to nicotine dependence including carbon monoxide levels, or craving for cigarettes (assesssed with the Questionnaire for Smoking Urges-Brief), nor did it affect withdrawal symptoms (assessed with the Minnesota Nicotine Withdrawal Scale). In a subjective evaluation, there was a trend towards an overall reduction in cigarette use during the study (main effect of time), but no group effect, indicating a lack of efficacy of that dose of NAC on tobacco use. In a separate double-blind placebo-controlled study, 22 students at least twenty years old smoking for an average of 6 years, received NAC (1800 mg twice daily) or placebo for 4 days (Schmaal et al., 2011). None of the subjects reported smoking during the 4 days of treatment. At the end of the experiment, NAC did not affect craving for cigarettes (assessed with the Questionnaire for Smoking Urges-Brief) or withdrawal symptoms (assessed with the Minnesota Nicotine Withdrawal Scale). However, compared to placebo, NAC reduced the subjective rewarding effect of a cigarette smoked at the end of the experiment, suggesting a potential preventative impact of the treatment on relapse.

4.5 NAC and alcohol dependence

NAC has just been evaluated for an 8-week treatment of alcohol dependence, but the results are not yet published (NCT00568087). NAC has only been fully assessed in humans for its antioxidant properties, with some results in combination with corticosteroids and enteral nutrition in the treatment of severe acute alcoholic hepatitis (for review see Reep and Soloway, 2011), while a recent study shows minimal benefits of the combination therapy by prednisolone plus NAC in terms of survival among patients with this indication (Nguyen-Khac et al., 2011). Finally, preliminary findings in rats suggest NAC may also be helpful in the prevention of alcohol-induced heart disease (Seiva et al., 2009). Clearly, further work regarding the potential of NAC treatment for alcohol dependence needs to be conducted.

4.6 NAC and opiates dependence

To our knowledge, NAC has not yet been evaluated in the treatment of opiate dependence in humans.

4.7 NAC and pathological gambling

NAC treatment has been shown to reduce pathological gambling. In an open-label study (Grant et al., 2007), 27 subjects who engaged in pathological gambling, with a mean age of 50.8 ± 12.1 and a mean age of onset of problem gambling of 37.1 ± 12.8, were treated for 8 weeks with NAC (increased dose from 600 mg daily to 1800 mg daily every 2 weeks). Twenty-three patients (85.2%) completed the study for which the primary outcome was the effect of NAC treatment on the pathological gambling score, an adaptation of the Yale-Brown Obsessive-Compulsive Scale (PG-YBOCS), measuring the severity and change in severity of pathological gambling symptoms (Pallanti et al., 2005). Of those that completed the study, 16 patients (69.6%) were responders on the PG-YBOCS, showing a 30% or greater reduction in total score at end-point compared with baseline. Ten patients reported total abstinence from gambling. The total score on the PG-YBOCS decreased during the treatment phase from 20.3 ± 4.1 to 11.8 ± 9.8. On the overall severity and change in clinical symptoms (assessed by the Clinical Global Impression-Improvement scale, a 7 point scale that requires the clinician to assess how much the patient's illness has improved or worsened relative to a baseline state at the beginning of the intervention), 59.3% of patients were 'much' or 'very much' improved at the end of the study. Urge, thought, and self-reported gambling symptoms were improved after NAC treatment. In a second phase, 13 of the patients who completed the open-label study and were considered responders were included in a double-blind placebo-controlled study with NAC treatment at the highest dose or placebo for another 6 weeks. At the end of the 6 weeks, 83.3% of active treatment patients vs. 28.6% of placebo patients still met responder criteria on the PG-YBOCS.

4.8 NAC and impulsive-compulsive spectrum disorders

Finally, NAC has been assessed in several impulsive-compulsive spectrum disorders other than addictions, including trichotillomania, obsessive-compulsive disorder (OCD), and nail-biting in patients suffering from bipolar disorder. In a double-blind placebo-controlled study (Grant et al., 2009), 50 patients with trichotillomania (compulsive hair-pulling), with a mean age of 34.3 ± 12.1 and a mean age of onset of 12.1 ± 5.0 years, were treated for 12 weeks with NAC (1200 mg daily for 6 weeks, then 2400 mg daily) or placebo. Eighty-eight percent of all patients completed the study regardless the group assignment. In a subjective evaluation, NAC-treated patients, as compared to those treated with placebo, displayed significant reductions in the severity of trichotillomania symptoms according to the patient self-rating (using the Massachusetts General Hospital Hair Pulling Scale) and the physician-assessment (with the Psychiatric Institute Trichotillomania Scale), associated with a significant improvement of the severity and the resistance and control dimensions of the disorder. On the severity and change in global clinical symptoms (assessed by the CGI-improvement scale), 56% of NAC patients were 'much' or 'very much' improved at the end of the study compared with 16% of those taking placebo. In a report series, NAC used as an add-on therapy in the treatment of bipolar disorder was associated with a dramatic reduction in nail-biting behavior in three cases (Berk et al., 2009). NAC efficacy on this behavior may be due either to an anti-impulsive action of NAC or to an effect on anxiety or stress. In a case report, NAC has been used in conjunction with fluvoxamine (a serotonin-reuptake inhibitor agent) treatment in a refractory OCD patient. During a total period of 12 weeks, including 7 weeks at the total daily dose of 3000 mg, Y-BOCS scores decreased dramatically and the patient was able to resist her compulsive symptoms during the treatment period (Lafleur et al., 2006).

These findings attest to the promise NAC treatment has for treating the behavioral symptoms of impulsive/compulsive disorders. Three double-blind placebo-controlled studies are currently being carried out, demonstrating the recent interest for NAC in the treatment of impulsive-compulsive spectrum disorders. The first one is evaluating the efficacy of NAC (3000 mg twice daily for 12 weeks) in adult Serotonin Reuptake Inhibitor-refractory obsessive-compulsive disorder and depression (NCT00539513). The second one is evaluating the efficacy of NAC (1600 mg twice daily for 2 weeks then 2600 mg capsules twice daily for the remaining 10 weeks) for the treatment of pediatric obsessive-compulsive disorder (NCT01172275), and the third one is assessing the efficacy of NAC (from 1200 mg daily to 3000 mg daily, during 12 weeks) in pathologic skin picking (repetitive, ritualistic, or impulsive picking of otherwise normal skin leading to tissue damage, personal distress, and impaired functioning; NCT01063348). Moreover, NAC is currently being evaluated in a double-blind placebo-controlled study for children with Tourette syndrome (childhood-onset neuropsychiatric disorder characterised by multiple and chronic motor and vocal tics; NCT01172288).

5. Conclusion

In laboratory studies, NAC has been shown to prevent escalation of cocaine use during long access (6h/day) to the drug (an animal model of loss of control over drug intake, a hallmark feature of addiction) without affecting drug use during short access (1h and 2h/day). NAC also prevents relapse behaviors, reducing drug-associated cues-, cocaine-, and heroin-priming-induced reinstatement after extinction and abstinence protocols (animal models of relapse, when a drug-addicted individual is exposed to different triggers of drug craving and relapse after a period of abstinence). Finally, NAC reduces cocaine seeking, when drug seeking has become habitual (an animal model of the daily behavior of drug foraging, as it can be seen in individuals who spend great deal of time in activities necessary to obtain and prepare the substance, rather than only during relapse following an extinction or abstinence period). These preclinical data resonate well with the human literature which shows overall promising results from clinical trials on drug addiction and impulsive-compulsive spectrum disorders. More specifically, the efficacy of NAC treatment for cocaine addiction appears relevant, with improvement of withdrawal symptoms, attenuation of subjective and objective craving for the drug (during laboratory experiments, NAC attenuates environmental and cocaine-induced urges to use), and persistent reduction in cocaine use even after the end of the treatment. Results in cannabis addiction are less marked but also hold promise, notably due to the absence of available treatment for addicted young adults, who are particularly vulnerable to the development of other, stronger, addictions and psychotic comorbid disorders (Gray et al., 2010). Promising but mitigated results in methamphetamine and nicotine addiction should make us remember that the pathology of addiction may be quite different across drugs of abuse and that a single pharmacotherapy may not be sufficient for all drugs (cf. Badiani et al., 2011). Even if the small sample size of these studies may have precluded the identification of statistically significant differences between groups, negative results may also be attributable to the implication of other biological and psychological factors in methamphetamine and nicotine dependence and craving. In particular, learned contextual associations and context-induced relapse (Crombag et al., 2008) may not be affected by NAC treatment. Indeed, interesting preliminary results in other behavioral disorders including pathological gambling and impulsive-compulsive disorders, which appear alleviated with NAC treatment, may suggest that NAC is not necessarily working to treat these behavioral disorders at the same level of the drug of abuse.

At the neurobiological level this suggests that NAC-induced re-regulation of the homeostatic extrasynaptic glutamate levels in the brain may be affecting the behavioral component of 'seeking' - whether that be drug, a poker game, or the anxiety-alleviation provided by compulsive hair pulling. Preclinical studies using models in rats that specifically address the development of habitual drug seeking behavior, compulsive seeking and taking behavior, or addiction-like behavior (Belin et al., 2011) may help to elucidate the main psychological and associated neural substrate whereby NAC exerts its action and so in the different addictions, as it has been shown, for example, that opiate and stimulants addiction are behaviorally and neurobiologically distinct (for review see Badiani et al., 2011). Studies evaluating the efficacy of NAC on neuropsychological processes that contribute to the development of drug addiction, (e.g., decision-making or impulsivity) may also prove useful. In humans, clinical studies should take interest in assessing efficacy of NAC as a cognitive enhancer (Brady et al., 2011), as it has been shown that improvement of inhibitory control, attentional and decision-making processes may help individuals perform better in face of stressful and complex environmental situations.

6. References

Ahmed SH, Koob GF (1998) Transition from moderate to excessive drug intake: change in hedonic set point. Science 282:298-300.

Amen SL, Piacentine LB, Ahmad ME, Li S-J, Mantsch JR, Risinger RC, Baker DA (2011) Repeated N-acetyl cysteine reduces cocaine seeking in rodents and craving in cocaine-dependent humans. Neuropsychopharmacology 36:871-878.

American Psychiatric Association (2000) Diagnostic and Statistical Manual of Mental Disorders DSM-IV-TR. Washington DC.

Arroyo M, Markou A, Robbins TW, Everitt BJ (1998) Acquisition, maintenance and reinstatement of intravenous cocaine self-administration under a second-order schedule of reinforcement in rats: effects of conditioned cues and continuous access to cocaine. Psychopharmacology 140:331-344.

Badiani A, Belin D, Epstein D, Calu D, Shaham Y (2011) Opiate versus psychostimulant addiction: the differences do matter. Nat Rev Neurosci 12:685-700.

Brady KT, Gray KM, Tolliver BK (2011) Cognitive enhancers in the treatment of substance use disorders: clinical evidence. Pharmacol Biochem Behav 99:285–294.

Baker DA, Xi Z-X, Shen H, Swanson CJ, Kalivas PW (2002) The origin and neuronal function of in vivo nonsynaptic glutamate. J Neurosci 22:9134-9141.

Baker DA, McFarland K, Lake RW, Shen H, Toda S, Kalivas PW (2003a) N-acetyl cystine-induced blockade of cocaine-induced reinstatement. Ann N Y Acad Sci 1003:349-351.

Baker DA, McFarland K, Lake RW, Shen H, Tang X-C, Toda S, Kalivas PW (2003b) Neuroadaptations in cystine-glutamate exchange underlie cocaine relapse. Nat Neuro 6:743-749.

Bannai S (1986) Exchange of cystine and glutamate across plasma membrane of human fibroblasts. J Biol Chem 261:2256-2263.

Belin D, Everitt BJ (2008) Cocaine seeking habits depend upon dopamine-dependent serial connectivity linking the ventral with the dorsal striatum. Neuron 57:432-441.

Belin D, Economidou D, Pelloux Y, Everitt BJ (2011) Habit formation and compulsion. In: Animal Models of drug addiction. Olmstead, MC, ed. pp 337–378. Neuromethods, vol. 53. Springer.

Belin D, Everitt BJ (2010) The Neural and Psychological Basis of a Compulsive Incentive Habit. In: Handbook of basal ganglia structure and function, Steiner, H, tseng, K, eds) Elsvier, ACADEMIC PRESS.

Belin D, Jonkman S, Dickinson A, Robbins TW, Everitt BJ (2009a) Parallel and interactive learning processes within the basal ganglia: Relevance for the understanding of addiction. Behavioural Brain Research, 199(1):89–102.

Belin D, Dalley JW (2012) Animal models in addiction research. In: Drug Abuse & Addiction in Medical Illness: causes, consequences and treatment, Vester, J, ed, Totowa: Humana Press Inc.

Belin D, Besson M, Bari A, Dalley JW (2009b) Multi-disciplinary investigations of impulsivity in animal models of attention-deficit hyperactivity disorder and drug addiction vulnerability. In: Endophenotypes of Psychiatric and Neurodegenerative Disorders in Rodent Models, Granon, S, ed, New York: Oxford University Press.

Berk M, Jeavons S, Dean OM, Dodd S, Moss K, Gama CS, Malhi GS (2009) Nail-biting stuff? The effect of N-acetyl cysteine on nail-biting. CNS Spectr 14:357–360.

Bouton ME (2002) Context, ambiguity, and unlearning: sources of relapse after behavioral extinction. Biol Psychiatry 52:976-986.

Briguori C, Quintavalle C, De Micco F, Condorelli G (2011) Nephrotoxicity of contrast media and protective effects of acetylcysteine. Arch Toxicol 85:165–173.

Chen BT, Bowers MS, Martin M, Hopf FW, Guillory AM, Carelli RM, Chou JK, Bonci A (2008) Cocaine but not natural reward self-administration nor passive cocaine infusion produces persistent LTP in the VTA. Neuron 59:288-297.

Chen BT, Hopf FW, Bonci A (2010) Synaptic plasticity in the mesolimbic system. Ann N Y Acad Sci 1187:129-139.

Crombag HS, Bossert JM, Koya E, Shaham Y (2008) Context-induced relapse to drug seeking: a review. Philos Trans R Soc Lond B Biol Sci 363:3233–3243.

Dauletbaev N, Fischer P, Aulbach B, Gross J, Kusche W, Thyroff-Friesinger U, Wagner TO, Bargon J (2009) A phase II study on safety and efficacy of high-dose N-acetylcysteine in patients with cystic fibrosis. Eur J Med Res 14:352-358.

Dean O, Giorlando F, Berk M (2011) N-Acetylcysteine in psychiatry: current therapeutic evidence and potential mechanisms of action. J Psychiatry Neurosci 36:78-86.

Decramer M, Rutten-van Molken M, Dekhuijzen PN, Troosters T, van Herwaarden C, Pellegrino R, van Schayck CP, Olivieri D, Del Donno M, De Backer W, Lankhorst I, Ardia A (2005) Effects of N-acetylcysteine on outcomes in chronic obstructive pulmonary disease (Bronchitis Randomized on NAC Cost-Utility Study, BRONCUS): a randomised placebo-controlled trial. Lancet 365:1552–1560.

Decramer M, Janssens W (2010) Mucoactive therapy in COPD. Eur Respir Rev 19:134-140.

Dietrich D, Kral T, Clusmann H, Friedl M, Schramm J (2002) Presynaptic group II metabotropic glutamate recepotrs reduce stimulated and spontaneous transmitter release in human dentate gyrus. Neuropharmacology 42:297-305.

de Wit H, Stewart J (1981) Reinstatement of cocaine-reinforced responding in the rat. Psychopharmacology 75:134-143.

Dodd S, Dean O, Copolov DL, Malhi GS, Berk M (2008) N-acetylcysteine for antioxidant therapy: pharmacology and clinical utility. Expert Opin Biol Ther 8:1955–1962.

Dringen R, Hirrlinger J (2003) Glutathione pathways in the brain. Biol Chem 384:505-516.

Economidou D, Dalley JW, Everitt BJ (2011) Selective norepinephrine reuptake inhibition by atomoxetine prevents cue-induced heroin and cocaine seeking. Biol Psychiatry 69:266-274.

EMCDDA (2009) The state of the drugs problem in Europe (annual report 2009).

Everitt BJ, Robbins TW (2000) Second-order schedules of drug reinforcement in rats and monkeys: measurement of reinforcing efficacy and drug-seeking behaviour. Psychopharmacology 153:17-30.

Everitt BJ, Robbins TW (2005) Neural systems of reinforcement for drug addiction: from actions to habits to compulsion. Nat Neurosci, 8:1481–1489.

Goldberg SR (1973) Comparable behavior maintained under fixed-ratio and second-order schedules of food presentation, cocaine injection or D-amphetamine injection in the squirrel monkey. *J Pharmacol Exp Ther* 186:18-30.

Grant JE, Kim SW, Odlaug BL (2007) N-acetyl cysteine, a glutamate-modulating agent, in the treatment of pathological gambling: a pilot study. Biol Psychiatry 62:652–657.

Grant JE, Odlaug BL, Kim SW (2009) N-acetylcysteine, a glutamate modulator, in the treatment of trichotillomania: a double-blind, placebo-controlled study. Arch Gen Psychiatry 66:756–763.

Grant JE, Odlaug BL, Kim SW (2010) A double-blind, placebo-controlled study of N-acetyl cysteine plus naltrexone for methamphetamine dependence. Eur Neuropsychopharmacol 20:823–828.

Gray KM, Watson NL, Carpenter MJ, Larowe SD (2010) N-acetylcysteine (NAC) in young marijuana users: an open-label pilot study. Am J Addict, 19:187–189.

Hall G (2002) Associative structures in Pavlovian and instrumental conditioning. In Gallistel R & Pashler H (Eds.) Stevens' Handbook of Experimental Psychology 3rd Edition: Learning, Motivation, and Emotion, Volume 3 (pp.1-45) John Wiley & Sons, Inc: New York.

Haugeto O, Ullensvang K, Levy LM, Chaudhry FA, Honoré T, Nielsen M, Lehre KP, Danbolt NC (1996) Brain glutamate transporter proteins form homomultimers. J Biol Chem 271:27715-27722.

Ito R, Dalley JW, Robbins TW, Everitt BJ (2002) Dopamine release in the dorsal striatum during cocaine-seeking behavior under the control of a drug-associated cue. J Neurosci 22:6247-6253.

Janáky R, Ogita K, Pasqualotto BA, Bains JS, Oja SS, Yoneda Y, Shaw CA (1999) Glutathione and signal transduction in the mammalian CNS. J Neurochem 73:889-902.

Kalivas PW (2009) The glutmate homeostasis hypothesis of addiction. Nat Rev Neurosci 10:561-572.

Kampman KM, Volpicelli JR, McGinnis DE, Alterman AI, Weinrieb RM, D'Angelo L, Epperson LE (1998) Reliability and validity of the Cocaine Selective Severity Assessment. Addict Behav 23:449–461.

Kampman KM, Volpicelli JR, Mulvaney F, Rukstalis M, Alterman AI, Pettinati H, Weinrieb RM, O'Brien CP (2002) Cocaine withdrawal severity and urine toxicology results from treatment entry predict outcome in medication trials for cocaine dependence. Addict Behav 27:251–260.

Kau KS, Madayag A, Mantsch JR, Grier MD, Abdulhameed O, Baker DA (2008) Blunted cysteine-glutamate antiporter function in the nucleus accumbens promotes cocaine-induced drug seeking. Neuroscience 155:530-537.

Knackstedt LA, LaRowe S, Mardikian P, Malcolm R, Upadhyaya H, Hedden S, Markou A, Kalivas PW (2009) The role of cystine-glutamate exchange in nicotine dependence in rats and humans. Biol Psychiatry 65:841-845.

Knackstedt LA, Melendez RI, Kalivas PW (2010a) Ceftriaxone restores glutamate homeostasis and prevents relapse to cocaine seeking. Biol Psychiatry 67:81-84.

Knackstedt LA, Moussawi K, LaLumiere R, Schwendt M, Klugmann M, Kalivas PW (2010b) Extinction training after cocaine self-administration induces glutamatergic plasticity to inhibit cocaine seeking. J Neurosci 30:7984-7992.

Koob G, Kreek MJ (2007) Stress, dysregulation of drug reward pathways, and the transition to drug dependence. Am J Psychiatry 164:1149-1159.

Kory RC, Hirsch SR, Giraldo J (1968) Nebulization of N-acetylcysteine combined with a bronchodilator in patients with chronic bronchitis. Dis Chest 54:504-509.

Lafleur DL, Pittenger C, Kelmendi B, Gardner T, Wasylink S, Malison RT, Sanacora G, Krystal JH, Coric V (2006) N-acetylcysteine augmentation in serotonin reuptake inhibitor refractory obsessive-compulsive disorder. Psychopharmacology 184:254–256.

LaRowe SD, Mardikian P, Malcolm R, Myrick H, Kalivas P, McFarland K, Saladin M, McRae A, Brady K (2006) Safety and tolerability of N-acetylcysteine in cocaine-dependent individuals. Am J Addict 15:105–110.

LaRowe SD, Myrick H, Hedden S, Mardikian P, Saladin M, McRae A, Brady K, Kalivas PW, Malcolm R (2007) Is cocaine desire reduced by N-acetylcysteine? Am J Psychiatry 164:1115–1117.

Leshner AI (1997) Addiction is a brain disease, and it matters. Science 278:45-47.

Lüscher C, Malenka RC (2011) Drug-evoked synaptic plasticity in addiction: from molecular changes to circuit remodelling. Neuron 69:650-663.

Madayag A, Lobner D, Kau KS, Mantsch JR, Abdulhameed O, Hearing M, Grier MD, Baker DA (2007) Repeated N-acetylcysteine administration alters plasticity-dependent effects of cocaine. J Neurosci 27:13968-13976.

Manzoni O, Michel J-M, Bockaert J (1997) Metabotropic glutamate recepotrs in the rat nucleus accumbens. Eur J Neurosci 9:1514-1523.

Mardikian PN, LaRowe SD, Hedden S, Kalivas PW, Malcolm RJ (2007) An open-label trial of N-acetylcysteine for the treatment of cocaine dependence: a pilot study. Prog Neuropsychopharmacol Biol Psychiatry 31:389–394.

Martin M, Chen BT, Hopf FW, Bowers MS, Bonci A (2006) Cocaine self-administration selectively abolishes LTD in the core of the nucleus accumbens. Nat Neuro 9:868-869.

McFarland K, Lapish CC, Kalivas PW (2003) Prefrontal glutamate release into the core of the nucleus accumbens mediates cocaine-induced reinstatement of drug-seeking behavior. J Neurosci 23:3531-3537.

Monti PM, MacKillop J (2007) Advances in the treatment of craving for alcohol and tobacco. In, P. M. Miller and D. Kavanagh, Eds. Translation of Addictions Science into Practice, Elsevier Science, New York, pp. 211-237.

Moran MM, McFarland K, Melendez RI, Kalivas PW, Seamans JK (2005) Cystine/glutamate exchange regulates metabotropic glutamate receptor presynaptic inhibition of excitatory transmission and vulnerability to cocaine seeking. J Neurosci 25:6389-6393.

Moussawi K, Pacchioni A, Moran M, Olive MF, Gass JT, Lavin A, Kalivas PW (2009) N-Acetylcysteine reverses cocaine-induced metaplasticity. Nat Neurosci 12:182-189.

Moussawi K, Zhou W, Shen H, Reichel CM, See RE, Carr DB, Kalivas PW (2011) Reversing cocaine-induced synaptic potentiation provides enduring protection from relapse. PNAS 108:385-390.

Murray JE, Belin D, Everitt BJ (in press) Double dissociation of the dorsomedial and dorsolateral striatal control over the acquisition and performance of cocaine seeking. Neuropsychopharmacology.

Murray JE, Everitt BJ, Belin D (2012) N-Acetylcysteine reduces early- and late-stage cocaine seeking without affecting cocaine taking in rats. Addict Biol 17:437-440.

Nguyen-Khac E, Thevenot T, Piquet MA, Benferhat S, Goria O, Chatelain D, Tramier B, Dewaele F, Ghrib S, Rudler M, Carbonell N, Tossou H, Bental A, Bernard-Chabert

B, Dupas JL; AAH-NAC Study Group (2011) Glucocorticoids plus N-acetylcysteine in severe alcoholic hepatitis. N Engl J Med 365:1781-789.

Niaura RS, Rohsenow DJ, Binkoff JA, Monti PM, Pedraza M, Abrams DB (1988) Relevance of cue reactivity to understanding alcohol and smoking relapse. J Abnorm Psychol 97:133-152.

O'Brien CP, Childress AR, Ehrman R, Robbins SJ (1998) Conditioning factors in drug abuse: can they explain compulsion? J Psychopharmacol 12:15-22.

O'Brien CP, Childress AR, McLellan AT, Ehrman R (1992) Classical conditioning in drug-dependent humans. Ann N Y Acad Sci 654:400-415.

O'Connor EC, Chapman K, Butler P, Mead AN (2011) The predictive validity of the rat self-administration model for abuse liability. Neurosci Biobehav Rev 35:912-938.

Olive MF, Cleva RM, Kalivas PW, Malcolm RJ (2012) Glutamatergic medications for the treatment of drug and behavioral addictions. Pharmacol Biochem Behav 100:801-810.

Olmstead MC, Lafond MV, Everitt BJ, Dickinson A (2001) Cocaine seeking by rats is a goal-directed action. Behav Neurosci 115:394-402.

Pallanti S, DeCaria CM, Grant JE, Urpe M, Hollander E (2005) Reliability and validity of the pathological gambling adaptation of the Yale-Brown Obsessive-Compulsive Scale (PG-YBOCS). J Gambl Stud 21:431–443.

Panlilio LV, Goldberg SR (2007) Self-administration of drugs in animals and humans as a model and an investigative tool. Addiction 102:1863-1870.

Panlilio LV, Yasar S, Nemeth-Coslett R, Katz JL, Henningfield JE, Solinas M, Heishman SJ, Schindler CW, Goldberg SR (2005) Human cocaine-seeking behavior and its control by drug-associated stimuli in the laboratory. Neuropsychopharmacology 30:433-443.

Pierce RC, Bell K, Duffy P, Kalivas PW (1996) Repeated cocaine augments excitatory amino acid transmission in the nucleus accumbens only in rats having developed behavioural sensitization. J Neurosci 16:1550-1560.

Pittenger C, Krystal JH, Coric V (2005) Initial evidence of the beneficial effects of glutamate-modulating agents in the treatment of self-injurious behavior associated with borderline personality disorder. J Clin Psychiatry 66:1492–1493.

Prescott LF, Park J, Ballantyne A, Adriaenssens P, Proudfoot AT (1977) Treatment of paracetamol (acetaminophen) poisoning with N-acetylcysteine. Lancet 2:432–434.

Reep GL, Soloway RD (2011) Recent and currently emerging medical treatment options for the treatment of alcoholic hepatitis. World J Hepatol 3:211–214.

Reichel CM, Bevins RA (2009) Forced abstinence model of relapse to study pharmacological treatments of substance use disorder. Curr Drug Abuse Rev 2:184-194.

Reichel CM, Moussawi K, Do PH, Kalivas PW, See RE (2011) Chronic N-Acetylcysteine during abstinence or extinction after cocaine self-administration produces enduring reductions in drug seeking. J Pharmacol Exp Ther 337:487-493.

Rohsenow DJ, Martin RA, Eaton CA, Monti PM (2007) Cocaine craving as a predictor of treatment attrition and outcomes after residential treatment for cocaine dependence. J Stud Alcohol Drugs 68:641–648.

Russo SJ, Dietz DM, Dumitriu D, Morrison JH, Malenka RC, Nestler EJ (2010) The addicted synapse: mechanisms of synaptic and structural plasticity in nucleus accumbens. TINS 33:267-276.

Saal D, Dong Y, Bonci A, Malenka RC (2003) Drugs of abuse and stress trigger a common synaptic adaptation in dopamine neurons. Neuron 37:577-582.

Sandilands EA, Bateman DN (2009) Adverse reactions associated with acetylcysteine. Clin Toxicol (Phila) 47:81–88.

Sansone RA, Sansone LA (2011) Getting a Knack for NAC: N-Acetyl-Cysteine. Innov Clin Neurosci 8:10–14.

Scalley RD, Conner CS (1978) Acetaminophen poisoning: a case report of the use of acetylcysteine. Am J Hosp Pharm 35:964-967.

Schindler CW, Gilman JP, Panlilio LV, McCann DJ, Goldberg SR (2011) Comparison of the effects of methamphetamine, bupropion, and methylphenidate on the self-administration of methamphetamine by rhesus monkeys. Exp Clin Psychopharmacol 19:1-10.

Schindler CW, Panlilio LV, Goldberg SR (2002) Second-order schedules of drug self-administration in animals. Psychopharmacology 163:327-344.

Schmaal L, Berk L, Hulstijn KP, Cousijn J, Wiers RW, van den Brink W (2011) Efficacy of N-acetylcysteine in the treatment of nicotine dependence: a double-blind placebo-controlled pilot study. *Eur Addict Res* 17:211-216.

Schmidt LE, Dalhoff K (2001) Risk factors in the development of adverse reactions to N-acetylcysteine in patients with paracetamol poisoning. Br J Clin Pharmacol 51:87–91.

Seiva FR, Amauchi JF, Rocha KK, Ebaid GX, Souza G, Fernandes AA, Cataneo AC, Novelli EL (2009) Alcoholism and alcohol abstinence: N-acetylcysteine to improve energy expenditure, myocardial oxidative stress, and energy metabolism in alcoholic heart disease. Alcohol 43:649–656.

Shadel WG, Martino SC, Setodji C, Cervone D, Witkiewitz K, Beckjord EB, Scharf D, Shih R (in press) Lapse-induced surges in craving influence relapse in adult smokers: an experimental investigation. Health Psychol. doi: 10.1037/a0023445

Siegel S, Ramos BMC (2002) Applying laboratory research: drug anticipation and the treatment of drug addiction. Exp Clin Psychopharmacol 10:162-183.

Stamm SJ, Docter J (1965) Clinical evaluation of acetylcysteine as a nucolytic agent in cystic fibrosis. Dis Chest 47:414-420.

Steensland P, Simms JA, Holgate J, Richards JK, Bartlett SE (2007) Varenicline, an alpha4beta2 nicotinic acetylcholine receptor partial agonist, selectively decreases ethanol consumption and seeking. Proc Natl Acad Sci U S A 104:12518-12523.

Stuber GD, Hnasko TS, Britt JP, Edwards RH, Bonci A (2010) Dopaminergic terminals in the nucleus accumbens but not the dorsal striatum corelease glutamate. J Neurosci 30:8229-8233.

Substance Abuse and Mental Health Services Administration (2010) Results from the 2009 National Survey on Drug Use and Health: Volume I. Summary of National Findings (Office of Applied Studies, NSDUH Series H-38A, HHS Publication No. SMA 10-4856Findings). Rockville, MD.

Taylor JR, Olausson P, Quinn JJ, Torregrossa MM (2009) Targeting extinction and reconsolidation mechanisms to combat the impact of drug cues on addiction. Neuropharmacology 56:186-195.

Ungless MA, Whistler JL, Malenka RC, Bonci A (2001) Single cocaine exposure in vivo induces long-term potentiation in dopamine neurons. Nature 411:583-587.

Vanderschuren LJ, Di Ciano P, Everitt BJ (2005) Involvement of the dorsal striatum in cue-controlled cocaine seeking. J Neurosci 25:8665-8670.

Weeks, JR (1962) Experimental morphine addiction: method for automatic intravenous injections in unrestrained rats. Science 138:143-144.

Wilson, MC, Hitomi M, Schuster CR (1971) Psychomotor stimulant self administration as a function of dosage per injection in the rhesus monkey. Psychopharmacologia 22:271-281.

Witkiewitz K, Masyn KE (2008) Drinking trajectories following an initial lapse. Psychol Addict Behav 22:157-167.

World Health Organization (2010) *ATLAS on Substance Use – Resources for the Prevention and Treatment of Substance Use Disorders*. WHO Press: Geneva, Switzerland.

Zapata A, Minney VL, Shippenberg TS (2010) Shift from goal-directed to habitual cocaine seeking after prolonged experience in rats. J Neurosci 30:15457-15463.

Zhou W, Kalivas PW (2008) N-Acetylcysteine reduces extinction responding and induces enduring reductions in cue- and heroin-induced drug-seeking. Biol Psychiatry 63:338-340.

Zimmer BA, Dobrin CV, Roberts DCS (2011) Brain-cocaine concentrations determine the dose self-administered by rats on a novel behaviourally dependent dosing schedule. Neuropsychopharmacology 36:2741-2749.

Section 4

Therapeutic Strategies – Behavioural, Social and Analytical Approaches

13

Proposals for the Treatment of Users of Alcohol and Other Drugs: A Psychoanalytic Reading

Cynara Teixeira Ribeiro[1,2,3] and Andréa Hortélio Fernandes[4,5]
[1]*Pontifícia Universidade Católica de São Paulo (PUC/SP)*
[2]*Universidade Federal da Bahia (UFBA)*
[3]*Universidade Federal Rural do Semi-Arido (UFERSA)*
[4]*Université de Paris VII*
[5]*Universidade Federal da Bahia*
[4]*France*
[1,2,3,5]*Brazil*

1. Introduction

Currently, the harmful use of alcohol and other drugs is recognized as a serious public health problem in many countries (WHO, 2002). However, it has not always been so. The reason is because, for quite a long time, the prevention and treatment related to the use of psychoactive substances were neglected in the context of public health policies, and delegated to other institutions such as justice and public safety. This fact gave rise to initiatives of total character attention[1] and to therapeutic practices that aimed mainly at the abstention from psychoactive consumption. Hence, traditionally, the great majority of treatments offered to users of alcohol and other drugs was based on the abstinence proposal (Marlatt; Larimer & Witkiewitz, 2012).

Nevertheless, a worldwide discussion about the difficulties that alcohol and other drug addicts have to drastically stop consuming such substances identified the need for the development of other treatment models as an alternative to the abstinence proposal (Brasil, 2005; Paes, 2006). As a consequence, many countries all over the world adopted the approach of harm reduction as the official strategy for prevention, treatment and education of people who use psychoactive substances in a harmful way (Brasil, 2001).

Another existing perspective in the treatment of alcohol and other drug users is the psychoanalysis proposal (Director, 2005; Laxenaire, 2010; Loose, 2000; Valentine & Fraser, 2008). Its main specificity lies in recognizing the different ways in which the subject relates to the toxic substances and consequently, understanding that drug use is anchored in the subjective dimension. Besides, psychoanalysis points to the fact that certain types of relationship to drugs can provide a kind of paradoxical and deadly satisfaction, called

[1] The term "initiatives of total character attention" is a mention to the term "total institutions", coined by Erving Goffmann (1985/2001).

jouissance (enjoyment)[2] (Lacan, 1969/1992; Laxenaire, 2010; Melman, 2000; Olievenstein, 2002), which is articulated to the unconscious and the death drive.

Thus, taking into consideration the abstinence proposal, the damage reduction proposal and the psychoanalytic proposal, this chapter will discuss the particular features of each one of these treatment models. Besides, it will also analyze the controversial and convergent points that exist among them, paying special attention to the debate between psychoanalysis and harm reduction. Finally, the chapter will briefly consider how the treatments of drug users can be optimized, as the result of the 'approximation' between these proposals.

2. The treatment proposals of drug use

In order to start a discussion on the treatments offered to users of alcohol and other drugs, first it is necessary to emphasize the historical character of the phenomenon of psychoactive substance use. As several authors have pointed out, the human practice of drug consumption is universal and ancient. In fact, in nearly all civilizations and human societies, the consumption of drugs capable to promote changes in what are considered as the human beings' states of consciousness has been a resource of great social and subjective importance (Mcrae, 2001; Seibel & Toscano Jr., 2001; Carneiro, 2006).

Although this consumption was historically widespread, it is important to highlight that, until a certain moment in history, it was restricted to small groups and happened in connection to collective ceremonies and sacred rituals, according to socially shared norms and conventions, which gave a predominantly symbolic value to the use of these substances. For instance, some ancient people believed that the consumption of certain substances made it possible for the spiritual representatives of certain groups to incorporate supposedly supernatural powers. This association between psychoactive substances consumption and religion lasted for quite a long time, including the medieval period, when the use of drugs was condemned because it was considered a hedonistic and sinful behavior.

However, this conception was strongly challenged from the seventeenth century on, with the development of medical studies, when certain vegetal products that have psychoactive effect started to be valued as a source of energy, stamina, humor and temper balance. As examples, we can mention the opium, originated from the poppy, which was for a long time prescribed as a painkiller, antitussive and antidiarrheal medication, and the marijuana, prescribed as a general sedative, for the specific treatment of rheumatism, neurosis, insomnia, headaches, diarrhea, seizures and anorexia as well as in the therapy of tetanus and cholera (Carneiro, 2006).

Furthermore, with the isolation of the active principles of the psychoactive substances in the eighteenth century, trade was established and certain products started to be available to the general population. Simultaneously, there was the weakening of the socio-cultural regulation strategies for the use of these substances, as well as the rise of a number of social issues that contributed to the large dissemination of drugs consumption, both for therapeutic and recreational ends. This dissemination, in turn, revealed the capacity of these substances to cause physical and psychological dependence in some users.

[2] 'Jouissance' means 'pleasure' or 'enjoyment', but the terms in English lack the sexual connotation that the word has in French. Hence, in consonance with the majority of the English translations of Lacan's works, the original term was adopted in this text.

Thereafter, the phenomenon of drug use was regarded both as a social and health problem, leading many scholars to devote themselves to the systematic investigation of the several types of addiction originated from the consumption of psychoactive substances. Consequently, especially from the nineteenth century on, the use of drugs has become the object of study in the field of psychiatry and started to be considered a psychopathology, and as such, it needed to be treated (Conte, 2000). This was the context in which several treatments for drug dependence appeared, which, in a first moment, focused mainly on the detoxification and/or the isolation of drug users.

In a review of the existing treatments, it is noticeable that the field of drug addiction presents a great variety of offers. These offers can be classified as: medicamental treatments, with or without internment (especially through pharmacological interventions aimed at detoxification); non-medicamental treatments with internment (in therapeutic communities, recovery program farms, etc); non-medicamental treatments through the engagement in mutual help groups (such as Alcoholics Anonymous and Narcotics Anonymous, based on the Minnesota Method, also known as the Twelve-Step Model); cognitive-behavioral therapies (with emphasis on counseling techniques, motivational interviewing, relapse prevention and skill training); psychoanalysis (through individual and/or group psychotherapy care) and more recently, harm reduction (which provides services of drop-in, needle exchange, target delivery of healthcare, outreach and drug consumption rooms) (Stevens, Hallam & Trace, 2006).

According to Queiroz (2001), except for psychoanalysis and harm reduction, the other treatments are predominantely grounded in the principle of abstinence. Hence, as previously mentioned, in the scope of drug addiction treatments at least three different proposals can be identified: abstinence, harm reduction and psychoanalysis.

3. The proposal of treatments that aim at abstinence

Considering that drug abuse treatments appeared mainly due to the recognition of drug addiction as a psychopathology by the psychiatry field, it is not difficult to understand why these treatments have been developed based on assumptions originated from psychiatry. Being a branch of medicine, initially psychiatry incorporated the hegemonic biomedical model and its strong emphasis on the organic and biological aspects of both physical and mental diseases (Pratta & Santos, 2009; Rothshild, 2010). Thus, due to the strong influence of the biomedical model on the psychiatry field, especially during the nineteenth and twentieth century, in many countries the treatments for drug use were led to adopt the same logic implemented in the therapies of other psychopathologies.

Therefore, traditionally, these treatments had as their main feature the hospitalocentric model, with predominantly pharmacological therapies aiming at healing, which in general, in the case of psychoactive substance users, was considered equivalent to the abstention of drug use (Faria & Schneider, 2009; Rothschild, 2010; Valentine & Fraser, 2008). Although this fact was more evident in some countries, such as the USA, who have lived under the aegis of a real 'war on drugs', in a way it did have, and still has, effects upon how certain organizations around the world deal with the drug addiction phenomenon[3] (Marlatt,

[3] An example of the influence of the prohibitionist concept on worldwide agencies were the three International Conventions organized by the UN Commission of Narcotic Drugs, that aimed at

Larimer & Witkiewitz, 2012). The concept underlying this type of this viewpoint about drug use was that drug addiction would be a neurochemical dysfunction caused by the use of drugs (Freda, 1989/1993; Khantzian, 1995; Olievenstein, 2002).

In the mid-nineteenth century, a moral model of religious or spiritualist origin was added to this classic psychiatric view of psychopathology and treatment (Marlatt & Witkiewitz, 2010). This model proposed that drug use was the result of character deviation, and rehabilitation, correlated to abstinence, was of divine nature (Faria & Schneider, 2009; Stevens, Hallam & Trace, 2006). This moral model is still adopted by some therapeutic communities and by a great part of the self-help groups, which propose that chemical dependence is an incurable physical, mental and spiritual disease.

In fact, according to Bastos (2009), there are still remaining practices of these ideas of morality in current treatment for drug users. Such practices determine that drug use treatments inserted into this logic take the strand of reward and punishment, to mould the drug users' behavior into the one desired by the public health service, that usually is the abstinent behavior. This way, it is noticeable that both treatments, the one originated from the classic psychiatry and the one originated from the moral model, have as their common objective to make the user abandon the use of drugs and reach the goal of abstinence.

In this sense, one may say that abstinence consists of a treatment proposal that is influenced by these two models, in that both establish the total abstention of consumption as the easiest way to avoid drug users to lose control in face of psychoactive substances. As a consequence, many countries that adopt abstinence based treatments (for examples, USA, Japan, Singapore, Malaysia, and others) favoring the therapeutic models based on the isolation of users (Alves, 2009; Pratta & Santos, 2009). It is worth mentioning that this preference for treatments with internment reveals the influence of the asylum model in mental health, which has been sharply questioned by the anti-psychiatry movement[4] (Marchant, 2010).

Among other reasons, this preference comes from the belief that inpatient care allows for better surveillance and control of the users, which would assure the abstention of drug consumption, at least while under treatment. However, one of the main criticisms to treatments in closed institutions lies in the fact that the patient's isolation from society creates an artificial environment which characteristics cannot be reproduced outside the institution's walls. Hence, once the treatment ends, the patient's reintegration to the family and social environment tends to be disturbing, favoring the occurrence of numerous relapses (Alves, 2009; Brasil, 2005; Marlatt; Larimer & Witkiewitz, 2012; Rothschild, 2010).

This idea of making users' access to psychoactive substances difficult is justified by the basic assumption that grounds the abstinence treatment proposal, which is that the drug makes the drug addict (Freda, 1989/1993). According to this viewpoint, drugs are seen as having a

---

implementing a common program to combat drugs in all its member states (Alves, 2009). In 1998, this same Organization devised an action plan, ratified in 2003, whose title was "A drug free world: We can do it," establishing the year 2008 as the deadline to reach this goal in several countries.

[4] It is important to emphasize that, in some countries such as France and Switzerland, due to the influence of psychoanalysis, historically the psychiatric treatments were not so subordinated to the biomedical model. However, a steady increase of an organicist perspective in mental health has been perceived lately, even in these countries (Decker, 2008).

supposedly intrinsic power of getting subjects addicted to them. Thus, the idea conveyed is that anyone who uses drugs will compulsorily become, sooner or later, a drug addict. This is considered especially true in regard to those drugs viewed as more powerful, such as cocaine, heroin and crack. But in a way, this is a belief that is extended to the remaining psychoactive substances - mainly in cases in which the consumption of these drugs goes beyond the socially established standards. However, this viewpoint ends up favoring the pharmacological aspect of drugs, and ignoring the individual, subjective, social and cultural aspects implied by the phenomenon of drug abuse and addiction.

Thus, in the perspective of treatments that aim uniquely and exclusively at abstinence, drug abuse is generally considered as a problem that concerns the disease, not the subject (Dufour, 2004; Olievenstein, 2002; Passos & Souza, 2011). By doing this, it is not taken into consideration the possibility that the use of drugs represents a way the subject found to deal with his/her conflicts and with the pain of existing, that is, the discontent that, in some measure, affects all human begins (Freud, 1930/1996)[5].

Therefore, in the abstinence proposal, it is assumed that the only means to prevent or treat drug addiction would be the non-use of drugs. This is one of the reasons why many drug addicts that are treated by the abstinence proposal say that they are permanently in recovery, regardless how long ago the last drug use was, and affirm that they are 'clean just for today'. The explanation for this type of discourse is based on the fact that relapses are seen as a great threat in the horizon of those who undergo this model of treatment. And since relapses are considered the total treatment failure, abstinence is thus placed as the objective to be pursued daily and for the whole life.

This conception favors the idea that once a drug addict, forever a drug addict. As a consequence, the abstinence proposal ends up promoting an imaginary collage of drug users to the signifiers 'addict', 'toxicomaniac', 'sick', etc. In turn, this collage makes it difficult for the user to get out of the subjective position of dependence on psychoactive substances. This is because the former user who structures his/her life around the abstinence from drugs continues to delegate to the drug a central role in his/her life, and to live under the aegis of an imperative: it is as if he/she had simply replaced the statement "I have to consume" for "I have to *not* consume", thus remaining in the same subjective position of being subjected to toxic substances. In this case, the patient, whether using drugs or not, continues to use the resource to the toxic as a subterfuge to avoid confronting his/her psychic issues, so that his/her submission to the external imperative of abstinence ends up exempting him/her from the need to make his/her own choices and be responsible for them (Rothschild, 2010).

Another criticism to drug treatments that aim exclusively at abstinence is the fact that they don't generally consider the different modalities of drug use and consequently, the fact that

---

[5] The concept that drug use is tied to a subjective need of the user was strongly advocated by Khantzian (1995), who, from the perspective of ego psychology, proposed that the intoxication practices were a type of self-medication which the subject used in an attempt to better deal with his torments. However, the association between the use of certain substances and the existence of specific psychological problems, proposed by this author, did not resist empirical tests and clinical experience. On the other hand, the hypothesis of self-medication ended up contributing to the spread of the adoption of the psychoanalytical approach in the treatment of drug users, which will be explained in more detail in following sessions.

not every drug user becomes what is considered a drug addict. This view ignores that most users of drugs do so for recreational or occasional purposes, but never come to a dependency relationship with them (Araújo, 2007; Nery Filho & Torres, 2002; Rezende, 2000; Stevens, Hallam & Trace, 2006)[6].

Nevertheless, the differences among the types of drug consumption are acknowledged in several fields of knowledge. In this respect, the UNESCO, for example, distinguishes four types of drug users: the experimenter, who tries one or several types of drugs, but limits this contact to the first experience; the occasional user, who occasionally uses one or several drugs, but is not a drug dependent; the habitual user, that frequently uses drugs, but still functions socially; and the dependent user (also called a drug addict or toxicomaniac), who lives by and for the drugs, and has his/her social bonds severely hampered or even broken by them (Rezende, 2000). Hence, the definition of drug addiction does not include the modalities of drug use in which the subject, although he/she uses the drug, does not place it at the center and as a destructive element in his/her life, and manages to preserve the social ties.

As a result of the various criticisms to the abstinence proposal, many authors have considered that, given the impossibility or great difficulty to maintain abstinence and eradicate drugs, the most interesting posture to be adopted is to try to manage the effects of drug use and minimize the damage caused by it, as proposed by the harm reduction strategy (Rezende, 1999; Queiroz, 2001; Pratta & Santos, 2009). And in fact, although the zero-tolerance policy to drug use still prevails in some countries, many other, especially in the European Union, adopt the harm reduction approach in the prevention and treatment of drug addiction as well as in the problem arising from it (Marlatt & Witkiewitz, 2010; OEDT, 2011).

4. The proposal of the harm reduction strategy

Harm reduction[7] is currently defined as a public health strategy that targets at reducing the damage caused to the individuals' health and controlling the possible adverse consequences that result from the adoption of risk practices (Marlatt; Larimer & Witkiewitz, 2012). In the specific context of alcohol and other drugs, harm reduction implies a set of interventions with the purpose of preventing the negative consequences of the consumption of psychoactive substances, without the requirement of immediate and automatic abstinence.

Among these interventions, it is worth of notice the distribution of syringes, needles and pipes, the presentation of educational lectures and the referral of users that are outside the health services to specialized institutions. Besides, the harm reduction approach is also dedicated to teach the patient the supposedly most efficient way to deal with the variety of risk factors that lead to the abuse of psychoactive substances, in order to help the patient to reach the goal he/she established for him/her, be it the total abstinence or moderate consumption. Hence, harm reduction presents an alternative perspective to treatments based on the abstinence logic, when it considers possible to prevent the negative effects of drug addiction without its compulsory interruption.

---

[6] According to the report published by the UM in 2007, approximately 200 million people use drugs worldwide, and only one-eighth of these have dependence problems. The remaining are occasional users (Araújo, 2007).

[7] In some places, the term harm reduction is replaced by risk reduction, and these two terms are often used as synonymous, although they are not.

The harm reduction approach, as a general guideline for action, was originated in England in 1926, through the development of the Rolleston Report (Stevens, Hallam & Trace, 2006). A ministerial committee chaired by the UK Ministry of Health established that the most adequate treatment for certain patients would be the maintenance of the use of certain substances, thereby regulating the right of British doctors to prescribe opiates to addicts of this type of drug. In the same Report, it was established that the criterion adopted for this prescription should be the need, after several failed attempts at abstinence, to manage the syndrome caused by the abstention of certain substances, besides the observation that the patient would not be able to lead a normal and productive life without a minimal dose of the drug administered regularly (Brasil, 2001).

This procedure was known as substitution treatment, and until today is one of the harm reduction strategies used (Marlatt & Witkiewitz, 2010; Stevens, Hallam & Trace, 2006). It consists of changing the substance which the user is dependent on for another substance that will offer lower risk. The most common strategy is the substitution of heroin by methadone, a synthetic opioid agonist with long half-life, which is consumed orally, helps to relieve some of the heroin withdrawal symptoms, causes less organic and psychological damage and is considered a substance with lower addictive power. Although this model of treatment appeared in a context different from the current, it is still in use in several countries such as England, Holland, Croatia and Norway, among others, especially in the European Union (Alves, 2009; OEDT, 2011).

Thus, the initial objectives of the harm reduction approach were to make it possible for users who were psychoactive dependents to lead a more stable and useful life, and to minimize the harmful health effects of drug use. However, after the 1980's, with the spread of the HIV/AIDS virus due to the large contamination originated from the sharing of needles, the harm reduction strategies also aimed at preventing this contamination among the users of injectable drugs.

As a consequence, due to some positive results obtained in the prevention of contamination in several countries such as Belgium, Australia, Germany, Switzerland, France and others (Brasil, 2001; Paes, 2006), many harm reduction programs appeared as public health strategies. Brazil was one of the countries that has most recently adopted this approach, when in 1994 the harm reduction model was embraced as the official policy by the Health Ministry (Brasil, 2005), resulting from the recognition of the harmful use of alcohol and other drugs as a serious public health problem. In addition, the observation that the majority of drug users are not capable or do not want to stop consuming such substances weighed heavily on this decision[8]. However, it is important to point out that despite all the incentives created by the Brazilian government, there has not yet been a significant adherence to this strategy that would allow for the institutionalization of the harm reduction policy in the entire public health system (Passos & Souza, 2011).

From a public health perspective, the adoption of harm reduction as a strategy for the treatment of addiction to psychoactive substances aims to recover the users' self-regulating

---

[8] One of the reasons why drug users do not want and/or do not manage to interrupt the consumption is the fact that they have already incorporated the drugs they use to their personal and relationships routine (Rothschield, 2010). Besides, in most cases, such substances are a source of jouissance, which they are not willing to do without (Laxenaire, 2010; Olievenstein, 2002).

role and citizenship, while stimulating their inclusion and mobilization in the society, through the expansion of their social relationships and the increase of the chances within the society in which they live. Theoretically, the objectives of the harm reduction proposal can be reached through the adoption of certain strategies of action, namely those that seek to reach users who, due to their socio-economic characteristics (lack of permanent housing, close relationship with illegal practices, lack of health concerns, etc), are generally excluded from health services (Marlatt & Witkiewitz, 2010; Pinheiro, 2002; Stevens, Hallam & Trace, 2006). Furthermore, there are other strategies that intend to promote drug users' moderation of consumption, such as drug consumption rooms and target delivery of healthcare.

As a consequence, the harm reduction proposes that, with the implementation of this new treatment model, users of alcohol and other drugs can receive counseling and adequate treatment in order to avoid the most serious consequences of drug abuse, such as deaths by overdose, organic damages and virus contamination. This way, there is the hope of contributing to a safer drug use and a global and less prejudicial understanding of this phenomenon.

In fact, many authors argue that the treatment of drug users with the harm reduction approach is not only more efficient but also less costly, when compared to the abstinence model policies of drug use combat, because it contributes to decrease the number of deaths and illnesses associated to the use of drugs and to improve the social functioning of psychoactive substances users (Marlatt & Witkiewitz, 2010; OEDT, 2011; Stevens, Hallam & Trade, 2006). Nonetheless, this effectiveness is difficult to be supported by statistical data, partly because, although abstinence and harm reduction are grounded in apparently opposite philosophies, many drug users that start treatment with the objective of achieving abstinence end up redefining their goals during the process and begin to seek moderation in consumption (Neale, Nettleton & Pickering, 2010). From this perspective, in a number of health services, abstinence and harm reduction become part of the same treatment strategy, and can actually be used together (McKeganey, 2011). Besides, because studies on efficacy, effectiveness, and cost-effectiveness of the varied types of treatment have often employed methods and research designs of varied quality (such randomized controlled trials, clinical trials, case series, reviews, meta-analysis, etc), it is difficult to make a direct comparison of the different interventions. These are the reasons why there is a growing need for the development of more research focusing on these issues (CIAR, 2008).

In spite of this, it is possible to state that, because it places lower demands, the harm reduction proposal seems more attractive to many users, and decreases the number of patients that give up treatment (Alves, 2009; Rothschild, 2010). In addition, some authors defend that the rampant increase in the consumption of illicit drugs and the growth of the progression from the use of least to most powerful drugs are less frequent in countries and areas that adopt the harm reduction perspective (Alves, 2006; OEDT, 2011).

Especially because of these reasons, harm reduction is considered an "ethical landmark" in the field of prevention and treatment of disorders associated with the use of alcohol and other drugs. From this perspective, the proponents of harm reduction programs defend that this approach "recognizes each user in his/her *singularities*, designing with him/her the strategies to defend his/her life" (Brasil, 2005, p.42)[9].

[9] All the translations from the Portuguese original versions were made by the author.

However, it is worth debating whether the ethic that the harm reduction strategy deals with actually takes into account the subjectivity of each user. Regarding this aspect, it is important to highlight that, in mental health practices based on harm reduction, the place occupied by the subjective aspects of the one who resorts to intoxication remains open to questioning. In this respect, it is valid to inquire whether this approach considers the dimension of *jouissance* coupled with the intoxication practices[10].

This issue deserves a thorough, deep discussion, to avoid falling in the empty promise of change, which will lead us to trade a practice that just considers the use of drugs as a disease, either physical or spiritual, for another practice that takes the drug use in its exclusively social dimension. Hence, it is important to note that drug addiction is a complex and multifaceted phenomenon. Thus, it is not possible to adopt a reductionist position, be it biological, moral, social or psychological, in relationship to it. This reservation derives from the assumption, advocated by some authors, that social inclusion and citizenship recovery in mental health, though important, tends to neglect the subjective nature entailed by the psychic suffering and the mode of *jouissance* of each subject (Kyrillos Neto, 2007; Rinaldi, Cabral & Castro, 2008).

The request for the inclusion of the singularities and the listening of the patient in mental health practices is strongly considered by some psychoanalysts (Figueiredo & Tenório, 2002; Valentine & Fraser, 2008), who, although recognizing the advances obtained by psychosocial rehabilitation, highlight that the emphasis on the citizen of rights can lead the current mental health practices to a new kind of subjective dismissal (Fernandes & Freitas, 2009). This is because there is a contemporary perspective in psychoanalysis that adverts that any rehabilitation proposal can only succeed if it follows the subject's discourse, since the rehabilitation that denies the clinic will inevitably fall into the trap of re-education (Viganó, 1999).

In this way, to psychoanalysis, the emphasis is placed on the subject, which makes the psychoanalytical practice different from the other approaches that are centered on the social determinants of the phenomena considered psychopathological, in spite of the agency and subjective choices (Valentine & Fraser, 2008). Thus, the psychoanalytical treatment focuses attention on what the patient says about him/herself, since the meaning of the symptoms, and consequently, the production of what Freud (1905/1996) called 'talking cure', will only be possible to emerge from the elements that the subject him/herself brings. Hence, the importance of psychoanalysis lies in the fact that this approach opens a space in which the patient's talking can be listened to, interpreted and analyzed.

5. The psychoanalysis proposal

Thus, psychoanalysis also presents a specific proposal for treating users of alcohol and other drugs. This psychoanalytical proposal for the understanding and treatment of drug addictions was outlined along psychoanalysis' own history. For, in this field, it was Freud who first became interested in this phenomenon, laying the conceptual foundations that

[10] It is important to emphasize that, from the psychoanalytical perspective, every type of drug use provides some kind of jouissance. However, in the case of drug addiction, the jouissance provided invades and dominates the user, in such a way that the subject remains subjected to the psychoactive substances.

made possible the subsequent development of psychoanalytical-based propositions on drug use such as the ones developed by Abraham (1908), Rado (1933), Krystal (1975), Lacan (1976), McDougall (1978), Wurmser (1995), Khantzian (1995), among others. Although all the theories formulated by these authors refer to the conceptual field of psychoanalysis, they are very different. Explaining each one of them is beyond the scope of this chapter, so the following considerations are embedded in the framework of Lacanian psychoanalysis, which stands out for having remained faithful to the Freudian doctrine and for being the only one that can explain why, in the use of drugs, pleasure and harm are inexorably interwoven (Loose, 2000).

Nevertheless, it is important to highlight that, despite the existence of so many psychoanalytical readings on drug use, "the association between psychoanalysis and drug addiction is not common" (Laxenaire, 2010, p. 524). One reason is the fact that there is currently a strong demand for evidences of cost-effectiveness of the several existing treatments. And psychoanalysis is usually assessed as a long-term treatment, which proofs of efficacy are still insufficient (CIAR, 2008; Harrison et al, 2003). One of the main explanations for this assessment is the fact that psychoanalysis does not work on the same efficacy parameters that are adopted by other fields. Because the therapeutic efficacy is always related to a certain conception of cure and the psychoanalytical view of cure differs from the other fields, since psychoanalysis recognizes the existence of something incurable in the subject, and hence, is warned that it is not possible to ensure a full state of well-being, for suffering, to some extent, is at the core of human existence (Freud, 1930/1996; Lacan, 1966/1998; Loose, 2000). Even so, many psychoanalysts have published works that demonstrate promising effects of the psychoanalytical treatment for drug addiction through the reports of clinical cases[11] (Rothschield, 2010; Loose, 2000; Marlo & Kalinian, 2002).

To start discussing the treatment proposal oriented by psychoanalysis, it is crucial to highlight that the psychoanalytical treatment operates under a view that is radically different from the therapeutic proposal originated in the medical-psychiatric field and from the one derived from the moral field as well (Silva, 2010). This is because psychoanalysis works with the notion of the subject of the unconscious, conceived as being beyond the individual and beyond the illness.

The psychoanalytical concept of the unconscious refers to a psychic system that runs parallel to the conscious system, and that operates in a determined way, having an order and structure of its own (Fink, 1995). But, unlike the conscious system, the unconscious can only appear as a stumble, just in the gaps of the conscious manifestations, in what Lacan (1957/1999) coined as the formations of the unconscious: dreams, lapses, faulty actions (Freudian slips), jokes and symptoms, which reveal a meaning that so far had been hidden to the subject him/herself. By doing this, the unconscious indicates to the self the existence of an instance which is, at the same time, inside and conflicting with it.

Whereas the consciousness operates in articulation with the reality principle, the unconscious operates in articulation with the pleasure principle, and, most importantly,

[11] This method of demonstration of results is justified because, as psychoanalysis emphasizes the singularity and the subject, it would be absolutely incoherent to expect that its efficiency could be demonstrated by statistical evidence. Hence, what can be expected from further research in this field are meta-analysis based studies that provide within-subject measures related to drug consumption, demonstrating the improvement of drug users that have undergone psychoanalytical treatment.

with the beyond pleasure principle. Whereas the reality principle, because it is articulated to the material reality, makes detours and delays in search of satisfaction, the pleasure principle seeks satisfaction in the shortest and most direct way (Freud, 1911/1996). The beyond pleasure principle, in turn, is articulated to the death drive, which Freud (1920/1996) defined as a certain tendency, inherent to all living beings, to seek the pacification of all the tensions - which ultimately can only be achieved with death.

This is why, in psychoanalysis, the resource to intoxication is understood as a choice of the subject who, moved by the unconscious laws, searches actively for a *jouissance* that is extended towards death. To psychoanalysis, this search does not happen despite the subject, as other psychotherapeutic approaches propose. Yet, it is a choice[12] made by the subject him/herself, but a choice that does not come from rational and logic elements alone, but also results from desires that many times escape rationality, since they resort to the unconscious and are articulated to the death drive.

In fact, according to Laxenaire (2010), the unconscious search for death is well evidenced in drug addiction. Thus, one of the main particularities of the psychoanalytical proposal in comparison to the other treatment modalities lies on the emphasis given to the subjective structure at the expense of the pathological phenomenon. This is so much true that, while the medical-psychiatric diagnosis is most of the times phenomenological and based on a set of previously defined signs, the psychoanalytic diagnosis is structural and is from this structural diagnosis that the psychoanalytical treatment will develop.

The structural diagnosis refers to the differentiation of the three clinical structures: neurosis, psychosis and perversion, which concern the mode of the resolution of the Oedipus Complex. This diagnosis results from the evaluation of the position assumed by the subject before the Other (Figueiredo & Tenório, 2002). This is explained by the fact that, to psychoanalysis, what marks out the structuring of the human psychism is the relationship with the Other, understood not as another person, but as the whole symbolic universe to which the individual finds him/herself referred to (the discourses, rituals, codes, beliefs, etc). Although this symbolic universe is initially transmitted by one primordial other (such as the mother or the one who is in charge of the child's insertion in the world of language), in the Lacanian theory the Other represents the entire culture, and is considered an indispensable element for the human subject constitution, in that it makes it possible for the individual not to be a mere biological representative of the human species, but to become a being provided with thoughts and feelings, and inserted into social bonds (Lacan, 1939/1985). From this perspective, every human subject is dependent on the Other, since no subject can engender him/herself on his/her own (Laxenaire, 2010).

From this viewpoint, addiction would be a posterior dependence, but anchored exactly in the mode of relationship the subject established with the world around him/her (Laxenaire,

[12] The term choice is used by psychoanalysis not in the sense of a pondered decision, but as something that is chosen because it relates to what is most intimate to the subject, his/her unconscious. Hence, to psychoanalysis the choices are overdetermined by his/her psychic reality. In other words, psychoanalysis refers to choices that are not always rational, such as for example, the choice of abusive intoxication that many times threatens the subject. However, despite the sometimes hazardous effects caused by the subjective choices, psychoanalysis emphasizes how important it is for health professionals who work with drug addiction issues to keep alert to the fact that, in some way, users make the choice of intoxication.

2010). This is why the structural diagnosis is of paramount importance in the psychoanalytical treatment of drug addiction, keeping in sight that it will enlighten the reasons why the inexorable dependence on the Other was transmuted into the dependence on a fixed object, which may give access to a kind of *jouissance* that is steady and repetitive, and to which the subject, from a certain moment on, becomes subordinated.

Thus, psychoanalysis defends that if, in the beginning, the consumption of drugs has basically a recreational function, it is during its use that the drug, for some users, turns into a product that acquires a vital and indispensable role, configuring thereby an addiction. Several reasons converge to explain why addiction happens only in a subgroup of drug users. Among them are individual, social, economic, cultural and family factors. However, the psychoanalytical treatment emphasizes the subject that resorts to drugs, and consequently, to the particular function that drugs have in the psychism of each drug user and/or addict, and also highlights the importance of a diagnosis that differentiates between drug consumption and drug addiction.

Hence, from a psychoanalytical perspective, "it is necessary to differentiate the simple uses of stupefiers from the imperative of treatment of the organism by a toxic drug, when this becomes the only means to shelter, on a daily basis, the body from an intolerable pain" (Kaufmann, 1996, p. 542). Thus, to psychoanalysis, drug addiction is defined as an "intense and exclusive relationship, in which the use of drugs has already been established as a function in the subject's psychic life" (Conte, 2000, p. 11).

For this reason, from a psychoanalytical viewpoint, the drug is not a problem in itself, since what can become problematic is certain types of drug use that some subjects make, which can turn into a form of the subject's own destruction. This means that, in the psychoanalytical treatment of drug addiction, it is a matter of removing the biological characteristic from the drug (although not denying its existence), to give value to something else, converting it in something other than a simple object that produces psychological or physiological effects, which, by the way, can only be apprehended by the signifier, by what the patient reports. In this sense, if the treatment modalities based on abstinence claim that the drug makes the addict, to the extent that drugs are considered as having the supposedly intrinsic power to get the subjects addicted, psychoanalysis states that the drug addict makes the drug (Freda, 1989/1993), because it understands that this is a private relationship between the subject and the object, that grants to the latter the power to become a source of satisfaction which the subject himself cannot do without.

From a psychoanalytical point of view, then, the addictions and the symptom have similar forming mechanisms, insofar as they both are a solution to an underlying conflict, but a solution that is not perfect, since it does not solve everything. But even being imperfect, it is a repeated solution, because there is something in it that the subject is not willing to give up, despite all the suffering that it brings (Loose, 2000). Hence, in the psychoanalytical treatment for drug addiction, it is understood that the subject's choice to use drugs, the relapses and the excessive use of the psychoactive substance will only stop being an escape for the subject when the treatment enables him/her to find other forms of symbolization that allow him/her to abstain from drugs, in cases when this outcome is possible – for there are cases in which, due to a extremely unstable psychic configuration, the addiction is simply the one and only way the subject finds to manage to continue living.

Thus, in the psychoanalytical treatment, it is necessary to take into account the function and the meaning of the drug use to each subject, in order to make possible the identification of the relationship established between the subject and the drug. And to psychoanalysis, this identification is only viable when it comes from the knowledge produced by the subject him/herself during the treatment. According to this perspective, the role of the psychoanalyst in toxicomania treatments is to conduct a quality listening of the subject, enabling the emergence of the unsaid, of what is not obvious, of what is beyond the pleasure principle, which, by nature, point at the subject of the unconscious. In other words, if addictions result from the choice for a *jouissance* in the body, a *jouissance* that does not express itself through language, so the psychoanalytic treatment objective is to enable the subject to make a movement "from ad-diction to diction" (Loose, 2000, p. 80).

According to Loose (2000), drugs and alcohol can only exert massive and extreme effects on the subject because they work pushing him/her out or against the language domain. In this sense, re-inserting him/her in the symbolic chain, in the diction domain, means going exactly in the opposite direction of the drug effects. Thus, the main difference from the psychoanalytical treatment is due to the ethic that guides psychoanalysis, which is radically different from any moralizing perspective. This is because, similarly to the medical-psychiatric treatments, the treatments originated from the moral model assume to know, *a priori*, about the subject and what is supposed to be the best for him/her. This characteristic results from the fact that the moral model aims at responding to a social demand of standardization and adaptation of deviant behaviors, rather than fulfilling the users' needs. Hence, the treatments based on this model end up promoting the subject's orthopedic framing or re-education, to the extent that they intend to teach him/her what is considered as the adequate behavior, which is, in this case, the social ideology of sobriety and aims at a certain preservation of the other citizens' life.

Still in regard to the moral model of treatment, psychoanalysis advises that, when the professional embodies the position of knowing about the subject, there is no room for the subject to produce any knowledge about him/herself (Bastos, 2009). And in a context in which the subject is not given the means to produce his/her own knowledge, it is very likely that he/she will remain at the mercy of the professionals or institutions, being unable to make his/her own choices and/or to be responsible for them. Consequently, instead of becoming responsible, the subject under treatment remains in a state of tutelage, in which there is an attempt to remove all of his/her possible responses that do not conform to the expectations of the health professionals and institutions. In sum, the great contribution that psychoanalysis offers to the treatments of drug abuse and addiction is to call the attention to the fact that, if the subject choses his/her addiction as a solution that makes him/her suffer and at the same time brings him/her *jouissance*, then, only the subject him/herself is able to, through treatment, choose what to do with what affects his/her body and life so radically.

6. Psychoanalysis and harm reduction: controversies and convergences

Reviewing the literature, it is possible to confirm the extent to which psychoanalysis, while a specific field of knowledge, has long adopted a critical position with regard to the existing drug use treatments based on the mandatory abstinence (Conte, 2004; Melman, 2000; Queiroz, 2001; Rothschield, 2010). For this reason, in the first instance, it would be possible to identify an approximation between psychoanalysis and harm reduction proposals, insofar as they both problematize the model of treatment guided by the logic of abstinence.

In fact, according to Paes (2006), "the literature on drugs that has psychoanalytical basis has often been used by technicians who work on the training of harm reducers" (p. 129). Since the 1970s, there has been an increase in the number of professionals with a psychoanalytical focus, who offer chemical dependents a different kind of treatment and express serious criticism to the existent models of treatment (Paes, 2006). One of the main psychoanalysts that represent this viewpoint is the psychiatrist Claude Olievenstein, who, in the 1970s, founded the Centre Médical Marmottan, an institution for the treatment of drug addicts in Paris that became a benchmark and was inspirational for many treatment centers worldwide (Freda, 1989/1993; Marchant, 2010).

Queiroz (2001) also believes that it is possible to consider an approximation between the psychoanalytical assumptions and the harm reduction approach, insofar as the programs that adopt the latter introduce the "dimension of the particularity of the subject" (p. 3) and therefore, acknowledges "drug users as particular subjects and citizens, who have the right to health and to a treatment that is in fact effective and produces meaning" (Queiroz, 2001). In this case, the production of meaning refers to the fact that both the harm reduction policies and the psychoanalytical approach grant drug users the right to use drugs, which makes possible for them to build significations for this use without necessarily having to interrupt it (Marchant, 2010; Rotschild, 2010).

Adopting a similar perspective, Conte (2004) states that not only the harm reduction approach but also the advances achieved by the psychosocial rehabilitation paradigm do come close to psychoanalysis. According to the author, in both of them "there is the common refusal to flatten the subject to a passiveness that asks for social assistance or to a subject-body condition (organic and biologic) that asks for a "medicamental solution" (Conte, 2004, p.26).

On the other hand, Conte (2004) warns that the principles that underlie the harm reduction proposals are not the same that guide psychoanalysis, and in this respect, adverts that "the differences are due to *the ethic*, the objectives of the interventions and those who they turn to" (p. 27). Hence, this proposal of conciliation between the singularity dimension, represented by the subject's clinic and grounded in psychoanalysis, and the universal dimension, represented by the perspective of social rehabilitation and consequently, harm reduction, is not consensual.

In this respect, Dufour (2004) presents a more critical position regarding the social emphasis given by some mental health policies, and advocates that "it is not about encouraging carelessness - as one is soon blamed when one shows the slightest reservation about the humanitarian conduct - but observing the effects, opposed to the desired ones, caused by the coercive kindness" (p.37). Therefore, the author indicates the existence of a certain amount of coercion in the psychosocial rehabilitation practices in mental health, and makes sure to explicitly include the harm reduction proposal under this view.

When referring to the movement that he coined as "to limit the damage" or "reduce the harm", Dufour (2004) states that:

the surprising fact in this type of proposal is that it does not take into consideration the opinion of the ones involved. It searches for their happiness and health, regardless of them. Some rebel against it. For example, a patient who lived with an HIV-positive woman used to say about precautions: 'you know, for me, making plastified love is not my business' (p.37).

It is important to pinpoint that, as previously mentioned, because it is a public health strategy, harm reduction is inserted in the psychosocial rehabilitation logic. Then, the harm reduction objectives are to reduce the damage caused by the use of psychoactive substances, and promote the bio-psychosocial well being of the health service users, having for main focus of attention the citizen of universal rights. Therefore, harm reduction aims to provide a treatment for everyone, and is thus based on the principle of equal rights and connected to the universal dimension. This universalizing perspective in public health and in harm reduction may bring a number of complicating factors in regard to the possibility of approximation with psychoanalysis, which points to the singularity of each subject's treatment.

Henceforth, although psychoanalysis and harm reduction may initially come close, because they both oppose the abstinence model, the possibilities of convergence between these two fields need to be more deeply investigated. Whereas psychoanalysis adopts an ethic that foregrounds the subjective position and the modality of *jouissance* achieved by the intoxication practices, the harm reduction approach, being a public health strategy, advocates in its principles the bio-psychosocial well being of the health service users.

7. Final considerations

In the mental health field, it is possible to outline the existence of at least three prevalent models: the exclusively biomedical or pharmacological, the exclusively sociological and the subjective (Rigter at al, 2004; Kyrillos Neto, 2007). The exclusively organicist model has as its object the mental disorders, taken as a "biologizing degradation of nosology", that ignores the subjective, political and social aspects of the psychic suffering, and has the purpose of treating them exclusively through the psychopharmaceutical sovereignty. In the specific context of alcohol and drug abuse, it would be possible to state that this model guides its treatments by abstinence, insofar as they do not consider the subjective and social issues that the use of psychoactive substances imply, and seem to give importance only to the neurochemical effects caused by toxic drugs.

On the other hand, the exclusively sociological model takes as its object the man in his suffering existence, and is guided by the notion of individual originated from the liberal ideology and the human rights advocated by the constitution of the democratic regime. This model draws attention to the need for development and empowerment of individuals and communities so that, thereafter, they become able to have democratic participation in the actions devised to protect and promote their own health (Duggan, Cooper & Foster, 2002). It is possible to approximate this sociological model to some proposals derived from the psychosocial rehabilitation perspective, insofar as these place the emphasis on the citizen of universal rights and on the socio-political dimension. Thus, in the realm of the treatments offered to drug users, we can assume that this exclusively sociological model would be represented by the harm reduction approach.

Finally, the subjective model has as its object the "subject of desire", defined by Lacan (1969/1992) as constituted from its position before the Other. Among the existing proposals for the treatment of drug abuse, this subjective model is almost exclusively represented by psychoanalysis.

According to Kyrillos Neto (2007), it is noticeable that, unfortunately, these three models are considered mutually exclusive in most health mental services. However, it is important to highlight that overcoming the impasses that arise daily in these services depends on an approach that does not rely only on the exclusive considerations of the social determinations nor on a purely clinical focus, but rather on the articulation of these important factors.

Consequently, it is necessary that the harm reduction strategies, when proposed as a mental health policy, be able to reach these multiple sides that outline the complexity of the phenomenon of drug abuse and addiction. In this respect, psychoanalysis has great contributions to offer, since the psychoanalytical treatment aims at promoting the articulation between the universal aspect of the structure and the singular nature of the psychic reality of each individual, allowing the treatment of the universal (the structure) through the singular (the subject).

Hence, despite the recognized need for more research in the field of treatments offered to drug users, it is important to ponder that any proposed treatment cannot leave out the consideration for the psychic aspects involved in the phenomenon of drug addiction (OEDT, 2011). This is why current reports have demanded more studies analyzing the effects generated by the several types of existing psychological interventions, considering that, until now, the collected data are not sufficient to show evidence of the compared efficacy of each intervention. However, many studies suggest that such interventions are fundamental to act upon both the causes and the psychological consequences associated to drug use, especially when combined with other treatments, such as, for instance, the substitution treatments (CIAR, 2008; Marlatt; Larimer & Witkiewitz, 2012). And it is precisely in this context that psychoanalysis becomes a treatment proposal that, for placing the subject as the focus of any therapeutic action, presents itself as extremely promising.

8. References

Abraham, K. (1908/1927). The psychological relations between sexuality and alcoholism. *Selected Papers on Psychoanalysis*. London: Karnac.

Alves, V. S. (2009). Modelos de atenção à saúde de usuários de álcool e outras drogas: discursos políticos, saberes e práticas. *Cadernos de saúde pública*, 25 (11), p. 2309-2319.

Araújo, T. (2007). Drogas: proibir é legal? *Revista Superinteressante, 244*, p. 62-71. São Paulo: Ed. Abril.

Bastos, A. (2009). *Considerações sobre a clínica psicanalítica na instituição pública destinada ao atendimento de usuários de álcool e/ou drogas*. (MA Dissertation). Universidade do Estado do Rio de Janeiro, Rio de Janeiro, RJ.

Brasil (2001). *Manual de Redução de Danos*. Brasília: Ministry of Health.

Brasil (2005). *Reforma Psiquiátrica e Política de Saúde Mental no Brasil*. Brasília: Ministry of Health.

Carneiro, H. (2006). As drogas no Brasil: entre o delírio e o perigo. *Revista Nossa História, 33,* p. 12-26. São Paulo: Ed. Vera Cruz.

Conte, M. (2000). *A clínica psicanalítica com toxicômanos: o corte & costura no enquadre institucional*. (PhD Thesis). Pontifícia Universidade Católica de São Paulo, São Paulo, SP.

Conte, M. (2004). Psicanálise e redução de danos: articulações possíveis. *Revista da Associação Psicanalítica de Porto Alegre, 26,* p. 23-33.

Decker, S. H. (2008). *Drug Smugglers on Drug Smuggling: lessons from the inside*. Philadelphia: Temple University Press.

Director, L. (2005). Encounters with omnipotence in the psychoanalysis of substance users. *Dialogues,* 15 (4), p. 567-584.

Dufour, A. (2004). Opiacidade. *Revista da Associação Psicanalítica de Porto Alegre,* 26, p. 34-57.

Duggan, M.; Cooper, A. & Foster, J. (2002). *Modernising the social model in mental health: a discussion paper*. England: SPN by Topss.

Faria, J. G. & Schneider, D. R. (2009). O perfil dos usuários do CAPS ad-Blumenal e as políticas públicas em saúde mental. *Psicologia e Sociedade, n. 21,* vol. 3, pp. 324-333.

Fernandes, A. & Freitas, L. (2009). Tempos de reforma psiquiátrica: a clínica da recepção e a direção do tratamento no Hospital Juliano Moreira de Salvador - Bahia. *Psicologia: Teoria e Prática, n. 11,* vol. 1, 2009, p. 97-109.

Figueiredo, A. C. & Tenório, F. (2002). O diagnóstico em psiquiatria e psicanálise. *Revista Latinoamericana de Psicopatologia Fundamental, vol. 5,* n. 1, p. 29-43, mar/ 2002.

Fink, B. (1995). *The Lacanian Subject: between language and jouissance*. Princeton: Princeton University Press.

Freda, H. (1989/1993). Quem lhe disse isso? *Coletânea de textos sobre toxicomania e alcoolismo do Centro Mineiro de Toxicomania* (p. 1-13). Belo Horizonte: Centro Mineiro de Toxicomania.

Freud, S. (1905/1996). Fragmento da análise de um caso de histeria. In: *Edição Estandard Brasileira das Obras Psicológicas Completas* (Vol. VII.). Rio de Janeiro: Imago.

Freud, S. (1911/1996). Dois princípios do funcionamento psíquico. In: *Edição Estandard Brasileira das Obras Psicológicas Completas* (Vol. XII.). Rio de Janeiro: Imago.

Freud, S. (1920/1996). Além do princípio do prazer. In: *Edição Estandard Brasileira das Obras Psicológicas Completas* (Vol. XVIII.). Rio de Janeiro: Imago.

Freud, S. (1930/1996). O Mal-estar na Civilização. In: *Edição Estandard Brasileira das Obras Psicológicas Completas* (Vol. XXI.). Rio de Janeiro: Imago.

Goffmann, E. (1985/2001). *A representação do eu na vida cotidiana*. Petrópolis, RJ: Vozes.

Harrison, L.; Cappello, R.; Alaszewski, A.; Appleton, S. & Cooke, G. (2003). *The effectiveness of treatment for substance dependence within the prison system in England: a review*. Canterbury, Kent: Centre for Health Services Studies.

Kaufmann, P. (1996). *Dicionário Enciclopédico de Psicanálise*. Rio de Janeiro: Jorge Zahar Ed.

Khantzian, E. (1995). Self-regulation vulnerabilities in substance abusers: treatment implications. In: Dowling, S. (Ed.). *The psychology and treatment of addictive behavior*, Madison, CT: International Universities Press.

Krystal, H. (1975). Affect tolerance. *Annual of Psychoanalysis*, 3, p. 179-219.

Kyrillos Neto, F. (2007). *Efeitos de circulação do discurso em serviços substitutivos de saúde mental*. (PhD Thesis). Pontifícia Universidade Católica de São Paulo, São Paulo, SP.

Lacan, J. (1939/1985). *Os complexos familiares na formação do indivíduo*. Rio de Janeiro: Jorge Zahar Ed.

Lacan, J. (1957/1999). *O Seminário, Livro V: As formações do inconsciente*. Rio de Janeiro: Jorge Zahar Ed.

Lacan, J. (1966/1998). A ciência e a verdade. *Escritos*. Rio de Janeiro: Jorge Zahar Ed.

Lacan, J. (1969/1992). *O Seminário, Livro XVII: o avesso da psicanálise*. Rio de Janeiro: Jorge Zahar Ed.

Lacan, J. (1976). Journées des cartels de l'École Freudienne de Paris. *Lettres de l'École Freudienne*, Paris, 18, p. 263-270.

Laxenaire, M. (2010). Psychanalyse et addictions sans substances. *Annales Médico-Psychologiques*, 168, p. 524-527.

Loose, R. (2000). The addicted subject caught between the ego and drive: the post-freudian reduction and simplification of a complex clinical problem. *Psychoanalytische Perspectieven*, 41/42.

Marchant, A. (2010). Answering drug epidemic at the beginning of the 1970s: experimenting new patterns, creating new practices, building standardization in matters of help care policy. *Conference Standardizing and Marketing the Drugs in the XXth Century*. History of Medicine University La Charité: Berlin (Allemagne), 7-8th October, 2010.

Marlatt, G. A. & Witkiewitz, K. (2010). Update on Harm-Reduction Policy and Intervention Research. *Annual Revue Psychology*, 6, p. 591-606.

Marlatt; G. A.; Larimer, M. E. & Witkiewitz, K. (2012). *Harm reduction: pragmatic strategies for managing high-risks behaviors*. New York: The Guilford Press.

Marlo, H. & Kalinian, H. (2002). Utilizing psychoanalytic psychotherapy in the treatment of substance abusers. *Clinical Psychology and Psychotherapy*, 9, p. 211-223.

McDougall, J. (1978). *Plea for a measure of abnormality*. New York: International Universities Press.

McKeganey, N. (2011). Abstinence and harm reduction: can they work together? *International Journal of Drug Policy*, doi: 10.1016/j.drugpo.2011.04.001.

Mcrae, E. (2001). Antropologia: aspectos sociais, culturais e ritualísticos. In: Seibel, S. & Toscano JR., A. (Eds.). *Dependência de drogas*. São Paulo: Atheneu.

Melman, C. (2000). *Alcoolismo, delinqüência e toxicomania – uma outra forma de gozar*. São Paulo: Escuta.

Nery Filho, A. & Torres, I. M. A. (Eds.) (2002). *Drogas: isso lhe interessa? Confira aqui.* Salvador: CETAD/UFBA/CPTT/PMV.

OEDT (2011). *Relatório anual 2011: a evolução do fenômeno da droga na Europa.* Luxemburgo: Serviço das Publicações da União Européia.

Paes, P. (2006). *Ensino e aprendizagem na prática da Redução de Danos.* (PhD Thesis). Universidade Federal de São Carlos, São Carlos, SP.

Passos, E. H. & Souza, T. P. (2011). Redução de danos e saúde pública: construções alternativas à política global de "guerra às drogas". *Psicologia & Sociedade,* 23 (1), p. 154-162.

Pinheiro, R. (2006). Redução de Danos e psicanálise aplicadas à toxicomania. In: Cirino, O. & Medeiros, R. (Eds.). *Álcool e outras drogas: escolhas, impasses e saídas possíveis.* Belo Horizonte: Autêntica.

Pratta, E. M. M. & Santos, M. A. (2009). O processo saúde-doença e a dependência química: interfaces e evolução. *Psicologia: Teoria e Pesquisa, n. 2,* vol. 25, p. 203-211.

Queiroz, I. (2001). Os programas de redução de danos como espaços de exercício da cidadania dos usuários de drogas. *Psicologia: ciência e profissão, 21,* 4, dez/ 2001.

Rado, S. (1933/1984). The Psychoanalysis of Pharmacothymia. *Journal of Substance Abuse Treatment,* I, p. 59-68.

Rezende, M. (1999). *Tratamento com dependentes de drogas: diálogos com profissionais da área de saúde mental.* (PhD Thesis). Universidade Estadual de Campinas, Campinas, SP.

Rezende, M. (2000). Uso, abuso e dependência de drogas: delimitações sociais e científicas. *Revista Psicologia & Sociedade, 12,* 144-155.

Rigter, H.; Van Gageldonk, A.; Ketelaars, T. & Van Laar, M. (2004). *Treatment of problematic use of drugs. State of the art for evidence based treatments and other interventions.* Utrecht (Niederlande): Trimbos Institute.

Rinaldi, D.; Cabral, L. & Castro, G. (2008). Psicanálise e reabilitação psicossocial: limites e possibilidades de articulação. *Revista Estudos e Pesquisas em Psicologia, vol. 8,* n. 1, jan./abr. 2008.

Rothschild, D. (2010). Partners in treatment: relational psychoanalysis and harm reduction therapy. *Journal of Clinical Psychology: In Session,* 66 (2), p. 136-149.

Seibel, S. & Toscano Jr., A. (Eds.). *Dependência de drogas.* São Paulo: Atheneu.

Schulte, B.; Thane, K.; Rehm, J.; Uchtenhagen, A; Stöver, H.; Degkwitz, P & Reimer, C. (2008). *Review of the efficacy of drug treatment interventions in Europe.* Hamburg: Centre for InterdiscipIinary Adicction Research (CIAR).

Silva, J. R. (2010). *A clínica psicanalítica das toxicomanias.* (MA Dissertation). Universidade do Estado do Rio de Janeiro, Rio de Janeiro, RJ.

Stevens, A.; Hallam, C. & Trace, M. (2006). *Treatment for dependent drug use: a guide for policymakers.* Beckley: The Beckley Foundation Drug Policy Programme.

Viganó, C. (1999). A construção do caso clínico em saúde mental. *Curinga - Psicanálise e Saúde Mental, n. 13,* set./1999.

Valentine, K. & Fraser, S. (2008). Trauma, damage and pleasure: rethinking problematic drug use. *International Journal of Drug Policy,* 19, p. 410-416.

WHO (2004). *Neurociências: consumo e dependência de substâncias psicoativas*. Genebra: WHO Library Cataloguing-in Publication Data.

Wurmser, L. (1995). *The hidden dimension: psychodynamics of compulsive drug use*. New Jersey: Jason Aronson Inc.

14

The Interactional Approach in the Treatment of Cocaine Addicts

Andrea Leonardi, Sonia Scavelli and Gianluca Ciuffardi
Fondazione Franceschi Onlus,
Italy

"A living system, due to its circular organization, is an inductive system and functions always in a predictive manner; what occurred once will occur again. Its organization (both genetic and otherwise) is conservative and repeats only that which works."
Humberto Maturana

1. Introduction

Over the last few years cocaine use has spread considerably to all social levels. According to statistical data currently available, cocaine is the psychoactive substance most frequently used in Europe, after cannabis (European Monitoring Centre for Drugs and Drug Addiction [EMDDA], 2011). Italy is one of the European countries where such consumption is more frequent: about 7% of the population report to have used cocaine at least once in their lifetime (Presidenza del Consiglio dei Ministri, 2007).

Cocaine is an alkaloid substance obtained from coca leaves, which acts on the central nervous system, especially on the dopamine system, compromising its functions. Cocaine use contributes to increased concentration of dopamine, a neurotransmitter that is present in different brain areas that governs cognition, emotional processes, motivation and associative processes related to feelings of pleasure. Normally, this neurotransmitter is released by neurons in response to a salient, pleasant stimuli, and then it is absorbed by the same cells that have produced it. Cocaine acts on these cells by blocking the recovery of dopamine, resulting in an accumulation of the neurotransmitter between synapses.

Repeated cocaine use damages the normal communication between neurons, leading to alterations in brain circuits for pleasure that is thought to contribute to the development of dependence. In addition, the brain needs progressively higher doses of the psychoactive substance to achieve the same effects and it needs increasing use in order to achieve the same levels of pleasure originally experienced (National Institute on Drug Abuse [NIDA], 2008).

The psychological effects of cocaine depend both on the amount consumed and on the route and modality of administration (Braglia et al., 2004): these effects consist mainly of sensations of euphoria, increased libido, reduction of hunger and thirst, and in the impression of increased perceptual abilities, but they may also generate panic attacks, mood disorders, paranoid ideation and induction of psychotic states with auditory, visual and tactile hallucinations (Braglia et al., 2004). Among the various routes of administration, the intravenous injection and the cocaine smoke are those causing a more rapid and intense action, while sniffing cocaine determines longer lasting effects, up to 30 minutes versus the 10 minutes of the smoke (NIDA, 2008).

Based on currently available data, cocaine addiction is a complex phenomenon in which various factors interact; there are those that are dependent on the central nervous system and therefore biological and those that are related to a certain lifestyle that from the point of view of the cocaine addict would encourage new opportunities for social meetings, sexual gratification and friendship (Rigliano, 2004).

2. Main therapeutic intervention protocols

Despite the considerable and ever increasing spread of cocaine, therapeutic intervention protocols that exist today in Europe are unfortunately still being tested and often result from treatment of other forms of addiction, such as heroin (EMCDDA, 2007a).

The pharmacological approach intervenes with the neurobiological systems involved in reinforcement and the long-term effects of drugs, thereby reducing the symptoms of abstinence. Most recently, some vaccines have also been developed based on the principle of using the properties of the immune system to counteract cocaine effects, preventing it from reaching the brain (Pirona & Hendrich, 2009).

The pharmacological approach, although representing a significant step forward in the care and treatment of cocaine dependence, has not proven sufficient to effectively treat cocaine addiction. The reason for this is that cocaine addicts continue to remember the pleasurable effects and states of arousal produced by the substance, and the attempt to reduce any pre-existing states of discomfort through the use of the psychoactive substance. Therefore, it is essential to integrate the pharmacological approach into a psychosocial and psychological treatment.

Among the various psychological orientations that have been proposed, those which have demonstrated a good level of effectiveness are as follows:

2.1 Cognitive Behavioural Therapy

Cognitive Behavioural Therapy (CBT) (Carroll, 1998) that treats cocaine addiction as a problematic behaviour depending on cognitive and environmental factors. Treatment is usually delivered on an outpatient basis and it lasts from 12 to 16 sessions, usually over 12 weeks. An individual format is preferred, because it makes possible to fit the treatment to the needs of each patient.

According to CBT, the learning processes are important factors for the development and the maintenance of cocaine use, but the same processes may be useful for helping the patient stop his drug use. So, CBT tries to assist the patient to recognize the situations in which he most probably takes cocaine, to avoid these circumstances if it is possible and to manage the difficulties and the problematic behaviours related to the cocaine use. CBT has two important components:

- *functional analysis*, that is, the identification of the patient's thoughts, feelings and circumstances before and after cocaine use. The functional analysis is helpful to assess the factors, or high-risk situations, that are likely to lead to cocaine consumption and it can gives insights into some of the causes of this use;

- *skills training*, aimed at unlearning the patient's habits associated with cocaine use and learning healthier skills and habits. At the beginning the skill training focuses on the practical and mental abilities which are useful to stop cocaine use. Then, the training is extended to other possible problems with which the patient may have difficulty facing (Carroll, 1998).

So, CBT encourages subjects to assume alternative behaviours than those associated with substance use (EMCDDA, 2007a).

2.2 Contingency Management Therapy

Contingency Management Therapy (Petry, 2002), based upon the principles of behaviour modification. This consists of providing positive reinforcement (in the form of clinic privileges, vouchers or payment) when the patient achieves given behaviours or treatment goals. In particular, for cocaine users this reinforcement is related to the urine tests carried out periodically (Higgins et al., 2000).

This therapy has four main values:

- *defining a target behaviour*, that is, what outcome the patient has to achieve. For example, drug abstinence and undertaking clinic and social activities related to a drug-free lifestyle;
- *regular monitoring of target behaviour* that has to be unequivocally assessed (for example, regular urine analysis would be undertaken to verify the patient's abstinence);
- *reward contingent on achievement of target behaviour*: at pre-established levels and frequencies, rewards are given to or retained by the patient depending on whether or not the target behaviours are achieved;
- *reinforcement* by brief counselling to reinforce the positive effects of the rewards (Weaver et al., 2007).

2.3 The Motivational Interview

The Motivational Interview (MI) (Miller & Rollnick, 2002) approach is a client-centred, directive method aimed at understanding the motives the patients have for addressing their substance use problems, to gather the clinical information needed to plan their care and to build and reinforce their readiness for change. The MI approach consists of short-term intervention to help the person in the changing process towards a healthier lifestyle through the resolution of ambivalence, that is, the tendency to provide opposite emotional responses to cocaine.

According to the MI, the patient can be in one of the following four stages of change:

- *pre-contemplation stage*, in which the patient does not want to change his behaviour;
- *contemplation stage*, when the patient would like to change, but he does not know how to do it;
- *preparation stage*, in which the person shows explicitly the intention to change;
- *action stage*, in which the patient realizes practical changes to feel better (Di Clemente & Velasquez, 2002).

2.4 Modified Dynamic Group Therapy

Modified Dynamic Group Therapy (MDGT) (Khantzian et al., 1990) aims to solve the problems of low self-esteem that lead the subjects to consume the substance. According to this theory, low self-esteem produces a "psychological vulnerability" which can predispose a person to drug use and decrease impulse control. The purpose of MDGT consists of helping patients become aware of their psychological vulnerability. This approach has four main therapeutic focuses:

- developing a better affective tolerance;
- improving self-esteem;
- improve interpersonal relationships;
- development of appropriate strategies of "self-care".

MDGT lasts about 6 months and has 3 main stages:

- during the first stage therapy consists of encouraging patients to address their vulnerability through better confidence resulting from the support of other members of the therapy and mutual listening;
- in the middle stage the attention is on members' attachment to the group, taken as a whole;
- in the last stage the older members take on the role of "co-therapists" and explain aspects of MDGT to new members.

So, the MDGT intervenes not only on drug use, but also in the self and on the relationship between some personality aspects and problems that can lead to relapse (Khantzian et al., 1990).

3. The interactional approach

The Interactional Approach (IA) is a type of psychological intervention that includes specific therapeutic techniques and procedures for the treatment of cocaine addiction.

Attempting to solve the problem of cocaine addiction, our research group has developed a short-term psychotherapeutic model, directed to increase the patient's interpersonal and communicative skills, to improve emotional control and the use of meta-cognitive resources, to adopt a healthy lifestyle, leading eventually to reduced risk of relapse. The proposed outpatient treatment has led to good results both in terms of effectiveness and efficiency (Leonardi et al., 2006, 2009; Leonardi & Velicogna, 2009).

At the basis of the psychological intervention there are studies on the processes of persuasive communication (Erickson et al., 1976; Erickson & Rossi, 1981), as well as theoretical models derived from constructivism (von Foerster, 1982; von Glasersfeld, 1984), the interactional approach (Jackson, 1961, 1965; Fisch et al., 1982; Watzlawick et al. 1967, 1974, 1984, 1997) and those derived from action research (Lewin, 1946).

Constructivism is a theoretical approach that challenges the idea that knowledge can be "objective", arguing that each man builds his own reality through cognition, sensory perception and communication processes. What the person sees and knows is a construction based on his own experiences. Therefore, from a psychological point of view it becomes essential to try to understand the meaning that individuals attribute to their experiences, how they organize their knowledge and the expectations they have about what will happen to them. Other authors who have contributed to develop this approach were Maturana and Varela (1980), who studied the way in which living systems are regulated and organized in their environment.

The interactional model is applied to relational aspects and it is based on the concept that psychological disorders depend on the interaction between the subject and his own perception of reality: the aim of the therapy is to facilitate the change through appropriate strategies, so that individuals can look at their problems in a different way and take the best solutions.

It often happens that just the *attempted solutions*[1], implemented by the person, contribute to complicate the problem inadvertently, while with appropriate strategies it becomes possible to change the patient's *perceptive-reactive system*, as well as his perspectives which are too rigid. The perceptive-reactive system is defined as the way a person constructs the three fundamental relationships: with himself, the others and the world. Thus, by intervening it is possible to change the processes of attribution of meaning to things over the perception of the problem (Nardone & Watzlawick, 1990).

In accordance with Franz Alexander (Alexander & French, 1946), the change is due to the *corrective emotional experience* that helps to modify initially set perceptions and in doing so engaging a virtuous process of learning new skills and competencies in the social sphere. Therefore, the scope of the interactional and constructivist therapy is to get the patient to change his perceptive-reactive system, through the experimentation with new and different strategies.

With regard to the interactional aspects, *injunctive and evocative language* is also really important: its aim is not to describe the surrounding reality, but to prescribe certain behaviours within a therapeutic relationship full of suggestion. Such injunctions can be very useful to interrupt the patient's dysfunctional patterns. The *injunctive and evocative language* is used to persuade the other to engage in specific tasks. Through the execution of such tasks the patient may perceive reality in a different way (Watzlawick, 1978).

Finally, our methodology of psychological treatment takes into consideration some aspects such as the neurological functional difference between the two hemispheres of the human brain. The left hemisphere uses a logical-analytical coding system and it specializes in the perception and in language, while the right one is involved in non-linguistic tasks such as recognition of their own and others' emotions or in activities that involve analogical processing such as the perception of images, configurations and contexts in their overview (Gazzaniga, 1972). The study of different functional specializations has been possible thanks to research on patients suffering from epilepsy and who had the corpus callosum surgically sectioned, a brain structure that represents the most important area linking the two hemispheres. Those studies revealed that the two hemispheres work in close synergy with each other, although responding to specific stimuli to their functional area, and that they are also highly integrated and complementary (Sperry, 1968).

According to Watzlawick (1978), a specific language is able to communicate and influence each of the two hemispheres, in order to activate one at the expense of the other: for example, evocative language and *hypnosis without trance*[2] (Erickson et al., 1976) are communicative modalities that can influence the right hemisphere. The purpose of these

---

[1] The *attempted solutions* are actions that a person does to try to solve his problem. If they do not lead to the resolution of the problem and if repeated, these solutions further complicate the situation preventing the change (Watzlawick et al., 1974). From the perspective of the therapist, the attempted solutions function as reducing complexity in the assessment of the clinical case examined.

[2] Without using formal hypnosis, Milton Erickson (Erickson et al., 1976) states that it is possible to realize a communicative exchange characterized by persuasion, control of attention and suggestion, which is able to bypass resistance to change.

communicative approaches consists of evoking certain images in the patient, as with the storytelling of metaphors, aphorisms and anecdotes. As a point of fact, these communicative modalities serve to bypass the normal resistance to change and provide easier access to unconscious psychological resources (Erickson et al., 1976).

In the therapeutic relationship, the use of suggestion, as well as the evocation of images, allows patients to gradually change their behaviours.

The experience "on their skin" of such behaviours allows the persons to realize that new ways of handling their problems are possible. The cognitive restructuring of these new experiences contributes to maintaining over time the modifications that have progressively occurred.

4. The five phases of the interactional model for the treatment of cocaine addiction

Our model is applied to both individual and group therapy. It can be divided into five phases of intervention that are interconnected with many levels of communication: each of these five phases is characterized by specific objectives and the achievement of each one allows access to the next level (Leonardi et al. 2006, 2009; Leonardi & Velicogna, 2009).

4.1 Evaluation-intervention

The purpose of the first phase is to collect useful information to explain how cocaine addiction has been established, to evaluate the level of motivation and to begin simultaneously the intervention aimed at changing.

Unlike what happens with other therapeutic approaches, such as Cognitive Behavioural Therapy (CBT) (Carroll, 1998), which uses more linear intervention strategies, our model consists of a sequence of self-corrective operations aimed at progressively increasing the effectiveness of care, which is accompanied by a circular type system of interaction with the patient. This happens from the first stage, in which there is no distinction between diagnosis and intervention. This distinction characterizes the traditional approach to the problem of cocaine addiction, where the time of diagnosis is considered free from possible communication influences.

During this initial phase, the therapist:

- investigates and assesses the overall situation;
- recalls situations associated with cocaine use;
- plans the most effective communication strategies to change the way the patient relates to the substance.

After collecting information on a person's life, the therapist identifies those elements that may have influenced the development of cocaine dependence (anamnesis). In parallel, he also seeks to assess the patient's level of motivation to change, which generally falls into one of the following categories:

- the person is motivated to seek help;
- the person is slightly motivated to seek help and forced into treatment by the family;

- the person is not motivated to change at all.

The elements of this scheme are additional to the already described usual resistance to change of the dysfunctional systems (Haley, 1963; Nardone, & Watzlawick, 1990).

The start time of problematic cocaine use and whether it coincided with a traumatic event should be assessed carefully (Leonardi & Velicogna, 2009).

It often happens that people who have occasionally used cocaine for fun or curiosity, increase their use considerably as a result of difficult situations that need to be addressed (such as bereavements, emotional loss, work problems, etc.), until the onset of a real physical and psychological dependence. Therefore, the therapist has to not only take care of the drug addiction behaviour, but he must attend also to the potential event that made things worse. Finding the possible reason that has contributed to the subsequent loss of control by the cocaine addict allows him to address the "real" problem that caused the suffering that he has tried to quell using cocaine (Leonardi & Velicogna, 2009).

Another important factor to take into consideration concerns modes of taking cocaine (which can be sniffed, smoked or injected into veins), because the therapeutic intervention must be calibrated depending on the method of intake of the substance. For example, in the case of cocaine injected into veins, in our experience we are often in the presence of a former heroin consumer that, maybe after years of abstinence, has decided to switch to cocaine and this must be taken into account in the psychological intervention. In the case of smoked and sniffed cocaine the sensory, perceptive and imagination techniques change, although the process of therapeutic intervention is similar.

During this first phase (see Table 1), the therapist adopts a style of communication aimed at increasing the level of the patient's motivation to overcome his natural resistance to change: through questions that explore the problem, we aim to change both the perceptions and reactions to the substance.

First phase of treatment	First level of therapeutic communication
• History and evaluation of general areas • Motivational levels • Outset • Intensity • Modality • Frequency	• Persuasive communication • Hypnosis without trance

Table 1. The evaluation-intervention.

For example, if a patient has just conjured up feelings of isolation and loneliness in relation to cocaine use, the therapist could explain this perception by means of a metaphor, comparing the patient to a person who is locked in by himself inside a cold and dark cell. This image evokes a painful sensation, but, at the same time, it produces a very refined restructuring because if a person has been able to enclose himself within a cell, he is also able to open it and to get out. As stated above, according to constructivist theory, the person may know and interact with the world around him through his own actions. Thus, an "objective" knowledge of reality is not possible, it depends upon the observer's point of view. But often the person is not aware of that building process. Rather, for that person knowledge has the value of "objective" truth and strongly influences his thoughts and actions (Nardone & Watzlawick, 1990).

On the one hand the interactional intervention works on the problem, on the other it has the aim of helping the patient to gradually build a different reality (De Shazer, 1985).

4.1.1 First clinical interviews

The first clinical interviews with cocaine users are crucial in order to explore the ways to develop the treatment. They serve to gather a preliminary knowledge of the individual and to lay the groundwork for increasing motivation to change: the patient describes in detail his problematic situation, which is compounded by drug-induced automatisms and compulsions.

Generally, people who seek psychological help for a problem of abuse and cocaine addiction have three levels of complexity that prevent the change:

- at the first level there is the inevitable resistance that occurs in this clinical setting, (Mascetti & Strepparola, 2006);
- at the second level lie the neurobiological modifications induced by cocaine use that render the brain less susceptible to changes (Shaham & Hope, 2005a; Edwards & Koob, 2010);
- finally, at the third level there is a lack of motivation of those who have been forced by family to undergo treatment.

Because of these difficulties, which are added to by the specific problems due to cocaine use, in this preliminary stage the use of the persuasive communication mode reaches noteworthy levels. In fact, by only "capturing" the attention of the patient it is possible to change his behaviour first and then, subsequently, also his perceptive-reactive system.

At this stage, the first question should be: "What is the problem?". According to our model, this simple question already contains an initial restructuring message, since the patient is not considered as a chronically ill patient, but he is treated as an individual who has a problem which can still be given a solution.

This is also the time to try to understand how the perceptive-reactive system works in relation to the problem of drug addiction. On the basis of our clinical experience gained over the years, we have found that cocaine users usually act like *sensation seekers* (Zuckerman, 1979), that is as people who actively and constantly seek strong pleasurable experiences.

Often, the first cocaine consumption happens randomly in a fun and entertaining context, such as in a club with friends. After a number of takings, which may vary from individual to individual, there is the loss of control leading to the emergence of a vicious circle which tends only to worsen (Serpelloni & Bertoncelli, 2006; Pavarin & Dionigi, 2009).

It is of the utmost importance to ask the patient to relive those first experiences of use: this re-enactment aims to make the patient conscious of the act of taking cocaine so that it ceases to be a mainly automatic process.

Generally, at the first interview the individual states that, after an initial phase characterized by extremely pleasurable sensations, side and opposite effects occurred (*paradox effect*). At this stage the therapist adopts a communication style characterized by suggestion and persuasion, emphasizing that cocaine has caused unpleasant effects which are opposite to those originally experienced and it is now those unpleasant effects that the patient wants to stop as soon as possible (Leonardi & Velicogna, 2009). To do that the therapist may use an analogy such as that of the cage, already mentioned above, to get the best view of the situation and to evoke the unpleasant feelings associated with cocaine use. The therapist ends the sentence with a post-hypnotic message: "The more you use it, the more you feel sick and the more you feel sick, the more you would like to free yourself of it."

The next step is to survey the attempted solutions that the patient uses to address cocaine addiction. Generally, there are three:

- appeal to the patient's willpower to resist the temptation to give in to drug use;
- avoid risk situations;
- try to not think about the substance.

In order to achieve the goal of getting out of vicious circles established by the failed attempts to solve problems, the questions asked by the therapist act as keys that unlock the ability to change. For example, at this stage a question feature is: "Now that you have decided to change your ways by coming here, what would you do to implement this?". This question prompts the person to feel *as if* he is actually changing and he is trying hard to do it, thus creating a prophecy that has a sensible hope of self-fulfilment[3].

Another category of questions is the one that puts the illusion of creating alternatives between two opposing choices. An example of this sequence of funnel-shaped questions could be the following: "Do you take more cocaine when you are with other persons or when you are alone?" If the answer is "alone", the therapist continues asking if this taking is usually done at home or outside. In this way we proceed with other questions of the same type, until the therapist summarizes all the collected information into a single sentence which aims to make the patient relive the intense feeling of loneliness that the drug causes every time, thus using the patient's arguments.

Change can be induced by other tools, such as metaphors, analogies and citations, because they have the advantage over the hedges of the analytical processes (Watzlawick, 1980), as well as having a strong educational and evocative component.

Towards the end of the first session, the therapist applies a *therapeutic double bind*[4] (Bateson et al., 1956), thus constraining the individual to be even more motivated to change. An example of a double bind is when the therapist at the end of the interview states that "usually the treatment works, but I don't know if it is so in your case. We'll see...". If the patient wants treatment to work, here he must commit to belonging to that category of people for whom the treatment was successful.

[3] The *self-fulfilling prophecy* is a prediction that, because it has been formulated, sooner or later it will be fulfilled. People who are convinced that a certain event will happen in the future, in the short or medium-term, tend to alter their behaviour in a way that ends in causing the events that they had expected (Watlawick et al., 1967).

[4] The concept of the *therapeutic double bind* was formulated by Bateson to describe a contradiction at the level of communication, both verbal and non-verbal.

Finally, we give the *prescriptions*[5], which can be direct or indirect behavioural injunctions formulated by means of a strongly suggestive language, so that the patient performs the task assigned between sessions. The behavioural prescriptions are intended to unhinge the attempted solutions used until then.

4.1.2 Psychological assessment

Although the interactional model is not planned to frame people by the diagnosis, however, our team has used a series of psychological assessment instruments to obtain statistically valid measures for research purposes.

The assessment procedure aims to evaluate personality elements and those related to self-esteem, cognitive processes and social skills. Therefore, diagnostic tools used in the research project investigate the relationship between behaviour, personality factors and attitudes.

The survey instruments are:

- the Eysenck Personality Questionnaire Revised Short Form (EPQ-RS) (Eysenck et al., 1985), which measures some personality traits like introversion and extroversion;
- the Parental Bonding Instrument (PBI) (Parker et al., 1979), which provides a reliable and valid evaluation about the relationship with both parents, especially with regard to the level of care received and the feelings of security;
- the Basic Self-Esteem Scale (SE-BASIC) (Forsman et al., 2003), which consists of a rating scale of self-esteem in adulthood, seen as a stable personality trait over time and whose score is independent of the skills and feedback received from others.
- other indices of cognitive and behavioural assessment that have been extrapolated during the psychological observation of patients, with particular reference to verbal and non-verbal communication factors.

4.2 Motivational intervention

In the second phase we address the problem of dependence, encouraging the patient to speak freely about the difficulties encountered in the relational and family field, which may have favoured the use of cocaine. This work is important not only because it allows defining the possible critical areas for the person, but also because it helps to shift attention from the main problem, cocaine, and it helps to decrease obsessive ideation about the dependence on the substance.

In fact, two seemingly contradictory phenomena can be detected in the problem of cocaine addiction: obsessive ideation about the substance and mental dissociation that occurs during the use. To counter these two aspects of the problem, patients should be stimulated in sensory, perceptual and cognitive awareness (Main, 1991; Bara et al., 2005; Leonardi & Velicogna, 2009; Belin et al., 2011) of the occurrence of the abuse of cocaine.

---

[5] *Direct prescriptions* are clear instructions to carry out specific actions. They are aimed at the resolution of the problem or at reaching one of a series of goals on the road to change. *Indirect prescriptions* are behavioural injunctions whose real objectives are hidden. The therapist prescribes an action that will produce a different result from the one that was seemingly being specified (Nardone & Watzlawick, 1990).

To effectively achieve the treatment objectives, it is necessary to establish a relationship with the patient geared to the understanding of the problem and to mutual cooperation. The therapist must try to convey the message to the patient that he is not judging him by the fact of being dependent on a substance. In addition, rather than commiserate or treat him as an incompetent, the therapist encourages the patient to take responsibility and develop better decision-making capacity. Depending on different situations, the relationship with the patient can take directive or non-directive aspects.

At this stage (see Table 2), we use specific intervention techniques to re-enact sensations and perceptions induced by cocaine on the imaginative level, thus increasing the patient's capacity to recall the context in which the drug abuse developed and to prevent a possible relapse.

Second phase of treatment	Second level of therapeutic communication
• Further evaluation-intervention	• Therapeutic capture
• Intervention on the use of cocaine	• Sensory and perceptual intervention

Table 2. The motivational intervention.

A special technique was developed called the transformational re-enactment technique (Leonardi & Velicogna, 2009). This re-enactment is much more intense than just simple memory recalling, because it becomes possible to highlight the unpleasant moments connected with the use of the substance.

Here now we provide an example of a case study to explain how this technique is structured, based on our previous publication (Leonardi & Velicogna, 2009, p. 48):

(…) Gaetano, 35 years, has had a problem of cocaine addiction for about five years. He is a building contractor by profession, married and childless. In the past, he had abused heroin from the age of fifteen, but he was able to solve this problem after a period of one year in a drug rehabilitation centre. Abstinent for a long time, then he begins to take cocaine underestimating the risks and he loses control very quickly.

During the motivational phase, the therapist applies the transformational re-enactment technique, asking the patient to recall a typical situation of cocaine abuse. Despite encountering some difficulties in the initial stage, the patient gradually achieves very satisfactory results: in fact, Gaetano claims to perceive a certain aversion in reviewing that situation, underlining that he had never thought previously about the specific moment of cocaine use.

Continuing with the treatment, the therapist puts a new element in, representative configuration of use, which takes advantage of the discomfort the patient feels in "seeing" himself during the action of using cocaine (principle of use, Erickson et al., 1976). In fact, the patient tries to live again the moments immediately preceding the situation of abuse, during cocaine use and then after, as if he was reviewing them in front of a mirror. The effect obtained is very strong, because it completely changes the perception that the person had so far: whereas before the use was associated only with pleasure, now painful and negative feelings appear. Taking advantage of the difficulty of see himself, the therapist assists in leading to a greater fear in the patient, through the dual action to see the scene and to be able to review his actions.

The next step was to create an alternative sequence in which Gaetano was able to avoid the situation of abuse, reviewing with satisfaction: him reducing the use until complete cessation and then focusing his attention on relationship problems and the lack of self-esteem that had led him to cocaine addiction.

Using the transformational re-enactment technique, the therapist achieves three different objectives:

- to avoid automatisms. This technique allows the patient to review, at sensory and perceptual level, three fundamental aspects of cocaine consumption: what happens before, during and after use. It has, also, the *prescription of the symptom*[6] function, because it forces the patient to re-think in detail something that until now escaped control: the dependence;
- to insert in the patient's memory of cocaine use minimal elements with an aversive content against the substance. Thus, the patient lives painful and unpleasant sensations at perceptual level, every time he thinks about the substance;
- the modification of the patient's mental patterns into more adaptive ones, so that he can imagine himself doing affirmative actions for his mental and physical health.

Patients treated with this technique have gradually reduced cocaine use, often eventually complete cessation of using the drug, so that in a short time they were able to focus on their relationship problems and lack of self-esteem (Leonardi & Velicogna, 2009).

4.3 Development and consolidation.

The third stage is used to consolidate the results achieved in the previous two phases, proceeding in this way to restructure the cognitive level, in terms of less rigid alternatives in the perception of the reality.

In this phase, which may occur during group or in individual sessions, we try to ensure that the patient thinks of new skills acquired through the therapeutic treatment. The course within a group has some advantages in terms of learning, because the person interacts with other individuals who share similar problems. Many circular exchanges occur in a group and they can improve the patient's capacity to communicate with himself, the others and the world. So, the thought moves from the main problem: cocaine. In this way the mobilization of meta-cognitive resources helps to control the impulsivity that is typical of drug addicts and has been shown to contribute to compulsivity (Belin et al., 2008; Dalley et al., 2011). The ability of meta-communication (Sluzki, 1966; Watzlawick et al., 1967; Bateson, 1972; Belin et al., 2011) about cocaine addiction also helps the individual to reflect on interactions with his social environment.

The development and consolidation phase (see Table 3) serves also to decrease the risk of relapse that may occur after several months or even years after cessation of use. Indeed, the prolonged use of cocaine produces changes at the neurobiological level (Huang et al., 2009; Dobi et al., 2011, for review see Belin et al., 2009), which likely involves the formation of a

---

[6] The prescription of the symptom is a type of paradoxical prescription. The patient has to perform voluntarily actions that were previously involuntary and uncontrollable, and that he had always tried to avoid. The voluntary performance of the symptom eliminates it, as it is no longer spontaneous and uncontrollable (Nardone & Watzlawick, 1990).

long-term memory trace (Lee & Dong, 2011) about the pleasurable effects caused by cocaine, even after a single exposure (Ungless et al., 2001). Thus, working on meta-cognition it becomes possible to act on the mechanisms of impulsivity that may promote relapse in cocaine addiction.

Third phase of treatment	Third level of therapeutic communication
• Therapy admission	• Increased collaboration
• The seven therapeutic topics	• Decrease in the evocative language

Table 3. Development and consolidation.

4.3.1 The seven learning topics

The intervention we propose acts on the specific problem of addiction and on the possible situations that led to its appearance. For this reason, we use seven learning topics that are connected to each other and relate to many psychological areas. Considering and confronting each other about these topics we invite the patients to act in a more constructive way (O'Connell & Palmer, 2003).

4.3.1.1 Choosing a healthy lifestyle

The difficulties that a person normally encounters in the management of his lifestyle can be exacerbated by cocaine addiction (Serpelloni & Bertoncelli, 2006). At this phase, the focus of the therapy is on the possible choices which the patient can make to improve his own life. The purpose of this topic is to increase the ability to organize and direct daily activities towards healthier life choices. Adherence to more balanced rules of life, such as living by time schedules, eating a healthy diet and doing sport, allows individuals to build a healthier lifestyle.

4.3.1.2 Avoidance of relapses

Through group discussion assisted by the facilitator, we focus on the reasons that led to the patient using cocaine in the past. These may be different, such as difficulties in managing specific emotional states, the problems related to significant emotional relationships or risk underestimation in certain circumstances.

Awareness of the factors that can lead to relapse may be increased through reflection on the choices made, on automatic thoughts[7] and on emotional experiences occurring in certain circumstances. In accordance with the principle of use, we try to exploit even possible relapses in a positive way: instead of judging them as failures, they are redefined as opportunities to move on with greater and renewed commitment. According to Milton Erickson (Erickson et al., 1976), the principle of use is based on identifying the patient's available resources, on the understanding of his belief system, on connecting the resources to deal with the problem and on conveying confidence to the patient about the fact that the present problems will soon be overcome.

[7] *Automatic thoughts* are ideas and unexpected images that the patient has when their beliefs related to addiction are activated. These thoughts may act to trigger and increase drug withdrawal (Newman & Ratto, 1999). Through repeated observations, the patient is able to consider objectively their automatic thoughts and recognize their possible unreliable and non-adaptive features. Beck (1975) calls this process *distancing*.

4.3.1.3 Increasing social skills

Cocaine tends to alter the state of consciousness, distorting the perception and, therefore, it worsens the person's ability to significantly relate to others. The experience of being part of a group is a powerful tool by which he constructs a network of shared meanings with other members. The facilitator helps group members to focus on the present moment, inviting them to feel the emotions that they are experiencing during the dialogue with others.

4.3.1.4 Development of communication and meta-communication skills

The communication can never be separated from the interactional aspects: the person learns to communicate through the discussions that take place in the group, drawing on the resources of the verbal and non-verbal sphere. The development of communication skills helps to contrast feelings of isolation that often accompany the experience of cocaine addiction.

4.3.1.5 Increasing meta-cognitive resources

Meta-cognition is the ability to reflect on your thought processes, because it is assumed that an increase of this ability may encourage the person to make global changes in his lifestyle and in the management of feelings evoked by the use of cocaine. The group facilitator invites the members to meta-communicate and reflect on their and others' thinking, in order to stimulate greater awareness in emotion management.

4.3.1.6 A more balanced emotion management

Group members are instructed to recognize their own emotions and those of others: in other words, everyone is invited to wonder what he feels and what the others feel. To do this, the group members are invited to observe their sensations here and now and to realize the emotions of others. The same process can be referred also to remember particular events, such as the cocaine use situation. Observation and acceptance of their emotional states play important roles in the recognition of unpleasant emotions associated with the use of the substance.

4.3.1.7 Increasing problem solving skills

Increasing the capacity to solve problems effectively is obtained by assigning to the group members problem solving exercises to stimulate learning more appropriate strategies. This capacity can also improve the perceived sense of self-efficacy and thus the level of self-esteem of the person.

The self-efficacy refers to all the beliefs the person has about their ability to organize and execute the necessary actions to achieve their goals (Bandura, 1997).

4.4 Gradual release

Once you have completed the phase of development and consolidation, the next step requires the patient to acquire greater autonomy and self-confidence. The therapeutic session takes place during this phase with a collaborative attitude, in order to monitor any signs which could have anticipated the risk of relapse in cocaine addiction. At this stage, the patient has gained a greater autonomy and confidence in his ability to continue alone down the road of change. In this regard, it is interesting to focus on the concept of deutero-learning, introduced by Bateson (1972), to indicate the learning level higher than that of the basic stimulus-response scheme: briefly, it describes the process by which an individual "learns to learn".

This step is essential to encourage the patient to develop a greater degree of autonomy (see Table 4), as well as a greater sense of security, such as he becomes able to deal with various difficult situations.

Fourth phase of treatment	Fourth level of therapeutic communication
• Increasing autonomy • Increased complexity of the arguments of the group • Deutero-learning	• Demonstration-rational language • Perceptual and sensory forms of intervention

Table 4. Gradual release.

During this phase, the therapist also aims to improve the quality of inner dialogue, for example, through a specific training technique called inner conversation (Leonardi & Velicogna, 2009), whereby the patient imagines himself thinking as speaking aloud, focusing so that his linguistic performance is as correct as possible. This exercise leads to a progressive increase in reflective ability (self-regulation of thought) with a corresponding decrease in impulsivity, which is one of the reasons of possible relapse in cocaine use, as demonstrated by preclinical studies (Economidou et al., 2009).

4.5 Follow-up

After treatment, the phase of periodic review of results begins and it is realized by monitoring urine tests and follow-up interviews. This is the time (see Table 5) to understand whether or not the therapy has reached its objectives: the patient should become more cooperative towards the therapist, as well as more inclined to discuss any other issues that have occurred in other areas of his life.

In order to avoid possible relapses, at this stage the therapist also uses training techniques and imaginative simulation procedures, similar to the transformational re-enactment technique described above.

Fifth phase of treatment	Fifth level of therapeutic communication
• Verification, development and consolidation of achievements	• Increased collaboration • Collaborative language

Table 5. Follow-up.

5. Evaluation of the effectiveness and efficiency of treatment

Cocaine addiction is a highly complex field of study, in which communicative, interpersonal and neurobiological processes act. In order to collect data about the *effectiveness* (that means to cease cocaine use) and *efficiency* (to reach this goal as soon as possible) of the interactional approach, our research group has used both quantitative tools, such as urinary tests, and qualitative tools, such as self-evaluation questionnaires completed by the patients directly.

Through these evaluations indexes, given before, during and after treatment, we think it is possible to obtain a reliable evaluation of the treatment outcome.

Data collected are used:

- to assess whether treatment produces concrete results and if it responds adequately to the initial expectations;
- to identify which aspects of the treatment are valid and which ones are ineffective and, therefore, modifiable;
- to improve further those treatment components that have shown to be effective.

One of the rules of scientific method is to never be satisfied with the results achieved, because in another context or with other patients the same results achieved in the past may not be obtained. So we need a constant monitoring of these activities, in order to modify certain aspects of the psychological intervention, if necessary.

In a previous article (Leonardi et al., 2006), we underlined the importance of this *circular deepening principle* which derives from Lewin's Action Research model (1946). According to this model, the research and intervention phases are interconnected and constantly changing thanks to a feedback mechanism. After theoretically defining the working hypotheses, the real finding phase, during which data are collected, follows. Through the analysis of these data it becomes possible to effectively coordinate the intervention. The evaluation of achievements generates new working hypotheses, thus determining the beginning of a circular process whereby it becomes possible to make corrections and changes to the treatment itself.

This cycle also allows us to adjust the treatment to very different realities compared to the initial sample which has been processed. As Trombetta and Rosiello (2000) claimed, the circularity of this process is characterized by a collection of new material to be analysed, which is then used in constructing and implementing new strategies and action plans.

The principle of circularity just described is consistent with systemic theory (von Bertanlaffy, 1971), which underlines the importance of feedback mechanisms that act through the different phases: in our case, these feedback processes concern the continuous analysis of clinical individual and group interviews, as well as observation of results achieved (urinary tests, remission of symptoms and change in behavioural style).

Over the years, this circular process has meant continuous improvements to the treatment protocol, thus increasing the final effectiveness.

The research process can be divided into three macro areas:

- observation of individual and group interviews;
- quantitative and qualitative monitoring of the results obtained, and the administration of cognitive and personality tests;
- theoretical study in the field of general psychology and drug addiction.

The evaluation of therapeutic work mainly consists of studying the interviews or the group meetings carried out, with particular reference to the interactional aspects which occur between the therapist and the patient.

As noted elsewhere (Leonardi et al., 2006), monitoring of the clinical situation through periodic urine tests represents an element of fundamental importance and is the primary tool to verify the abstinence from cocaine and thus, indirectly, to obtain an *objective evaluation index* on the effectiveness of treatment.

According to our intervention protocol, urine tests should be carried out twice a week during treatment. These data provide an objective parameter for achieving and maintaining abstinence from cocaine, and they are also used to detect the possible occurrence of relapses. The statistical analysis of urine test results also allows the detection of the presence of some critical periods during the course of treatment, when abstinence from the drug is relatively more likely to be established (see Leonardi et al., 2006, for more details).

To monitor the validity of the therapy we also use some *subjective evaluation indices* that refer to how the patients views the therapeutic activity, the skills that they believe they have acquired during the treatment and the personal areas where they would require further therapeutic intervention. These evaluations are obtained through semi-structured interviews.

Finally, the study of general psychology and drug addiction literature has allowed expanding the existing knowledge, implementing it with new ways to observe and act on the person. The updating of bibliographic material is designed to deepen knowledge about the neurological, cognitive and social aspects related to the phenomenon of cocaine addiction.

6. Conclusions

Solving the problem of cocaine addiction presents considerable difficulties because of frequent relapses in the use of the substance. For this reason, a gradual change of subjective models for the construction of reality should also be combined with the psychological change, which begins to develop from the first session.

The interactional model has allowed us to reach good levels of effectiveness and efficiency of treatment. For example, as reported in Leonardi et al. (2006), in a group of 22 subjects who finished the treatment successfully, 73% resulted in abstinence from cocaine after 12 weeks. A 12 week outpatient study of Carroll et al. (1991), comparing the effectiveness of CBT with Interpersonal Psychotherapy or IPT (Klerman et al., 1984), reported that in a group of 42 subjects, 57% of the patients assigned to CBT and 33% of those assigned to IPT attained three or more continuous weeks of abstinence.

Our results (see Leonardi et al., 2009, for more details) were achieved by continuous research and correction of what was not fully satisfactory for the purpose of the therapy. On the basis of the results and data collected over time, we have developed a specific protocol for dealing with the problem of cocaine addiction, characterized by the following principle: try constantly to adapt the treatment to changes occurring during the therapeutic work.

7. References

Alexander, F. & French, T.M. (1946). Psychoanalytic Therapy: Principles and Applications, Ronald Press Company, New York.

Bandura, A. (1997). Self-Efficacy: the exercise of control, W.H. Freeman & Company, ISBN 978-0716726265, New York.

Bara, G.B., Colle, L., Bosco & F.M. (2005). Metacognizione: aspetti rilevanti per la clinica, In: Bara, B.G. (Ed.), Nuovo manuale di Psicoterapia Cognitiva, Vol. I, Bollati Boringhieri, ISBN 978-8833957685, Torino.

Bateson, G. (1972). Steps to an Ecology of Mind: Collected Essays in Anthropology, Psychiatry, Evolution, and Epistemology, University Of Chicago Press, ISBN 0226039056, Chicago.

Bateson, G., Jackson, D.D., Haley, J. & Weakland, J. (1956). Toward a Theory of Schizophrenia, *Behavioural Science*, 1(4): 251-264.

Belin, D., Daniel, M.L., Lacoste, J., Belin-Rauscent, A., Bacconnier, M. & Jaafari, N. (2011). Insight: perspectives étiologiques et phénoménologiques dans la psychopathologie des désordres obsessionnels compulsifs. *Annales Médico-psychologiques, revue psychiatrique*, 169(7): 420-425.

Belin, D., Mar, A., Dalley, J., Robbins, T. & Everitt, B. (2008). High Impulsivity Predicts the Switch to Compulsive Cocaine-Taking. *Science*, 320(5881):1352–1355.

Belin, D., Jonkman, S., Dickinson, A., Robbins, T.W. & Everitt, B.J. (2009). Parallel and interactive learning processes within the basal ganglia: Relevance for the understanding of addiction, *Behavioural Brain Research*, 199(1):89–102.

Bertalanffy, Von, L. (1969). General System Theory. Foundations, development, applications, George Braziller, ISBN 978-0807604533, New York.

Beck, A.T. (1975). Cognitive Therapy and the Emotional Disorders, International Universities Press, ISBN 978-0823609901, New York.

Braglia, D., Gerra, G., Mezzelani, P., Quaglio, G., Timpano, M.E., Zaimovic, A. & Zambelli., U. (2004). Cocaina: Farmacocinetica, abuso, dipendenza, detossificazione e trattamento. In: Trattato completo degli abusi e delle dipendenze, Nizzoli, U. & Pissacroia, M. (Eds.), Piccin, ISBN 978-8829916481, Padova.

Carroll, K.M., Rounsaville, B.J. & Gawin F.H. (1991). A comparative trial of psychotherapies for ambulatory cocaine abusers: relapse prevention and interpersonal psychotherapy, *The American Journal of Drug and Alcohol Abuse*, 17(3):229-247.

Carroll, K.M. (1998). A Cognitive-Behavioural Approach: Treating cocaine addiction, NIH Publication 98-4308, National Institute on Drug Abuse, Rockville, Retrieved from archives.drugabuse.gov/TXManuals/CBT/CBT1.htm

Childress, A.R., Mozley, P.D., McElgin, W., Fitzgerald, J., Reivich, M. & O'Brien, C.P. (1999). Limbic activation during cue-induced cocaine craving, *American Journal of Psychiatry*, 156: 11-18.

Dalley, J.W., Everitt, B.J., Robbins, T.W. (2011) Impulsivity, compulsivity, and top-down cognitive control, *Neuron*, 69(4):680–694.

De Shazer, S. (1985), Keys to Solutions in Brief Therapy, W.W. Norton & Company, ISBN 978-0393700046, New York.

Di Clemente, C.C., & Velasquez, M. (2002). Motivational Interviewing and the Stages of Change, In: Miller, W.R. & Rollnick, S. (Eds.), Motivational Interviewing: Preparing People to Change, The Guilford Press, ISBN 978-1572305632, New York.

Dobi, A., Seabold, G.K., Christensen, C.H., Bock, R. & Alvarez, V.A. (2011). Cocaine-induced plasticity in the nucleus accumbens is cell-specific and develops without prolonged withdrawal, *The Journal of Neuroscience*, 31(5): 1895–1904.

Economidou, D., Pelloux, Y., Robbin, T.W., Dalley, J.W. & Everitt, B.J. (2009). High impulsivity predicts relapse to cocaine-seeking after punishment-induced abstinence, *Biological Psychiatry*, 65(10): 851-856.

Edwards, S. & Koob, G.F. (2010). Neurobiology of dysregulated motivational systems in drug addiction, *Future Neurology*, 5(3): 393-401.

Erickson, M.H. & Rossi, E. (1981). Experiencing Hypnosis. Therapeutic Approaches to Altered States, Irvington Publishers, ISBN 0829002464, New York.

Erickson, M.H., Rossi E. & Rossi S. (1976), Hypnotic Realities: The Induction of Clinical Hypnosis and Forms of Indirect Suggestion, Irvington Publishers, ISBN 978-0829001129, New York.

European Monitoring Centre for Drugs and Drug Addiction, (2007a), EMCDDA Literature reviews - Treatment of problem cocaine use: a review of the literature, European Monitoring Centre for Drugs and Drug Addiction, ISBN 9291682748, Lisbon, Retrieved from
http://www.emcdda.europa.eu/attachements.cfm/att_44787_EN_cocainetreatment_literature_review.pdf

European Monitoring Centre for Drugs and Drug Addiction, (2011), 2011 Annual report on the state of the drugs problem in Europe, European Monitoring Centre for Drugs and Drug Addiction, ISBN 978-9291684700, Lisbon, Retrieved from http://www.emcdda.europa.eu/attachements.cfm/att_143743_EN_EMCDDA_AR2011_EN.pdf

Eysenck, S.B.G., Eysenck, H.J. & Paul Barrett, P. (1985) A revised version of the psychoticism scale, *Personality and Individual Differences*, 6(1):21-29.

Forsman, L., Johnson, M., Ugolini, V., Bruzzi, D. & Raboni, D., (2003), Basic SE. Basic self-esteem scale. Valutazione dell'autostima di base negli adulti, Edizioni Erickson. ISBN 978-8879465304, Trento.

Fisch, R., Weakland, J. & Segal, L. (1982). The Tactics of Change. Doing Therapy Briefly, Jossey-Bass, ISBN 978-0875895215, San Francisco.

Foerster, Von, H. (1982). Observing systems, Intersystems Publications, ISBN 978-0914105190 Seaside.

Gazzaniga, M.S. (1972). One brain - two minds?, *American Scientist*, 60(3): 311-317.

Glasersfeld, Von, E. (1984). An Introduction to Radical Constructivism, In: The invented reality: How do we know what we believe we know? (Contributions to Constructivism), Watzlawick, P. (ed.), pp. 17-40, W.W. Norton & Company, ISBN 978-0393017311, New York.

Haley, J. (1963). Strategies of psychotherapy, Grune & Stratton, ISBN 0808901680, New York.

Higgins, S.T., Wong, C.J., Badger, G.J., Odgen, D.E. & Dantona, R.L. (2000). Contingent reinforcement increases cocaine abstinence during outpatient treatment and 1 year of follow-up, *Journal of Consulting and Clinical Psychology*, 68(1): 64-72.

Huang, Y.H., Lin, Y., Mu, P., Lee B.R., Brown T.E., Wayman, G., Marie, H., Liu, W., Yan, Z., Sorg, B.A., Schlüter, O.M., Zukin, R.S., & Dong, Y. (2009). In vivo cocaine experience generates silent synapses, *Neuron*, 63(1): 40–47.

Jackson, D. (1961). Interactional psychotherapy, In: Contemporary Psychotherapies, Stein, M. (Ed.), pp. 256-271, The Free Press of Glencoe, New York.

Jackson, D. (1965). The study of the family, Family Process, 4(1): 1-20.

Khantzian, E.J., Halliday, K.S. & McAuliffe, W.E. (1990). Addiction and the vulnerable self: Modified Dynamic Group Therapy for drug abusers, Guilford Press, ISBN 978-0898621723, New York.

Klerman, G.L., Weissman, M.M., Rounsaville, B.J., & Chevron, E.S. (1984). Interpersonal Therapy of Depression, Basic Books, New York.

Lee, B.R. & Dong, Y. (2011). Cocaine-induced metaplasticity in the nucleus accumbens: silent synapse and beyond, *Neuropharmacology*, 61(7): 1060–1069.

Leonardi, A., Fioravanti, P., Scavelli, S. & Velicogna, F. (2006). Programma Conoscenza: trattamento psicoeducativo integrato ed evoluto per problemi di cocaina. In: Cocaina. Manuale di aggiornamento tecnico scientifico, Serpelloni G., Macchia T., Gerra G. (Eds.), Progetto "START" del Dipartimento Nazionale per le Politiche Antidroga, ISBN 978-8895149004, Retrieved from http://iport.dronet.org/com/filedownloadlink/allegatoA.php?key=116&lingua=1

Leonardi, A., Fioravanti, P., Scavelli, S. & Velicogna, F. (2009). Programma Conoscenza. Psycho-educational, integrated and evolved treatment for cocaine addiction. *International Journal of Mental Health and Addiction*, 7(4):513–529.

Leonardi, A. & Velicogna, F. (2009). Cocaina: dipendenza e trattamento. Un modello di intervento psicologico, Franco Angeli, ISBN 987-8856812848, Milano.

Lewin, K. (1946), Action Research and minority problems, *Journal of Social Issues*, 2(4):34-46.

Main, M. (1991). Metacognitive knowledge, metacognitive monitoring and singular (coherent) vs. multiple (incoherent) models of attachment: findings and directions for future research, In: Parkes, C., Stevenson-Hinde, C.M & Marris, P. (Eds.), Attachment across the life cycle, Tavistock & Routledge, ISBN 0415056519, London.

Mascetti, W. & Strepparola, G. (2006). I disturbi da uso di sostanze, In: Bara, B.G. (Ed.), Nuovo manuale di Psicoterapia Cognitiva, Vol. III, Bollati Boringhieri, ISBN 978-8833957708, Torino.

Maturana, H.R. & Varela, F.J. (1980). Autopoiesis and Cognition: the realization of the living, D. Reidel Publishing Company, ISBN 978-9027710161, Boston.

Miller, W.R. & Rollnick, S. (2002), Motivational Interview: Preparing people to change, Guilford Press, ISBN 978-1572305632, New York.

Nardone, G. & Watzlawick, P. (1990). L'arte del cambiamento, Ponte alle Grazie, ISBN 978-8879284653, Firenze.

National Institute on Drug Abuse, (2008). Cocaine, NIDA InfoFacts, Retrieved from http://www.nida.nih.gov/pdf/infofacts/Cocaine08.pdf

Newman, C.F. & Ratto, C.L. (1999). Cognitive therapy of substance abuse. In: Comparative treatments of substance abuse, Dowd, E.T., Rugle, L. (Eds.), Springer Publishing Company, ISBN 0826112765, New York.

O'Connell, B. & Palmer, S. (2003). Handbook of Solution-Focused Therapy, Sage Publications, ISBN 978-0761967842, London.

Parker, G., Tupling, H., & Brown, L.B. (1979). A Parental Bonding Instrument, British *Journal of Medical Psychology*, 52(1):1-10.

Pavarin, R.M. & Dionigi, A., (Eds.), (2009). Cocaina. Percezione del danno, comportamenti a rischio e significati, CLUEB , ISBN 978-8849133325, Bologna.

Petry, N.M. (2002). Contingency management in addiction treatment, *Psychiatric Times*, 19(2): 52-56.

Pirona, A. & Hedrich, D. (2009). Treatment of cocaine use - a short update, European Monitoring Centre for Drugs and Drug Addiction, Retrieved from http://www.emcdda.europa.eu/attachements.cfm/att_76877_EN_EMCDDA-cocaine%20treatment-update.pdf

Presidenza del Consiglio dei Ministri (Eds.). (2007). Relazione sullo stato delle tossicodipendenze in Italia anno 2007, Retrieved from http://www.governo.it/GovernoInforma/Dossier/relazione_droga_2007/Relazione_2007.pdf

Rigliano, P. (2004). Piaceri drogati. Psicologia del consumo di droghe, Feltrinelli, ISBN 978-8807817908, Milano.

Serpelloni, G. & Bertoncelli, S. (2006). Cocaina: profili dei soggetti in base alle modalità d'uso, agli aspetti comportamentali e sociali, In: Cocaina. Manuale di aggiornamento tecnico scientifico, Serpelloni G., Macchia T., Gerra G. (Eds.), pp. 637-653, Progetto "START" del Dipartimento Nazionale per le Politiche Antidroga, ISBN 978-8895149004, Retrieved from http://iport.dronet.org/com/filedownloadlink/allegatoA.php?key=141&lingua=1

Shaham, Y. & Hope, B.T. (2005a). The role of neuroadaptations in relapse in drug seeking, *Nature Neuroscience*, 8(11): 1437-1439.

Sluzki, C. (1966). Seminario sobre metacomunicacion: nota, *Acta Psiquiatrica y Psicologica de América Latina*, 12:119.

Sperry, R.W. (1968). Hemisphere deconnection and unity in conscious awareness, *American Psychologist*, 23(10): 723-733.

Ungless, M.A., Whistler, J.L., Malenka, R.C. & Bonci, A. (2001). Single cocaine exposure in vivo induces long-term potentiation in dopamine neurons, *Nature*, 411(6837): 583-587.

Watzlawick, P. (1978). The Language of Change: elements of therapeutic communication, Basic Books, ISBN 978-0465037926, New York.

Watlawick, P. (Ed.)(1984). The invented reality. How do we know what we believe we know? (Contributions to Constructivism), W. W. Norton & Company, ISBN 978-0393017311, New York.

Watzlawick, P., Beavin, J. & Jackson, D. (1967). Pragmatics of human communication. A study of interactional patterns, pathologies and paradoxes, W. W. Norton & Company, ISBN 978-0393010091, New York.

Watlawick, P. & Nardone, G. (1997). Terapia Breve Strategica, Raffaello Cortina Editore, ISBN 978-8870784718, Milano.

Watlawick, P., Weakland, J., & Fisch, J. (1974). Change. Principles of problem resolution. W. W. Norton & Company, ISBN 978-0393011043, New York.

Weaver, T., Hart, J., Fehler, J., Metrebian, N., D'Agostino, T. & Benn, P. (2007), Are contingency management principles being implemented in drug treatment in England?, National Treatment Agency for Substance Misuse, Retrieved from

http://www.drugsandalcohol.ie/11939/1/NTASM_rb33_contingency_management_summary.pdf
Zuckerman, M. (1979). Sensation seeking: beyond the optimal level of arousal, L. Erlbaum, ISBN 978-0470268513, Hillsdale.

15

Research and Intervention for Drug-Addicted Mothers and Their Children: New Perspectives

Paolo Stocco[1], Alessandra Simonelli[2],
Nicoletta Capra[3] and Francesca De Palo[2]
[1]*Therapeutic Community "Villa Renata", Venice,*
[2]*Department of Developmental and Social Psychology, Padua University,*
[3]*Mother-Child Therapeutic Community "Casa Aurora e Villa Emma," Venice,*
Italy

1. Introduction

According to research carried out by the EMCDDA, drug-addicted women in Europe account for at least one quarter of the total European population consuming illicit substances (Emcdda, 2006a). A specific research platform entitled "Women and Drugs" was created within the context of the second European project "Democracies, Cities and Drugs." This platform is focused on what characterizes and distinguishes female substance addiction from male substance addiction: its manifestation, its attributes, and the interventions or services which can be put into effect while devoting special attention and offering specialized care to this phenomenon. Our findings confirm that women substance users are exposed to a great number of risks such as medical, social, economic, familial and psychopathological risks requiring intervention through specific tools and aimed responses (see Brentari, Hernandez, Tripodi, 2011). The investigated factors included pregnancy, parenthood and the well-being as well as development of the child, while taking into account institutional and ethical reflections regarding this complex theme.

The substance abuse phenomenon indeed affects a high number of fertile women. When drugs are consumed during pregnancy, they can have serious, direct and indirect effects on the postpartum development with subsequent effects on the child (OTIS, 2010). Substance abusing mothers represent an at-risk parenting situation which, in turn, profoundly influences the quality of the mother-child relationship. The awareness of these at-risk situations for children along with the widely accepted notion that ideally, children should always be raised by their mothers led to the introduction of residential treatment in Italy. These services deal with maternal pathologies and provide care and assistance for children; in fact, these therapeutic communities accommodate addicted mothers as well as their children.

Up until recently, therapies for children (particularly medical ones) were administered by institutions outside of the community, while no therapeutic treatment was mandated for minors. The first therapeutic communities for drug addicted mothers and their children appeared in Europe in the early nineties. These institutions must provide assistance to children and assure them the greatest possible social, psychological and physical well-being. In addition to the funds available for each mother, funds for each individual minor are made available on a daily basis. Our project: "Research and intervention on minors in communities for addicted mothers and their children: from at-risk parenting to child well-being" was promoted within this specific intervention framework. The project aims to secure child well-being by assessing maternal parenting as well as by carrying out direct and indirect observations of the child, his/her caregivers and the caregiver-child relationship. At the same time, the most suitable intervention for each single subject is put into effect.

2. Female substance addiction, pregnancy and parenthood

As stated above, there is an ever increasing interest towards defining characteristics which are specifically related to substance abuse in the female population, with specific reference to the following two crucial aspects.

a. general differences, in terms of individual and relational characteristics, life history and family history which single out addicted women as subjects with experiences of trauma, abandonment or neglect, from either a physical or psychological standpoint (Parsec Association, 2004; Stocco et Al., 2000, 2002; Studio VEdeTTE, 2007). These subjects suffer also for their specific medical problems (HIV, sexually transmitted pathologies, etc.), for their social situation (prostitution, access to the job market, etc.) and institutional difficulties (organization and access to services). From this point of view, the interest is to detect and realize any available data projections referring to female substance addiction and feasible interventions from the legislative and health perspective (Home Ministry Government, 2010).
b. specific issues related to pregnancy and parenthood in substance abusing women from the medical-gynecological perspective, including all psychological aspects which might have an impact on the subsequent relationship with a child.

2.1 Substance abuse

All international data confirm a commonly shared view according to which male drug users outnumber women drug users by far (UNODC, 2004). However, recent research suggests that the gender gap may be narrowing, at least with reference to some types of drugs (EMCDDA 2006a). For example, for cannabis use and binge drinking, differences in drug use between men and women have substantially narrowed, at times showing an almost equal consumption between the genders. Another trend indicated a higher percentage of female rather than male students using tranquilizers or sedatives which are bought without prescription. Patterns of drug use based on gender differences are illustrated by the percentage of patients entering treatment services in Europe. The percentage of female patients is around 20% (EMCDDA 2005): among those receiving drug treatment, problems relating to amphetamine-type stimulant drugs (ATS) are most common among young people (under 20 years old), whereas problems relating to the use of sedatives or pharmaceutical drugs are most widespread among older patients (over 39 years old) (EMCDDA 2005).

With reference to intravenous drug use (IDU), the WHO reported a rapid increase in the rate of female IDUs in recent years, especially in Eastern Europe and Asia (Pinkham and Malinowska-Sempruch, 2007). According to available epidemiological data, women are more likely than men to abuse and become dependent on substances such as tranquilizers and sedatives when used without prescription (Simoni-Wastila et. al, 2004). It has also been shown that women typically become dependent on substances more quickly than men: this holds good for cannabis, cocaine and other stimulants, as well as opioids, inhalants and hallucinogens (UNODC, 2004).

With respect to "binge drinking"[1], an EMCDDA gender perspective report underlines that male predominance in general is lower in those countries where the prevalence of binge drinking is highest. Gender correlation with respect to cannabis use and binge drinking increases proportionally according to the increased use of those substances (EMCDDA, 2006a). Other studies show that in recent years, risky alcohol consumption has increased among young girls and adolescents (Anderson, Baumberg, 2006; O.N.Da, 2008).

Several studies suggest that women are more likely to use and abuse prescribed psychoactive drugs such as painkillers, sleeping pills and tranquillizers (EMCDDA, 2006a). This remark applies especially to opioids and depressants of the central nervous system. Sleeping-pill and anti-anxiety drug abuse is less visible than other, more common forms of addiction among women (PNS, 2008; Stocco, 2000). Actually, this seems related to the high incidence of depression or anxiety disorders in women (WHO, 2000). It is important to note that a lifetime prevalence of benzodiazepine use (for sleep or anxiety problems) without medical prescription among school students between the ages of 15 and 16 is significantly higher in females than in males (EMCDDA, 2006a).

2.2 Mental health and dual diagnosis

A high percentage of women substance users suffer from mental disorders. This specific type of diagnostic comorbidity, called *dual diagnosis*[2] was defined as the co-existence, in one

[1] Binge drinking is defined as a dangerous practice of consuming large quantities of alcoholic beverages in a single session. More specifically, experts agree that binge drinking occurs when one consumes 5 or more alcoholic drinks within a couple of hours.

[2] The term "comorbidity" was introduced by Feinstein and further specified by Klerman (1990) who used it to denote two or more disorders occurring at the same time or in the life course of one and the same subject. Cloninger (1990) stated that comorbidity implied the likeliness for a subject with a specific index disorder to develop a second disorder. Finally, Golberg (1996) very interestingly pointed out that it was only possible to talk of comorbidity when the assessed disorders were clearly distinct entities: symptoms of interrelated domains should not be classified as comorbidity. This clarification must be kept in mind since comorbidity only occurs when two different disorder categories can be recognized and described: however, it cannot be considered irrelevant that a "disorder" should be accompanied by symptoms or clusters of symptoms belonging to domains that are to a greater or lesser extent interrelated with the psychopathological domain of the index disorder. Rather, this reveals a "specific vulnerability" for a psychopathological development of the interrelated domain to reach disorder level and, therefore, comorbid condition (Di Sciascio, Nardini, 2005).

and the same subject, of a disorder related to psychoactive substance abuse and another psychiatric disorder (World Health Organization, WHO, 1995). As far as addiction is concerned, co-morbidity refers to the co-presence of a serious mental disorder and a disorder caused by substance abuse/dependence when such causality can be demonstrated (De Leon, 1989; Buckley, Brady, Hermann, 2010; Bobes, Casas, Szerman, 2009).

Dual diagnosis is more frequent among women than among men, particularly with regard to affective and anxiety disorders. Affective disorders (especially depression, moodiness and low self-esteem, loss of interest or pleasure in enjoyable activities) and anxiety disorders (excessive anxiety with physical and emotional effects such as apprehension, nervousness or fear) are common and serious pathologies to be treated in addicted women. A recent comprehensive study in United States confirmed that feelings of depression, hopelessness, sadness and suicidal ideation are more frequent in high school girls than in boys and that these feelings are more likely associated with a high risk for drinking and other drug use in girls (CASA 2003, cit. in Brady, Back, Greenfield, 2009). Also personality disorders (mostly Cluster B), posttraumatic stress disorders, suicide attempts and eating behavior disorders have to be treated in addict women. Schizophrenia and other psychotic symptoms are also frequent in women (Stocco et al., 2000, Instituto de la Mujer, 2007).

Particularly, exposure to trauma is a very frequent condition in drug-addicted women and it is the environmental basis for a posttraumatic stress disorder: sexual assault is the most frequent type of trauma experienced by women, but all different kinds of abuse are suffered by women before or during drug addiction. All in all, women are four times more likely to develop this disorder than men after exposure to traumatic events (Ciechanowski, 2010; Instituto de la Mujer, 2007)

Moreover, a lifetime prevalence of eating disorders (such as anorexia and bulimia) was found in women misusing substances: these disorders are thought to be behavioural patterns stemming from emotional conflicts that need to be solved so that the patient can develop a healthy relationship with food (Charles & Pull, 2004). Among psychiatric disorders, these are serious mental illnesses with a high incidence of co-morbidity and also with a high mortality rate (Ibidem).

Causes for high co-morbidity between substance misuse and mental health issues are not known and prevalence varies among different populations. Etiological theories in dual diagnosis include factors that are common to both disorders: a substance use disorder secondary to mental illness; a mental illness secondary to substance use, as well as bidirectional models. Women have more difficulties than men when treated for dual pathologies: these difficulties are related to drug addiction and mental illness. Drug addiction damage in a woman's body occurs earlier and more intensely than in men. Women seek treatment later than men, and addiction treatments do not often include a suitable program for dual diagnosis cases. In addition to this, women with mental illness usually suffer from some degree of impaired cognition. This makes them feel embarrassed, and contributes to a lack of compliance and difficulties when confronted with the need to change their lifestyle. Moreover, these women don't seek specific services: on the contrary, they usually prefer to see general practitioners. Women typically don't ask for mental or addiction treatments nor for social help. As a result, doctors that are unprepared to treat these cases may delay assistance (Instituto de la Mujer, 2007).

Finally, reference should be made to the co-dependence phenomenon (also called bi-dependence): more often than not, drug-addicted women experience problematic relationships with multi-problematic partners who also have drug- or alcohol-addiction problems (Moral Jiménez & Sirvent Ruiz, 2007).

2.3 Medical implications

Drug use, particularly intravenous drug use (IDU) remains one of the major risk factors for acquiring blood-borne infections for both men and women. With reference to the risk of infections related to sharing needles and other drug paraphernalia, it has been demonstrated that a significant number of women begin using drugs in the context of a sexual relationship (Unodc, 2004; Price & Simmel, 2002). Women are also more likely than men to borrow or share injection equipment, particularly with their sexual partners. They also often rely on men to acquire and inject them with drugs (Doherty et al. 2000; Vidal-Trecan at al, 1998, Pinkham et al. 2007). Women share needles with more people in their social network than men do (Sherman et al. 2001). This leads to an increased risk for acquiring blood-borne infections, particularly HIV and hepatitis C, which is generally very high among intravenous drug users.

Biological and social factors contribute to the increase of women drug users' risks for HIV. The overall data available for 25 European countries in 2005 showed that 35% of newly diagnosed cases of HIV were among women, reaching 41% in Eastern Europe, where the epidemic was mainly concentrated among IV drug users (Euro-HIV, 2007). Studies in nine EU countries showed that the average HIV prevalence was more than 50 percent higher among women IV drug users than among their male counterparts (EMCDDA, 2006). The correlation of IV drug use, sex work and unsafe sexual practices led to a significantly increased risk of HIV infection among women (UNODC, 2004).

Risk behaviour for infections needs to be considered not only with reference to HIV, but also to other blood-borne diseases such as Hepatitis C and B. Hepatitis C is the most common infectious disease among IV drug users, since it is transmitted through the sharing of needles, syringes and, unlike HIV, other injection-related equipment (Eurasian Harm Reduction Network (2007b). In 2006, the EMCDDA reported that median sero-prevalence of hepatitis C virus (HCV) is quite similar in male and female IV drug users: 58.1 % in males and 56.4 % in females. It is generally understood that it is more difficult to acquire HCV through sexual transmission than it is to acquire HIV. Infection among IV drug users will therefore be almost exclusively the result of sharing syringes and other injecting paraphernalia (EMCDDA, 2006).

2.4 Gender violence and social conditions

Neglect and abuse in childhood are common trends in the personal backgrounds of many female substance users.

European data estimates that one in five women experiences some form of physical or sexual violence (European Women's Lobby, 2001; Stocco, Llopis et al., 2000). In England and Wales alone, there were over 1 million female victims of domestic violence between 2009-2010. In the same area, every year over 300,000 women are sexually assaulted and 60,000 women are raped. Overall in the UK, more than one in four women experience domestic abuse during their lifetime (Home Minister Government, 2010)[3].

These women tend to define their substance use as the best coping mechanism available to them. Parental negligence and lack of attention in addition to the trauma of physical or sexual abuse make women more vulnerable to developing problems with substance abuse. In the absence of adequate support, such conditions can become a descending spiral (EMCDDA, 2009).

The link between substance use and gender violence/domestic abuse is complex. There is no reliable evidence of a cause-effect link between the two. However, where problems with substance use exist, domestic abuse is often present as well. Physical or sexual abuse on women is often perpetrated by a male partner or other male family members. Studies show that women with substance use problems are more likely than men to have experienced physical and/or sexual abuse (UNODC, 2004). A history of violence can have an impact on a woman's experience with substance abuse and mental health problems. Women who use substances are also more likely to live in environments where violence or sexual abuse is a common pattern: a study by Vogt (1998) and Zenken et Al. (2003) found that a significant background variable for female drug addiction are past experiences of violence, especially sexual exploitation. In line with this view, some Italian research studies have shown that about 50 % of young female drug users with anti-social behaviour and one-third of female psychiatric patients were victims of untreated sexual abuse during childhood (Gelinas, 1983; Malacrea, 2006).

Social, physical and psychological deprivations expose women to the influence and exploitation of male partners. Substance use can also drive women into sex work as a source of income (EMCDDA, 2009).

2.5 Pregnancy and parenthood

Women drug users who become pregnant form an additional sub-group requiring specific attention and care, both for them and for their babies (EMCDDA, 2006a). Drug use is associated with direct and indirect complications throughout pregnancy, postnatal morbidity and developmental delays (Hunter and Powis 1996): for instance, within the groups studied by Aronica et al. (1987) and by Palmieri (1991), 50% of the subjects were pregnant women with one or more children. Alleged reproduction difficulties in this population were attributed both to neuroendocrine alterations induced by substances such as heroin and opioids and to an irregular and inconstant lifestyle, alimentary deficits and poor hygienic, sanitary habits (Genazzani, 1987). However, neither of the two classes of factors seem to significantly reduce the chances for these subjects to bear children (Ibidem).

These women usually report deep feelings of anguish and dismay which build up their inner world, always suspended between impotence and manipulative, boundless omnipotence. Actually, addicted women often wish to get pregnant and bear a child as a form of vital defense or a redemption experience, even though this idealized view does not prevent the emergence of phases of anguish which are tied to the clashing of evidence against the ever incumbent denial of the event (Tempesta, et al., 1987). Evidence of this

[3] Figures from 2009/10 British Crime Survey data http://rds.homeoffice.gov.uk/rds/

denial can be found in the failed acknowledgement of a delayed period as a "sign" of pregnancy, the delay with which they finally resolve to taking a pregnancy test and, later on, their carelessness towards the fetus' needs (Tempesta et al., 1987). Moreover, these women often keep on using drugs during pregnancy while keeping their lifestyle unchanged for as long as possible, in homage to drug addiction homeostasis (Di Cagno et al., 1985). Even when drug consumption is discontinued during pregnancy, it is often resumed after delivery or during the postpartum period in an attempt to feel up to the new task and soothe the sense of guilt and failure.

In fact, for an addicted woman, delivery may imply having to cruelly realize what she was not able to do for her child and her negligence towards him/her: when real life needs become too hard, either because of the child's or the mother's difficulties or else for lack of a support network, the dream embodied in the fetus/child is shattered and heavy, depressive feelings may ensue which, up to that point, had been kept at bay by a megalomaniac investment on the child and on an idealized maternal image (De Zordo, 1997; Tempesta, et al., 1987).

No matter whether these women remain abstinent or else resume drug consumption, their difficulties in carrying out parenting functions emerge fairly early. Generally speaking, these mothers seem to find it difficult to build and maintain gratifying interpersonal relationships (with their partners and their families of origin), they tend to adopt a lifestyle leading to isolation and, above all, they have trouble in recognizing and satisfying their children's needs (Fiks, Johnson, Rosen, 1985). Their more or less conscious inadequacy in performing the parenting function has been suggested to derives from their early feelings and experiences: affective deprivation, losses, separations, lack of affective continuity in their families of origin (Johnson, Cohen, Brown, et al., 1999; Ravndal, Lauritzen, Frank, Jansson, Larsson, 2001). This inadequacy seems to be at the root of their educational style which is often characterized by an authoritarian overinvolment of the child: any external influence is rejected with a tendency to isolation, while the child is urged to become independent as quickly as possible and communication is controlled and avoided (Wellisch, Steinberg, 1980). Moreover, ambivalence seems to be a complex and typical feature of the relationships these mothers build with their children: they often expect them to take their mothers' expectations and wishes on themselves and consequently, they induce a role reversal and a process whereby these children are forced to think and act like adults, something they also experimented during their infantile past (Malagoli Togliatti, Mazzoni, 1993).

Finally, becoming a mother to a newborn does not coincide with a renewed motivation to seek counselling and/or treatment, rather, it strictly depends on a wide range of variables (McMahon, Luthar, 2000): according to the data available in the literature, mothers seem to be more prone to entering a detoxification and drug treatment when they are in young age, have more than one child, have got financial and legal problems, have suffered physical mistreatment and, above all, when they join advanced therapeutic programs (Grella et Al., 2006).

3. Children of drug-addicted mothers

It is indisputable that the development of children born from drug-addicted parents is highly at risk already before their birth, because the interaction of personal, relational and social factors does not support the individual's adjustment to his/her environment (see Nicolais, 2010). In this respect, Cicchetti and Rizley (1981) identify two categories of developmental risk factors: endogenous risk factors, such as physical or behavioral anomalies and psychological disorders, which make it difficult for the parent to take care of the child; exogenous risk factors, related to the environmental context in which the child is raised, such as features of his/her parents' personal histories, their psychological characteristics as well as ecological aspects of his life context or the one of the whole family. Both categories have become the subject of interest in several studies on this special children population.

3.1 Endogenous risk factors

Many research studies on children of addicted mothers, originally from US, focused on the harmful effects on the fetus following exposure to psychotropic substances, since recent data indicate that around 5% of all pregnant women aged between 15 and 44 years use substances (Substance Abuse and Mental Health Service Administration, 2005) which leads to the birth of approx. 375,000 babies with withdrawal symptoms every year.

In fact, psychoactive substances can have various harmful perinatal effects. Among others, the authors listed: rupture of the placenta and premature birth, low weight at birth and APGAR[4] scores below normal, low cranial circumference, the occurrence of perinatal stroke, congenital deformities and neurobehavioral disorders in newborns who had been exposed to cocaine and heroin during pregnancy (Lutinger, Graham, Einarson, Karen, 1991; Mayes, Granger, Bornstein, Zuckermann, 1992; Zuckerman, Bresnahan, 1991; Zuckerman et al., 1989). Moreover, the fetus can develop a dependency to the substances used by the mother: after delivery, when drug intake is abruptly discontinued, the baby runs the risk of undergoing real withdrawal crises (Foetal Drug Syndrome, FDS) which intensity may vary according to the used substance and its intake method (Finnegan, 1986; Zacchello, Giaquinto, 1997; Zuckerman, Brown, 1993).

Finally, it must be pointed out that many of these children test HIV-positive at birth: in most cases, remission occurs during the first months of life but for some of them, it is indicative of infection. Similar data are reported also for other infective pathologies such as hepatitis, syphilis, toxoplasmosis, cytomegalovirus (Zacchello, Giaquinto, 1997).

Later on, some studies report rhythm irregularities in the sleep-awake state and in food intake, as well as a tendency to hyperactivity (Zuckerman, 1994) already in early infancy. Learning difficulties, low attentive capacities and a higher degree of aggressiveness in

[4] Apgar: Abbreviation for the Apgar score, a practical method of evaluating the physical condition of a newborn infant shortly after birth. The Apgar score is a number arrived at by scoring the heart rate, respiratory effort, muscle tone, skin color, and response to a catheter in the nostril. Each of these signs can receive 0, 1, or 2 points. A perfect Apgar score of 10 means an infant is in the best possible condition. An infant with an Apgar score of 0-3 needs immediate intensive care. The Apgar score is measured routinely 60 seconds after delivery and then it is repeated after 5 minutes. In the event of a difficult resuscitation, the Apgar score may be done again at 10, 15, and 20 minutes. An Apgar score of 0-3 at 20 minutes of age is predictive of high morbidity (disease) and mortality (death). <http://www.medterms.com/script/main/art.asp?articlekey=2302>

preschool and school age (Cavazzuti, Frigieri, Finelli, 1987; Fundaro, Salvataggio, 1987; Oloffson, Buckley, 1983; Sanderegger, Zimmermann, 1978; Wilson, McCreary, Kean, Baxter, 1979) are also reported in these children, even if, compared to controls, neither differences in IQ levels nor alterations of intellectual functions are to be found (Azuma, Chasnoff, 1993). In this respect, Lester and Tronick (1994) offer an outlook on the effects of prenatal drug exposure which takes into consideration functional difficulties in the "4A" childhood areas (attention, arousal, affectivity and action). However, we should also remember the results of a research by Alessandri, Bendersky and Lewis (1998) revealing a correlation between the severity of the child's developmental deficit and the amount of substance (in their specific research, heroin) consumed by the mother during pregnancy. The neurobehavioral vulnerability which is typical of children who were exposed to drugs *in utero* must, therefore, be considered within a wider context including relational and environmental aspects too, two factors which also have an influence upon child development immediately after birth.

The clinical presentation of the "addicted babies" depends on the type of substances used by the mother during pregnancy, by value, frequency and time since last use / abuse. Substances commonly used by drug addicts are Alcohol, Nicotine, Marijuana, Tranquilizers, Cocaine and opioids in general, as well as 'heroin and methadone (Johnson & Kate, 2000; Lester & Barry, 2000). It was found that if the mother has made extensive use of drugs such as alcohol, hypnotics, or heroin–that could be considered "not exciting" the nervous system–the infant will manifest respiratory depression problems immediately after birth. Expressions of neonatal abstinence syndrome could be constant irritability, tremors and stiffness of muscle tone. Other possible symptoms include: irritability of the nervous system, gastrointestinal disorders, vomiting, diarrhea, hysterical crying, sleep disturbances, rapid breathing.

When we consider the effects of the substance exposure on the development of the child, the researches reveal that the global development is slowed and more in deficit at the cognitive level but not completely destroyed. In general, the child exposition to heroin and methadone during intrauterine development, is already evident after 48 hours of birth, while the exposure to the Alcohol leave marks immediate developing a real withdrawal syndrome. With reference to the specific symptoms related to different substances, many studies are interested to the exposure to Cocaine, that is a stimulant causing the blood vessels : this substance decreases the oxygen supply to the fetus and, consequently, the infant is at risk of suffocation. Also, the infants exposed to cocaine in the last gestational period reveal a state of reduced alertness and reduced responsiveness to external stimulation, when compared with controls.

In the table below are classified as such direct effects, distinguishing them according to the type of substance used by the mother (Wright & Walker, 2001).

3.2 Environmental factors: the attachment contribution

In addition to the various aspects highlighted in the studies mentioned above, we should not forget the multiple postnatal factors which contribute to determine the developmental outcomes of children who were born from drug-addicted parents.

The effect of drugs on mother and baby				
Drug	**Antepartum**	**Intrapartum**	**Post-partum**	**Long term**
Smoking	Growth restriction	Fetal Distress	Increases in Infant deaths	
Alcohol	Fetal Alcohol Syndrome		Maternal withdrawal symptoms	Fetal Alcohol syndrome Mental Impairment
Heroin / Opiates	Preterm Labor Growth restriction	Problem with analgesis	Neonatal abstinence syndrome	Probably not
Cocaine	Placental Pathology Growth Restriction Impaired brain development Abruption	Placental Pathology Low birth weight Fetal distress	Prolonged fetal withdrawal (3 days - 3 weeks) Chaotic lifestyle	Aggressive children Neurodevelopmental delay
Amphetamine	Growth restriction Maternal hypertension Antisocial behavior	Maternal cardiovascular disturbances	Chaotic lifestyle	
Ecstasy	Congenital defects			
Benzodiazepines	Cleft lip and palate			Neurodevelopmental delay

Table 1. The effect of drugs on mother and baby. Source: Wright & Walker, 2001

A large part of research in this domain have focused interest on the role of the quality of the proximal environmental factors on child development and well being; one of the most important factors that have an impact on child's early development is the quality of interactions and relations between child and the significant adults who play a protective role for him (the mother and/or other caregivers). In this perspective, the "Attachment theory" (Bowlby, 1969-1980) has provided useful theoretical and methodological tools to study the affective-relational development during the first years of life both in normal as well as in "at-risk" populations, in order to study the role of the quality of early interactions on the child well being and adaptation to the context.

According to this theoretical model, feeling safe and secure is the first and most important, early developmental task during the child's first year of life and one major protection factor in the process of adjusting himself/herself to the environment. Various research studies investigated the parent and child role and how they influenced the quality of the attachment bond: however, the contribution of each of the two parties is still not clear.

Van IJzendoorn, Goldberg, Kroonenberg, and Frenkel (1992) carried out a meta-analytical work on the influence of the child's and/or the parents' problems on the development of attachment during the first year of life. Attachment was assessed using the Strange Situation

Procedure[5] (Ainsworth, Blehar, Waters, Wall, 1978): researchers found a lower percentage of Secure attachment (B) and an increase in the Disorganized/Disoriented (D) category among samples of mother-child dyads at risk which differentiated them from the distributions observed in the general population. Moreover, a prevalent influence of maternal problems and difficulties rather than of children's endogenous risk factors came to light affecting the quality of infant-mother attachment. In fact, attachment distributions within groups of children of mistreating mothers (Carlson, Cicchetti, Barnett, Braunwald, 1989; Crittenden, 1985; Schneider-Rosen, Braunwald, Carlson, Cicchetti, 1985), mentally disturbed mothers or drug addicted mothers (Rodnig, Beckwith, Howard, 1989) revealed high divergence when compared to normative samples, more so than in case of problems coming from the child's side only. In fact, the child's problems did not seem to jeopardize the process of creating a secure attachment bond with the mother (van JIzendoorn et al., 1992).

Research studies with groups of parents suffering from psychiatric disorders, behavioral disorders or else mistreating their children seem to proceed along the same direction: once again, they reveal a high percentage of insecure attachment and, more specifically, entangled attachment (E) and unresolved attachment (U) tied to experiences of trauma and bereavement. These subjects seem to have difficulties in working through life experiences which they went through during childhood while their caregivers only proved to be scarcely adequate and supportive (van IJzendoorn, Bakermans-Kranenburg, 1996). Therefore, parents belonging to clinical populations do not seem to be emotionally secure, which represents a potential risk factor for their children, because of the process of intergenerational transmission of attachment, according to which the mother's representational world has got a fundamental role in the co-construction of a bond with the

[5] The Strange Situation is a standardized observation procedure (Ainsworth et al., 1978; Ainsworth, Wittig, 1969) which aims at activating and intensifying the child's attachment behavior towards his/her parent by exposing the child to a moderately, yet increasingly stressful situation. In fact, the Strange Situation takes place within a context – an observation laboratory – which is not familiar to the child: it foresees the presence of an unfamiliar adult and a series of two separations and reunions with the mother (or any other adult figure we might be interested in studying the child's attachment relationship with). This procedure is applicable to children between 12 and 24 months of age: between two subsequent administrations, a time interval of at least 6 months must be respected, so that the child can forget the situation and the stressful feelings tied with it (Ainsworth, 1985; Ainsworth, Bell, Stayton, 1971). The procedure is subdivided into eight short episodes, each of them lasting approximately three minutes and following one another according to a fixed order and a clearly stated consignment.
The SSP coding is based on the observation of the overall organization of a child's attachment behavior and foresees two assessment levels: the first one is based on graduated ordinal scales on a 7-point Likert scale (range 1 – 7), which refer to specific behavioral sequences the child can display in the various episodes. They can be applied to each procedure episode at 15-second intervals. The second level leads to the assignment of an attachment pattern according to four categories. It is based on the observation of the way in which the behavioral systems of attachment and exploration are organized during the whole procedure both towards the caregiver, as well as the stranger, while various stress elements are introduced, one after the other. The four categories are (Scheme 3): secure attachment (B) – research studies referring to "non-clinical" United States children show that between 54.9% and 67% of the population fall into this category; avoidant attachment (A) is observed in an average range of 20.5% - 22.9% of the population. Resistant attachment (C) is less frequent among the population (7.5% -12.5%), while disorganized/disoriented attachment (D) is observed in 14.7% of the children (van IJzendoorn, Goldberg, Kroonenberg, Frenkel, 1992).

child (Benoit, Parker, 1994; Fonagy, Steele, Steele, 1991; Ward, Carlson, 1995; van IJzendoorn, Bakermans-Kranenburg, 1997; Zeanah, 1992).

4. Therapeutic communities and the intervention model in Italy: an overview

In Europe, during the past years, referral to Juvenile Court was the most commonly applied procedure to drug-addicted mothers (Pomodoro, 1993, 1996). More often than not, these cases resulted in the suspension or revocation of parental rights, until the mother or both parents passed examinations which were required by the Court and administered by services in charge of evaluating and following the case. In case of substance addiction, a common solution during evaluation period was to separate the child from the mother (or both parents) and relocate him/her elsewhere, that is, for instance, at the grandparents' home, or else, at other out-patients services'. The first TC for mothers and children were founded in Switzerland, Germany and Italy in the early 1990s, then also in Spain and Portugal. Further solutions included admitting the child to family crisis intervention homes or placing the child in an extra-familial home or elsewhere, depending on the resources available in the territory. As for Italy, the juvenile judges' reluctance to place children in therapeutic communities - even though this would guarantee the presence of their mothers at their side - was justified by the fact that this environment - although run by professionals - did not seem to guarantee adequate attention to the child, nor did community workers seem to possess adequate training and the right methodological tools to operate for the well-being of the child and the mother-child couple. Therefore, more often than not, judges would take steps towards a separation of the mother-child dyad. These measures clearly indicated a lack of alternative possibilities within the enlarged network of fostering services but also un underlying prejudice towards drug-addicted parents who were considered "irredeemable" with regard to their capability to offer adequate care and protection to their children, especially in the very first years of their lives (Pomodoro, 1993, 1996). Confiding the child to his/her grandparents in foster care has become the most frequently adopted measure when one or both parents are drug-addict, even though this measure is still considered controversial as for its outcomes (Cirillo, 1996; Ghezzi, 1996). More specifically, criticism is raised towards its generalized and almost automatic use: if it is true, on the one hand, that it can provide an answer to the child's immediate need for protection, on the other hand it can turn into a very heavy obstacle against a possible recovery of the child's parents (Cirillo et Al., 1996). For this reason - as well as many others - the need has arisen for new intervention paths to be sought and experimented.

4.1 Therapeutic communities for drug-addicted women and their children

Over the past twenty years, the Veneto region has radically modified the functions of therapeutic communities for addicted mothers and their children, rethinking assessment and intervention measures in case of female drug addiction while paying special attention to children's well-being and to the results obtained in the short and long run. Communities for drug-addicted women and their children offer residential care to the mother-child dyad (sometimes to the father too) and provide a comprehensive rehabilitation program which takes place during a two-year stay. Many of these facilities are now present on the whole national territory: they greatly differ from each other in terms of constituent aspects which have now been included into a complex and articulated regulation that also leaves room for autonomous regional organization and definition (available places, internal arrangement, monthly fee etc.). These facilities can accommodate up to 10-12 dyads: as for the children's age, the range spans from few-months-old babies (but more and more often, pregnant women are admitted too) up to school age children. In the first place, communities give hospitality to drug-addicted women (already detoxified or on methadone therapy and followed by the "Ser.T.", territorial services), who are offered a comprehensive rehabilitation path.

One further aspect of paramount importance is that, within a mother-child therapeutic community, addicted mothers are offered parenting support. Admitting the mother-child dyad into the community means guaranteeing an adequate intervention for the adult, while providing a protective environment for the child. Indeed, many of the problems associated with child development when a mother suffers from addiction can be addressed more easily and eventually solved once these children are offered an appropriate and stable relational context (Chasnoff, 1992). Moreover, a direct admittance of the mother-child dyad satisfies the need to overcome barriers between generations, since both the addicted woman's and her partner's families of origin are often not willing to help looking after the child. Moreover, it has been demonstrated how implementing assistance tools for children and families with a family-based approach prevents treatment dropouts (McComish, et al., 2000; Grella, et al., 2000). In fact, a droupout risk exists from the very first moment addicted mothers enter a therapeutic community, which is for them a very difficult step to take. These mothers fear that they might be labeled as incapable of caring for their children and consequently, that they have to be separated from them (National Institute on Drug Abuse, 1996; Stevens, et al., 1989).

As for the intervention methods, a combined treatment (that is, for the parent and the child together) is carried out on an intensive basis (the dyads are in residential care): in other words, it is typical of these communities to offer a therapeutic rehabilitation program which is centered on the family-parent-child system taken as a whole (Meisels, Dichtelmiller, Fong-Ruey Liaw, 1993). Usually, the mother is the primary focus of the intervention: however, special attention is given to the mother-child relationship too in all facilities offering support to the dyad. An intervention on the child is carried out only when it becomes clear that there is a need for it: in fact, in most cases, these children are physically and psychologically healthy but their caregiving environment reveals a symptomatology which must be tackled and solved. However, in recent times, greater and greater attention has been paid to ensuring the well-being of children living in therapeutic communities, since having a drug-addicted parent is indeed considered as a sort of risk factor in relation to the child's evolutionary path (Capra, 2011). The length of time mothers have to devote to their rehabilitation program actually affects children too. At a very early stage in their lives, when many new experiences should be made and new things should be learnt, they spend a long time at a therapeutic community's. Actually, already during the gestation period, they were exposed to the drugs consumed by the mother and often had to endure their mother's irregular alimentation and burdensome life rhythms. Even when delivery and the post partum period went well and without complications, during the first months of life most of these children experienced multiple separations from their mothers or closest caregivers, who were often scarcely respectful of their rhythms and needs. Others had to confront themselves with new people and environments: for instance, with specialized health care services, or else they had to meet social workers, psychologists or community workers.

Finally, some of them had to endure sudden changes in their daily life and moved to another house or a different town etc. Because of all this, one of the primary interventions in favor of children residing at a community's is to offer them stable life conditions, deep affective experiences as well as sound routine practices. With reference to the last mentioned aspect, communities seem to work as a place of physical and psychological attachment within which it becomes possible to create new and adequate affective relationships: all this is made possible thanks to the "holding" function supplied by the community as a context of early caregiving and a guarantee of protection from danger, as well as a secure base for the exploration of the environment. This concept of community allows us to consider it, all in all, as a parenting environment where the a growth towards motherhood can be followed and supported, where mothers are no longer blamed or punished for their inadequacy and difficulties but rather are offered a very important chance to experience regression to the role of daughters and children in need (who are taken care of by community workers, psychologists etc.). The chance to experience mixed feelings towards their institutional "parents" seems to make it possible for these women to trace down the relational and representational bonds which were cut short during their infancy and adolescence favoring a review of their own past which is very beneficial to the relationship with their children.

5. A research and intervention project on minors in therapeutic communities for addicted mothers and children

Until a few years ago, in Italy, communities for drug-addicted mothers and their children provided treatments to disintoxicate mothers and favour their rehabilitation into society, while also ensuring overall medical and social support for their children's development, for whom no specialized health treatment was foreseen (in case of need, treatment would be carried out by facilities outside of the community). However, in the last few years, a radical and much needed-for reorganization has come into effect in the field of residential and semi-residential services for drug-addicts and alcohol-addicts. More specifically, during the years 2006-2007 in North-Eastern Italy, new service units have been defined for addiction treatment, among others: swift admission services, semi-residential services, residential services (type A - B - C), type C1 (for drug-addicted mothers with minor children) and C2 (for drug-addicted minors). Moreover, requirements and standards authorizing socio-sanitary and social facilities to offer assistance have been redefined so as to bestow them recognition at institutional level. Over the years, especially in the Veneto region, it became clear that it was necessary to better define professional competences together with the methodological and organizational pre-requisites which are at the root of the intervention procedures in these specialized services. Treatment paths and management procedures within these services were redefined, whereby treatment must include a parallel series of medical-pharmacological, psychological and socio-educational interventions which are offered not only to the mother, but to the child too. Therefore, since 2008, the mother-child dyad and the quality of the caregiving relationship which develops between the two in the course of time have acquired prominent focus in the assessments and interventions by professionals who work in this specific field. The combination of all these assessment procedures is extremely important in order to arrange the best therapeutic and rehabilitation path for the mother who, up to that point, had been considered the sole subject to be taken therapeutic charge of in the community.

However, when minors are sent to therapeutic communities together with their mothers, this usually happens following a decree by a tutelary judge of the juvenile court so as to make sure that they receive protection and their psycho-physical health condition is assessed. For this reason, it was necessary to reconsider all areas of competence within direct and indirect interventions in favour of minors. Following this path, as of 2010, new socio-sanitary services for children in therapeutic communities type C1 have received official recognition. They are conducted by health professionals and technicians and foresee individualized interventions (individual psychological support, psychomotility , pet therapy), group psychomotility, clinical observation and assessment of the father-child and mother-child relationship, neuropsychiatric observation and assessment, mother-child relationship supervision and relational psychotherapy. Therefore, nowadays, not only are mothers but also their children officially considered clients of a community, where they are offered specific interventions of socio-psycho-physical health care.

It is not easy to combine clinical and rehabilitation activities with research. The authors have striven to set innovative research projects in motion which methodological principles are going to be described in the following pages. In so doing, we hope to stimulate cultural growth while improving care giving practices. The first, preliminary results are presented in this chapter.

The project "Research and intervention on minors in communities for drug-addicted mothers and their children: from at-risk parenting to child wellbeing" is the result of joint work carried out by the Psychology Department of the University of Padua and two therapeutic communities for addicted mothers and their children, *Villa Emma* and *Casa Aurora,* located in Venice and its mainland (Mestre) and run by the social cooperative *Villa Renata.*

The project provides a multi-method evaluation through a longitudinal approach aimed at programming and monitoring the interventions performed by parents while following the development of children living in therapeutic communities. Developmental risk factors and/or clinically relevant, real life symptoms are identified as they emerge. Our theoretical and methodological points of reference are based on the study of parenting and development according to the current, dynamic, multi-factor models of influence (Belsky, 1984; Gabble, Belsky, Crnic 1992; De Palo, 2010).

The setting of the project is the therapeutic community and its complex caregiving system. The focus of the assessment is set on three areas, each of which is investigated at different levels: (a) evaluation of the mother's psychic condition, in terms of personality and individual characteristics, assessed through interviews (such as the Adult Attachment Interview[6], SCID-II[7]), questionnaires and dynamic tests (Rorchach[8]); (b) evaluation of the

[6] **The Adult Attachment Interview** (AAI) developed by George, Kaplan and Main (1985) is a semi-structured interview assessing attachment in adolescence and adult age. The interview includes a series of questions through which a subject is asked to recall his/her attachment history and attachment experiences with his/her caregivers during infancy. The AAI coding scheme foresees two distinct phases: a first phase during which text content and form are analyzed through Evaluation Scales (Scales of Subjective Experience and Scales of the State of Mind) and a second phase during which the interview is analyzed as a whole in order to formulate a categorical classification of the subject's attachment.

mother's parenting capabilities as well as those of the father's (if present), through the observation of their interactions with the child both in daily routine exchanges and/or in structured settings (Attachment Q-Sort[9], Lausanne Trilogue Play[10], Emotional Availability Scales[11]); (c) evaluation of the child's development and adjustment through assessment measures for the developmental age (Vineland Scales[12], Child Behavior Check List[13], Attachment Story Completion Task[14]), aimed at identifying a developmental diagnosis according to the indications of the current 0-3 classification system for early infancy; (d) a comprehensive analysis of the progressive and current context of relations between caregiver and child, exploring limits and points of strength; (e) data obtained at various observational levels are shared by a professional team striving to achieve data integration so as to guarantee a very careful and comprehensive evaluation. Thanks to these organized data, it is possible to acquire a deeper knowledge and a better understanding of the

---

[7] **The Structured Clinical Interview for DSM-III-R** . The SCID-II (First, Gibbon, Spitzer, Williams, & Benjamin, 1997) allows diagnostic evaluations of a potential personality disorder such as the ones included on Axis II of DSM-IV, passive-aggressive and depressive disorders (Appendix B of DSM-IV) and unspecified personality disorder (UPD). The Italian version of the SCID for DSM-IV was published in 2003.

[8] **The Rorschach Test** (Rorschach, 1921) is a perception, projective, psycho-diagnostic instrument. It is composed of 10 standardized cards out of 23 (5 black and grey, 2 red and grey and 3 multi-coloured), each of them carrying a symmetric ink-blot. With this test, it is possible to observe both stable personality traits as well as a possible psychopathology or possible affective disorders. Moreover, this test offers very valuable information on the subject's intelligence and cognitive processes. As for data analysis and interpretation, they are carried out both at quantitative and at qualitative level.

[9] **The Attachment Q-Sort** (Waters, & Deane, 1985) allows repeated data acquisition over one single week, so as to compare the attachment bonds created by the child with his/her caregivers, as well as a measurement of children's attachment over a longer period of time (from 1 to 5 years). The AQS comprises 90 items which describe a child's attachment behaviours in his/her natural, everyday home environment.

[10] **The Lausanne Trilogue Play** (LTP, Fivaz-Depeursinge, Corboz-Warnery, 1999) is a semi-standardized, laboratory, play procedure during which mother, father and child interact. This procedure allows observation and evaluation of the quality of interactions within the mother-father-child family system during a play interaction where all three partners are involved at the same time. The coding scheme of the LTP procedure is made up of 10 scales, each of them defining an observation variable (Lavanchy, Cunnet, Favez, 2006). They are graduated on a 5-point Likert Scale (range 1 – 5) and coded for each of the four parts of the procedure.

[11] **Emotional Availability Scales** (EAS, Biringen Robison Emde, 1998) Interactive adult-child video-recordings are observed and evaluated according to the adult's sensitivity, his/her capacity to frame the environment, his/her non-intrusiveness and non-hostility. The child's involvement and his/her replies to the adult are evaluated too.

[12] **The Vineland scales** allow measurement – by means of a semi-structured interview –of 4 main dimensions (scales) and 11 sub-dimensions (subscales). They can find application in various clinical, educational and research settings: they are particularly useful to observe adaptive behaviours and to investigate to what degree a disability, if present, can have an impact on the subject's everyday performances.

[13] **Child Behavior Check List Achenbach CBCL** (1991, 1992) This scale allows to investigate social competencies and behavioural problems in children aged 18 months - 18 years. Its items favour a description of the child's behavioural and emotional repertoire through the narratives supplied by parents, teachers and/or educators supporting the evaluation of a potentially problematic conduct as listed in the behavioural scales.

[14] The **Attachment Story Completion Task** (ASCT; Bretherton, Ridgeway, Cassidy, 1990) was designed to assess attachment style in preschool and school age. Five story stems referring to attachment-relevant family themes are presented to the child who is asked to complete them freely using a set of dolls and props.

1st PHASE	**Assessment of mother's parental capabilities**		
OBJECTIVE	Investigate mother's personality characteristics and her attachment history since these are indexes of her parental competence.		
INVESTIGATED AREAS	Personality ↓	Pathology self-perception ↓	Attachment ↓
MEASURES	Rorschach Test	SCID II (Structured Clinical Interview for DSM-IV)	AAI (Adult Attachment Interview)

2ndPHASE	**a) Indirect assessment of the child (through mothers/educators)**		
OBJECTIVE	1) Evaluation of the child's relational and developmental competencies and psychopathological aspects 2)Give mothers a chance to compare and share their perceptions of their children with those of the educators, so as to find a common language on the main topics referring to the children		
INVESTIGATED AREAS	Development ↓	Symptomatology ↓	Attachment relationship ↓
MEASURES	VABS (Vineland Adaptive Behavior Scales)	CBCL (Child Behavior Checklist)	AQS (Attachment Q-Sort)

	b) Assessment of adult-child relationships			
OBJECTIVE	1) Observation and evaluation of the mother-child dyadic relationship (if possible, the father-child relationship too) then comparison with the educator-child dyadic relationship 2) If possible, observation and evaluation of the mother -father -child triadic relationship			
OBSERVED RELATIONSHIPS	Mother-Child ↘	Educator-Child ↓	Father-Child ↙	Mother-Father-Child ↓
MEASURES	EAS (Emotional Availability Scales)			LTP (Lausanne Trilogue Play).

3rdPHASE	**Direct assessment of the child**
	This investigation is only carried out on children who show dysfunctional or pathological characteristics during screening phase 2

OBJECTIVE	Observation and evaluation of the child's development, symptomatology and relationships. If any of these fields prove to be dysfunctional, it is possible to carry out a direct diagnostic investigation on the child.			
INVESTIGATED AREAS	Development ↓	Symptomatology ↙ ↓ ↘		Attachment relationship ↓
MEASURES	VABS (see phase 2)	Rorschach Test (see phase 1)	CBCL (see phase 2)	ASCT
		N.B. If CBCL results provide evidence of cognitive problems, WPPSI-III/WISC-III and BSID-III are administered.		
4th PHASE	**Intervention**			
	According to the child's age and needs as identified during the assessment phase, the offered intervention and support can be organized as follows:			
	Group: Therapeutic support is offered to the child. Intervention mainly focused on the relational dynamics with peers	Dyadic: Therapeutic support is offered to the mother-child dyad. Intervention on the relationship	Individual: Therapeutic support is offered to the child. Individual intervention	
	Psicomotility: individual - group			

Table 2. Phases of our research project: "A model of research and intervention on minors in communities for drug-addicted mothers and their children: from at-risk parenting to child wellbeing".

caregiver, the child and their relationship: these data also help professionals to more clearly identify the therapeutic and pedagogical objectives to be suggested to the dyad, which can then be supported and monitored over time. These objectives can be modified and re-elaborated according to each individual project but also to the changes observed during the intervention. In fact, the same evaluation procedure is administered at different times during the mother-child residential period. It aims at monitoring the interventions and any possible change as well as identifying eventual aspects of danger and/or increased risk that may require the use of further community facilities. A continuous assessment of the intervention is a powerful instrument to reflect, both clinically and ethically, on the opportunity to go on providing care to mother-child pairs featuring elements of danger and pathology. This assessment also examines the presence of prejudicial clinical manifestations of the child and any developmental difficulties related to inadequate maternal care which can arise in spite of the protective and rehabilitative intervention provided by the community and its comprehensive setting. In 2010, we started gathering data which are presently being processed and which will be described in depth in this chapter.

6. Conclusions

Our project started in 2009: the following, preliminary results are now available (De Palo, Simonelli, Capra, 2010). Twenty-four mothers took part to the program: they were evaluated according to the 1st phase protocol. The reported data refer to the first twelve of them, whom data have already been processed for. Generally speaking, 31 is their mean age: they entered the community at different times from 2007 to 2010. Most of them started consuming substances during pre-adolescence/adolescence (12-19 years).

The first aspect refers to personality diagnosis: 10 subjects were diagnosed a structure of personality with borderline features (polydrug use of psychotropic substances with heroin as the main substance of abuse). This characteristic shows a clinically significant association with some other investigated aspects, particularly, with an insecure attachment style which is prevalent within the group and which seems to be rooted in experiences of traumatic and/or doleful events during these women's infancy, especially physical and sexual abuse which most of them experienced in intra-familial environments. Moreover, their attachment style, which developed on the basis of their infantile experiences with their caregivers, is associated to disorganization characteristics and a difficulty to work through early experiences of loss or trauma. The educational style they experienced in their families of origin was predominantly coercive. To sum up, at exploratory level we can say that, in the mothers accommodated at the community, we notice associations between early traumatic events (coercive educational style and abuse) experienced within their families of origin, an insecure working-through of their own attachment history and borderline personality features. These results urge us towards a reflection on feasible intervention methods for patients presenting similar clinical pictures where drug-addiction almost seems just a symptom of a more complex pathology. At the same time, this reflection seems of paramount importance to globally re-think interventions in favor of minors living in the community: in fact, shouldn't the fact of being born to mothers with similar characteristics be considered in itself a vulnerability factor which shall issue to psychopathology?

We believe that a possible answer can be found within the described project, since the main objective of our research and intervention model is to observe the child's level of development and the risk and protective factors characterizing his/her growth so as to plan taylor-made interventions to satisfy each single minor client's needs and support each single mother-child relationship. Therefore, within the model we presented in this paper, attention is focused on the well-being of minors who were born to drug-addicted mothers. Reason for this choice is the unavoidable need to carefully and realistically consider the condition of these children: their drug-addicted mothers present an at-risk parenting function and are therefore supported by educators who play the role of more adequate, alternative caregivers. The "adolescent" aspect of drug-addicted women can be a major risk factor against the assumption of their parental role: these mothers are often envious of the therapeutic support which is given to the child and which develops in a situation of conflict between mother and child. Moreover, these patients often have great difficulties in acknowledging limits, even physical ones, between their child and themselves: these mothers often find it hard to distinguish themselves from their child, especially if it is a female child, and they mix up their thoughts, actions and feelings with those of their daughters. When they have a male child, they find it difficult to differentiate their sons from their own fathers or partners. Therefore, by choosing to set up a project on minors' health, all research objectives are focused on the viable, most adequate actions to be taken in order to achieve the set goal, that is, the well-being of children born to adults with parenting function at risk.

To this extent, a parallel administration of evaluation measures both to the mother and to the educator makes it possible to investigate what is the latter's (and the community's) image of the child. Carefully monitoring the idea the community has of a child makes it possible to create a univocal perception of him/her which otherwise gets lost in the various circumstances characterizing the community environment. The attention educators continuously devote to the child is shared with the mother, with whom they strive to create a univocal, shared image of the minor. Actually, within a community for drug-addicted mothers and their children, both educators and the very treating team perform the function of secure base which neither the mother nor the child have found elsewhere: they offer an alternative and vicarious relational model both to women and their children. Since educators possess characteristics that are typical of early caregivers (closeness, continuous presence, responsiveness etc.), they often find themselves emotionally involved in the relationship with the child: for this reason, their continuous training and supervision aim at helping them to stick to their professional role, without wanting to replace the mother's role.

7. References

Achenbach, T.M. (1991). Manual for the Child Behavior Check List/4-18 and 1991 Profile. Burlington: University of Vermont.

Achenbach, T.M. (1992). Manual for the Child Behavior Check List/2-3 and 1992 Profile. Burlington: University of Vermont.

Ainsworth, M. D. S. (1985). Patterns of infant-mother attachment: antecedents and effects on development. Bulletin of the New York Academy of Medicine, 61, 771-791

Ainsworth, M. D. S, Wittig B. A. (1969). Attachment and exploratory behavior of one-year-olds in a strange-situation. In B. M. Foss (Eds), Determinants of infant behavior IV, Methuen, London, 113-136.

Ainsworth, M. D. S., Bell, S. M., Stayton, D. J. (1971). Infant-mother attachment and social development: socialization as a product of reciprocal responsiveness to signals. In M. P. M. Richards (Eds) (1971). The integration of a child into a social world, Cambridge University Press, London, 99-135

Ainsworth, M. D. S., Blehar, M. C., Waters, E., & Wall, S. (1978). Patterns of attachment: A psychological study of the strange situation. Hillsdale, NJ: Erlbaum.

Alessandri S. M., Bendersky, M., Lewis, M. (1998). Cognitive functioning in 8- to 18-month-old drug-exposed infants, Dev Psychol. 1998 May;34(3):565-73. Retrieved from <http://www.ncbi.nlm.nih.gov/pmc/articles/PMC1531636/?tool=pubmed>

Anderson, P., & Baumberg, B. (2006). Alcohol in Europe. A public health perspective. Analysis for the European Commission. Institute of Alcohol Studies, UK. Retrieved from <http://ec.europa.eu/health/ph_determinants/life_style/alcohol/documents/alcohol_europe.pdf >

Aronica E. et Al. (1987). Il rapporto tra donna e droga. Alla ricerca di possibili differenze e specificità. Atti del Convegno "La donna e l'eroina". Torino: CIC Ed. Internaz.

Associazione Parsec (2004, April, 16). In-Dipendenza Donna: Workshop su Tossicodipendenza e Maternità, Paper presented at meeting of Istituto Superiore di Sanità, Roma.

Azuma, C.D., & Chasnoff, I. J. (1993). Outcome of children prenatally exposed to cocaine and other drugs: A path analysis of three-year data. Pediatrics, 92(3), 396-402.

Belsky, J. (1984). The Determinants of Parenting: A Process Model. Child Development, 55, 83-96.

Benoit, D., & Parker, K.C.H. (1994). Stability and Transmission of Attachment across Three Generations. Child Devolopment, 65, 1444-1456.

Biringen, Z., Robinson, J., & Emde, R.N. (1998). The emotional availability scales (3rd ed.). Unpublished manuscript, Department of Human Development & Family Studies, Colorado State University, Fort Collins, CO.

Bobes J., Casas M., Szerman N. et al. (2009). "Manejo clínico del paciente con patología dual. Recomendaciones de expertos". In Socidrogalcohol. Valencia. Retrieved from <www.socidrogalcohol.org>

Bowlby, J. (1969). Attachment: Attachment and Loss (Vol. 1). New York: Basic Books (trad. it. Attaccamento e perdita (Vol. 1): L'attaccamento alla madre, Boringhieri, Torino 1972.)

Bowlby, J. (1973). Separation: Anxiety & Anger: Attachment and Loss (Vol. 2). London: Hogarth Press (trad. it. Attaccamento e perdita (Vol. 2): La separazione dalla madre, Boringhieri, Torino, 1975).

Bowlby, J. (1980). Loss: Sadness & Depression: Attachment and Loss (Vol. 3). London: Hogarth Press (trad. it. Attaccamento e perdita (Vol. 3): La perdita della madre, Boringhieri, Torino, 1983.)

Brentari, C., Herrera Hernandez, B., Tripodi, S. (2011, in press). Attention to Women Drug Users in Europe, Guidelines of the "Democracy, Cities and Drugs II" Project. A Public Health Executive Agency project. Retrieved from <www.democitydrug.org>

Bretherton, I., Ridgeway, D., & Cassidy, J. (1990). Assessing internal working models of the attachment relationships: An Attachment Story Completion Task for 3-year-olds. In M.T. Greenberg, D. Cicchetti, & E.M. Cummings (Eds.), Attachment in the preschool years: Theory, research, and intervention (pp. 273-308). Chicago: University of Chicago Press.

Buckley, P., Brady, K., & Hermann, R.. (2010). Dual diagnosis: Severe mental illness and substance use disorders. UpToDate, Inc. MA. Online 18.2:, Retrieved from <www.uptodate.com>

Capra, N. (2011). Presentazione del progetto terapeutico di presa in carico residenziale in comunità per madri tossicodipendenti e i loro figli. Paper presented at International conference "L'esposizione dei minori alle droghe: dalla vita prenatale all'adolescenza", February 24-26 2011 Padova, Italy.

Carlson, V., Cicchetti, D., Barnett, D., & Braunwald, K. (1989). Disorganized/disoriented attachment relationships in maltreated infants. Developmental Psychology, 25, 525-531.

Cavazzuti, G.B., Frigieri, G., & Finelli, P. (1987). Il follow up del bambino nato da madre farmacodipendente. Bollettino per le farmacodipendenze e l'Alcolismo, 10(6), 20-28.

Charles Pull, C.B., (2004). Binge Eating Disorder. Current Opinion in Psychiatry, 17(1), 43-48.

Chasnoff, I.J. (1992). Cocaine, pregnancy, and the growing child. Current Problems in Pediatrics, 22, 302–321.

Cicchetti, D., & Rizley, R. (1981). Developmental perspective on the etiology,Intergenerational trasmission and Sequelae un Child Abuse and Neglect. Journal of American Accademy of Child Adolescent Psychiatry, 34, 541-565.

Ciechanowski, P., Katon W., Stein, B.M., & Hermann R. (2010), Post-traumatic stress disorder: Epidemiology, pathophysiology, clinical manifestations, and diagnosis, UpToDate, Inc. MA. Retrieved from <www.uptodate.com>

Cirillo S. et Al., (1996), La famiglia del tossicodipendente, Cortina, Milano

Cloninger, C. (1990). The empirical structure of psychiatric comorbidity and its theoretical significance. US: American Psychiatric Association.

Crittenden, P.M. (1985). Maltreated infants: Vulnerability and resilience. Journal of Child Psychology and Psychiatry, 26, 85-96.

De Leon, G. (1989). Psychopathology and substance abuse and psychiatric disorders: what is being learned from research in therapeutic community. Journal of psychoactive drugs, 21, 177/188.

De Palo, F. (2010). The trasmission gap: quali influenze familiari e contestuali nel passaggio tra rappresentazioni dell'adulto e comportamenti di attaccamento del bambino. Ph.D. Thesis. Milan University

De Palo, F., Simonelli, A., & Capra, N. (2010). Madri tossicodipendenti: attaccamento personalità e trattamenti possibili. Paper presented at "Congresso Nazionale dell'Associazione Italiana di Psicologia (AIP) - Sezione di psicologia clinica" September 24-26 2010. Università degli Studi di Torino.

De Zordo, M.R. (1997). Genitori e bambini: genitori-bambini. In G. Fava Vizziello & P. Stocco (Eds.), Tra genitori e figli la tossicodipendenza (pp. 103-120). Milano: Masson.

Di Cagno, L., et al. (1985). Distorsione della relazione oggettuale e persistente della tossicodipendenza. Giornale di Neuropsichiatria dell'Età Evolutiva, 5,(2) 133-138.

Di Sciascio, G., & Nardini, M. (2005). Comorbidità fra disturbi mentali e dipendenze patologiche: il problema della cosiddetta "Doppia Diagnosi". DITE-Edizioni Scientifiche.

Doherty, M.C., Garfein, R.S., Monterroso, E., Latkin, C., & Vlahov, D. (2000). Gender difference in the initiation of injecting drug use among young adults. Journal of Urban Health, 77(3), 397

Eurasian Harm Reduction Network. (2007). Hepatitis C among Injecting Drug Users in the New EU Member States and Neighboring Countries. Situation, Guidelines and Recommendations. Vilnius: Eurasian Harm Reduction Network.

EuroHIV. (2007). HIV / AIDS Surveillance in Europe, Mid-year report 2006, No. 74. French Institute for Public Health Surveillance, Saint-Maurice.

European Monitoring Centre for Drugs and Drug Addiction (EMCDDA). (2005). Differences in patterns of drug use between women and men. Paper presented at meeting of European Drug Situation, Lisbon. Retrieved September 10, 2010 from <http://www.emcdda.europa.eu/html.cfm/index34278EN.html>

European Monitoring Centre for Drugs and Drug Addiction (EMCDDA) (2006). The state of the drugs problem in Europe. Annual report. EMCDDA. Luxembourg: Publications Office of the European Union.

European Monitoring Centre for Drugs and Drug Addiction (EMCDDA) (2006a). A gender perspective on drug use and responding to drug problems. Paper presented at meeting of European Drug Situation, Lisbon.

EMCDDA (European Monitoring Center for Drugs and Drug Addiction) (2009). The State of the Drugs Problems in Europe. Annual Report. Luxembourg: Publications Office of the European Union, 2009 – ISBN 978-92-9168-384-0

European Women's Lobby (2001), Young Women's Guide to Equality between Women and Men in Europe, EWL- LEF, Brussels, Retrieved from <http://www.womenlobby.org>

Ficks, K.B., Johnson, H.L., & Rosen, T.S. (1985) Methadone-Mantained Mothers: Three-Year Follow-up of Parental Functioning. The international journal of the addiction, 20(5), 45-57.

Finnegan, 1986. Neonatal Abstinence Syndrome (NAS) Clinical Presentation and Management.

First, M.B., Gibbon, M., Spitzer, R.L., Williams, J.B.W., & Benjamin, L.S. (1997). Structured Clinical Interview for DSM-IV Axis II Personality Disorders, (SCID-II). Washington: American Psychiatric Press.

Fivaz-Depeursinge, E., & Corboz-Warnery, A. (1999). The Primary Triangle: A develompmental system view of fathers, mothers and infants. New York: Basic Books. (Trad. it. Il triangolo primario: Le prime interazioni triadiche tra padre, madre e bambino, Cortina, Milano, 2002).

Fonagy, P., Steele, M., & Steele, H. 1991, Maternal representation of attachment during pregnancy predict the organisation of infant-mother attachment at one year of age. Child Development, 62, 891-905.

Fundaro, C. & Salvataggio, E. 1987, Lo sviluppo del bambino di madre tossicodipendente. Bollettino per le Farmacodipendenze e l'Alcolismo, X, 6.

Gable, S., Belsky, J., & Crnic, K. (1992). Marriage, Parenting, and Child Development: Progress and Prospects. Journal of Family Psychology, 5, 276-294.

Ghezzi, D., & Vadilonga, F.1996, (Eds.) La tutela del minore. Milano: Raffaello Cortina Editore.

Gelinas, D. (1983). "The persisting negative effects of incest". Psychiatry, 46, p. 312-332

George, C., Kaplan, N., & Main, M. (1985). Adult Attachment Interview. Unpublished manuscript, Department of Psychology, University of California, Berkeley.

Genazzani, A.R., Santoro, V., Carino, M., Golinelli, S., Maietta Latessa, A., & Volpe, A. (1987). Riproduzione e farmacodipendenza. Bollettino Farmacologico e Alcol, 6, 609-615.

Goldberg, D. (1996), A dimensional model for common mental disorders, British Journal of Psychiatry, Vol 168 (Suppl 30), Jul 1996, 44-49.

Grella, C.E., Joshi, V., & Hser, Y.I. (2000). Program variation in treatment outcomes among women in residential drug treatment. Evaluation Review, 24(4), 364–383.

Grella, C.E., Hser, Y,I., Huang, Y.C. (2006). Mothers in substance abuse treatment: differences in characteristics based on involvement with child welfare services, Child Abuse Neglect, Jan; 30(1), 55-73.

Home Ministry Government (2010). Call to End Violence against Women and Girls, ISBN: 978-1-84987-377-2, London, Retrieved from <http://www.homeoffice.gov.uk/publications/crime/call-end-violence-women-girls/vawg-paper?view=Binary>

Hunter G and Powis B., (1996). Women drug users: barriers to service use, and service needs. The Centre for Research on Drugs and Health Behaviour: Executive Summary, 47, 1996

Instituto de la Mujer. (2007). Ministerio de Trabajo y Asuntos Sociales. Intervención en drogodependencias con enfoque de género. Nipo: 207-07-132-8. Madrid. Retrieved from <http://www.mtas.es/mujer>

Ijzendoorn M. H. Van, Goldberg S., Kroonenberg P. M., Frenkel O. J. (1992). The relative effects of maternal and child problems on the quality of attachment: a meta-analysis of attachment in clinical samples, Child Development , 63, 840-858

Johnson, J., G., Cohen, P., Brown, J., et al. (1999). Childhood maltreatment increases risk for personality disorders during early adulthood. Archives of General Psychiatry, 56, 600-606.

Johnson, K. (2000). Prenatal Cigarette, Cocaine Exposure Tied to Language Problems. OB GYN News, 35, 13.

Klerman, G.L. (1990). Approaches to the phenomena of comorbidity. American Psychiatric Association, US

Lavancy, C., Cuennet & Favez, N. (2006). Coding manual for Family Alliance Assessment Scale (Evaluation grid of the Lausanne Triadic Play). Fourth version. Manoscritto non pubblicato. Centre d'Etude de la Famille (CEF). Lausanne.

Lester, B. M. & Tronick, E. Z. 1994, The effects of prenatal cocaine exposure and child outcome. Infant Mentaal Health Journal, 15(2), 107-120.

Lester, Barry. (2000). Drug-addicted Mothers Need Treatment, Not Punishment. Alcoholism & Drug Abuse Weekly, 12, 5.

Malacrea, M., (2006). Caratteristiche, dinamiche ed effetti della violenza su bambini e bambine", In: Bianchi, D., Moretti, E., (2006). Vite in bilico. Indagine retrospettiva su maltrattamenti e abusi in età infantile. Ministero della Solidarietà Sociale, Centro Nazionale Documentazione e Analisi per l'Infanzia e l'Adolescenza. Retrieved from <http://ems.cilea.it/archive/00000763/01/Vite_in_bilico_Q40.pdf>

Malagoli Togliatti, M., Mazzoni, S. (1993). Maternità e tossicodipendenza. Milano: Giuffrè

Mayes, L. C., Granger, R. H., Bornstein, M. H., & Zuckerman, B. 1992, The problem of prenatal cocaine exposure: A rush to judgment. Journal of the American Medical Association, 267, 406-408

McComish, J.F., Greenberg, R., Ager, J., Chruscial, H., & Laken, M. (2000). Survival analysis of three treatment modalities in a residential substance abuse program for women and their children. Outcomes Management for Nursing Practice, 4(2), 71-77.

McMahon, T.J., Luthar, S.S. (2000). "Women in Treatment: Within-Gender Differences in the Clinical Presentation of Opioid-Dependent Women", In Journal of Nervous & Mental Disease: October 2000 - Volume 188 - Issue 10 - pp 679-687

Meisels, S. J., Dichtelmiller, M., & Fong-Ruey L. (1993). Un'analisi multidimansionale dei programmi di intervento per la prima infanzia. In C.H. Zeanah (Ed.), Manuale di salute mentale infantile (pp.317-339). Milano: Masson.

Ministero della Salute (2010). Rilevazione attività nel settore tossicodipendenze: Anno 2008. Retrieved October 3, 2010, Retrieved from <http://www.salute.gov.it/imgs/C_17_pubblicazioni_1306_allegato.pdf>

Moral Jiménez, M., Sirvent Ruiz, C. (2007). Codependence and Gender: exploratory analysis in differences in tds- 100 symptomatic factors. 8° Congreso Vrtual de Psiquiatría. Interpsiquis Febrero 2007. Psiquiatria.com, Retrieved from <http://www.fispiral.com/wp/wp-content/uploads/2012/01/21.pdf>

National Institute on Drug Abuse (NIDA) (1996). National pregnancy and health survey: Drug Use Among Women Delivering Livebirths. Rockville, MD: National Institutes of Health Publications.

NSW Department for Women, Young Women's health: depression and risk taking behavior. Retrieved from <www.women.nsw.gov.au/pdf/young_womens_health>

Oloffson, M. & Buckley,W. (1983). Investigation of 85 children born by drug-addicted mothers. II Follow up 1-10 years after birth. Acta Pediatr. Scand., 72, 407-413.

O.N.Da. (Osservatorio Nazionale sulla salute della Donna). (2008). La Salute della Donna. Proposte, strategie, provvedimenti per migliorarla. Libro verde, FrancoAngeli Milano

OTIS (Organization of Teratology Information Specialists) (2010), O.T.I.S. Fact Sheets ©. Retrieved from <http://www.otispregnancy.org/otis-fact-sheets-s13037#6>

Palmieri, V. (1991). Osservazione e analisi del tossicodipendente detenuto. Progetto carcere: Quaderni della Fondazione Villa Maraini, 1, Roma.

Pinkham S., Malinowska-Sempruch K. (2007). Women, Harm Reduction, and HIV. New York: International Harm Reduction Development Program of the Open Society Institute. Retrieved from <http://www.idpc.net/sites/default/files/library/IHRD_WomenHRHIV_EN.pdf>

Pomodoro, L. (1993). Aspetti giuridici. In M. Malagoli Togliatti & S. Mazzoni (Eds.), Maternità e tossicodipendenza (pp.13-24). Milano: Giuffrè.

Pomodoro, L. (1996). Introduzione. In D. Ghezzi & F. Vadilonga (Eds.), La tutela del minore (pp.1-13). Milano: Raffaello Cortina Editore.

PNS: Ministerio del Interior (Delegación del Gobierno para el Plan Nacional sobre Drogas) (2000 – 2008). Estrategia Nacional Sobre Drogas. España. NIPO: 126-99-041-3.

Price A. and Simmel C. (2002). Partners' Influence on Women's Addiction and Recovery: the Connection Between Substance Abuse, Trauma and Intimate Relationships (Berkeley, California, National Abandoned Infants Assistance Resource Center, School of Social Welfare, University of California at Berkeley, 2002). Retrieved from <http://aia.berkeley.edu/media/pdf/partners.pdf>

Ravndal, E., Lauritzen, G., Frank,O., Jansson, I., Larsson, J. (2001). "Childhood maltreatment among Norwegian drug abusers in treatment". In International Journal of Social Welfare, 10, 142-147.

Rorschach, H. [1921] (1932). W. Morgenthaler (Ed.), Psychodiagnostik (2nd ed.). Bern-Berlin: Hans Huber (trad. it. Psicodiagnostica, Kappa, Roma, 1981).

Rodning, C., Beckwith, L., & Howard, J. (1989). Characteristics of attachment organization and play organization in prenatally drug-exposed toddlers. Development and Psychopathology, 1, 277-289.

Sanderegger,T. & Zimmermann, E. 1978, Adult behavior and adrenocortical function following neonatal morphine treatment in rats. Psychopharm., 56, 103-109.

Schneider-Rosen, K., Braunwald, K. G., Carlson,V., & Cicchetti, D. (1985). Current perspectives in attachment theory: Illustration from the study of maltreated infants. In I. Bretherton & E. Waters (Eds.), Growing points of attachment theory and research. Monographs of the society for research in child development, 50(209), 194-210.

Sherman, S. G., Latkin, C. A., & Gielen, A.C. Social factors related to syringe sharing among injecting partners: a focus on gender, Substance Use and Misuse, vol. 36, No. 14 (2001), pp. 2113-2136.

Simoni-Wastila, L., Ritter, G., & Strickler, G. (2004). Gender and other factors associated with the nonmedical use of abusable prescription drug. Substance Use and Misuse, 39(1), 1-23.

Stevens, S., Arbiter, N., & Glider, P. (1989). Women residents: Expanding their role to increase treatment effectiveness in substance abuse programs. International Journal of the Addictions, 24, 425-434.

Stocco, P., Llopis Llacer, J.J., De Fazio, L., Calafat, A., & Mendes, F. (2000). Women drug abuse in Europe: Gender identity. Palma de Mallorca: European Institute of Studies on Prevention (IREFREA). Retrieved April 8, 2010 from <http://www.irefrea.org/uploads/PDF/Stocco%20et%20al_2000_Women%20Drug%20Abuse.pdf>

Stocco, P., Llopis Llacer, J.J., de Fazio, L., Facy, F., Mariani, E., Legl, T., et al. (2002). Women and opiate addiction: A European Perspective. Palma de Mallorca: European Institute of Studies on Prevention (IREFREA). Retrieved April 08, 2010 from <http://www.irefrea.org/uploads/PDF/Stocco%20et%20al_2002_Women%20Opiate.pdf>

Studio VEdeTTE (2007). Monografia n. 7: Differenze di genere nello studio VEdeTTE. Spoleto (PG): Litografia Spoletina-Del Gallo.

Substance Abuse and Mental Health Services Administration (2005), Overview of Findings from the 2004 National Survey on Drug Use and Health, Office of Applied Studies, NSDUH Series H-27, DHHS Publication No. SMA 05-4061. Rockville, MD.

Tempesta, E., et al. 1987, Storia psichica della gravida tossicodipendente. Bollettino delle Farmacodipendenze e Alcoolismo, 6, X, 602-607.

United Nations Office on Drug and Crime (2004, August). Substance abuse treatment and care for women: Case studies and lessons learned. Wien. Retrieved September 11, 2010 Retrieved from <http://www.unodc.org/pdf/india/womens_corner/sustance_abuse_treat_care.pdf>

van IJzendoorn, Bakermans-Kranenburg, (1996). Attachment representations in mother, fathers, adolescents, and clinical groups: a meta-analytic search for normative data. Journal of Counseling and clinical psychology, 64.

van IJzendoorn, M. H. & Bakermans-Kranenburg, M. J. (1997). Intergenerational transmission of attachment: A move to the contextual level. In L. Atkinson, & K. J. Zuckerman (Eds.), Attachment and psychopathology (pp. 135-170). New York: Guilford Press.

van IJzendoorn, M. H., Kroonenberg, P. M., & Frenkel, O. J. (1992). The relative effects of maternal and child problems on the quality of attachment: A meta analysis of attachment in the clinical samples. Child Development, 63, 840-858.

Vidal-Trécan, G, Coste, J, Coeuret, M, Delamare, N, Varescon-Pousson, I, Boissonnas, A (1998). Risk behaviors of intravenous drug users: are females taking more risks of HIV and HCV transmission? Rev Epidemiolo Sante Publique; 46(3):193-204

Vogt, I., Gender and drug treatment systems. In Klingemann H, Hunt G (eds), Drug Treatment Systems in an International Perspective: Drugs, Demons and Delinquents. Sage, London, 1998

Ward, M. J. & Carlson, E. A. 1995, Association among adult attachment representations, maternal sensibility, and infant-mother attachment in a sample of adolescent mothers. Child Development, 66, 69-79.

Waters, E., & Deane, K. E. (1985). Defining and assessing individual differences in attachment relationships: Q-methodology and the organization of behavior in infancy and early childhood. In I. Bretherton & E. Waters (Eds.), Growing points of attachment theory and research. Monographs of the Society for Research in Child Development, 50(1-2), 41-65.

Wellish, D.H. & Steinberg, M.R. 1980, Parenting Attitudes of Addicts Mothers. The International Journal of Addictions, 15, 6.

WHO (1995). The World Health Report 1995. Bridging the gaps, Geneva, World Health Organization, Retrieved from <http://www.who.int/whr/1995/en/whr95_en.pdf>

WHO (2000). Women's Mental Health: An Evidence Based Review, WHO, Geneva.

WHO (2007a), Interventions to address HIV in prisons: HIV care, treatment and support. Geneva, World Health Organization (Evidence for Action Technical Papers; Retrieved from <http://www.who.int/hiv/pub/advocacy/idupolicybriefs/en>

Wilson, G. S., McCreary, R., Kean, J., & Baxter, J. C. 1979, The developmental of preschool children of heroinaddicted mothers: A controlled study. Pediatrics, 63(1), 135-141.

Wright A., Walker J. (2001). Drugs of abuse in pregnancy. Best Practices Res Clin Obstet Gynaeco, 1, pp. 987-998.

Zacchello, F. & Giaquinto, M. (1997). Figlio di madre tossicodipendente. Problemi clinici e assistenziali. In G.M. Fava Vizziello & P. Stocco (Eds.), Tra genitori e figli la tossicodipendenza (pp.161-168). Milano: Masson.

Zeanah, C.H. (1992). L'esperienza soggettiva nella relazione di attaccamento: la prospettiva di ricerca. In M. Ammaniti & D. N. Stern (Eds.), Attaccamento e psicoanalisi, Roma: Laterza.

Zenker ,C., Bammann, K.and Jahn, I., (2003). Genese und Typologisierung der Abhängigkeitserkrankungen bei Frauen. Baden-Baden, Schriftenreihe des Bundesministeriums für Gesundheit, Nomos.

Zuckerman, B. (1994). Prenatal Cocaine Exposure - 9 Years Later. Mosby-Year Book Inc.

Zuckerman, B. & Bresnahan, K. (1991). Developmental and behavioral consequences of prenatal drug and alcohol exposure. Pediatric Clinics of North America, 38, 1387-1405.

Zuckerman, B., & Brown, E.R. (1993). Maternal substance abuse and infant development. In Zeanah C.H. (Ed.), Handbook of infant mental health (pp. 143–158). New York: Guilford Press.

Zuckerman, B., Frank, D. A., Hingson, R., Amaro, H., Levenson, S. M., Kayne, H., Parker, S., Vinci, R., Aboagye, K., Fried, L. E., Cabral, H., Timperi, R., & Bauchner, H. (1989). Effects of maternal marijuana and cocaine use on fetal growth. New England Journal of Medicine, 320, 762-768.

16

HCV and Drug Use – What Can Be Learned from the Failure to Control This Epidemic?

Philippe Chossegros
UHSI Lyon, Hospives Civils de Lyon,
French National Coordination of Healthcare Networks,
France

1. Introduction

Around 10 million intravenous drug addicts (IDUs) have been infected by the virus of hepatitis C (HCV) and around 1.2 million are HBsAg positive. Clear geographical differences exist in prevalence ranging in Western Europe between 37 and 98 % (1). At WHO's 63rd World Health Assembly in May, 2010, a resolution was passed to establish "goals and strategies for disease control, increasing education and promoting screening and treatment of people infected with HBV and HCV". In 2011, the WHO argued that injecting drug users (IDUs) are a key group that needs to be specifically targeted for prevention and treatment of viral hepatitis. At a time when a worldwide significant reduction in the HIV epidemic among drug users (DU) is observed, the spread of HCV infections is not controlled. If large variations are observed between countries and regions, prevalence of HCV infection of more than 70 % has been reported among recent-onset DUs (2) and, in 2009, in a city, Vancouver, with one of the most diversified and publicized panel of care services for substance users, Grebely et al. could make the statement that "overall, the rate of new HCV seroconversions in this cohort in the study period was about 25 times the rate of HCV treatment uptake. There are extremely low rates of HCV treatment initiation and very limited effectiveness, despite a high prevalence of HCV infection in this large community-based cohort of inner city residents with access to universal healthcare". It underlines the limits of the risk reduction policy which has been advocated and promoted for the last 20 years (3).

This quasi universal observation may be explained by differences between the viral epidemics of HIV, HBV, HCV and HDV and between their local management. I will confront my own experience and what I have understood of this epidemic in France to a selection of the international literature to propose what, I believe, could improve the care not only of hepatitis but of DUs themselves.

2. A scientific look at the HCV epidemic among DUs

An attempt at understanding the HCV epidemic can be considered as an object of science and discussed as such.

2.1 What is known of HCV hepatitis?

Our knowledge of HCV has grown tremendously since its discovery in 1988. However, gray areas persist. To develop effective control strategies, it is crucially important to determine how epidemiological significant organisms infect us, what is their natural history and what efficacy for its treatment. In most cases these evaluations are not easy.

2.1.1 HCV transmission among DUs: A reappraisal

In 2008, Rhodes et al. observed that "there was much confusion and uncertainty concerning HCV knowledge, including its medical and transmission risks" among drug injectors. Most IDUs viewed HCV prevalence as high and HCV transmission as an inevitable consequence of injecting, HCV risk was perceived as ubiquitous and unavoidable" (4). Is this confusion and uncertainty to be assigned to the messages they receive or our limited understanding of this disease and of its communication?

2.1.1.1 Drug use and HCV: the mystery of the contamination of non injecting drug users (NIDU)

The discovery of HCV followed a search for a viral cause of the remaining post-transfusion hepatitis after HBV had been excluded. Injections make a difference:

- Blood borne transmission through syringe and needle sharing (NSS) has never been questioned and the evidence linking drug injection and NSS to HCV infections are overwhelming. However the level of infectivity of the HCV containing blood remaining in a needle or a syringe after injecting is not known. It is likely that the viral load will be a limiting factor and it is obvious that HCV is able to survive in the environment but we do not for how long? HCV infection is robustly associated with the duration of injections, the number of receptive injecting episodes and of needles and syringes exchanges (NSS), but despite these associations, IDUs may remain hepatitis free after years of risks and others may be contaminated after a unique exchange The observation of Smyth and al. that accidental and unnoticed sharing of injecting equipment may be an important contributor to an IDU's increasing risk of infection over time (5) tallies with my own experience.
- The incidence of contamination through other drug paraphernalia is still debated. Cross-sectional studies have given conflicting results, but cohort studies were able to show significant relations between HCV contamination and sharing drug cookers and filtration cottons among IDUs who did not share syringes (6,7).
- Despite a much higher HCV prevalence (35.3 %) in non injecting drug users (NIDUs) than in non-drug users in some studies (8), the role of equipment (straws, bills, pipes,…) in HCV transmission remains unclear since statistical correlation has never been consistently found, since some misclassification of previous injectors could have occurred and since other possible modes of contamination such as tattooing or sexual transmission were often present (8). However, in some other studies, this prevalence was in the low range observed in individuals living in the same household as HCV carriers. Since it is obvious that every contact is not infectious, a comparison relating their number, the state of the nasal and buccal mucosa (cocaine, heroin) and the lips (crack) (9,10) at the time of sharing , as well as the HCV status of the DUS with whom the equipment was shared could help to understand the cause of these staggering discrepancies.

2.1.1.2 Possible modes of HCV contamination: blood but what else?

An early assimilation to HBV and to HIV, led to the hypothesis that HCV was a sexually transmitted disease. In 1990, a study conducted in Barcelona, in an AIDS clinic, found that 11 % of the partners of infected drug users and 16 % of the partners of infected homosexuals were seropositive for HCV (11). In 1999, using HCV genotypes, Neumayr et al., exploring heterosexual transmission of hepatitis C, finding no other cause of contamination concluded that sexual intercourse could be the cause of contamination in half of the cases (2,5 %) despite any significant relationship with any sexual practice (12). The same year, a metaanalysis computed an order of 1-3 % probability of being found infected among sexual partners of HCV carriers with no other known risk of contamination. The authors had no clue to counsel on their sexual practice viremic HCV carriers with a long term relationship who had not transmitted their infection (13). Overall, since the allocation of these contaminations to sexual intercourse was not significantly related with any history of particular sexual practice, room is left for other possible but never proven modes of contamination such as sharing razor or toothbrushes or, once every other suspected modes of contamination have been excluded, the mysterious "household" transmission (14).

Recent studies rediscovered the risk of sexual transmission among men who have sex with men (MSM) with high-risk sexual behavior (15–17). The HIV epidemic with its mortality and its transient behavioral changes may have hidden its existence for a while, but a Canadian cohort study of HIV positive MSM was able to trace their first contaminations to 1996, with an increase in the incidence of HCV contamination from 0.9 to 2.2 per 1000 person-year to 23.4 and 51.1 % in 2007 which could be related to an increase in the HCV prevalence among MSM as well as an increased level of risks taken during sexual intercourse (18).

Needles are used to perform tattoos and piercings. They are an obvious risk of transmission of HCV and they have been involved in small epidemics. Today, sterile material is used in professional parlors. Thus it is not surprising that non professional tattooing may be associated with a significant risk of HCV transmission among high-risk groups (19). However, like snorting drug, these contaminations, if possible, remain epidemiologically marginal when compared with NSS (20).

2.1.1.3 New insights and new tools could change our understanding of the HCV epidemic

- A consensual belief that HCV antibodies can always be detected years after a contamination has been recently contradicted. If a previous contamination with HCV gives usually rise to antibody production (humoral response) 45–68 days after HCV infection, the presence of a cellular immunity in absence of antibodies has been known for more than 10 years but its epidemiological implication has been ignored until recently (21,22). The discovery that some acute HCV hepatitis could occur and be spontaneously cured without any detection of anti HCV through sequential studies of new expositions has confirmed this hypothesis. It was observed in as many as 33 % of RNA positive cases (23). HCV has also been found in the liver or lymphoid tissue despite the absence of detectable HCV RNA and, even, of HCV antibodies. These occult infections could be the cause of some cases of persistently elevated transaminases (24). However, the clinical meaning of these silent forms which include persistence of HCV in the tissue after clearance of HCV viremia is still a subject of debate (24,25). There was no difference in the prevalence of HCV markers between family members of patients with occult HCV infection and family members of patients with a chronic hepatitis C (26).

Among IDUS different profiles have been described: but existing data are too scarce and sometimes contradictory to decide what is the real occurence of these evolutions:

- In IDUs engaging in risky behaviors for years without being infected by HCV, the prevalence of HCV-specific T cell response was significantly higher than that of healthy controls in an English study (58/19 %, p=.004) (27). In another study, this response reached 62 % of at risk IDUs lacking antibodies (28). The authors report a 100 % positive response for subjects who indicated that they had shared syringes during the previous 6 months as compared to 50 % who had not, implying a possible disappearance of cellular immunity with time.
- The studies of reinfections occurring in IDUs followed up with repeated blood testing added a new understanding to the clearance of HCV infections: When the rate of NSS remains high and if the tests are repeated at short intervals, a significant incidence of reinfections is observed with a new clearance of HCV RNA observed in more than 40 % of the cases (29,30). It confirms the well known notion of an absence of a total protection by a previous immunization against HCV, as well as the possible immunity in some cases (31,32), but points out a high prevalence of repeated HCV clearance which was not known.
- At last, genotyping HCV core sequences may identify phylogenic clusters and help to better understand HCV transmissions among IDUs and NIDUs (33).

These notions could be of use to explain some of the confusing observation of dissimilar serological status among couples and IDUs with the same risky behaviors in the same neighborhood.

2.1.2 The evolution of HCV chronic hepatitis: A lottery governed by genes?

Currently, HCV, a positive-strand RNA virus distantly related to the Flaviviriadae family, is classified in 6 major genotypes and multiple subtypes. An excellent description of the disease can be found online in the 2004 EMCDDA monography (34).

2.1.2.1 What prognosis for the HCV infections of IDUs?

If some chronic HCV infections progress to cirrhosis, liver cancer and death, this evolution is still unpredictable:

- It is assumed that, after an acute infection, 20 % of the subjects will clear spontaneously the virus. Using antibody screening followed by RNA amplification, 20 % of the cases occurring among IDUs following an acute infection resolve spontaneously (35,36) with a lower clearance rate in HIV infected and African-Americans (37). This prevalence of viral clearance is not significantly different from the general population.
- Progression toward cirrhosis of HCV hepatitis has been studied by two meta-analysis, the second selecting DUs (38,39). The first concluded that cirrhotic progression was comprised between 7 and 18 % after an evolution of 20 years, the second was more precise with a progression rate of 14,8 % with a confidence interval of 7.5 to 25.5 %. Male sex and alcohol consumption added an additional 5 % each. However, when the original studies were independently considered the progression rate could vary from

0.3 to 34.9 %, and the computation was performed using the data of 47 papers selected out of 764 potentially relevant articles and 6 679 abstracts. Significant bias could explain these ranges such as a selection of symptomatic patients or the different proposal to perform liver biopsies and their acceptance. In my own series of 650 DUs recruited through my addiction network and in prison with liver biopsies proposed and performed (acceptance 98 %) whenever HCV RNA was present independently of the level of transaminases, after 20 years, the prevalence of cirrhosis was 10,5 % (alcoholics non alcoholics 3.6 %; alcoholics 12.5 %). In a study conducted in the general population in Italy, HCV infection was associated with a severe liver disease in less than 50 % of the cases (40). In these studies as well as in a study of DUs, a high daily intake of alcohol (3 or more drinks) explained most early progression to cirrhosis in DUs (36).

- The prognosis of post-transfusional hepatitis mortality has been the first to be studied. They are characterized by their high rate of early death, their old age at contamination and the one-shot infection. It is believed that infections occurring at a younger age have a more benign evolution. Nurses infected by contaminated gammaglobulins had a 1 % prevalence of cirrhosis with no death after 25 years (41). This benign evolution has been confirmed by others (42). In 5 transfusion retrospective studies, 25 years after exposure all-cause mortality was not different between cases with an history of acute hepatitis and controls and the liver-related death significantly higher than controls was lower than 3 % (42). 16 years after contamination, a national cohort had no excess mortality compared to controls, but the risk of death directly from liver diseases was higher (Hazard ratio: 2.71, 95% CI 1.09-6.75). An excessive alcoholic consumption was present in 30 % of those deaths (43) Progression after 20 years is "less" known but the overall mortality of HCV liver diseases is usually considered to be in a range of 20 to 30 %. The higher rate of death observed among veterans. infected by HCV by Butt et al in 2009 could be related to the presence of other comorbidities such as alcohol, tobacco, violence… since the cause of death was not recorded (44). However, modelisation of the impact of C hepatitis treatment on patients' survival should consider the high rate of other causes of death among IDUs. They represent a significant proportion of infected people (44) : In a cohort of acute HCV hepatitis followed 25 years, if 8 % were cirrhotic, the death rate by overdose was eight times higher than the risk of dying of a liver disease (45) suicide, violence are common and, in older DUs, cardiovascular or pulmonary diseases compete with HIV and HCV (46–4).. In a more recent study conducted in of long-term heroin addicts in California, premature mortality was high, but "only" 14 % of the deaths were related to liver diseases (50).

A search of prognosis markers of progression in hepatitis C has led to the identification of modifiable and non-modifiable factors which influence its evolution. An older age at infection, a longer evolution, being male or African-American (cancer), viral genotype 3 are non-modifiableOn the contrary, an alcohol consumption greater than 30-50 g/day, smoking (cancer), iron overload, coinfection in HBV and/or immunocompromised HIV positive patients, presence of a metabolic syndrome (obesity, steatosis, insulin resistance) can be acted upon to improve individual prognosis (51). More recently, a search for more accurate predictors of progression to cirrhosis led to genome-wide association studies (GWAS), screening the entire human genome. They identified single nucleotide polymorphisms (SNP) which are not often responsible for functional effects but serve as tag for the causal variant that is not genotyped:

- The study of patients resistant to HCV infection has shown that multiple independent protective genetic factors could explain their diverse evolution: clearance of HCV remaining anti HCV positive (52,53) and "protection" against HCV without production of antibodies (53).
- A link between fibrosis progression and genetic predisposition has been considered after the observation of familial clusters of HCV-related cirrhosis (54). An independent GWAS identified a genetic variant, already associated with alcoholic and non-alcoholic fatty liver disease (55), associated with steatosis and fibrosis severity in HCV related hepatitis (56). The screening of host genetic factors has led to a selection of seven single-nucleotide polymorphisms used to compute a Cirrhosis Risk Score (CRS) which could be able to stratify patients' cirrhosis risk prior to liver biopsy (57). This CRS was able to predict progression to cirrhosis in male patients at a F0 stage of fibrosis, result which could lead to treat them early without having to wait for the development of a significant liver disease. The prognosis value of the CRS held true even in patients who abused alcohol (58).

2.1.2.2 Coinfections of HCV hepatitis with other viruses have worse disease progression and outcome

Since high risk practices are common among IDUs, concomitant or successive contaminations by HBV, HCV and HDV, as well as HIV may be observed:

- HBV is a partially double stranded, enveloped DNA virus of the Hepadna family and HDV is a defective RNA virus which requires the presence of an active HBV infection for its multiplication. The evolution of coinfections is dependent of the innate and adaptative immune host response. The results of their interactions are unforeseeable, but it seems that the newcomer will act as a dominant virus which can lead to the clearance of preexisting infections. Acute HBV, HDV or HCV coinfections or superinfection of HBV or HCV may be the cause of fulminant or subfulminant hepatitis. These interactions may also lead to occult, serologically silent HBV or HCV infections. Coinfections are believed to result in worse disease progression with a higher risk of cirrhosis and hepatocellular carcinoma when compared to HBV or HCV alone (46,59,60).
- Up to one-third of HIV-infected patients are infected with hepatitis C virus. The advent of Highly Active Antiviral treatment (HAART) has transformed the prognosis of HIV infected patients with the occurrence of significant liver related death related to the prolongation of their life expectancy. A meta-analysis of 17 studies including 3567 individuals confirmed that chronic hepatitis C outcomes are worse among coinfected individuals with a prevalence of cirrhosis of 49 % (40 to 59 %), twice the rate observed in monoinfected patients (21 %; 16-28 %). This acceleration is mainly observed in immunocompomised patients and could be acccentuated by an immune reactivation occurring after the introduction of HAART. On the other hand, HAART might lessen progression of chronic liver disease and improve response to anti-HCV therapy without fully correcting the adverse effect of HIV infection on HCV prognosis (61-63) . If hepatic side effects of antiretroviral treatments are common, they do not seem to have a significant effect on the progression of liver fibrosis (64).

2.1.3 Hepatitis C management: Toward a potential Copernician revolution (at a price)

2.1.3.1 Less invasive diagnosis tools

Medical tools have also evolved with less invasive tests for the diagnosis and the follow-up of HCV hepatitis:

- Individuals who perform a test are eager to know its result without waiting for days. Blood access of IDUs is often problematic. Rapid tests answer these problems. After HIV, they have become available for HCV diagnosis. They can be performed using saliva, whole blood, serum or plasma. The frame of their use is controversial. In France, they can only be used by healthcare professionals with a complementary traditional test as confirmation. In the United-states where HIV auto-tests are available, in a DTP 24 % of preferred to remain anonymous, preference which reached 38 % if the test was free (65).
- To detect an ongoing infection, an amplification of the viral RNA is performed which is prone to contamination and false positive results. HCV core antigen detection, easily automated, and requiring less technical skill, has been advocated. Its limitations are noted in some HBV/HCV coinfections (66–68).
- Liver biopsy is often believed to be dangerous and painful by some patients and most general practitioners becoming a barrier to the care of hepatitis C patients. Non invasive tests are proposed: either scores computed from the results of different blood tests or a measure of the elastance (fibroscan) of the liver. Diverse algorithms have been proposed to improve their results but they are today an indisputable alternative to liver biopsy even in HIV/HCV coinfected patients (69,70). The fibroscan does not need a blood sample and gives immediate results (71).

2.1.3.2 Treat all, cure all?

- For 10 years, the treatment of HCV hepatitis has been an association of a long lasting form of alpha interferon with ribavirine. It is able to reduce significantly HCV related mortality (71) Today, there is a clear-cut difference of the response rate to treatment between the types of HCV viruses. Among the 6 genotypes, 2 and 3 need only 6 months of treatment with 80 to 90 % sustained viral response (SVR) whereas, genotype 1 and 4 usually need 12 months for a SVR of 50 %. Response rate of DUs are in the same range as the general population (72). Our finding of a significantly better SVR of genotype 1 infected DUs treated by buprenorphine as compared to methadone remains to be explored in a prospective study exploring that difference (73). An "à la carte" adaptation of the duration of treatment has been proposed for genotype 1 following the time of RNA clearance at 4, 12 or 32 weeks followed by respective treatment duration of 24, 48 or 72 weeks which has been confirmed for HIV/HCV coinfections (74,75). For patients with advanced diseases, treatment has been completed thanks to the use of growth factors which improved their tolerance (76)).
- This individual response could be predicted before treatment prescription: A better knowledge of the immune response against hepatitis C gives a central role to regulatory T lymphocytes which are present in the necroinflammatory infiltrate of the liver. By studying a single nucleotide polymorphisms (SNPs) linked to the IFN-lambda 3 (IL28B) gene it is now possible to predict a better prognosis for patients infected with genotype 1 with the CC genotype. They are more than twice as likely to respond to 48 weeks of treatment than non-CC genotypes (CT,TT) (77,78). This association has also been found in hepatitis C virus genotype 2 or 3 patients (79) and in HIV coinfected patients (80), but not in genotype 5 (81).

- However, new drugs which have been specifically tailored to HCV will improve these results. The first antiproteases on the market, Telaprevir and boceprevir improved the SVR for genotype 1 from 50 to 70 % for naïve patients and improved significantly SVRs of previous relapsers or non-responders (82,83). Since these drugs are added to interferon/ribavirine side–effects are more frequent and severe with serious cutaneous reactions (telaprevir) or a need for more growth factors (boceprevir). Early responder could benefit of shorter treatments. Other drugs are in the pipeline which could still have better results. The combination of two antivirals to the association of interferon/ribavirine led to a 100 % viral response, 12 weeks after the completion of treatment in previous non responders of a classical bitherapy. In a near future, association of 2 antivirals tailored for HCV should be able to cure almost every infected patient. This improvement has a cost: A full treatment course of telaprevir (12 weeks fixed-duration) will cost £30 000, whereas a full treatment course of boceprevir will range from to €22 000 to €40 000 (84) which should be added to the €16 000 of 48 weeks of bitheray by interferon and vidarabine for a genotype 1 (for a genotype 2 or 3, 24 weeks of a classic bitherapy are usually sufficient) and to the €1 000, annual cost of the care. The latest communications in international hepatology meetings promise a second generation of antivirals more effective with less side-effects which could be used in association without interferon and, in some cases, ribavriine in a near future. They should be able to cure almost all the hepatitis whatever their genotype. We do not know yet what will be their cost.
- Among HCV/HIV coinfected DUS at risk for liver disease progression a combination of interferon and ribavirin, is not highly effective; it has lower rates of SVR than monoinfected patients, especially for coinfected patients with HCV genotype 1 and those of African descent. Direct-acting antivirals might overcome factors such as immunodeficiency that can reduce the efficacy of IFN with the additional problem of interaction with antiretrovirals which should lead to early treatment independent of the stage of the liver disease, before the introduction of an HIV antiviral treatment (85).
- Most of the infectious epidemics observed in humans have been controlled by vaccination campaign. Novel vaccine candidates have been studied based on molecular technology such as recombinant proteins (E1 and/or E2 glycoprotein), poly peptides, virus-like particles, plasmid DNA and recombinant viral vectors which can be combined with novel adjuvants. Some of them have reached Phase I/II human clinical trials with, in some cases, production of robust antiviral immunity but the challenge is to move to test their efficacy in at-risk of infected population to prevent new infections. Their cost has led to preferential studies of their efficacy as adjuvant for existing treatment (86,87).

2.1.4 Conclusion: DUs confusion and uncertainty are founded (they are not alone in that situation)

We may know for certain that HCV infection follows conditions or practices causing blood transmission whether through contaminated needles or through mucosal traumatism and/or bleeding during hetero or homosexual intercourse. However, the studies of HCV transmission explore only the expected associations the researchers believe to be relevant. One must be cautious not to mix up low statistical significant association with causal relationship and remember that our inability to explain some HCV contamination may be related to, until now, unknown or overlooked modes of contamination: Animal bites were found significantly related to HCV infections (88) and a model of transmission of HCV by biting arthropods could explain the maintenance of long-term endemic transmission of HCV in Africa and South-East Asia (89). The route of contamination of patients on hemodialysis has not yet been understood leading to a debate on the interest of their isolation (90).

Today, our prevention messages are "simple"!!!:

- Do not inject and if you do, never share syringes, needles or any injecting paraphernalia.
- Never share bills and straws you use for sniffing or pipes you use to smoke cocaine.
- Use condoms for every sexual intercourse.
- Choose a reliable professional to perform your tattoos or piercings
- Never share your toothbrush and your razor.
- If, despite these counsels, you have taken some risks make a blood test.
- If positive for HCV, ask to be treated.

But, even if a DU could follow these very restricting recommendations, it is not possible to guarantee an absence of contamination. Confusion and indetermination are not gone. We are not on the eve of a simple training course for professionals as well as for the public at large which would explain hepatitis C and give coherent and always effective recommendations for prevention. We have to wait for effective vaccines.

2.2 The epidemic of HCV hepatitis among DUs is not controlled

More than 20 years after the discovery of the hepatitis C virus, much of the ongoing epidemic is attributable to unsafe drug injections. An evaluation of the drug consuming population and of the DUs infected with HCV is recognized as an arduous exercise. One can consider snapshots taken at one time or can study a trend in a cohort. Both approaches must consider the evolution of:

- The population of DUs and the nature of drug consumption. Younger addicts cannot be treated as the older ones minus ten or twenty years. The French OFDT study "le matos" (the works), interviewing a panel of injectors, has been documenting these changes since the nineteen seventies. These different attitudes may coexist in different age groups (91). Despite globalization, each country and, even, each region, has its own history and market. I have described its course in France in a short overview in 2007 (92). A series of publications relevant to the French drug consumption can be downloaded from the site of the Observatoire Français des Drogues et des Toxicomanies (OFDT) in free acess (http://www.ofdt.fr/ofdtdev/live/publi.html).
- Illegal drugs' use has cycles. Cocaine will succeed heroin, designer drugs will find a new public. A new drug is detected each week in the European market (93). Recently, high levels of amphetamine injection have been reported around the Baltic, as well as Slovakia and Hungary…. A tremendous growth of the drug business occurred since the beginning of a war on drugs and the repressive laws of the 1970s. It is related to the huge profitability of the trafficking and the increasing demand of new consumers for psychoactive drugs, licit or illicit.

2.2.1 How many (intravenous) drug users and what proportion is infected by HCV?

Despite these recognized problems, figures are none the less produced: in counties of Western Europe, HCV prevalence among IDUs fall in a range comprised between 47.1 % (Austria) and Netherland (86.2 %) (94). The number of infected DUs in Western Europe could reach 727 500 (95% CI 497 000 - 1018 000).

France is the only country were different approaches have been used at different times to estimate the number of DUs and of people infected by HCV. A comparison of their results gives an idea of the accuracy of these estimations:

- The OFDT recently produced and discussed an estimation of the prevalence of problem drug users in France following a methodology shared by all the European countries: 5,4 to 6,4 /1 000 hab 15-64 years old. This estimate is almost twice that of Germany but lower than Italy, Spain and UK which had the highest prevalence. It has certain limits which are listed in the publication with a rare honesty (95):
    - First, the changing definition of the subject of the estimate. In 1993, "heroin addicts" were, at least, 160 000. In 1995, the estimate was of 142-172 000 "opiate problem users". In 2006, a new definition, taking into account the change in the drug market, considered "intravenous drug users or regular users of opiates, cocaine or amphetamines", led to an increase of 44 %. The change in these estimates may be more related to a difference in definition than to a real change in the size of the population.
    - Second, the proposed estimate of 230 000 problem users (210 to 250 000) cannot hide the fact that the real range computed through the four different methods before its narrowing by the experts to a definite number, without convincing arguments explaining their choice, was 147 000 to 367 000.
    - Third, these approaches ignored the users who have not been and will not be in contact with one of the information sources used (arrest, treatment, health problems, death, etc.)". For cocaine which is considered to be one of the most "addictive" drugs, no more than 20 % of users become addicted after 20 years of use, 80 % may not be accounted for by these evaluation (Wagner 2002). This statement is of importance, since this population is not negligible and can influence the evaluation of the number of patients infected by HCV through their drug use (96,97). In the nineties, most patients 30 to 40 years old, carriers of HCV, who came in our unit without any history of a possible contamination, confessed that 10 years before, on one or two "festive" occasions, they had injected drugs with friends and shared their syringes. They were not "addicts" and they did not consider themselves as such.
- The Veille Sanitaire (VS), the French organization studying public health, conducted 4 different surveys leading to four different results:,
    - Starting from HCV prevalence in the general population, two successive studies were conducted ten years apart (1994-2004) (98,99). Both addressed people covered by the French public welfare system (only 9 % of the recruited population agreed to make a test. They differed only by their scope. The second being much larger than the first. The interval of the first estimate was 500 000 to 600 000. Among IDUs, HCV prevalence was 78 %. Ten years later, what was presented as a more accurate

estimation of 367 000 was given with 65 % of viremic patients. The only explanation given to this spectacular decrease was the better methodology of the second study. Among the 0,38 % who recognized a previous history of injecting drugs, HCV prevalence was 55,5 % which would lead to a total of 150 000 French people with an history of at least one drug injectors in 2004, 82 500 of whom would be infected by HCV.

- In 2003, the number of DUs infected by HCV and of the incidence of new contaminations started with an hypothesis of a number of active injectors ranging from 80 to 100 000, given, at the time, by the OFDT and a prevalence of 60 to 70 %. The proposed number of infected IDUs was 48 000 to 70 000 and the number of new infections ranged from 2 700 to 4 400 for an estimated yearly new contaminations of 11 % (100).
- The fourth study was a cross-sectional multicenter survey of DUs having injected or snorted drugs at least once in their life conducted in 2004, the same year as the second population prevalence study (101). It was a two stage random survey of DUs selected to represent the diversity of drug use. Fingerprick blood samples were collected on blotting paper in 75 % of the screened population. The overall prevalence of HIV and HCV were respectively 10.8 (0.3 % under 30 years of age) and 59.8 % (NIDUs 27.9 %; IDUs 73,8 %; under 30 years 28%). In multivariate analysis, factors independently associated with HCV seropositivity were age over 30, HIV seropositivity, having ever injected drugs, opiate substitution treatment (OST), crack use, and precarious housing. HIV seroprevalence was not related to an history of injecting, but increased with age with a geographic difference of prevalence.

Contrary to the OFDT, no explanation was given of these discrepancies: a decrease of one third of the number of people infected by HCV between 1994 and 2004, and, the same year, 2004, a discrepancy of 18.3 % between two estimations using different methodologies to assess HCV prevalence among IDUs.

2.2.2 Is it possible to know HCV prevalence and incidence among DUs and what is the efficacy of harm reduction programmes?

2.2.2.1 Cohorts the incidence and risk factors of new infections can only be studied in cohorts of IDUs initially seronegative

Ideally, these cohorts should begin when IDUs start to inject and no drop out should occur or, at least, the drop outs should not differ from the rest of the cohort. Of course, these requirements are almost impossible to fulfill. In some cases, infection incidence rate was even computed from a retrospective selection of patients who had at least two serum samples available and found initially seronegative (102–104). In a prospective study in the north and east of France, 28.6 % were lost to follow-up and differed significantly from the others who remained in the study (6). These studies can inform on the modes of contamination. They can never accurately predict the true HCV incidence among all the DUs. However, the incidence rate of new HCV contaminations among NIDUs remained low in the few cohort studies which included them: 1/422 (0.4/100 PY (95 % CI 0.0-1.2) (105), none in those who did not start injection (106).

The four randomized studies of the impact of interventions to prevent hepatitis C infection among IDUs were not able to show significant differences (106–108). Despite an exclusion of severe psychiatric or somatic illnesses, which represent a significant bias, the drop-out rates were high. For example, Abou-Saleh et al. explored behavioral interventions among DUs already followed by drug treatment services. Among the 206 IDUS (initially 1354) who remained after exclusion of HCV positivity, of severe mental or physical illnesses or serious legal problems, 54 % refused or dropped out during the inclusion process, 95 were randomized, 82 % and 65 % were followed at six months and 12 months. In a per-protocol approach, the rate of contamination was higher at the end of six months (18 %) than after 12 months (12 %) and there was no significant difference between the two interventions even if the trend was "in the anticipated direction" (108). In an intention to treat, drop-outs would have been considered as possible contaminations raising the contamination rate over 50 %.

Hagan et al. (109), mixed up these studies with different other interventions from bleach disinfection of syringes to behavioral interventions, in a report with strong methodological bias. First, the majority of the 26 studies were not intended to assess the efficacy of an intervention but to measure the rate of new infections among a cohort of IDUs. Then, they included the univariate odds-ratios of seroconversion even if they were not retained in multivariate analysis. For example, in the French study, a 60 % reduction in HCV incidence was observed between the patients treated with oral substitution treatment (OST) and the others. However, once the level of cotton and syringe sharing were included, this difference disappeared because these levels were not equally distributed between the two groups.

These observations explain why the quality of evidence of intervention impacts is found to be lacking and why it is so difficult to prove the efficacy of any harm reduction procedures. At best they can show that DUs retained in a programme fare better than those who stay outside or who quit. But they cannot prove that the decision to take part in the programmes does not select less risky behaviors and, most of all, that the proposal of these programmes to every DU would result in a significant decrease of new contaminations, which, of course, should be their aim.

2.2.2.2 Cross sectional studies

The results of repeated cross-sectional studies have the advantage of not being dependent of the retention rate in a programme. However, the population recruitment must be representative of the population studied and its modalities must not change from one period to the next. An incidence survey has been added to the cross-sectional approach in some cases. The community based study by Mehta et al. in Baltimore (110) and the study of IDUs attending Needle and Syringe Programs (NSP) in Autsralia by Falster et al. (111) can be considered as models:

- Mehta et al. studied a cohort of IDUs initially recruited in 1988-1989 and then added new IDUs in 1994-1995, 1998 and 2005-2008. They followed those who were seronegative for HCV and HIV and compared the new recruits. They observed a significant decrease in HIV infection from 5.5 cases/100 patient/year in 1988-1989 to 0/100 py in 2005-2008, whereas there was no significant change in HCV incidence. The prevalence study observed a decline in HCV prevalence among the youngest (39 years) and those who had a shorter injection history (<15 years). An increase in the duration of injection to reach a 80 % prevalence was observed between 1988-1989 (5-9 years) and

2005-2008 (15-19 years). After adjustment for demographic and time since injection, significant differences were observed between HCV prevalence in 1988-1989 and 1994-1995 on one hand and 2005-2008 on the other. A small proportion of this decline was explained by changes in drug-related risk behavior over time. It could be the consequence of a decrease of HCV prevalence.

- In Australia all IDUs attending a NSP site participating in the study were invited to complete an anonymous questionnaire and to provide a capillary blood sample (participation rate: 41 to 61 %) every year between 1995 and 2004 (Falster 2009). After adjustment for covariates, HCV antibody seropositivity remained associated with a longer duration of injecting, older age, participation in the state of New South Wales, opiates as the last drug injected, imprisonment in the last year, female sex, daily or more frequent injection, sharing needles and syringes in the last month, sex work, and survey participation in 2000–2004. An increase in HCV prevalence was found within injection initiation cohorts over time, with prevalence appearing to reach saturation around 90% in the older cohorts. An increase from 1895-1996 to 2003-2004 in the prevalence of HCV infection among IDUs who had injected less than 7 years could reflect an increase in the prevalence of HCV in that population.

2.2.2.3 France and Lyon: the course of an epidemic

Knowing the methodological limits of any evaluation of an HCV epidemic among DUs and of the effectiveness of harm reduction programs, I will present the results of the studies I conducted in Lyon and in France and, taking into account the other French evaluation on the subject and my experience of thirty years of care to DUs, I will give a tentative interpretation of the course of the epidemic in France.

2.2.2.3.1 Prison

I conducted studies in Lyon's prison because it was the only place, outside of complex snowball enquiries, were no bias was met, in the recruitment of IDUs, which could be related to a care demand. Every IDU entering Lyon's prisons between 19987-1989, 1997-1999 and 2009-2011 were asked to answer a questionnaire and to provide a blood sample. Acceptance was high (>90 %).

- Among DUs entering prison, before 1990, injection was the rule (90 %) and heroin was the main product. This study showed a sharp decrease of "indiscriminate" sharing from 65 % for those who had begun their drug use before 1980, to 15 % for those whose first use began after 1987. This change was related to the occurrence of the AIDS epidemic in 1984-1985 and predated the free access to sterile needles and syringes of 1987 which, nevertheless, had an additional impact. After 1985, an increasing number of pharmacists agreed to sell syringes answering an increasing demand of IDUs. Follow-up studies conducted in the same environment among injectors confirmed this trend in the change of behavior and of viral prevalence with a quasi disappearance of indiscriminate syringe sharing after 1992. Conversely, the absence of any sharing reported by less than 5 % of IDUs who had begun to inject before 1980, reached 70 % after 1990.
- In 2009-2010, a radical change in drug consumption had occurred from heroin injection associated by less than 10 % of DUs to cocaine in speedballs in the eighties to an almost equal number of heroin and cocaine consumers (cocaine 82 %; heroin 70 %; 52,6 % used

both drugs). Only one fourth had injected. These results underline the change in drug use observed at a national level (95). The prevalence of injection was higher (29.5 %) among heroin addicts than among cocaine abusers (18.3 %) but, among injectors syringe and needle sharing was not different. There was no difference in HCV prevalence between non drug users (2.4 %) and NIDU (3.9 %, OR 1.7 95 % CI=0.7-4.2). This prevalence rose to 48.6 % for IDUs who said they had never shared their needles (OR/NIDU 23.9 95 percent CI=8.0-65.8) and to 66.7 % for those who had (OR/NIDU 44.7 95 percent CI=13.6-167.4). HCV detection was also related to an older age and a longer drug use but had no relation, among injectors, with the nature (heroin or cocaine) of the drug used. One fourth (24,4 %) were nationals of countries belonging to the exUSSR which is in accordance with a trend observed in most French hepatitis units for some years.

- In a comparison of IDUs entering prison in 1987-1989, 1997-1999 and 209-2011, the decrease of syphilis infections among that population as soon as 1986 (11 % before to 4.7 % after) and its disappearance after 1990 demonstrated the decrease of the trade of sex for drug. In a multivariate analysis controlling for date of first injection, duration of injection, place of injection (for HIV alone) and risk sharing the Odds ratio of viral infection in 1987-1988 compared to 1997-1998 were 15,4 for HIV, 7,8 for HBV and 3,3 for HCV, indicating a decrease (certain for HBV and HIV, possible for HCV) in the prevalence of these infections among injecting drug users. On the contrary, no difference was observed between 1978-199 and 2009-2011.

2.2.2.3.2 Multicenter cross-sectional studies

In 1996 a multicenter study, at that time the largest state funded study of DUs, recruited 1302 DUs in 3 French towns (Lille, Lyon, Paris) among GPs and their referral hospitals. 120 data were collected. It confirmed the trend observed in Lyon's prison with a decrease of the indiscriminate needle sharing. A consistent increase in age for first drug use since the end of the eighties was observed. Before 1981 and after 1991, the prevalence of syringe sharing without precaution was divided by 8 while that for spoons was only divided by 1.4, for cotton wool by 1.6 and that for back loading by 1.3. Needle sharing was more frequent at night (60% versus 30 %). The proportion of nightly exchanges increased during periods when patients were "high" (59%), during withdrawal (61 %) and at the time of a relapse (76 %). This sharing at the time of relapse was unpredictable and represented approximately 25% of cases. Shared material other than syringes were in decreasing order: spoons (46%), filtration cotton (39%) and 'back loading' (20%). 9 years after the legalization of the purchase of needles and syringes in pharmacies and 5 years after the opening of the first NSP in Paris, a very small proportion attended NSPs (7%) or vending machines (2%). Socio-economic variables were not associated with the extent of needle sharing (a continuous professional activity was only found in 20% of cases but only 3% of drug addicts in this study did not benefit from any kind of social assistance). Gender, living with a partner and housing were not significant. Only the level of education and, to a lesser degree, professional situation was of importance. The prevalence of needle exchanges without precautions decreased from 29% in users who had primary level of education compared to 12 % in those who had started high school. Prostitution was seldom reported by men (3 %), but 29 % of women recognized this practice which declined from 33 % before 1980 to 21 % after 1990, most frequently observed in occasional "hookers" (28 to 16 %). The prevalence of cutaneous abscesses (23 %) and of overdoses (29 %) had not changed with time.

2.2.2.3.3 Discussion

These studies confirmed the disappearance of the HIV epidemic and, on the contrary, a persistence of the HCV epidemic. This observation is concordant with the results of national surveys. In 2008, the estimated French total number of new HIV infections among IDUs was 70 (95 % CI 0-190) with, for the first time, a majority of DUs newly discovered being born abroad (112)(Levu 2011). A credible story can be told:

- Before the AIDS epidemic, if hepatitis were known to be present among DUs, they was ignored since their symptoms were few, no treatment was available and their death rates (fulminant or subfulminant hepatitis) were exceptional, much lower than those of deaths by overdoses, violence or suicides. With the sudden onset of the HIV epidemic, everything changed. DUs wasted and died and as soon as 1984-1985 everybody knew that AIDS was an infectious disease transmitted through sexual intercourse and blood transmission. The message had all the characteristics which make a message "stick": it was simple (HIV infection led to death), unexpected (people paid attention), concrete (it was understood and remembered), credible (people agreed and believed), emotional (people cared) and led people to act (a credible story was told with a solution: condoms and sterile works). Paraphernalia use (the impact was obvious on needle and syringes, filters were mostly ignored) as well as sexual practices changed significantly. I observed a decrease in NSS which begun well before the law of 1987 on the free access to needle and syringes, sex for drug and the prevalence of syphilis declined at the same time and, furthermore, DUs died (those who took the most risks). As a result, the HIV epidemic disappeared in regions like Lyon were its prevalence had been low when the epidemic was discovered. In others (Paris, Bordeaux, the south of France), a small pool of DUs infected with HIV survived. They were slow progressors and were able to access HIV infectious specialists and wait until HAART were available. They remained a reservoir for some occasional contaminations (the respective role of injection and homo or heterosexual transmission in these new infections is unknown). This is in accordance with our multicenter study of 1996 and explains the discrepancy between the high rate of HIV prevalence observed in Marseille and the national observation of a very low incidence of new infections (113). Contrary to Jauffret-Roustide (101), I believe that the difference in HIV prevalence between Lille and Marseille in 2004, is not mainly related to a prevalence of injection, which was not significantly related to HIV seroprevalence in their survey, but to a difference in the course in the epidemic shown by our 1996 study: Marseille had already one of the highest HIV prevalence in the early eighties and the explosion of drug use in Lille occurred in the late eighties, when people were aware of the HIV epidemic, explaining the constant low HIV prevalence. However, recent changes are observed with the occurrence of new cases coming form countries were HIV prevalence is high among IDUs (today countries from the ex-USSR, maybe Africa were drug use is expanding tomorrow). The impact of this new epidemic on native DUs is still unknown.
- The course of the HBV epidemic followed that of HIV. To be infected, one must encounter a infectious carrier: 90 % of adults newly infected will spontaneously clear the virus and only a fraction of them will be infectious through sexual contacts and through NSS. If in the eighties and most of the nineties, a diagnosis of infection through drug use could be made when HBV together with HCV markers were detected, it was not the case anymore after 2000, or earlier with younger addicts only infected with

HCV. HDV, which needs an HBV coinfection, had disappeared at the end of the eighties, but comes back, sporadically, with eastern migrants.

- For HCV, the course of the epidemic is radically different. It is obvious that in the early eighties, HCV, like HBV prevalence was high among IDUs, in the range of 80 to 90 %. There was no difference between French regions. Harm reduction did not exist. The 3 surveys I conducted before 2000 give a coherent picture of their evolution. Before the discovery of the AIDS epidemic, the majority of IDUs took no precaution with their "works" (even if they injected only once in a recreational setting). Since most IDUs were infected the first year of injection, HCV prevalence among IDUs with an history of only few injections did not differ significantly from that of those who had been indiscriminate. A decrease in NSS occurred in the eighties resulting in a delay when duration of injection was considered, but the influence of the level of NSS, when it had occurred, was not significant, reflecting the persisting high HCV prevalence. The 1996 survey emphasizes the low access to harm reduction programs such as NSP or vending machines at a time when most of the changes in the course of the HIV and HCV epidemic had occurred. NSS occurred at a time when pharmacies were closed, at a place where vending machines were absent and when a sudden craving was felt. Behavior reported by most of the few IDUs I followed who seroconverted. This situation was not exceptional in DUs receiving OST after 1996. A small but significant trend was noted toward a reduction in the epidemic when comparing IDUs who had begun injecting before 1990 and between 1990 and 1999. This decrease was sustained in 2009 but the size of the sample is too small to make final conclusions. However, differences may exist between French regions. In Alsace, in a GP network, HCV prevalence among DUs under 30 years of age was only 7 % (114). This dissociation in the evolution of HIV and HCV epidemic has been observed in Vancouver (115) and in most countries were drug injection was present before 1980 (116,117).

2.3 From an addition of successive layers of harm reduction to the recognition of the complexity of the control of risky behaviors

A thorough synthesis and evaluation of harm reduction effectiveness has been published in an EMCDDA monograph in 2010 (118) following others (119–121) with the same conclusions: the absence of high-quality review evidence leading to question this efficacy. I will try to consider the respective impact of past harm reduction programmes and the improvement which could be implemented to improve their efficiency in the French context.

2.3.1 Prevention

2.3.1.1 Oral substitution treatment

The massive introduction of OST in France in 1996 was followed by an instantaneous and tremendous change in the care for DUs. In 2002, it was assumed that one third of problematic opiate users (52 000) were engaged in long-term treatment with an additional 22 000 receiving prescriptions on an irregular basis (122). OST introduction occurred at a time when the HIV epidemic among DUs was already controlled. Its impact is, thus, difficult to assess. However, OST in community setting is considered to reduce HIV seroconversion and to have a possible role in reducing the number of HCV seroconversions among DUs who remain in the programmes. From my experience and from the results of a study of the migration of IDUs inside Lyon's healthcare and penal institutions I conducted in 1989, OSTs have delayed the time of transition to injection among heroin users. But since many other variables have changed during that period, and since we still do not know the evolution of the prevalence of injectors, this assumption remains speculative. The problem which remains is what to do with the non compliant DUs, most at risk of infection or with those who do not attend OSTs? The change in the nature of the drugs consumed by DUs observed in the last years with an increase in cocaine/crack use could limit the impact of OST on these consumers and should lead to an evolution of the DPs even if, recently a disaffection for cocaine and a come-back of heroin through micronetworks of users-sellers (123) has been reported in France.

2.3.1.2 Reduction of syringe and needle sharing (NSS)

The first harm reduction programme implemented in France occurred in 1987 with a law allowing free access to needles and syringes in French pharmacies. The motivation behind this decision, like the decision, in 1996, to offer an easy access to OST, was more a protection of the heterosexual community from HIV and hepatitis viruses than an improvement of DUs' care. For someone who lived that period, it is obvious that, this decision increased significantly a preexisting trend and was significantly associated to a quasi disappearance of indiscriminate NSS among IDUs. From my study in prison and the national survey of 1996 as well as my own experience with the IDUs I followed at that time when no OST, beside neocodion, was available, it is "obvious" that it answered a demand of IDUs and decreased significantly NSS after they had discovered and realized the risk inherent to that practice. Following this first move, steribox containing needles, syringes, filters and condoms have been sold to IDUs for a low price or have been available through NSP which have been opened in the early nineties. In 1998, with an estimation of 2.8 injections per IDU per day, Lurie and al. estimated that between 920 million and 1.7 billion injections by IDUs took place each year in the United States (estimated 12 million in San Francisco and >80 million in New York City) (124). Using the same level of daily injections, with a conservative estimation of 80-100 000 IDUs, 80 and 100 000 million of injections could take place in France. An annual estimation of syringes sold to IDUs in France between 1996 and 2003 made by the INVS increased from 1996 to 1999 (14.7 to 17.7 M) and then decreased dramatically from 1999 to 2003 (10.9 M) (125). This decrease was ascribed to an increase in OST during the same period. NSP accounted for only 1.5 M exchanges with large differences in the number of steribox exchanged yearly (253-10 000) between as many as 129 programmes or vending machines. The observation that a syringe can be reused 10 times is not a surprise. Pharmacies after they began to give free steribox have been shown to quadruple in the first 6 months the number they dispensed to the same number of IDUs (126). In a survey of 35 large metropolitan areas in the US, the range of the number of syringes distributed was 2 per 10 injection events to 3 per 10 000 injection events (127). Sterile syringes for each shoot may be desired, but can this goal be reached and would it be sufficient to prevent receptive exchanges? For cocaine users, distribution of glass stems, rubber mouthpieces, brass screens, chopsticks, lip balm and chewing gum, reducing the harms associated with smoking crack, may decrease the number of injections (128).

Considering what is unknown about the number of IDUs, their access to harm reduction programmes (HRPs), the efficacy of theses HRPs and the modes of viral contamination, one can be surprised that models fitting strategies to control the HCV epidemic can be proposed.

However, models exist even if they are oversimple and if some (many) of their initial assumptions on the rate of viral transmission or the efficacy of NSP and OST to prevent infection, may be problematic. The conclusion that high-risk DUs are infected early and that the rate of infection among low-risk groups will continue for years are truisms (34). Percolation-based approximations can be highly biased when one incorrectly assumes that infectious periods and when deterministic models assume that every contact is with a new individual. Thus, models should be significantly improved, for example, with the use of stochastic models which take into account lasting relationships and inclusion in groups, but they should also use additional data on specific populations (129,130). Despite these limits, Vickerman et al. suggest that, in the UK, NSP and OST have been able to limit 50 000 new infections in the UK, but even with their initial optimistic assumptions, they conclude that a reduction by half in chronic HCV prevalence would need OST and 100% NSP to be scaled up to 80 % coverage for at least 20 years (131).

French results do not support a significant impact of harm reduction programmes on the course of the HIV and HCV epidemic outside of the free access to sterile needles and syringes in pharmacies (112).

2.3.2 Hepatitis treatment

The treatment of DUs' viral infections has been considered since the occurrence of the AIDS epidemic. In the nineteen eighties, our diagnosis tools were limited and available treatments were experimental. In Lyon we used the first anti HBV antiviral in continuous perfusions of four weeks durations for severe HBV hepatitis as early as 1979, then with beta interferon for HBV/HDV coinfections and NonA NonB hepatitis in 1984 and alpha interferon for both since 1989 after the first randomized trials of 1987. This know-how encompassed also HIV infections and at every step we treated active IDUs years before OST could be prescribed (1996) in France. Our recruitment was biased, but we were able to screen and treat most of the DUs who asked for heroin detoxification or hepatitis and HIV treatment. On another level, a national consultation in 1991, concluded that HIV infected DUs did not differ from the other patients. Compliance was related to housing problems whatever the modalities of infection. Having treated DUs for their HIV infections since 1984 and for their hepatitis since 1986, we did not agree with the recommendations of the French consensus conferences which denied the treatment of HCV hepatitis to active DUs in 1997. This position, initially controversial, has become the norm with an emerging consensus that DUs can be treated for their hepatitis on a case by case basis. In a study of the perception of their disease in 2000, 60 IDUs successively entering Lyon's prisons were interviewed. At least one liver biopsy had been performed in 49 (90 % of those whose hepatitis had been discovered more than 5 years earlier). 80 % of viremic DUs who had a significant fibrosis (> F1) had been treated and 50 % of the others on account of fatigue or a desire to be treated. The multi-disciplinary management we developed with success in the early nineteen nineties is now proposed as a possible solution to improve access to treatment (132–134). The possible impact of treating HCV infected DUs on the course of the epidemic has even been studied by different models which are the subject of debates (135,136).

In France when we proposed to study the possibility of treating HCV hepatitis to decrease HCV prevalence in a nationally funded Clinical Hospital Research Programme in 2002, few hepatitis units received IDUs. In 2004, in a national observational study of 40 hepatitis units, only two hepatitis reference centers treated a significant number of HCV hepatitis of drug users. In 2011, after three successive national plans, the situation has changed. 90 % of the 31 hepatitis reference centers who treat two third of French HCV hepatitis declared that DUs' hepatitis care was a strategic decision. Differences in history and location, as well as the size of the HCV specialist team (range 0.8-10) made each centre a special case. Various innovative solutions have been implemented, in some cases before the allocation of resources. A partnership was present with drug treatment programs (DTP) (85,2 %) and GPs' network (25.9 %). 44.7 % found that care for DUs hepatitis did not need a specific competence. Perceived problems were reported by only 34.3 % of HCV specialists (absenteeism) and 48.3 % of nurses (absenteeism, blood access). Waiting times were similar for DUs and non-DUs. Our results support collaboration between services involved in DUs' care. However their complete and complex integration may only be needed for the most precarious such as homeless adolescents.

3. HCV, drug use, and the world complexity

Biomedical knowledge of the HCV epidemic among DUs is obviously not enough to be able to control its course. My practice taught me that if objectification of DUs as well as of their hepatitis was inescapable, an understanding of its limits implies an integration of other aspects of our "being-here" (Dasein) such as the brain, society, social systems and ethics.

- The "rationality" of one's decision includes his lifetime experience, "being-here". The human brain constructs the world from gestation onward in an interaction with its environment. This process governed by genes and their expression (epigenetic) (137) leads to more and more complex "logical" choices following statistical "Bayesian inferences" (138), the results of which may be forgotten but still predetermine future decisions by limiting the scope of one's expectations. Its integrated complexity is mainly unconscious and organizes a memory which is more concerned by one's future efficiency than by an accurate memorization of past events. It leaves a small place to what we consider as consciousness which has to decide among a limited number of preselections networked through sleep and "mind wandering" (139–142). Brain exercise like meditation could improve its efficiency. The development of the brain is crucially sensitive in its first months and years to its relations with its human environment which will make up the limits of its future "creativity" through the secure basis of its attachment (143–145). At adolescence, the brain restructuration will settle its adult functional frame (146) . Drug use and addiction represent only one dimension of this complex adaptative interaction which cannot be "revolutionized" by a single logical argumentation. The impact of the initial AIDS epidemic, with its massive death toll, observed in France in the nineteen eighties will not occur anymore. It was "one shot". Prevention messages, treatment proposals have to take into account these changing individual ecologies. One can be immediately convinced by the description of the risk of NSS but will nevertheless engage in NSS when its result is an instant improvement in well being compared with an improbable success of hepatitis prevention over the future years of addiction and the high probability of dying before the advent of an improbable liver cancer.
- Modern society, faced with the management of its growing complexity, has organized itself functionally around social systems which rationally objectify the world (147).

They follow an initial selection of their missions through binary codes (health/disease for medicine, presence or absence of an hepatitis for HCV specialists) which makes them "blind" to what has been excluded (the complexity of the world) and gives them a meaning which is the basis of their communication with their environment. These self-referential systems fight to survive and extend their territories responding to stimulations (irritations) of their environment through the limited structural couplings they themselves made possible. Hepatologists will use scientific medical mathematics to modelize the HCV epidemic from scarce and improbable data to convince politics and economics to maintain and, even, increase their funding. Publication of these computations will improve the academic status of biostatisticians. The pharmaceutical industry will fund these studies which secure the outlet of their products and so on. For an hepatitis specialist DU exists first as a carrier of an HCV infection for an hepatitis specialists This practical discovery explains the absence of specificity of DUs' hepatitis management reported by French HRCs: The only limit of HCV treatment was compliance, problem which was not restricted to DUs and, in our French study of HRCs, did not need a specific management for consulting DUs. The question of the control of the HCV epidemic was irrelevant. The global failure of society faced with the problem of drug use and of its management, the awareness of its social complexity are the source of the demand by the professionals of an association in the same place of diverse services addressing belonging to multiple social systems: they would "have to" manage the failures of one particular service which, once its limits recognized, would not be considered as such.

- This organization ignores the complexity of one's "being-here" and is the source of a modern reactivation of the ethical debate (148–151). A DU does not exist as such outside its representation by society's Other. The practical success of HCV care cure but also prevention) is related to the capacity of each individual to recognize and make recognized the inscrutable "otherness" present in every human being. Rational objectification, which is at the core of every scientific approach, is supported by the emptiness of universal concepts which deny this recognition. This otherness is the source of an infinite demand which founds inter human relations. The limited offer which one can propose in return, leaves to this "neighbour", who is to be "loved like oneself ", the freedom to make the right choice. In its absence, the quenching of the scientific rational solution (see Descartes's discourse of a method), when it is implemented, may be transformed into an unbearable violence which will force one to step out of the symbolic order to express one's freedom and say no to an impossible but irrefutable proposal (see paragraph II.1.3.): "death drive" for Freud, "radical negativity" for German Idealism. This "acting-out" has its own inescapable rationality: the immediacy of one's (emotional and conscious) survival in the "death struggle" of the Hegelian demand for recognition. Care and cure cannot be summed up as an accurate diagnosis and prescription. In my practice, this (not so) simple recognition of the other's freedom had a constant practical impact. One of society's responses is the development of a "third sector", non-profit organizations outside of organized social systems which answer its latencies such as individual and social complexity but whose precarious survival depends on their perceived immediate social utility.

4. Finally, let us try to be creative

At the end of this general survey, limiting their scope to the HCV epidemic, four options are possible.

- The first would keep the status quo, leaving the community with the belief that harm reduction is efficient, efficiency which could be boosted by additional funding of each of these actions and a better collaboration between services leading to integration in drug treatment programmes which would encompass them all. The sole aim of many papers published in journals dedicated to drug use and DUs is to convince their reader of its validity. This position is held by each subsystem which, to survive and even grow has to convince its environment of its performance. In my opinion, it may appear as the less costly in energy and financial involvement, but I believe, in the long term, it will be the less efficient.
- The second is more ambitious. It considers HCV hepatitis as an epidemic which should be controlled and DUs as users of services supplied by the healthcare system which may not be spontaneously desired by DUs but which use such as the treatment of HIV and hepatitis should be implemented to control these epidemics. From a DU's stand point HCV hepatitis cannot be considered alone. It is never more than a part of his "being-here" for which society's goals of harm reduction may not be relevant. To succeed society has to propose an environment "good-enough" to enable him to live without a continuous help of drugs. This option depends on the assumption that a better knowledge and a better management could control the HCV epidemic. Today, it remains a "wishful thinking" of existing social systems:
  - The initial assumption would be that the control of the HCV epidemic should associate prevention of new infections to the treatment of "all" (at least a large majority) the infected DUs (even not in DTP) to decrease viral prevalence to a level which would, by itself, limit the new contaminations, passing from an epidemic to sporadic cases, evolution observed for HIV in most countries where the initial prevalence remained low.
  - The first step would design and conduct an ethno-epidemiological study of a population in a geographical delimited area relevant for the proposed intervention. It would collect its socio-demographics, health status, social networks, drugs consumed and risks associated to that consumption, viral status and use of social and health care as well as its motivations, desires and plans (152).
  - From that collection, an analysis would define potentially different subgroups which would be targeted for different interventions which would try to build a "cultural" environment including a positive vision of HCV care and the conscience of the necessity of a global commitment needed to control the HCV epidemic. It would try to understand its course among these different subgroups including the possible viral reservoirs among DUs who do not attend healthcare services. The first goal of these programmes would be to win the trust of the concerned DUs by proposing services answering their need (desires). Beside proposing substitution treatments or social help to find work or housing, considering the cost of harm reduction and HCV treatment, one could propose conditional cash transfer or vouchers which have been used successfully in many countries to improve access to school or healthcare programmes and which is one of the few incentives proven to be efficient in cocaine addiction (153,154). Heroin treatment should be considered. It has been shown to be significantly more effective than methadone for difficult to maintain patients (155,156). This efficacy was also present in DUs without previous maintenance treatments (157). It can be delivered intranasally or orally (158). It has been shown to be cost-effective (159).

HCV prevention and treatment would only come second, tailored to the course of the epidemic, targeting opinion leaders through peers' interventions explaining the ethical goal of the project which would not be limited to the individual gain of the cure of one's hepatitis but would want to control the HCV epidemic in the area, control which would benefit not only DUs but also their family, friends and neighbors. Their success would be conditioned by a complete appropriateness between the discourse and the means: To improve the impact of NSP, a significant rise would be mandatory to decrease significantly the occurrence of receptive exchanges. It could mean a tenfold increase in the number of syringes exchanged, but it would not be enough. NSP should shift from exchange to distribution (160) allowing IDUs to store sterile syringes for future use and "providers" to distribute syringes to other IDUs who are in need of sterile syringes and cannot access a NSP or a pharmacy (161) This would help to cover unexpected "craving" episodes in former IDUs at times when pharmacies and NSP are closed which represent, at least in my experience, a significant cause of new contaminations. Home self-test for the diagnosis of HIV and HCV infection should be an option (65). As long as the HCV prevalence remains high, to be efficient, NSP as well as potential consumption rooms should be located in the neighborhood of every drug scene (162-164) embedded within existing spatial and social relations of DUs (165). Outreach, bringing services to the DUs with the lowest social functioning can also decrease NSS). Open scenes, where users could come to buy their drugs, find NSP and meet harm reduction services, could reduce the level of NSSHCV screening could only be considered if a treatment could be proposed to every infected DU. Interventions should be adapted to the evolution of each case. Building trust takes time, even more when every partner (from customers to professionals) are concerned.

  - The simplistic idea that one would only need to bring potential actors together to carry out a community project is long overdue [166]. Understanding the implications of the affiliation of professionals to social sub-systems could help them as well as those responsible for leading and managing programs to consider the limits of their individual scope, the need for an evolution of their missions and for new cooperative programs. The evolution of the French care of DUs' hepatitis C bears witness of its feasibility. To reach these goals, time and specific resources must be allocated and a common will and trust between the different actors is mandatory to overcome the existing barriers to an effective integration of prevention and treatment of hepatitis C (167-169). The proposed approach makes the control of the HCV epidemic an example of a new health policy paradigm: efficient integrated services (medical and social) based on the knowledge of the health of a population in a designated area as advocated by most groups working on the improvement of clinical effectiveness. This multilevel approach to change should include the individual, group/team, organization, and larger environment/system level (170).

- The third alternative would be the legalization (not a simple depenalization) of drug consumption. Of course this proposal may appear heretic when one considers drug related deaths and comorbidities. However, the rational behind the "war on drugs" was its possible success. 40 year after its implementation, one is forced to observe its failure,

failure which has a precedent with alcohol prohibition in the United States (171-181). The belief that this legalization would result in a huge increase in drug consumption can be compared to the fantasy of an increase in sexual promiscuity induced by sexual education in the eighties, which was proven to be false. The obvious benefit would be the huge amount of taxes which escapes today every government. The drug market is still one of the most perfect examples of a free market economy adapting its products to its customers and one of the most profitable. Of course, it would mean a negative impact on many social sub-systems devoted to this war like justice, police, customs or, even, medicine with a significant reduction of state spending. They would not able to "understand" a proposal which would negate the mission which justifies their existence and reduce their "power". A global vision would be mandatory. One must also not forget drug dealers who have an interest in keeping their trade illegal and can spend large sums of money to bribe people who are able prevent that evolution. An initial transfer of marijuana market from organized crime to state management could assess the risks and benefits of this change of policy. Of course, its impact on the HCV epidemic would wait heroin and cocaine legalization which would only reduce the number of new contaminations.

- The fourth and last solution would be the development of a vaccine comparable to the HBV vaccine and which could be implemented on a population basis at least at adolescence. Of course this solution, when available, could improve each one of the previous solutions.

5. References

[1] Matheï C, Buntinx F, van Damme P. Seroprevalence of hepatitis C markers among intravenous drug users in western European countries: a systematic review. J.Viral. Hepat. 2002 May;9(3):157-73.

[2] Hagan H, Des Jarlais DC, Stern R, Lelutiu-Weinberger C, Scheinmann R, Strauss S, et al. HCV synthesis project: preliminary analyses of HCV prevalence in relation to age and duration of injection. Int. J. Drug Policy. 2007 oct;18(5):341-51.

[3] Grebely J, Raffa JD, Lai C, Krajden M, Kerr T, Fischer B, et al. Low uptake of treatment for hepatitis C virus infection in a large community-based study of inner city residents. J. Viral Hepat. 2009 mai;16(5):352-8.

[4] Rhodes T, Treloar C. The social production of hepatitis C risk among injecting drug users: a qualitative synthesis. Addiction. 2008 oct;103(10):1593-603.

[5] Smyth BP, Barry J, Keenan E. Irish injecting drug users and hepatitis C: the importance of the social context of injecting. Int. J. Epidemiol. 2005 feb;34(1):166-72.

[6] Maher L, Jalaludin B, Chant KG, Jayasuriya R, Sladden T, Kaldor JM, et al. Incidence and risk factors for hepatitis C seroconversion in injecting drug users in Australia. Addiction. 2006 oct;101(10):1499-508.

[7] Lucidarme D, Bruandet A, Ilef D, Harbonnier J, Jacob C, Decoster A, et al. Incidence and risk factors of HCV and HIV infections in a cohort of intravenous drug users in the North and East of France. Epidemiol. Infect. 2004 août;132(4):699-708.

[8] Scheinmann R, Hagan H, Lelutiu-Weinberger C, Stern R, Des Jarlais DC, Flom PL, et al. Non-injection drug use and Hepatitis C Virus: a systematic review. Drug Alcohol Depend. 2007 juin 15;89(1):1-12.

[9] Macías J, Palacios RB, Claro E, Vargas J, Vergara S, Mira JA, et al. High prevalence of hepatitis C virus infection among noninjecting drug users: association with sharing the inhalation implements of crack. Liver Int. 2008 juill;28(6):781-6.

[10] Nurutdinova D, Abdallah AB, Bradford S, O'Leary CC, Cottler LB. Risk factors associated with Hepatitis C among female substance users enrolled in community-based HIV prevention studies. BMC Res Notes. 2011;4:126.

[11] Tor J, Llibre JM, Carbonell M, Muga R, Ribera A, Soriano V, et al. Sexual transmission of hepatitis C virus and its relation with hepatitis B virus and HIV. BMJ. 1990 nov 17;301(6761):1130-3.

[12] Neumayr G, Propst A, Schwaighofer H, Judmaier G, Vogel W. Lack of evidence for the heterosexual transmission of hepatitis C. QJM. 1999 sept;92(9):505-8.

[13] G Rooney, Gilson RJ. Sexual transmission of hepatitis C virus infection. Sex Transm Infect. 1998 déc;74(6):399-404.

[14] Tsai P-S, Chang C-J, Chen K-T, Chang K-C, Hung S-F, Wang J-H, et al. Acquirement and disappearance of HBsAg and anti-HCV in an aged population: a follow-up study in an endemic township. Liver Int. 2011 août;31(7):971-9.

[15] Ghosn J, Thibault V, Delaugerre C, Fontaine H, Lortholary O, Rouzioux C, et al. Sexually transmitted hepatitis C virus superinfection in HIV/hepatitis C virus co-infected men who have sex with men. AIDS. 2008 mars 12;22(5):658-61.

[16] Urbanus AT, van de Laar TJ, Stolte IG, Schinkel J, Heijman T, Coutinho RA, et al. Hepatitis C virus infections among HIV-infected men who have sex with men: an expanding epidemic. AIDS. 2009 juill 31;23(12):F1-7.

[17] van de Laar T, Pybus O, Bruisten S, Brown D, Nelson M, Bhagani S, et al. Evidence of a large, international network of HCV transmission in HIV-positive men who have sex with men. Gastroenterology. 2009 mai;136(5):1609-17.

[18] van der Helm JJ, Prins M, del Amo J, Bucher HC, Chêne G, Dorrucci M, et al. The hepatitis C epidemic among HIV-positive MSM: incidence estimates from 1990 to 2007. AIDS. 2011 mai 15;25(8):1083-91.

[19] Tohme RA, Holmberg SD. Transmission of hepatitis C virus infection through tattooing and piercing: a critical review. Clin. Infect. Dis. 2012 avr;54(8):1167-78.

[20] Hwang L-Y, Kramer JR, Troisi C, Bull L, Grimes CZ, Lyerla R, et al. Relationship of cosmetic procedures and drug use to hepatitis C and hepatitis B virus infections in a low-risk population. Hepatology. 2006 août;44(2):341-51.

[21] Koziel MJ, Wong DK, Dudley D, Houghton M, Walker BD. Hepatitis C virus-specific cytolytic T lymphocyte and T helper cell responses in seronegative persons. J. Infect. Dis. 1997 oct;176(4):859-66.

[22] Bronowicki JP, Vetter D, Uhl G, Hudziak H, Uhrlacher A, Vetter JM, et al. Lymphocyte reactivity to hepatitis C virus (HCV) antigens shows evidence for exposure to HCV in HCV-seronegative spouses of HCV-infected patients. J. Infect. Dis. 1997 août;176(2):518-22.

[23] Kim JY, Won JE, Jeong S-H, Park SJ, Hwang SG, Kang S-K, et al. Acute hepatitis C in Korea: different modes of infection, high rate of spontaneous recovery, and low rate of seroconversion. J. Med. Virol. 2011 juill;83(7):1195-202.

[24] Pham TNQ, Coffin CS, Michalak TI. Occult hepatitis C virus infection: what does it mean? Liver Int. 2010 avr;30(4):502-11.

[25] MacParland SA, Pham TNQ, Guy CS, Michalak TI. Hepatitis C virus persisting after clinically apparent sustained virological response to antiviral therapy retains infectivity in vitro. Hepatology. 2009 mai;49(5):1431-41.

[26] Castillo I, Bartolomé J, Quiroga JA, Barril G, Carreño V. Hepatitis C virus infection in the family setting of patients with occult hepatitis C. J. Med. Virol. 2009 juill;81(7):1198-203.

[27] Thurairajah PH, Hegazy D, Chokshi S, Shaw S, Demaine A, Kaminski ER, et al. Hepatitis C virus (HCV)--specific T cell responses in injection drug users with apparent resistance to HCV infection. J. Infect. Dis. 2008 déc 15;198(12):1749-55.

[28] Mizukoshi E, Eisenbach C, Edlin BR, Newton KP, Raghuraman S, Weiler-Normann C, et al. Hepatitis C virus (HCV)-specific immune responses of long-term injection drug users frequently exposed to HCV. J. Infect. Dis. 2008 juill 15;198(2):203-12.

[29] Aitken CK, Lewis J, Tracy SL, Spelman T, Bowden DS, Bharadwaj M, et al. High incidence of hepatitis C virus reinfection in a cohort of injecting drug users. Hepatology. 2008 déc;48(6):1746-52.

[30] Osburn WO, Fisher BE, Dowd KA, Urban G, Liu L, Ray SC, et al. Spontaneous control of primary hepatitis C virus infection and immunity against persistent reinfection. Gastroenterology. 2010 janv;138(1):315-24.

[31] Mehta SH, Cox A, Hoover DR, Wang X-H, Mao Q, Ray S, et al. Protection against persistence of hepatitis C. Lancet. 2002 avr 27;359(9316):1478-83.

[32] Grebely J, Conway B, Raffa JD, Lai C, Krajden M, Tyndall MW. Hepatitis C virus reinfection in injection drug users. Hepatology. 2006 nov;44(5):1139-45.

[33] Sacks-Davis R, Daraganava G, Altken C, Higgs P, Jenkinson R, Tracy SI, Bawden S, Robins G, Pattison P, Grebely J, Barry AE, Helard M. Molecular epidemiolgical evidence that social network research can identify hepatitis C transmission pathways in people who inject drugs. Hepatology. 2011;54(S1):1164A.

[34] Jager JC, European Monitoring Centre for Drugs and Drug Addiction. Hepatits C and injecting drug use: impact, costs and policy options. Luxembourg: European Monitoring Centre for Drugs and Drug Addiction; 2004.

[35] Loomba R, Rivera MM, McBurney R, Park Y, Haynes-Williams V, Rehermann B, et al. The natural history of acute hepatitis C: clinical presentation, laboratory findings and treatment outcomes. Aliment. Pharmacol. Ther. 2011 mars;33(5):559-65.

[36] Page K, Hahn JA, Evans J, Shiboski S, Lum P, Delwart E, et al. Acute hepatitis C virus infection in young adult injection drug users: a prospective study of incident infection, resolution, and reinfection. J. Infect. Dis. 2009 oct 15;200(8):1216-26.

[37] Thomas DL, Astemborski J, Rai RM, Anania FA, Schaeffer M, Galai N, et al. The natural history of hepatitis C virus infection: host, viral, and environmental factors. JAMA. 2000 juill 26;284(4):450-6.

[38] Thein H-H, Yi Q, Dore GJ, Krahn MD. Natural history of hepatitis C virus infection in HIV-infected individuals and the impact of HIV in the era of highly active antiretroviral therapy: a meta-analysis. AIDS. 2008 oct 1;22(15):1979-91.

[39] John-Baptiste A, Krahn M, Heathcote J, Laporte A, Tomlinson G. The natural history of hepatitis C infection acquired through injection drug use: meta-analysis and meta-regression. J. Hepatol. 2010 août;53(2):245-51.

[40] Bellentani S, Tiribelli C. The spectrum of liver disease in the general population: lesson from the Dionysos study. J. Hepatol. 2001 oct;35(4):531-7.

[41] Kenny-Walsh E. The natural history of hepatitis C virus infection. Clin Liver Dis. 2001 nov;5(4):969-77.

[42] Seeff LB, Hollinger FB, Alter HJ, Wright EC, Cain CM, Buskell ZJ, et al. Long-term mortality and morbidity of transfusion-associated non-A, non-B, and type C hepatitis: A National Heart, Lung, and Blood Institute collaborative study. Hepatology. 2001 févr;33(2):455-63.

[43] Harris HE, Ramsay ME, Andrews NJ. Survival of a national cohort of hepatitis C virus infected patients, 16 years after exposure. Epidemiol. Infect. 2006 juin;134(3):472-7.

[44] Butt AA, Wang X, Moore CG. Effect of hepatitis C virus and its treatment on survival. Hepatology. 2009 août;50(2):387-92.

[45] Grønbaek K, Krarup HB, Møller H, Krogsgaard K, Franzmann M, Sonne J, et al. Natural history and etiology of liver disease in patients with previous community-acquired acute non-A, non-B hepatitis. A follow-up study of 178 Danish patients consecutively enrolled in The Copenhagen Hepatitis Acuta Programme in the period 1969-1987. J. Hepatol. 1999 nov;31(5):800-7.

[46] Amin J, Law MG, Bartlett M, Kaldor JM, Dore GJ. Causes of death after diagnosis of hepatitis B or hepatitis C infection: a large community-based linkage study. Lancet. 2006 sept 9;368(9539):938-45.

[47] Neal KR, Ramsay S, Thomson BJ, Irving WL. Excess mortality rates in a cohort of patients infected with the hepatitis C virus: a prospective study. Gut. 2007 août;56(8):1098-104.

[48] Guiltinan AM, Kaidarova Z, Custer B, Orland J, Strollo A, Cyrus S, et al. Increased all-cause, liver, and cardiac mortality among hepatitis C virus-seropositive blood donors. Am. J. Epidemiol. 2008 mars 15;167(6):743-50.

[49] Omland LH, Krarup H, Jepsen P, Georgsen J, Harritshøj LH, Riisom K, et al. Mortality in patients with chronic and cleared hepatitis C viral infection: a nationwide cohort study. J. Hepatol. 2010 juill;53(1):36-42.

[50] Smyth B, Hoffman V, Fan J, Hser Y-I. Years of potential life lost among heroin addicts 33 years after treatment. Prev Med. 2007 avr;44(4):369-74.

[51] Missiha SB, Ostrowski M, Heathcote EJ. Disease progression in chronic hepatitis C: modifiable and nonmodifiable factors. Gastroenterology. 2008 mai;134(6):1699-714.

[52] Dring MM, Morrison MH, McSharry BP, Guinan KJ, Hagan R, O'Farrelly C, et al. Innate immune genes synergize to predict increased risk of chronic disease in hepatitis C virus infection. Proc. Natl. Acad. Sci. U.S.A. 2011 avr 5;108(14):5736-41.

[53] Knapp S, Warshow U, Ho KMA, Hegazy D, Little A-M, Fowell A, et al. A polymorphism in IL28B distinguishes exposed, uninfected individuals from spontaneous resolvers of HCV infection. Gastroenterology. 2011 juill;141(1):320-325, 325.e1-2.

[54] Pagliaro L, Pasta L, D'Amico G, Madonia S, Pietrosi G. Familial clustering of (mostly) HCV-related cirrhosis. A case-control study. J. Hepatol. 2002 déc;37(6):762-6.

[55] Sookoian S, Pirola CJ. Meta-analysis of the influence of I148M variant of patatin-like phospholipase domain containing 3 gene (PNPLA3) on the susceptibility and histological severity of nonalcoholic fatty liver disease. Hepatology. 2011 juin;53(6):1883-94.

[56] Trépo E, Gustot T, Degré D, Lemmers A, Verset L, Demetter P, et al. Common polymorphism in the PNPLA3/adiponutrin gene confers higher risk of cirrhosis and liver damage in alcoholic liver disease. J. Hepatol. 2011 oct;55(4):906-12.
[57] Huang H, Shiffman ML, Friedman S, Venkatesh R, Bzowej N, Abar OT, et al. A 7 gene signature identifies the risk of developing cirrhosis in patients with chronic hepatitis C. Hepatology. 2007 août;46(2):297-306.
[58] Marcolongo M, Young B, Dal Pero F, Fattovich G, Peraro L, Guido M, et al. A seven-gene signature (cirrhosis risk score) predicts liver fibrosis progression in patients with initially mild chronic hepatitis C. Hepatology. 2009 oct;50(4):1038-44.
[59] Riaz M, Idrees M, Kanwal H, Kabir F. An overview of triple infection with hepatitis B, C and D viruses. Virol. J. 2011;8:368.
[60] Jamma S, Hussain G, Lau DT-Y. Current Concepts of HBV/HCV Coinfection: Coexistence, but Not Necessarily in Harmony. Curr Hepat Rep. 2010;9(4):260-9.
[61] Greub G, Ledergerber B, Battegay M, Grob P, Perrin L, Furrer H, et al. Clinical progression, survival, and immune recovery during antiretroviral therapy in patients with HIV-1 and hepatitis C virus coinfection: the Swiss HIV Cohort Study. Lancet. 2000 nov 25;356(9244):1800-5.
[62] Vallet-Pichard A, Pol S. Natural history and predictors of severity of chronic hepatitis C virus (HCV) and human immunodeficiency virus (HIV) co-infection. J. Hepatol. 2006;44(1 Suppl):S28-34.
[63] Weis N, Lindhardt BO, Kronborg G, Hansen A-BE, Laursen AL, Christensen PB, et al. Impact of hepatitis C virus coinfection on response to highly active antiretroviral therapy and outcome in HIV-infected individuals: a nationwide cohort study. Clin. Infect. Dis. 2006 mai 15;42(10):1481-7.
[64] Mehta SH, Thomas DL, Torbenson M, Brinkley S, Mirel L, Chaisson RE, et al. The effect of antiretroviral therapy on liver disease among adults with HIV and hepatitis C coinfection. Hepatology. 2005 janv;41(1):123-31.
[65] Skolnik HS, Phillips KA, Binson D, Dilley JW. Deciding where and how to be tested for HIV: what matters most? J. Acquir. Immune Defic. Syndr. 2001 juill 1;27(3):292-300.
[66] Morota K, Fujinami R, Kinukawa H, Machida T, Ohno K, Saegusa H, et al. A new sensitive and automated chemiluminescent microparticle immunoassay for quantitative determination of hepatitis C virus core antigen. J. Virol. Methods. 2009 avr;157(1):8-14.
[67] Mederacke I, Potthoff A, Meyer-Olson D, Meier M, Raupach R, Manns MP, et al. HCV core antigen testing in HIV- and HBV-coinfected patients, and in HCV-infected patients on hemodialysis. J. Clin. Virol. 2012 févr;53(2):110-5.
[68] Hosseini-Moghaddam S, Iran-Pour E, Rotstein C, Husain S, Lilly L, Renner E, et al. Hepatitis C core Ag and its clinical applicability: Potential advantages and disadvantages for diagnosis and follow-up? Rev. Med. Virol. 2012 mai;22(3):156-65.
[69] Ahmad W, Ijaz B, Gull S, Asad S, Khaliq S, Jahan S, et al. A brief review on molecular, genetic and imaging techniques for HCV fibrosis evaluation. Virol. J. 2011;8(1):53.
[70] Cacoub P, Carrat F, Bédossa P, Lambert J, Pénaranda G, Perronne C, et al. Comparison of non-invasive liver fibrosis biomarkers in HIV/HCV co-infected patients: the fibrovic study--ANRS HC02. J. Hepatol. 2008 mai;48(5):765-73.

[71] Lucidarme D, Foucher J, Le Bail B, Vergniol J, Castera L, Duburque C, et al. Factors of accuracy of transient elastography (fibroscan) for the diagnosis of liver fibrosis in chronic hepatitis C. Hepatology. 2009 avr;49(4):1083-9.

[72] Huckans MS, Loftis JM, Blackwell AD, Linke A, Hauser P. Interferon alpha therapy for hepatitis C: treatment completion and response rates among patients with substance use disorders. Subst Abuse Treat Prev Policy. 2007;2:4.

[73] Chossegros P, Mélin P, Hézode C, Bourlière M, Pol S, Fhima A, et al. A French prospective observational study of the treatment of chronic hepatitis C in drug abusers. Gastroenterol. Clin. Biol. 2008 oct;32(10):850-7.

[74] Moreno C, Deltenre P, Pawlotsky J-M, Henrion J, Adler M, Mathurin P. Shortened treatment duration in treatment-naive genotype 1 HCV patients with rapid virological response: a meta-analysis. J. Hepatol. 2010 janv;52(1):25-31.

[75] Martin-Carbonero L, Nuñez M, Mariño A, Alcocer F, Bonet L, García-Samaniego J, et al. Undetectable hepatitis C virus RNA at week 4 as predictor of sustained virological response in HIV patients with chronic hepatitis C. AIDS. 2008 janv 2;22(1):15-21.

[76] Falasca K, Ucciferri C, Mancino P, Gorgoretti V, Pizzigallo E, Vecchiet J. Use of epoetin beta during combination therapy of infection with hepatitis c virus with ribavirin improves a sustained viral response. J. Med. Virol. 2010 janv;82(1):49-56.

[77] Rauch A, Kutalik Z, Descombes P, Cai T, Di Iulio J, Mueller T, et al. Genetic variation in IL28B is associated with chronic hepatitis C and treatment failure: a genome-wide association study. Gastroenterology. 2010 avr;138(4):1338-1345, 1345.e1-7.

[78] Suppiah V, Gaudieri S, Armstrong NJ, O'Connor KS, Berg T, Weltman M, et al. IL28B, HLA-C, and KIR variants additively predict response to therapy in chronic hepatitis C virus infection in a European Cohort: a cross-sectional study. PLoS Med. 2011 sept;8(9):e1001092.

[79] Mangia A, Thompson AJ, Santoro R, Piazzolla V, Tillmann HL, Patel K, et al. An IL28B polymorphism determines treatment response of hepatitis C virus genotype 2 or 3 patients who do not achieve a rapid virologic response. Gastroenterology. 2010 sept;139(3):821-827, 827.e1.

[80] Neukam K, Nattermann J, Rallón N, Rivero A, Caruz A, Macías J, et al. Different distributions of hepatitis C virus genotypes among HIV-infected patients with acute and chronic hepatitis C according to interleukin-28B genotype. HIV Med. 2011 sept;12(8):487-93.

[81] Antaki N, Bibert S, Kebbewar K, Asaad F, Baroudi O, Alideeb S, et al. IL28B polymorphisms do not predict response to therapy in chronic hepatitis C with HCV genotype 5. Gut [Internet]. 2012 févr 16 [cité 2012 avr 23]; Available de: http://www.ncbi.nlm.nih.gov/pubmed/22345656

[82] Kwo PY, Lawitz EJ, McCone J, Schiff ER, Vierling JM, Pound D, et al. Efficacy of boceprevir, an NS3 protease inhibitor, in combination with peginterferon alfa-2b and ribavirin in treatment-naive patients with genotype 1 hepatitis C infection (SPRINT-1): an open-label, randomised, multicentre phase 2 trial. Lancet. 2010 août 28;376(9742):705-16.

[83] Sherman KE, Flamm SL, Afdhal NH, Nelson DR, Sulkowski MS, Everson GT, et al. Response-guided telaprevir combination treatment for hepatitis C virus infection. N. Engl. J. Med. 2011 sept 15;365(11):1014-24.

[84] Ramachandran P, Fraser A, Agarwal K, Austin A, Brown A, Foster GR, et al. UK consensus guidelines for the use of the protease inhibitors boceprevir and telaprevir in genotype 1 chronic hepatitis C infected patients. Aliment. Pharmacol. Ther. 2012 mars;35(6):647-62.

[85] Sulkowski MS, Benhamou Y. Therapeutic issues in HIV/HCV-coinfected patients. J. Viral Hepat. 2007 juin;14(6):371-86.

[86] Halliday J, Klenerman P, Barnes E. Vaccination for hepatitis C virus: closing in on an evasive target. Expert Rev Vaccines. 2011 mai;10(5):659-72.

[87] Habersetzer F, Honnet G, Bain C, Maynard-Muet M, Leroy V, Zarski J-P, et al. A poxvirus vaccine is safe, induces T-cell responses, and decreases viral load in patients with chronic hepatitis C. Gastroenterology. 2011 sept;141(3):890-899.e1-4.

[88] Bellentani S, Pozzato G, Saccoccio G, Crovatto M, Crocè LS, Mazzoran L, et al. Clinical course and risk factors of hepatitis C virus related liver disease in the general population: report from the Dionysos study. Gut. 1999 juin;44(6):874-80.

[89] Pybus OG, Markov PV, Wu A, Tatem AJ. Investigating the endemic transmission of the hepatitis C virus. Int. J. Parasitol. 2007 juill;37(8-9):839-49.

[90] Agarwal SK. Hemodialysis of patients with HCV infection: isolation has a definite role. Nephron Clin Pract. 2011;117(4):c328-332.

[91] Sous le signe du «MATOS» Contextes, trajectoires, risques et sensations liés à l'injection de produits psychoactifs.

[92] Chossegros P. [Management of drug addiction in France (a short history)]. Gastroenterol. Clin. Biol. 2007 sept;31(8-9 Pt 3):4S44-50.

[93] EMCDDA–Europol 2011 Annual Report on the implementation of Council Decision 2005/387/JHA.

[94] Nelson PK, Mathers BM, Cowie B, Hagan H, Des Jarlais D, Horyniak D, et al. Global epidemiology of hepatitis B and hepatitis C in people who inject drugs: results of systematic reviews. Lancet. 2011 août 13;378(9791):571-83.

[95] Prévalence de l'usage problématique de drogues en France - estimations 2006. Saint-Denis, OFDT, 2009,. OFDT;

[96] Kuebler D, Hausser D, Gervasoni JP. The characteristics of « new users » of cocaine and heroin unknown to treatment agencies: results from the Swiss Hidden Population Study. Addiction. 2000 oct;95(10):1561-71.

[97] Fontaine A, Fontana C. Drogues, activité professionnelle et vie privée. OFDT. 2003;

[98] Dubois F, Desenclos JC, Mariotte N, Goudeau A. Hepatitis C in a French population-based survey, 1994: seroprevalence, frequency of viremia, genotype distribution, and risk factors. The Collaborative Study Group. Hepatology. 1997 juin;25(6):1490-6.

[99] INVS. Estimation des taux de prévalence des anticorps anti-VHC et des marqueurs du virus de l'hépatite B chez les assurés sociaux du régime général de France métropolitaine, 2003-2004. Analyse descriptive [Internet]. 2005. Available on: http://www.invs.sante.fr/publications/2005/analyse_descriptive_140205/index.html

[100] Emmanuelli J, Jauffret-Roustide M, Barin F. Epidémiologie du VHC chez les usagers de drogues, France, 1993-2002. BEH. 2003;97-9.

[101] Jauffret-Roustide M, Le Strat Y, Couturier E, Thierry D, Rondy M, Quaglia M, et al. A national cross-sectional study among drug-users in France: epidemiology of HCV

and highlight on practical and statistical aspects of the design. BMC Infect. Dis. 2009;9:113.
[102] Villano SA, Vlahov D, Nelson KE, Lyles CM, Cohn S, Thomas DL. Incidence and risk factors for hepatitis C among injection drug users in Baltimore, Maryland. J. Clin. Microbiol. 1997 dec;35(12):3274-7.
[103] van Beek I, Dwyer R, Dore GJ, Luo K, Kaldor JM. Infection with HIV and hepatitis C virus among injecting drug users in a prevention setting: retrospective cohort study. BMJ. 1998 aug 15;317(7156):433-7.
[104] Smyth BP, O'Connor JJ, Barry J, Keenan E. Retrospective cohort study examining incidence of HIV and hepatitis C infection among injecting drug users in Dublin. J Epidemiol Community Health. 2003 avr;57(4):310-1.
[105] Fuller CM, Ompad DC, Galea S, Wu Y, Koblin B, Vlahov D. Hepatitis C incidence--a comparison between injection and noninjection drug users in New York City. J Urban Health. 2004 mars;81(1):20-4.
[106] Stein MD, Herman DS, Anderson BJ. A trial to reduce hepatitis C seroincidence in drug users. J Addict Dis. 2009 oct;28(4):389-98.
[107] Garfein RS, Golub ET, Greenberg AE, Hagan H, Hanson DL, Hudson SM, et al. A peer-education intervention to reduce injection risk behaviors for HIV and hepatitis C virus infection in young injection drug users. AIDS. 2007 sept 12;21(14):1923-32.
[108] Abou-Saleh M, Davis P, Rice P, Checinski K, Drummond C, Maxwell D, et al. The effectiveness of behavioural interventions in the primary prevention of hepatitis C amongst injecting drug users: a randomised controlled trial and lessons learned. Harm Reduct J. 2008;5:25.
[109] Hagan H, Pouget ER, Des Jarlais DC. A systematic review and meta-analysis of interventions to prevent hepatitis C virus infection in people who inject drugs. J. Infect. Dis. 2011 juill 1;204(1):74-83.
[110] Mehta SH, Astemborski J, Kirk GD, Strathdee SA, Nelson KE, Vlahov D, et al. Changes in blood-borne infection risk among injection drug users. J. Infect. Dis. 2011 mars 1;203(5):587-94.
[111] Falster K, Kaldor JM, Maher L. Hepatitis C virus acquisition among injecting drug users: a cohort analysis of a national repeated cross-sectional survey of needle and syringe program attendees in Australia, 1995-2004. J Urban Health. 2009 janv; 86(1):106-18.
[112] Jauffret-Roustide M, Emmanuelli J, Desenclos JC. [Limited impact of the harm-reduction policy on HCV among drug-users. The ANRS-Coquelicot survey example]. Rev Epidemiol Sante Publique. 2006 juill;54 Spec No 1:1S53-51S59.
[113] Cazein F, Le Strat Y, Pillonel J, Lot F, Bousquet V, Pinget R, Le Vu S, Brand D, Brunet S, Thierry D, Leclerc M, Benyelles L, Couturier S, Da Costa C, Barin F, Semaille C. Dépistage du VIH et découvertes de séropositivité, France, 2003-2010. BEH. 2011;(43/44):446-54.
[114] Di Nino F, Imbs JL, Melenotte GH, le réseau RMS3, Doffoel M. Dépistage et traitement des hépatites C par le réseau des microstructures médicales chez les usagers de drogues en Alsace, France, 2006-2007. BEH. 2009;
[115] Patrick DM, Tyndall MW, Cornelisse PG, Li K, Sherlock CH, Rekart ML, et al. Incidence of hepatitis C virus infection among injection drug users during an outbreak of HIV infection. CMAJ. 2001 oct 2;165(7):889-95.

[116] Skidmore CA, Robertson JR, Robertson AA, Elton RA. After the epidemic: follow up study of HIV seroprevalence and changing patterns of drug use. BMJ. 1990 janv 27;300(6719):219-23.

[117] Tempalski B, Lieb S, Cleland CM, Cooper H, Brady JE, Friedman SR. HIV prevalence rates among injection drug users in 96 large US metropolitan areas, 1992-2002. J Urban Health. 2009 janv;86(1):132-54.

[118] Harm reduction: evidence, impacts and challenges. EMCDDA, Lisbon, April 2010;

[119] Institute of Medicine (U.S.). Committee on HIV Screening and Access to Care. HIV screening and access to care exploring the impact of policies on access to and provision of HIV Care. Washington, D.C.: National Academies Press; 2011.

[120] Colvin HM, Mitchell AE, Institute of Medicine (U.S.). Committee on the Prevention and Control of Viral Hepatitis Infections, Institute of Medicine (U.S.). Board on Population Health and Public Health Practice. Hepatitis and liver cancer a national strategy for prevention and control of hepatitis B and C [Internet]. Washington, DC: National Academies Press; 2010 [cité 2012 juin 8]. Available on: http://site.ebrary.com/id/10395833

[121] Expertise collective. Réduction des risques infectieux chez les usagers de drogues. INSERM; 2010.

[122] Costes JM, Cadet-Tairo A. Drug maintenance treatments in France: recent results 2004. OFDT; 2004.

[123] Phénomènes marquants et émergents en matière de drogues illicites (2010-2011). OFDT; 2012.

[124] Lurie P, Jones TS, Foley J. A sterile syringe for every drug user injection: how many injections take place annually, and how might pharmacists contribute to syringe distribution? J. Acquir. Immune Defic. Syndr. Hum. Retrovirol. 1998;18 Suppl 1:S45-51.

[125] Emmanuelli J, Desenclos J-C. Harm reduction interventions, behaviours and associated health outcomes in France, 1996-2003. Addiction. 2005 nov;100(11):1690-700.

[126] Bonnet N. [Pharmacy syringe exchange program for injection drug users]. Presse Med. 2006 déc;35(12 Pt 1):1811-8.

[127] Tempalski B, Cooper HL, Friedman SR, Des Jarlais DC, Brady J, Gostnell K. Correlates of syringe coverage for heroin injection in 35 large metropolitan areas in the US in which heroin is the dominant injected drug. Int. J. Drug Policy. 2008 avr;19 Suppl 1:S47-58.

[128] Leonard L, DeRubeis E, Pelude L, Medd E, Birkett N, Seto J. « I inject less as I have easier access to pipes »: injecting, and sharing of crack-smoking materials, decline as safer crack-smoking resources are distributed. Int. J. Drug Policy. 2008 juin;19(3):255-64.

[129] Volz E, Miller JC, Galvani A, Ancel Meyers L. Effects of heterogeneous and clustered contact patterns on infectious disease dynamics. PLoS Comput. Biol. 2011 juin;7(6):e1002042.

[130] Kretzschmar M, Mangen M-JJ, Pinheiro P, Jahn B, Fèvre EM, Longhi S, et al. New Methodology for Estimating the Burden of Infectious Diseases in Europe. PLoS Med. 2012 avr;9(4).

[131] Vickerman P, Martin N, Turner K, Hickman M. Can needle and syringe programmes and opiate substitution therapy achieve substantial reductions in HCV prevalence? Model projections for different epidemic settings. Addiction (Abingdon, England) [Internet]. 2012 mai 7 [cité 2012 mai 11]; Available de: http://www.ncbi.nlm.nih.gov/pubmed/22564041

[132] Birkhead GS, Klein SJ, Candelas AR, O'Connell DA, Rothman JR, Feldman IS, et al. Integrating multiple programme and policy approaches to hepatitis C prevention and care for injection drug users: a comprehensive approach. Int. J. Drug Policy. 2007 oct;18(5):417-25.

[133] Sylvestre DL, Zweben JE. Integrating HCV services for drug users: a model to improve engagement and outcomes. Int. J. Drug Policy. 2007 oct;18(5):406-10.

[134] Wilkinson M, Crawford V, Tippet A, Jolly F, Turton J, Sims E, et al. Community-based treatment for chronic hepatitis C in drug users: high rates of compliance with therapy despite ongoing drug use. Aliment. Pharmacol. Ther. 2009 janv;29(1):29-37.

[135] Vickerman P, Martin N, Hickman M. Can Hepatitis C virus treatment be used as a prevention strategy? Additional model projections for Australia and elsewhere. Drug Alcohol Depend. 2011 janv 15;113(2-3):83-85; discussion 86-87.

[136] Zeiler I, Langlands T, Murray JM, Ritter A. Optimal targeting of Hepatitis C virus treatment among injecting drug users to those not enrolled in methadone maintenance programs. Drug Alcohol Depend. 2010 août 1;110(3):228-33.

[137] Keverne EB, Curley JP. Epigenetics, brain evolution and behaviour. Front Neuroendocrinol. 2008 mai;29(3):398-412.

[138] Perfors A, Tenenbaum JB, Griffiths TL, Xu F. A tutorial introduction to Bayesian models of cognitive development. Cognition. 2011 sept;120(3):302-21.

[139] Cichy RM, Chen Y, Haynes J-D. Encoding the identity and location of objects in human LOC. Neuroimage. 2011 févr 1;54(3):2297-307.

[140] Dijksterhuis A, Aarts H. Goals, attention, and (un)consciousness. Annu Rev Psychol. 2010;61:467-90.

[141] Kompus K. Default mode network gates the retrieval of task-irrelevant incidental memories. Neurosci. Lett. 2011 janv 10;487(3):318-21.

[142] Holyoak KJ, Cheng PW. Causal learning and inference as a rational process: the new synthesis. Annu Rev Psychol. 2011;62:135-63.

[143] Winnicott DW. Playing and Reality. 2e éd. Routledge; 2005.

[144] Bowlby J. Attachment and Loss: Separation - Anxiety and Anger v. 2. New Ed. Penguin Books Ltd; 1975.

[145] Wallin DJ. Attachment in Psychotherapy. 1er éd. Guilford Press; 2007.

[146] Schmithorst VJ, Yuan W. White matter development during adolescence as shown by diffusion MRI. Brain Cogn. 2010 janv;72(1):16-25.

[147] Luhmann N. Social Systems. 1er éd. Stanford University Press; 1996.

[148] Lacan J. Les psychoses, 1955-1956. Editions du Seuil; 1981.

[149] Critchley S. Infinitely Demanding: Ethics of Commitment, Politics of Resistance. Verso Books; 2008.

[150] Zizek S, Santner EL, Reinhard K. The Neighbor: Three Inquiries in Political Theology. New edition. University of Chicago Press; 2006.

[151] Dahlstrom DO. Heidegger's Concept of Truth. 1er éd. Cambridge University Press; 2009.

[152] Moore D, Dray A, Green R, Hudson SL, Jenkinson JL, Siokou C, Perez P, Bammer G, Maher L, Dietze P. Extending drug ethno-epidemiology using agent-based modeling. Addiction. 2009. 104(12):1991-7.

[153] Festinger DS, Marlowe DB, Dugosh KL, Croft JR, Arabia PL. Higher magnitude cash payments improve research follow-up rates without increasing drug use or perceived coercion. Drug Alcohol Depend. 2008 juill 1;96(1-2):128-35.

[154] García-Fernández G, Secades-Villa R, García-Rodríguez O, Sánchez-Hervás E, Fernández-Hermida JR, Higgins ST. Adding voucher-based incentives to community reinforcement approach improves outcomes during treatment for cocaine dependence. Am J Addict. 2011 oct;20(5):456-61.

[155] Schulte B, Schütt S, Brack J, Isernhagen K, Deibler P, Dilg C, et al. Successful treatment of chronic hepatitis C virus infection in severely opioid-dependent patients under heroin maintenance. Drug Alcohol Depend. 2010 juin 1;109(1-3):248-51.

[156] Rehm J, Frick U, Hartwig C, Gutzwiller F, Gschwend P, Uchtenhagen A. Mortality in heroin-assisted treatment in Switzerland 1994-2000. Drug Alcohol Depend. 2005 août 1;79(2):137-43.

[157] Haasen C, Vertheim U, Eiroa-Orosa FJ, Schäfer I, Reimer J Is heroin-assisted treatment effective for patients with no previous maintenance treatment? Results form the German randomized controlled trial Eur. Addict. Res 2010

[158] Dijkgraaf MGW, van der Zanden BP, de Borgie CAJM, Blanken P, van Ree JM, van den Brink W. Cost utility analysis of co-prescribed heroin compared with methadone maintenance treatment in heroin addicts in two randomised trials. BMJ. 2005 juin 4;330(7503):1297.

[159] Frick U, Rehm J, Zullino D, Fernando M, Wiesbeck G, Ammann J, et al. Long-term follow-up of orally administered diacetylmorphine substitution treatment. Eur Addict Res. 2010;16(3):131-8.

[160] Small D, Glickman A, Rigter G, Walter T. The Washington Needle Depot: fitting healthcare to injection drug users rather than injection drug users to healthcare: moving from a syringe exchange to syringe distribution model. Harm Reduction J. 2010 january;7(1): 10.1186/1477-7517-7-1

[161] Snead J, Downing M, Lorvick J, Garcia B, Thawley R, Kegeles S, et al. Secondary syringe exchange among injection drug users. J Urban Health. 2003 juin;80(2):330-48.

[162] Hutchinson SJ, Taylor A, Goldberg DJ, Gruer L. Factors associated with injecting risk behaviour among serial community-wide samples of injecting drug users in Glasgow 1990-94: implications for control and prevention of blood-borne viruses. Addiction. 2000 juin;95(6):931-40.

[163] Cooper HLF, Des Jarlais DC, Ross Z, Tempalski B, Bossak B, Friedman SR. Spatial access to syringe exchange programs and pharmacies selling over-the-counter syringes as predictors of drug injectors' use of sterile syringes. Am J Public Health. 2011 juin;101(6):1118-25.

[164] Parkin S, Coomber R. Injecting drug user views (and experiences) of drug-related litter bins in public places: a comparative study of qualitative research findings obtained from UK settings. Health Place. 2011 nov;17(6):1218-27.

[165] Rhodes T, Kimber J, Small W, Fitzgerald J, Kerr T, Hickman M, et al. Public injecting and the need for « safer environment interventions » in the reduction of drug-related harm. Addiction. 2006 oct;101(10):1384-93.

[166] Building knowledge about community change : moving beyond evaluation. The Aspen Institute; Roundtable on community change 2004.

[167] Sobeck J, Agius E. Organizational capacity building: Addressing a research and practice gap. Evaluation and Program Planning 2007;30:237–246.

[168] Baser H. and Morgan P. 2008. Capacity, Change and Performance Study Report. (ECDPM Discussion Paper 59B). Maastricht: ECDPM.

[169] Owen J., Cook T., Jones E. Evaluating the early excellence initiative: the relationship between evaluation, performance management and practitioner participation Evaluation 2005;11:331-349.

[170] Tooke J. 283028/Report of the High Level Group on Clinical Effectiveness A report to Sir Liam Donaldson Chief Medical Officer Department of Health 2007

[171] Wodak A. Drug prohibition: it's broke, now go and fix it. Int. J. Drug Policy. 2012 janv;23(1):22-3.

[172] Room R, Reuter P. How well do international drug conventions protect public health? Lancet. 2012 janv 7;379(9810):84-91.

[173] Bewley-Taylor D, Jelsma M. Regime change: re-visiting the 1961 Single Convention on Narcotic Drugs. Int. J. Drug Policy. 2012 janv;23(1):72-81.

[174] Okrent D. Last call: The rise and fall of prohibition. Scribner 2011.

[175] Drug war facts. Ed; McVay A. 2007. www.drugwarfacts.org.

[176] Marez C. Drug wars: the political economy of narcotics. Univ Of Minnesota Press 2004.

[177] Wyler LS, Cook N. Illegal drug trade in Africa: Trends and U.S. policy. CRS Report for Congress 2009.

[178] World drug reports –Global illicit drug trends UNODC 1999-2012. http://www.unodc.org/unodc/en/data-and-analysis/WDR.html

[179] MacCourt RJ. Reuter P. Drug war heresies: learning from other vices, times, and places (RAND studies in Policy Analysis). Cambridge University Press 2001.

[180] McCoy. The politics of heroin: CIA complicity in the global drug trade 1991

[181] Scott PD, American war machine: deep politics, the CIA global drug connection and the road to Afghanistan. Rowman & Littlefield Publishers 2010.